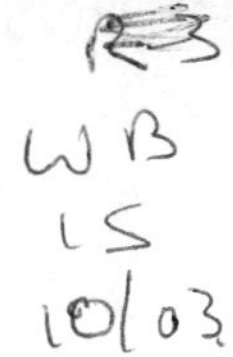

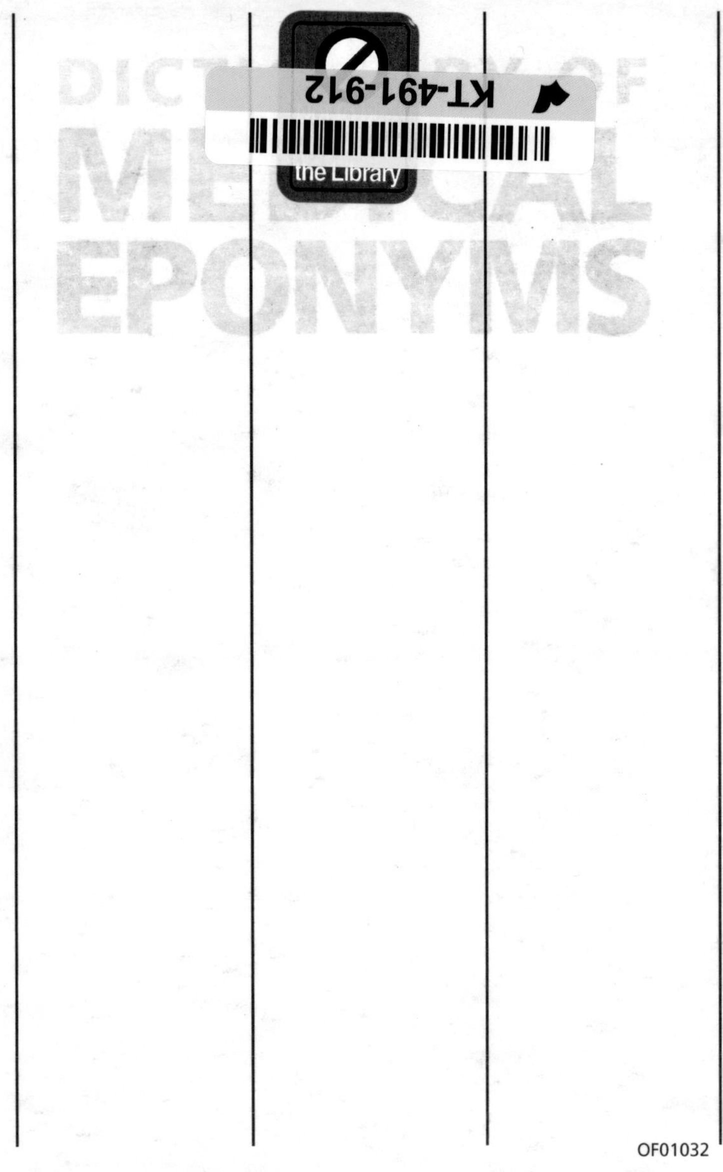

DICTIONARY OF MEDICAL EPONYMS

B.G. FIRKIN &
J.A. WHITWORTH

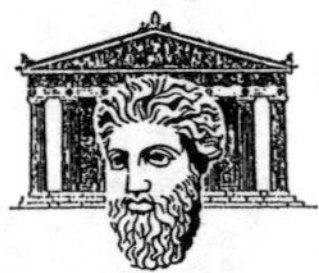

The Parthenon Publishing Group
International Publishers in Medicine, Science & Technology

A CRC PRESS COMPANY
BOCA RATON LONDON NEW YORK WASHINGTON, D.C.

Library of Congress Cataloging-in-Publication Data
Data available on request

British Library Cataloguing in Publication Data
Data available on request

ISBN 1850703337

Published in the USA by
The Parthenon Publishing Group Inc.
One Blue Hill Plaza
Pearl River
New York 10965, USA

Published in the UK and Europe by
The Parthenon Publishing Group Limited
23–25 Blades Court
Deodar Road
London SW15 2NU, UK

First edition published 1987
Second edition published 1996
This paperback edition published 2002

Typesetting by Keele University Press, Staffordshire, UK
Printed and bound by J. W. Arrowsmith Ltd., Bristol, UK

Introduction

In this second edition we have endeavored to correct spelling errors and incorrect assignation of eponyms. In the first edition Forssman antibodies were attributed to the Nobel Laureate, a German urologist who first developed the technique of cardiac catheterization, whereas their true discoverer was a distinguished Swedish scientist. The Fleischer of Kayser–Fleischer ring was not Richard Fleischer, the physician who described 'March' hemoglobinuria, but Bruno Fleischer, an ophthalmologist who in 1903 first described the phenomenon to which his name is attached. He recognized that this was a marker for a neuropsychiatric disorder associated with cirrhosis, but Kinnier Wilson's more definitive paper was published in the same year. The Bohr Effect was the work of the physiologist, Christian Bohr, and not his nephew the physicist, Nils Bohr. We have added a number of new entries and enlarged on others where further information has been obtained. A number of people have suggested that some of the discredited and/or antiquated syndromes or signs should be removed, e.g. Rosving sign, Horsley sign. We have retained them on the grounds that they are a part of the old medical literature and in many instances refer to colorful people who should not be forgotten. Of more concern to us were the requests of some to withdraw their name from an allocated eponym on the grounds that either someone else should have priority or that a more appropriate term was now available. Whilst we understand and respect these wishes, we believe that the listing of these names in current dictionaries, textbooks of medicine and in the literature past and present makes it mandatory that they continue to be listed.

A frequent criticism has been the lack of acknowledgment or indication of the source of each individual entry. The task of annotating each would add greatly to the bulk of the book and we have, therefore, continued to list the sources we have mainly used in collecting this material at the end of the introduction. We particularly acknowledge the help of Jan Waldenstrom in the revision of the first edition. He has made many invaluable suggestions as well as correcting a number of errors. Others from whom we have received enthusiastic help and encouragement include Hugh Dudley, Geraint James, Clark Nelson, George Stevenson and John Ludbrook as well as many others too numerous to identify. We hope this book will provide interest and insight into figures of medical history to show the more human aspects of the people who have advanced our profession so greatly. We continue, therefore, to be most interested to receive any anecdotes or 'human interest' stories that may be added to future editions. In conclusion, this revision would not have been possible without the dedication, persistence and sheer hard work by Mrs Marilyn Bushell, secretary to the Department of Medicine, Alfred Hospital, Monash University.

Additional references used in the 2nd Edition are:

1. *Butterworths Medical Dictionary*, Macdonald Critchley, Editor-in-Chief, 2nd Edition, 1978, reprinted 1990. (London: Butterworth and Co.)
2. *Churchill's Medical Dictionary*, Ruth Koenigsberg, Managing Editor, 1st Edition, 1989. (New York, Edinburgh, London, Melbourne: Churchill Livingstone)
3. Stanley Jablonski (1991). *Jablonski's Dictionary of Syndromes and Eponymic Diseases*. (Malabar, Florida: Krieger)
4. Peter Beighton and Greta Beighton. *The Man Behind the Syndrome*. (Berlin, Heidelberg: Springer-Verlag)
5. Harold L. Klawans (1982). *The Medicine of History from Paracelsus to Freud.* (New York: Raven Press)
6. Rowan Nicks (1984). *Surgeons All.* (Sydney: Hale and Iremonger)

The authors would welcome observations or further information that would be helpful in the preparation of a Third Edition. Please write to them via the Publishers at the address shown on page iv.

Introduction to the First Edition

Over the years many people have condemned the use of eponyms in medical practice, but eponyms are with us to stay whether the more fastidious like it or not, and will remain as long as medicine is practised in its present fashion. Some remain permanently whilst others vanish after a short moment of glory; their usage changes as much as fashion. Down syndrome for example was not used in the 1950s and only Mongolism was listed in the indices of textbooks at that time. Curious regional differences are noticeable within the same country; the cholecystogram in Melbourne is called the Graham test in Sydney. There is even greater variation from country to country. The Plummer-Vinson syndrome as it is known in the United States and Australia is referred to as the Patterson-Kelly syndrome in the United Kingdom and the Waldenström-Kjellberg syndrome in Scandinavia.

In some instances surnames are the sole eponym, in others Christian names are attached, e.g. Pierre Robin syndrome, Grahame Steell murmur, Marcus Gunn syndrome, etc.

It is also difficult to understand why certain names are attached to certain syndromes. Behçet disease was first described by Bluthe and Osler-Rendu-Weber telangiectasia by Babington, whilst Reiter syndrome was clearly described by Brodie and Kartagener syndrome by the Russian Siewert (Zivert), to name a few examples.

At times, efforts are made to rename the disease, but even when eponyms may be inappropriate, they remain despite efforts to change them. The great English epidemiologist of a decade or so ago, William Pickles, used the term Bornholm disease, which in Australia is still a common eponym attached to Coxsackie virus infections. Following approaches from his colleagues, Pickles tried to change the name of this disease to Sylvest disease, after his friend Enjar Sylvest, the general practitioner in Copenhagen whom he believed had contributed most to the identification and knowledge of this syndrome. However, in Australia, few use the term Sylvest disease.

In recent years there has been increasing usage, particularly in the fields of blood coagulation, of the name of the patient first described with this disorder. This method in terminology is not new. It was used by Hutchinson who described skin sarcoidosis, 9 years after Boeck in 1908, calling it Morbus Mortimer after his patient. Whilst this displays suitable modesty on the part of the investigator, it is unfortunate, since the use of such eponyms reveals little about the history of the disease, or the people associated with its initial description, one of the charms and perhaps one of the virtues of eponyms. It is true that some become very touchy about the use of an eponym. It is said that Guillain, when hearing the Guillain-Barré syndrome referred to as the Landry-Guillain-Barré syndrome remarked "c'est une confusion nosographique absolue"[1]. The further comment could be made that the authorship of the original paper was Guillain, G., Barré, J. and Strohl, A.: Sur un syndrome de radiculo-néurite avec hyperalbumose du liquide céphalo-rachidien sans reaction cellulaire. Remarques sur les caractères cliniques et graphiques des réflexes tendineaux. *Bull. Soc. Med. Hop. Paris 1916*, 14: 1462–1470. Somewhere along the line Strohl seems to have been forgotten!

In a letter to one of his friends whilst he was in Germany, Osler commented that the Goddess of Medicine was very happy in Germany, having moved there from Vienna. He remarked that she was unlikely to move because of the honor and respect which she had in Berlin and Germany. Possibly he was pointing to the time when the better features of German and British medicine would be combined in the United States, when with the advent of Nazi Germany she moved across the Atlantic. In reading through these eponyms, it has been interesting to note how she in fact has moved from Italy to France to England to Austria, to Germany and to the United States. This is reflected by the numbers of eponyms attributable to those countries and the date of their origin.

This book is an endeavor to list eponyms used in the practice of internal medicine in Australia and probably in most of the English-speaking countries in the world. While many eponymous terms in the subspecialities of medicine such as neurology, dermatology and pediatrics have been omitted, we have tried to include all those which are commonly encountered in internal medicine. Eponyms are unfortunately like the Joneses – no-one can keep up with them. It is hoped that it will help nurses and medical students as well as practitioners, not only to inform them as to the usage of these terms but wherever possible to indicate briefly a little of the person whose name is used eponymously.

These historical vignettes vary considerably from entry to entry. Sometimes this reflects ignorance on the authors' part, in others perhaps we have erred on too detailed an entry, reflecting our own bias. We have undoubtedly perpetrated errors of omission or commission, but feel sure our readers will alert us to any that have been made. In this book we have adopted the suggestion of a number of medical editors by dropping the use of the possessive in eponyms for clarity, e.g. Achard-Thiers syndrome, not Achard-Thiers' syndrome.

In conclusion, we would like to acknowledge the help of Jo Marshall and the Monash Biomedical Library staff, Marjorie Brown, Carolyn Bowes and Marjorie Grundmann, Monash University Department of Medicine, Alfred Hospital, Eric Pihl of the Monash University Department of Pathology, Chris Hale, Photography Department, Monash University, the late Hal Luke of the Radiology Department, Alfred Hospital and Susanne Firkin. Many other colleagues in this and other countries have also helped in gathering the information in this book, but they are too numerous to name.

[1] *Ann. Med. Paris 1953, 54: 81–149*

Reference books that we particularly relied upon were:

1. F.H. Garrison (1929). *History of Medicine*, 4th edition. (Philadelphia: W.B. Saunders & Co.)
2. R.H. Major (1954). *A History of Medicine*, 2 vols. (Oxford: Blackwell)
3. W. Haymaker and F. Schiller (1970). *The Founders of Neurology*, 2nd edition. (USA: Charles C. Thomas)
4. W. Haymaker (1953). *The Founders of Neurology*, 1st edition. (USA: Charles C. Thomas)
5. A. McGhee Harvey (1974). *Adventures in Medical Research*. (USA: Johns Hopkins University Press)
6. C.A. Birch. *Names We Remember.* (Beckingham, Kent, England: Ravenswood Publications)
7. S. Jablonski (1969). *Illustrated Dictionary of Eponymic Syndromes and Diseases and their Synonyms*. (Philadelphia: W.B. Saunders & Co.)
8. H. Bailey and W.J. Bishop (1959). *Notable Names in Medicine and Surgery*, 3rd edition. (H.K. Lewis)
9. W. Bulloch (1938). *The History of Bacteriology*. (Oxford: Oxford University Press)
10. K.E. Rothschuh (1973). *History of Physiology,* translated by G.B. Risie. (New York: R.E. Kreiger)
11. H. Speert (1958). *Obstetric and Gynaecologic Milestones*. (New York: The Macmillan Company)
12. L.T. Morton (1970). *A Medical Bibliography*, 3rd edition. (London: Andre Deutsch)
13. *Blakiston's Gould Medical Dictionary*, 3rd edition, McGraw-Hill, 1972
14. World Who's Who in Science. *From Antiquity to the Present*. Marquis Who's Who Inc., 1968
15. J.T. Crossey and L.C. Parish (1981). *The Dermatology and Syphilology of the Nineteenth Century*. (New York: Praeger)
16. J. Lourie (1982). *Medical Eponyms: Who was Coude?* (London: Pitman)
17. Obituaries appearing in a wide range of medical publications

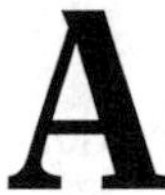

AAGENAES SYNDROME

Familial lymphedema with recurrent cholestasis.

Oystein Aagenaes (1925–) Norwegian pediatrician who graduated from the University of Copenhagen in 1952 and gained his M.D. with Dr Hagedorn at the Steno Memorial Hospital in 1962 thus commencing his life-long interest in diabetes. Currently he is chairman of the Department of Paediatrics at the Aken Hospital in Oslo. He is a keen yachtsman and cross-country skier.

ABADIE SIGN

1. Spasm of the levator palpebrae superioris in thyrotoxicosis.
2. Pinching or pressure of the Achilles tendon without resultant pain in tabes dorsalis.

Charles A. Abadie (1842–1932) French ophthalmologist at l'Hôtel Dieu who made contributions to surgical management of trachoma and medical treatment of glaucoma, and introduced alcohol injection of the Gasserian ganglion to treat trigeminal neuralgia.

ABDERHALDEN-KAUFFMAN-LIGNAC SYNDROME

Renal rickets with cystinosis (v. LIGNAC-FANCONI SYNDROME).

Emil Abderhalden (1877–1950) Swiss physiologist and biochemist, a Basel graduate, 1902, who studied with Emil Fischer, synthesized polypeptides containing up to 19 amino acids and became Professor of Physiology at Berne (1908) and then at Halle (1911). He wrote a number of textbooks including a "Text on Methodology". One of his first publications in 1904 was a complete review of the effects of alcohol and alcoholism and he remained an ardent promoter of the temperance movement. He founded a children's hospital in 1915 and promoted the evacuation of malnourished German children to Switzerland in the 1914–1918 war. He was a strong opponent of smoking and any student with nicotine stained fingers risked being failed by him. A deeply religious man, he founded two journals, one on enzymology and the other on ethics. In 1945 he and his family left Halle and he returned to Switzerland as Emeritus Professor in Zurich, where he died of a cerebral hemorrhage.

Eduard Kauffman (1860–1931) German physician who undertook the first study of cartilage changes in achondroplasia.

George O.E. Lignac (1891–1954) Dutch pathologist, born in Java (Indonesia) where his father was a civil servant. He studied medicine at Leyden, and then returned to the Dutch East Indies to teach pathology in Batavia (Jakarta). He succeeded Tendeloo as Professor of Pathology in Holland in 1934, contributed to knowledge of skin pigmentation, cystine metabolic anomalies and their effects on the kidneys, and tumors, especially the effects of benzol as a leukemogenic agent, and died in an air crash at Shannon Airport.

ACHARD-THIERS SYNDROME

Combined features of Adrenogenital syndrome and Cushing syndrome. Bearded female with diabetes (diabète des femmes à barbe).

Emile C. Achard (1860–1944) Paris physician, attached to Beaujon and Cochin Hospitals. He introduced one of the first tests of renal function (based on time of appearance of dyes in urine after injection), and coined the term paratyphoid fever. He wrote on many topics including encephalitis lethargica and edema in Bright disease. He was appointed Professor of General Pathology and Therapeutics and in 1919 Professor of Clinical Medicine.

Joseph Thiers (1885–) Paris physician born in Bastia, Corsica, and was schooled there and in Marseilles and then studied medicine in Paris, where he was trained by Professor Dieulafoy, Pierre Marie and Achard and became mainly interested in neurology, writing many papers on this subject. He was President of the French Neurology Society in 1949.

ACHILLES TENDON (Tendo calcaneus)

Tendon attaching gastrocnemius to the calcaneus.

Achilles (Greek mythology) was the son of Peleus and Phetus. His mother plunged him into the Styx to make him invulnerable, but held him by the heel. He was a hero of the Trojan War and slew Hector, but was himself slain by being wounded in his vulnerable heel by Paris.

ACKERMAN TUMOR

Verrucous carcinoma of the larynx – a rare locally malignant tumor which is malignant in behavior but whose pathology is relatively benign.

Lauren V. Ackerman Contemporary U.S. pathologist, Washington University, St. Louis. Some believe this was the tumor biopsied by Morel McKenzie and reported on by Virchow as benign which killed the liberal German Kaiser Frederick II and led to the accession of Wilhelm I to the German throne, probably changing the course of history. Ackerman was one of the most respected histopathologists of his day who was an authority in oncology and the interpretation of frozen sections. He had a keen interest in and collection of wines.

ADAMS

v. STOKES ADAMS ATTACKS

ADDIS COUNT

Quantitative estimation of urinary cellular excretion.

Thomas Addis (1881–1949) Born in Edinburgh, he graduated in medicine from the University of Edinburgh in 1905, gained his M.D. and M.R.C.P. in 1908 and then won a Carnegie Scholarship and studied in Berlin and Heidelberg (1909–1910). In 1911 he was invited to Stanford University and appointed Professor of Medicine in 1921.

He was one of the first to show that normal plasma could correct the defect in hemophilia, and made contributions on bile pigment metabolism. His major interest, however, was the kidney, and in 1916 he commenced studies on urea excretion with G. Barnett, which led him to the concept of clearance (so much blood "freed" of urea per unit time) and the birth of modern renal physiology. He published a textbook on the kidney with Jean Oliver and studied the effect of dietary protein on renal function and its importance in management of renal disease.

ADDISON ANEMIA

Pernicious anemia or megaloblastic anemia, secondary to vitamin B_{12} deficiency.

ADDISON DISEASE

Disorder resulting from destruction of the adrenal glands.

ADDISON-SCHILDER DISEASE

v. SCHILDER

Thomas Addison (1793–1860) English physician at Guy's Hospital, and a contemporary of Bright and Hodgkin. He was born at Long Benton near Newcastle and studied medicine in Edinburgh where he graduated in 1815. He commenced practice in London, started at Guy's in 1820 and was appointed as an assistant physician in 1824. In 1827 he was appointed lecturer in materia medica. He was a brilliant lecturer and diagnostician but a rather shy and taciturn individual and as a result had a small practice. He exerted a great deal of influence at Guy's and taught in a dogmatic and forceful manner. He was described as the type of doctor who is always trying to discover the rearrangement in a piece of machinery rather than one, who, like Babington (*v. infra*) regarded his patients as suffering, sensitive human beings. His monograph "On the constitutional and local effects of disease of the suprarenal capsule" was published in London in 1855 and represented the beginning of the study of the endocrine glands. This work was much debated in England and Scotland and largely discounted, H. Bennet in Edinburgh denying the existence of the disease. Trousseau in Paris, however, was quick to recognize adrenal failure and gave it the eponym Addison disease.

With Bright he was to write a textbook of Medicine, but only one volume was written and that by Addison. With Gull, Addison described xanthoma diabeticorum, and he also first described morphea (circumscribed scleroderma), which is sometimes called Addison keloid. He showed that pneumonia was a process occurring in the alveoli (air cells) and not in the interstitial tissue.

Addison had a number of episodes of severe depression which he greatly feared. He practiced and taught medicine in a most fastidious fashion and was an eloquent lecturer and at his best at the bedside, always moving to one side since he was slightly deaf in one ear. He used to tell his students that if he could not reach a diagnosis in a patient he would think of all the possible explanations for his patient's symptoms on his way to and from the hospital. His abilities to sift evidence and come up with a diagnosis were unrivalled in his day, but he did not devote the same energies to alleviation or cure. When he called in to see one patient he spent a long time in finally arriving at the diagnosis of an abdominal cancer and discussed this with the attending doctor and the patient's friends and relatives and was leaving when he was reminded that he had not written a prescription. He asked what he was already being given and when told a "magnesium mixture" he said "a very good medicine, go on with it". This probably explains why his practice was not as big as it might have been. He retired in 1860 because of an incipient cerebral disorder (depression) and probably committed suicide soon after, jumping from a window and fracturing his skull.

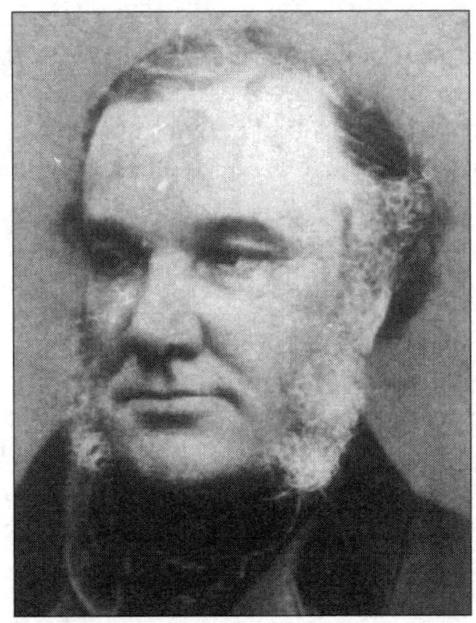

Thomas Addison (Courtesy of the Royal Society of Medicine, London, UK)

ADIE PUPIL

One pupil is usually larger than the other. They react slowly or not at all to light or accommodation; this is frequently associated with a decrease or loss of ankle jerks.

William J. Adie (1886–1935) English physician who also described narcolepsy. He was born in Geelong, Australia, but studied medicine at the University of Edinburgh, graduating in 1911. He fought in France in World War I and took part in the retreat from Mons, although a timely bout of measles kept him from the battle in which his regiment was decimated. He was mentioned in despatches for saving a number of soldiers in one of the early gas attacks in 1916 by improvising a mask of clothing soaked in urine! After the war he was a medical registrar at Charing Cross Hospital and eventually joined the staff of the National Hospital for Nervous Disease, Queens Square, and the Royal London Ophthalmic Hospital. He was a very able teacher and diagnostician, treating his students as he would his colleagues. A keen ornithologist and lover of snow sports, he died from a myocardial infarct.

v. HOLMES-ADIE SYNDROME

ADSON MANEUVER OR TEST

The left/right radial pulse is palpated, the patient's chin raised and the head rotated to the left/right on deep inspiration. In the presence of compression of the thoracic outlet, e.g. scalenus anticus syndrome, the radial pulse will disappear.

ADSON SYNDROME
(also called NAFFZIGER SYNDROME)

1. Scalenus anticus or cervical rib syndrome – compression of brachial plexus leading to unilateral sensory disturbance of the upper limb.
2. Adult amaurotic familial idiocy (v. TAY SACHS DISEASE).

Alfred W. Adson (1887–1951) Born in Terrill, Iowa, graduated University of Nebraska, 1912, B.Sc. and M.D. University of Pennsylvania. U.S. surgeon and pioneer of neurosurgery at the Mayo Clinic. He was one of the first to use sympathectomy for the treatment of hypertension, and cervical sympathectomy for Raynaud syndrome. Head of the section of neurological surgery at the Mayo Clinic from 1917 to 1946. One of his sons (M.A.) is currently head of the section of surgery at the Mayo Clinic.

ALAGILLE SYNDROME
(also called SYNDROMATIC PAUCITY OF INTERLOBULAR BILE DUCTS)

Multiple abnormalities associating neonatal cholestasis prolonged during childhood and adulthood due to paucity of interlobular bile ducts. There is a characteristic facial appearance noted from the first month with a prominent forehead, widely separated and deeply set eyes with a straight nose and a small pointed chin. Other features are butterfly-like vertebral arch defects, peripheral defects of pulmonary artery and growth and mental retardation. Other associated features include hypogonadism, bone manifestations, mesangiolipomatosis of the kidney and an unusual voice. Long-term prognosis is usually good, and biliary cirrhosis does not develop. It is essential to differentiate this syndrome from "non-syndromatic paucity of interlobular bile ducts" in which the anatomic defect of interlobular bile ducts is isolated.

Daniel Alagille Born in Paris in 1925. Graduated University of Paris 1954. Worked from 1954 to 1964 at the Hôpital Saint-Vincent-de Paul as an Assistant Professor. Since 1964, at the Hôpital de Bicêtre, as an Associate Professor, then as a Professor of Paediatrics and Clinical Genetics, University Paris-Sud (1970). Staff Physician and Chairman of the Department of Paediatrics, Hôpital de Bicêtre, since 1982. Chief of the Paediatric Liver Research Unit of the Institut National de la Santé et de la Recherche Médicale since 1964. He worked mainly on congenital bleeding diseases (1952–1964) and on liver and biliary tract disease in children since 1964. His hobbies are flying and roses.

ALBERS-SCHÖNBERG DISEASE
(Marble bone disease)

Osteopetrosis with accompanying leukoerythroblastic anemia and hepatosplenomegaly due to extramedullary hematopoiesis.

Heinrich E. Albers-Schönberg (1865–1921) German radiologist, who was born in Hamburg and graduated from Leipzig in 1891. He was initially a surgeon but in 1897 he started a private radiological institute. He was a pioneer radiologist who made a number of technical advances and founded a journal of radiology. He first described osteopoikilosis, discovered that irradiation damaged the reproductive organs and was the first Professor of Radiology at the University of Hamburg (1919). He died of radiation-induced cancer.

ALBRIGHT ANEMIA

Anemia seen in advanced hyperparathyroidism, secondary to osteitis deformans.

ALBRIGHT SYNDROME

1. Albright hereditary osteodystrophy-pseudohypoparathyroidism. Short stature, round face,

shortened metacarpals and metatarsals. Ectopic ossification of fascia and skin, but no abnormality of parathyroid function, but a resistance in end organ response. This is frequently due to an abnormality in the G proteins which regulate the adenyl cyclase system. Some members of the same family may lack the resistance to the hormone although phenotypically the same. These patients have been termed pseudopseudohypoparathyroidism. It is sometimes familial.

2. Polycystic fibrous dysplasia. Fibrous dysplasia of bone with skin pigmentations, characteristically localized over the bone lesion and on one side of the body.

ALBRIGHT-HADORN SYNDROME

Osteomalacia associated with hypokalemia.

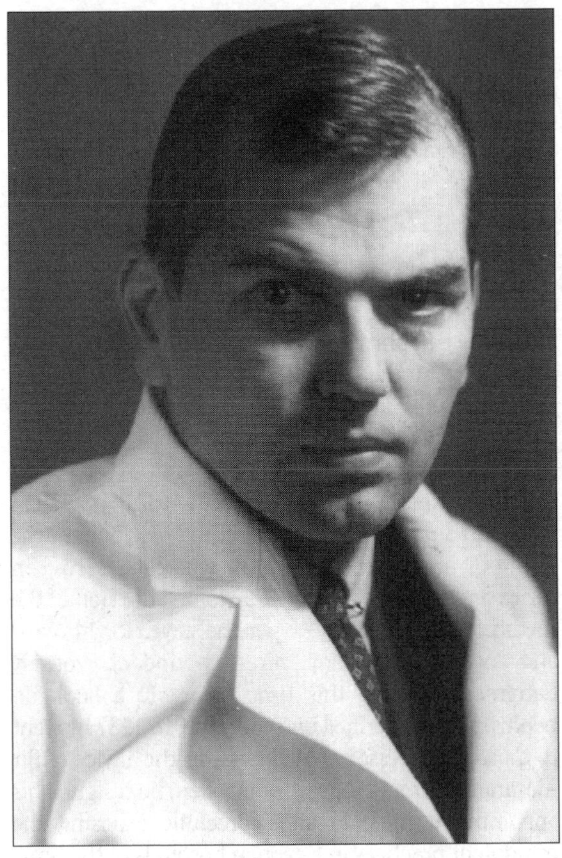

Fuller Albright (Courtesy of Dr Ann Forbes)

Fuller Albright (1900–1969) Graduated from Harvard in 1924 and was an intern with Aub and Bauer. His interest in calcium metabolism commenced in the famous Ward 4 of Massachusetts General Hospital. In 1927–28 he worked as an assistant resident with Ellsworth at Johns Hopkins and then went to Berlin, working with Zondek where he directed his attention to the pituitary.

He established a biological laboratory at M.G.H. on his return to the U.S. as well as an ovarian dysfunction clinic and a stone clinic (the Quarry), thus melding the laboratory and clinic. He won worldwide acclaim as a clinical investigator and popularized metabolic balance studies. He was famous for his circuit diagrams to establish working hypotheses – "any theory is better than no theory". He made major contributions to calcium metabolism and disorders of bone and his students included E. Reifenstein, H. Sulkowitch, Cockrill, Fred Bartter (Bartter Syndrome), Russell Fraser, W. Parson and C.H. Burnett (Milk-alkali syndrome), and Klinefelter (*v. infra*). In an article for his 25th anniversary class report in 1946 he wrote "For the past 10 years I have had the interesting experience of observing the development of Parkinson's syndrome on myself. As a matter of fact, this condition does not come under my special medical interests, or else I am sure I would have had it solved long ago. It interferes with one's locomotion and gives one a certain amount of rigidity which makes small talk appear somewhat forced. The condition has its compensations: one is not yanked from interesting work to go to the jungles of Burma ... one avoids all kinds of deadly committee meetings, etc." He concluded one of his papers as follows: "(1) I have told you more about osteoporosis than I know. (2) What I have told you is subject to change without notice. (3) I hope I have raised more questions than I have given answers. (4) In any case, as usual, a lot more work is necessary".

He became incapacitated with Parkinson disease and died many years after an unsuccessful surgical attempt at remedy.

Walter Hadorn (1898–1948) Swiss physician who was Professor of Internal Medicine in Berne. A highly regarded physician who had a large practice and was a connoisseur of painting with an excellent private collection of French Impressionists.

ALDER-REILLY ANOMALY

v. REILLY BODIES

ALDRICH SYNDROME

Sex-linked disease with increased susceptibility to infections, dermatitis and thrombocytopenia.

Robert A. Aldrich (1917–) U.S. pediatrician who is the son of another outstanding American pediatrician, C.A. Aldrich, who was Professor of Pediatrics at the Mayo Clinic. He graduated from Northwestern University in 1944 and held posts in pediatrics at the Universities of Minnesota (1950), Oregon (1951–53), and Washington, Seattle, from 1953. He became Professor of Pediatrics at University of Colorado, Denver in 1970, and has worked on heme synthesis, the biochemistry of porphyrins, and inborn errors of metabolism.

v. WISKOTT-ALDRICH SYNDROME

ALEUTIAN DISEASE

Plasma cell disorder of minks with some findings similar to multiple myeloma.

Aleutian Islands Chain of islands in the North Pacific Ocean over 1200 miles from the south west of Alaska towards Kamchatka Peninsula, Siberia.

ALEXANDER DISEASE

Leukodystrophy with megalocephaly.

William S. Alexander Contemporary New Zealand pathologist who described the condition whilst working with Professor Dorothy Russell at the London Hospital.

ALLEN TEST

Test of arterial supply to hand which involves compression and release of radial and ulnar vessels and observation of color change.

Edgar V. Allen (1900–1961) U.S. physician who was born in Cozad, Nebraska and graduated from the University of Nebraska in 1925. He worked thereafter at the Mayo Clinic where he became Professor of Medicine in 1947. He introduced coumarin anticoagulants into clinical practice and edited one of the first comprehensive textbooks on peripheral vascular disease in 1946.

ALPERS DISEASE

Progressive cerebral poliodystrophy (v. CHRISTENSEN-KRABBE DISEASE).

Bernard J. Alpers (1900–) U.S. neurologist. He was a student of Alfons Jakob, graduated from Harvard in 1923 and became Professor of Neurology and Chairman at Jefferson Medical College in Philadelphia. He wrote numerous books and papers on vertigo, dizziness and clinical neurology.

ALPORT SYNDROME

Hereditary nephritis with nerve deafness and infrequently a mild platelet defect and cataracts. Inheritance is autosomal dominant with variable penetrance.

Arthur C. Alport (1880–1959) South African physician who graduated in Edinburgh. He joined the R.A.M.C. in the Ist World War, where he served in Africa and England, and in 1922 joined the staff of the medical unit at St. Mary's where he stayed for 14 years, and became assistant director under Prof. F. Langmead. During this time he wrote a book on nephritis and described his syndrome. In 1937 he went to Cairo as Professor of Medicine, on the advice of Sir Alexander Fleming. Always outspoken, he resigned his appointment in 1944 after forcefully exposing the fraudulent practices in Egyptian hospitals of the time, and in particular the neglect of poor patients.

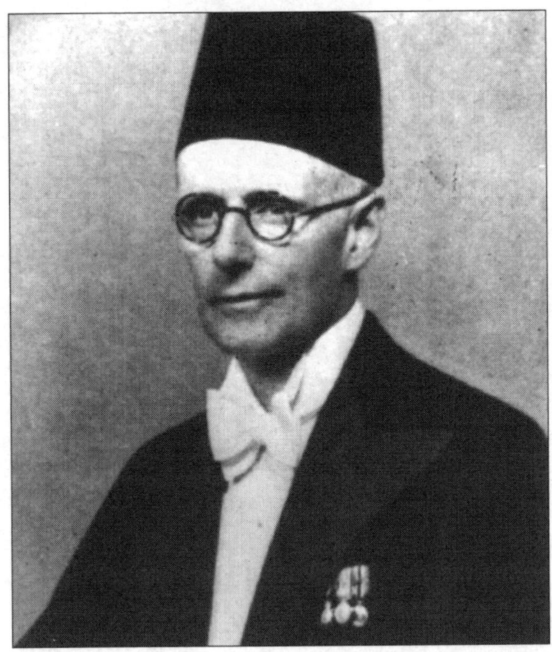

Arthur C. Alport (Reproduced from *"One Hour of Justice"*, Dorothy Crisp & Co. 1946/47)

This was the theme of his book "One Hour of Justice" which he dedicated to the twin gods of decency and justice, and ultimately resulted in a revision of medical practice in Egypt. He had a passion for golf and died at 79 in his old hospital in London.

ALSTRÖM SYNDROME

Similar to Laurence-Moon-Biedl syndrome. Autosomal recessive condition presenting as childhood obesity, with nerve deafness, primary hypogonadism in the male and atypical retinitis pigmentosa which often progresses to blindness. Diabetes and renal disease may develop. Skin manifestations include baldness and acanthosis nigricans. The patients are resistant to insulin, vasopressin and gonadotrophin. They rarely have mental retardation and digit abnormalities, characteristically seen in Laurence-Moon-Biedl syndrome.

Carl H. Alström Contemporary Swedish geneticist, Professor of Psychiatry at the Karolinska Institute. He has published widely on human genetics as well as psychiatry.

ALZHEIMER DISEASE

This is the commonest cause of presenile dementia. The age of onset is rarely before 45 and the patient may successfully hide the problem for a few years and be distressfully aware of the situation.

Alois Alzheimer (1864–1915) German psychiatrist and neurologist. He was born in the small Bavarian town of Marktbreit and went to medical school at Würzburg, Tübingen and Berlin, graduating in 1887. In 1889, Nissl (*v. infra*) joined him at a state institute in Frankfurt-am-Main. This began a lifetime association of friendship and collaboration. Nissl was regarded as the more innovative, but Alzheimer was the careful and dedicated laboratory worker who proved the observations histologically and who had a wonderful gift of description of his microscopical findings. Kraepelin invited him to Heidelberg in 1902 where he rejoined Nissl, who had been working there since 1895. In 1903 he again followed Kraepelin to Munich where he

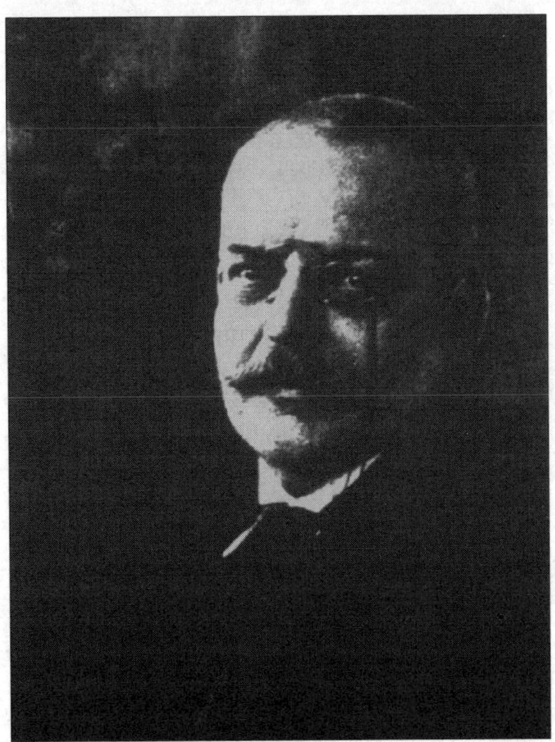

Alois Alzheimer
(Courtesy of the Royal Society of Medicine, London, UK)

became a well-loved figure to students from all over the world. He would spend hours with each one, explaining things as they shared a microscope, always with a cigar which would be put down as he commenced his explanations, and it is said that at the end of the day there would always be a cigar stump at every student's bench by the microscope. He was a close friend of W. Erb who had treated a banker for syphilis and at the end of the treatment the banker financed a scientific expedition to North Africa on the proviso that he and his wife would accompany the team. They had just arrived in Algeria when the banker had a mental breakdown! Erb contacted Alzheimer, who came to Algeria to bring the banker and his wife back to Germany. When the banker died Alzheimer married his widow and this made him financially independent so that he was able to supplement all the texts he wrote with numerous illustrations. He was appointed Professor of Psychiatry at the University of Breslau (Wroclaw) in 1912, but died shortly after of rheumatic endocarditis.

ANDERS DISEASE

Adiposa tuberosa simplex. Small subcutaneous fatty nodules which are tender to touch and are usually found in the extremities or on the abdomen.

James M. Anders (1854–1936) U.S. physician. Graduated M.D., PhD., in 1877 from the University of Pennsylvania, Philadelphia. He was Professor of Medicine at the Medico-Chirurgical College of Philadelphia which became the Graduate School of Medicine of the University of Pennsylvania. He wrote a successful textbook of medicine and amongst other honors was awarded Chevalier of the Legion of Honour of France in 1923.

ANDERSEN DISEASE

Type IV muscle glycogenosis due to a deficiency of the branching enzyme -1, 4-glucan, -1, 5-glucan 6-glucosyl transferase. Abnormal glycogen accumulates mainly in the liver, causing cirrhosis, but also in muscle. Presents with hepatomegaly and failure to thrive in infancy. Muscle hypotonia with portal hypertension (ascites and splenomegaly) secondary to hepatic cirrhosis are the characteristic clinical features.

ANDERSEN SYNDROME

Cystic fibrosis of the pancreas.

Dorothy H. Andersen (1901–1963) U.S. pediatrician and pathologist.

ANDERSON-FABRY DISEASE

Angiokeratoma corporis diffusum universale.

(For description v. FABRY DISEASE)

William Anderson (1842–1900) English surgeon and dermatologist, born in London, who was initially an art student at the Lambeth School of Art where he obtained a medal for artistic anatomy. He entered medical school at St. Thomas' Hospital in 1864, graduating with the Cheselden Medal for Surgery. He was house surgeon at St. Thomas' and later surgical registrar and demonstrator in anatomy. He was an excellent teacher, although somewhat shy and retiring. The Japanese Government founded a Naval Medical College in Tokyo and advertized for an English surgeon to act as Head. Anderson was appointed and remained in Japan for 7 years, lecturing firstly with the aid of an interpreter, and later in Japanese, on anatomy, physiology, surgery and medicine. He built up a superb collection of Japanese art, engravings, etchings and illustrated books, and these he sold to the British Museum. At the time they were considered to be the finest to be assembled in Europe and perhaps the world.

Anderson also wrote several authoritative texts on Japanese art. In 1880 he was invited back to St. Thomas' as assistant surgeon and lecturer in anatomy and in 1887 was placed in charge of the Dermatology Department where he described "angiokeratoma corporis diffusum universale" continuing to teach anatomy until he became a joint lecturer in surgery (1898). He became a full surgeon in 1891 and was an examiner for the Royal College of Surgeons for the Conjoint Board until his sudden death. He did not write voluminously but did make contributions to history of surgery, art in relation to medical science and on deformities of the fingers and toes, and also textbooks. He succeeded Professor Marshall as Professor of Anatomy to the Royal Academy (1891). He was a founder and President of the Japan Society and was honored by the Japanese Government which awarded him "Commander of the Order of the Rising Sun". Many Japanese doctors came to work with him at St. Thomas'. He had an eye for beauty and when failing a particularly handsome but ignorant student, drew the attention of his colleagues to the young Apollo and said "Some woman has spoilt him". On another occasion when discussing another – "His ugly face has soured his life and his manners. I should like to try the effect of a wig and a beard". He had believed he was suffering from indigestion but died suddenly from a ruptured cord of the mitral valve, presumably secondary to a coronary thrombosis.

ANGELUCCI SYNDROME

Vernal conjunctivitis, hyperexcitability, tachycardia and vasomotor lability.

Arnaldo Angelucci (1854–1933) Italian ophthalmologist who was Professor of Ophthalmology at Cagliari, then Messina, then Palermo and ultimately Naples where he remained until his retirement in 1929. Southern Italy had a high incidence of trachoma and he therefore had a wide experience and a life-long interest in this disease. Being multilingual he was a well-known international figure and President of the International Ophthalmological Congress in Naples in 1909.

ANGSTROM UNIT

1/10 000 of a micron.

Anders J. Angstrom (1814–1874) Swedish physicist and astronomer awarded the Rumford Medal of the Royal Society, England, in 1872. He discovered hydrogen in the solar atmosphere and published his map of the normal solar spectrum in 1868.

He demonstrated that thermal conductivity is related to electrical conductivity.

ANTON SYNDROME

Blindness, denial of blindness and confabulation.

Gabriel Anton (1858–1933) Austrian neurologist born in Graz. He graduated from the University of Prague in 1882 and in 1887 went to work in Vienna with Theodor Meynert whom he regarded as his greatest influence. In 1892 he was appointed as director of the University clinic in Innsbruck and later (1894) Graz. In 1905 he succeeded Wernicke in Halle an der Saale retiring in 1926. He contributed to the study of chorea describing scars in the lenticular nuclei. He linked brain pathology with psychology in his pioneering work on the lack of self perception of their deficits in patients with cortical blindness and deafness (1903). Schilde was his assisistant at Halle (1909–1912) and with him he analyzed choreic and athetoid movements.

APERT SYNDROME

v. CROUZON-APERT DISEASE

ARAN-DUCHENNE DYSTROPHY OR SYNDROME

Progressive spinal muscular atrophy involving mainly proximal musculature with onset in childhood so that the subject often does not reach adult life. Cardiomyopathy may occur and serum enzymes (creatinine kinase) are high. It is an X-linked recessive condition.

François A. Aran (1817–1861) French physician.

G.B.A. Duchenne French neurologist (*v. infra*).

ARGYLL ROBERTSON PUPIL

The pupil does not respond to light but reacts to accommodation. It is classically seen in syphilis but also in other conditions, e.g. Wernicke encephalopathy and diabetes.

Douglas M.C.L. Argyll Robertson (1837–1909) Scottish physician and ophthalmic surgeon. He studied in Berlin with A. von Graefe and returned to Edinburgh to found ophthalmology there and became President of the College of Surgeons of Edinburgh in 1886. A fine golf player whose studies on the effects of extracts of the Calabar bean (*Physostigma venomaos*) on the pupil began an important era in neuropharmacological research.

ARMANNI-EBSTEIN NEPHROPATHY

Glycogen vacuolation of the terminal portion of the proximal convoluted tubules in diabetes appears to be directly related to glycosuria.

Luciano Armanni (1839–1903) Italian pathologist.

Wilhelm Ebstein (1836–1912) German physician (*v. infra*).

ARNETH COUNT

A count of neutrophil lobes – the more mature the cell the greater the number of lobes. An increased number of lobes is termed a shift to the right and is seen in megaloblastic anemias.

Joseph Arneth (1873–1956) German physician, born in Bavaria, who studied medicine in Munich, Heidelberg and Würzburg, and was Director of the Department of Medicine at the Municipal Hospital in Münster from 1907–1944. He wrote extensively on blood disorders and pulmonary tuberculosis but much of his theoretical work was strongly criticized and gained little acceptance. He was nonetheless one of the pioneers of German hematology.

ARNOLD-CHIARI SYNDROME

Developmental abnormality often resulting in hydrocephalus and associated frequently with spina bifida and meningocele.

Julius Arnold (1835–1915) German pathologist who was Professor of Pathology at Heidelberg.

Hans Chiari (1851–1916) Austrian pathologist (v. BUDD-CHIARI SYNDROME).

ARNOLD PICK SYNDROME

Aperceptive blindness with central atrophy. The patient cannot fix reflexly on objects within his gaze.

Arnold Pick (1851–1924) Czechoslovakian physician.

v. PICK DISEASE

ARTHUS PHENOMENON

Inflammation resulting from antigen-antibody (IgE) combination in tissues with resultant local reaction and damage.

Nicholas M. Arthus (1862–1945) French physiologist, born in Angers and appointed Professor of Physiology at the University of Fribourg in Switzerland in 1895. After 5 years he returned to France to direct the Pasteur Institute at Lille. In 1902 he was put in charge of the physiology course at the School of Medicine in Marseilles and in 1907, following the death of Herzer, he was offered the Chair of Physiology at the University of Lausanne.

In 1890 he commenced working on the coagulation of milk and with Calixte Pageo showed that the conversion of caseinogen to casein required calcium, as had already been shown for blood coagulation. He introduced the use of sodium oxalate as an anticoagulant for blood and milk. He commenced working on anaphylaxis in 1903, following its demonstration by Portier and Richet who injected extract of marine animals into dogs. Arthus studied subcutaneous injections of horse serum into rabbits. After the fourth injection he noted that absorption was slow and a local edematous reaction occurred; after the fifth it became purulent and after the seventh gangrenous. Intravenous injection, however, produced characteristic anaphylaxis, with rapid respiration, hypotension and incoagulability of the blood and if a high enough dose was given, respiratory and cardiac death.

He also studied the actions of snake venoms, initially separating them into three types, the cobra (*Naja tripudiens*), causing death by respiratory arrest, the Russell viper, causing massive blood coagulation, and the *Crotalas adamanteus*, producing death by shock. Careful analysis of these effects in animals using small repeated doses of cobra venom made the animal resistant to muscular paralysis but resulted in death from shock. He then developed antivenene by treating the venom with formalin prior to injection into the animal.

His final years were devoted to study of physiological effects of the products of micro-organisms.

Arthus modelled himself on Claude Bernard – he was particularly critical of theories which could not be tested and insisted on distinguishing such from hypotheses which could be subjected to laboratory testing.

ASCHHEIM-ZONDEK TEST

Classical test for pregnancy involving injection of test urine into mice and observing ovarian changes.

Selmar Aschheim (1878–1965) German gynecologist, born in Berlin, who studied at Freibourg, Munich and Hamburg, and became a Professor at Berlin University in 1931. With the advent of Hitler he moved to France and became a naturalized French citizen and Director of the National Research Centre at the Hospital Beaujon. He made numerous contributions to the understanding of estrogen effects, especially at a histological level and demonstrated that anterior lobe pituitary implants into immature rodents produced sexual development.

Bernhard Zondek (1891–1966) German gynecologist, born in Wronke, he graduated from the University of Berlin in 1918 and became Associate Professor there in 1926, and Chief of the Department of Obstetrics and Gynaecology at the Municipal Hospital of Berlin-Spandau. When the Nazis came to power he was dismissed from his posts (1933) and he left Germany and moved to Jerusalem where he was appointed Professor of Obstetrics and Gynaecology at the Hebrew University, and Head of Obstetrics and Gynaecology at the Hadassah Hospital. He was one of the proponents of the interdependence of the endocrine glands under the guiding hand of the pituitary and his studies on pituitary-ovary interaction did much to establish this fundamental tenet. He established that the chorionic tissue of the placenta had endocrine capacity and this led to diagnostic techniques important for the recognition and treatment of hydatiform mole and chorionic carcinoma. He was devoted to Israel and many of his students and collaborators occupy key posts in that country.

ASCHOFF NODULES

Granuloma specific for rheumatic fever.

Karl A.L. Aschoff (1866–1942) German pathologist, graduated from the University of Bonn, 1889, and became Professor of Pathology at Marburg 1903 and later at Freiburg (1906–1936). He introduced the term reticuloendothelial system as well as writing classical histological descriptions of rheumatic conditions, and made contributions to appendicitis, gall stones and scurvy. He wrote an excellent text book on anatomical pathology.

ASHBY TECHNIQUES

Non-radioisotope techniques for determining red cell volume and red cell life-span by injecting red cells of a different blood group into the recipient.

Winifred Ashby (1879–1975) U.S. pathologist, born in London, U.K. and when 14 years old migrated with her parents to the U.S.A. She graduated B.S. from Chicago University in 1903 and M.S. from Washington University, St. Louis, in 1905, studied malnutrition in the Philippines and then returned to the U.S. where she taught school physics and chemistry. She began a Fellowship at the Mayo Clinic and there developed the Ashby technique for estimating red cell survival which was widely used before isotopic methods became freely available. She made contributions to diagnostic techniques in syphilis and studied carbonic anhydrase in the brain. She was a gifted musician and composed music. She left the Mayo Clinic in 1924 and worked at St. Elizabeth Hospital, Washington, D.C., until her retirement.

ASHERMAN SYNDROME

Secondary amenorrhea due to excessive curettage or damage to the endometrium.

Joseph G. Asherman (1885–1968) Czechoslovakian gynecologist who moved to Israel and worked in the Tel Aviv Municipal Hospital becoming director of Obstetrics and Gynaecology. He retired in 1963.

ASHKENAZI JEWS

Race of Jewish people who from the twelfth century onwards migrated and lived in Germany, Poland and Russia. Term derived from modern Hebrew referring to medieval Germany. Used to distinguish from Sephardic and Oriental groups.

AUBERGER BLOOD GROUP

Found in 82% of Caucasians. May be related to the Lutheran system.

Auberger A 59-year-old woman with esophageal varices. The name of the patient in which this blood group was first detected.

AUER RODS OR BODIES

Rod or crystalline shaped inclusions seen in myeloblastic and monoblastic leukemia due to faulty granule formation.

John Auer (1875–1948) Born in Rochester, N.Y. and graduated B.S. from Michigan University in 1898 and Johns Hopkins Medical School in 1902. He was Pharmacologist at the Rockefeller Institute and Chairman of Pharmacology at St. Louis University School of Medicine, and his research encompassed digestion and respiration as well as physiology of drug action. He published his article on Auer Rods in 1906, which resulted from his study of a patient admitted to Osler's service at Johns Hopkins, when Auer was Osler's house officer. He investigated the effects of magnesium on tetany while at the Rockefeller with S.J. Meltzer whose daughter he married. He introduced intra-tracheal intubation to give "continuous respiration without respiratory movement". He gave the first account of the physiological events associated with anaphylaxis in the guinea pig and this led Meltzer to propose it as a mechanism for asthma. A well-rounded scholar he read French, German and Latin authors. He sketched and was a keen gardener. He died with a coronary thrombosis.

AUERBACH PLEXUS

Autonomic nerve plexus in the esophagus.

Leopold Auerbach (1828–1897) German anatomist and Professor of Neuropathology at Breslau (Wroclaw). He was one of the first to investigate the nervous system using histological stains and reported the plexus in 1862.

AUSTIN FLINT MURMUR

Late diastolic mitral murmur heard in aortic incompetence in the absence of pathology of the mitral valve.

Austin Flint (1812–1886) American physician, from a medical family. Born in Petersham, Massachusetts. At Harvard he was influenced by a teacher, Jackson, who was a follower of Laennec. He graduated in 1832. He first practiced in Boston but moved to Buffalo where he helped to found the Buffalo Medical College to which he was appointed Professor of Medicine. He later held Chairs at Chicago, Louisville, New Orleans and New York. He was a superb teacher who wrote numerous books on medicine and physical examination, and first described the hepatorenal syndrome. His son, Austin Flint, Jr., became an eminent physiologist.

AUSTRALIAN ANTIGEN

Hepatitis B antigen which was first identified in the serum of an Australian aboriginal by B.S. Blumberg.

AVELLIS SYNDROME

Palatopharyngeal paralysis due to lesion of upper part of the nucleus of the Xth nerve.

Georg Avellis (1864–1916) German otolaryngologist.

AYERZA SYNDROME OR DISEASE *or* AYERZA-ARRILLAGA DISEASE

Intense cyanosis and polycythemia due to pulmonary insufficiency.

Abel Ayerza (1861–1918) Argentinian physician who described the condition in 1901 in clinical lectures "Cardiacosnegros". His student Arrillaga subsequently wrote a thesis in 1913 which correlated the clinical findings with sclerosis of the pulmonary artery.

AZOREAN DISEASE

v. JOSEPH DISEASE or JOSEPH-MACHADO DISEASE

B

BABESIOSIS DISEASE

Tick-borne protozoan disease which may be endemic in domestic and wild animals. Small malarial-like parasites are seen in the red cells. In man the condition has been most commonly reported in people who have had a splenectomy where it may be fulminant and fatal. It is characterized by fever, anemia, nausea, hemoglobinuria and jaundice proceeding to renal failure, hypertension and coma in fatal cases. Where the patient is not immune-compromised the infestation may be asymptomatic or self-limited with fever, myalgia, anemia and splenomegaly.

Victor Babès (1854–1926) He was born in Vienna but educated and worked for many years in Paris at the Pasteur Institute where he worked on rabies and with Lepp demonstrated the protective effect of serum from an immunized animal. He co-authored (with Cornil) one of the first bacteriology text books. He became Professor of Pathology at the University of Bucharest and the Director of the Antirabies Institute of Rumania. He first discovered *Babesia* in the red cells of Rumanian cattle in 1888.

BABINGTON DISEASE

v. OSLER DISEASE

Hereditary telangiectasia.

Benjamin G. Babington (1794–1866) Son of a physician, William Babington, he was educated at Charterhouse. He entered the Royal Navy as a midshipman and served at the Battle of Copenhagen and then entered the Indian service and published an Indian grammar. He returned to England because of ill health and studied medicine at Guy's Hospital and Pembroke College, Cambridge, and wrote on cholera, epilepsy and chorea, and was one of the first to suggest that fibrin was formed in blood from a more soluble precursor. He invented an instrument which he called the glottiscope in 1828 for examining the larynx and was probably the first person to introduce routine indirect laryngoscopy. He was very gifted in other fields, being a skilled sculptor and painter, as well as a linguist and translator of verse. He was a fine billiard player and a good shot. In 1834 he was appointed physician at Guy's ahead of Hodgkin (*v. infra*). This aroused a great deal of controversy and acrimonious debate. The treasurer of the hospital said he would have no one at Guy's Hospital who was seen in the company of a North American Indian – a reference to Hodgkin's well-known liberal tendencies – Hodgkin was a founder of the Aborigine Society. Babington was also probably helped by his family connections; his father had been a physician at Guy's and his sister was Richard Bright's first wife. Babington resigned in 1854 following a disagreement with the hospital administration over restriction of access of students to the hospital. He died from renal and bladder disease.

BABINSKI SIGN, TEST, REFLEX

A test for pyramidal tract disturbance. Stroking the lateral aspect of sole of foot normally results in the plantar flexion of the great toe. In upper motor neurone lesions involving the pyramidal tract, or in infancy, the toe dorsiflexes.

BABINSKI-NAGEOTTE SYNDROME

Lesions of pontobulbar or medullary bulbar region giving ipsilateral Horner syndrome, nystagmus and cerebellar ataxia with contralateral hemiparesis and sensory disturbance.

Josef F.F. Babinski (1857–1932) His parents were Polish political refugees who arrived in Paris in 1848 and he was brought up in Montparnasse. He was tall, massive and strikingly handsome. Babinski graduated from the University of Paris in 1884 with a thesis on multiple sclerosis, suggested to him by Vulpian, then worked under Charcot at the Salpêtrière and from 1890–1927 (after he failed his Agrégé exam) headed the Neurological Clinic at the Hôpital de la Pitié. Together with Brissaud, Pierre Marie, Dejerine, Soques and others, he founded the Société de Neurologie de Paris. He built up the systematic approach of physical examination which is currently used in neurology and introduced new techniques such as having the patient kneel to elicit the ankle jerk.

He described dystrophia adiposogenitalis in 1900 – a year before Frölich. He conceived that hysteria was produced by suggestion and could be cured by it. He drew attention to the asymmetry of movement caused by cerebellar disease and that it could be tested by asking the patient to perform rapidly alternating movements (sometimes called the Babinski Sign). As he failed in his examination for the title Professeur Agrégé, he did not have heavy teaching commitments. He lived with his brother Henri (a distinguished engineer) who was also a famous cook and published a recipe book under the pseudonym Ali-Bab, which was very popular in Paris. It is said that Babinski once interrupted his ward round when the nurse in charge whispered to him that the soufflé was nearly ready. He spent the evenings at the theater, opera and ballet. In the last years of his life he developed Parkinson disease.

Jean Nageotte (1866–1948) Was born in Dijon and studied medicine in Besançon and then Paris where he graduated in 1893 and was appointed physician to the Bicêtre in 1898. In 1912 he was appointed to the Salpêtrière and to the Chair of Comparative Histology in the College de France, following Ranvier. He placed the initial lesion of tabes dorsalis in the dorsal root component of the radicular nerve (the radicular nerve of Nageotte), described the boutons terminaux of spinal nerves, and with Babinski the lateral medullary syndrome. They combined to write a book on the cerebrospinal fluid. Nageotte did extensive work on the myelin sheath and nerve grafting. He loved literature and although somewhat sarcastic was admired by people such as Cajal and Babinski. Nageotte was a devoted clinician as well as an investigator, and his wife was a prominent pediatrician who became President of the Société de Pédiatre (v. MARFAN). He was left paralyzed following an accident in 1923.

BACHMANN BUNDLE

Longitudinally orientated atrial fibres which preferentialy conduct impulses from the sino-atrial node from right to left atrium.

Jean G. Bachmann (1877–) American physiologist.

BAGHDAD BOIL

Cutaneous leishmaniasis.

Baghdad Capital of Iraq.

BAHIMA DISEASE

Seen in Africa. It is characterized by (1) tower skull (2) X-ray showing "hair on end" appearance and widening of diploë (3) no evidence of thalassemia, sickle cell or other hemolytic anemia. Postulated that it is due to iron deficiency in children fed exclusively on a diet of cow's milk. Occurs in "Hamitic" Bahima people in Uganda.

BAINBRIDGE REFLEX

Increase in heart rate due to a rise in right atrial pressure.

Francis A. Bainbridge (1874–1921) was an English physiologist, born in Stockton-on-Tees, where his father was a pharmacist. He won a scholarship to study at Leys School, Cambridge, and from there went to Trinity College, Cambridge, where he took first class honors in the natural sciences tripos in 1897. He trained at St. Bartholomew's Hospital, London, and obtained his M.B. in 1901 and M.D., Cambridge, in 1904. In 1905 he became Gordon Lecturer in Pathology at Guy's Hospital and in 1907 became assistant bacteriologist to the Lister Institute of Preventive Medicine. He was appointed as Professor of Physiology at Durham University (1911), and in 1915 moved to the Chair of Physiology at St. Bartholomew's Hospital, which he occupied until he died. He was elected F.R.S. in 1919. His initial investigations were on the mechanism of lymph formation. Bainbridge showed, in studies on the submaxillary gland and liver, that lymph flow resulted from local production of metabolites by cells with a consequent rise of osmotic tension in the tissue fluid which attracted fluid from blood vessels. He made an important contribution in distinguishing different types of paratyphoid bacilli.

Bainbridge and A.P. Beddard repeated Nussbaum's experiments, examining the mechanisms of urine secretion, and added important evidence supporting Cushny's view of the glomeruli as filters. He worked with Henry Dale on the movement and innervation of the gall bladder. His most important contribution was to the physiology of exercise and his demonstration that an increase in pressure on the venous side of the heart resulted in an increase of heart rate due to the inhibition of vagal influences and the excitation of some accelerator mechanisms. This was the converse of Marey Law, which stated a rise in pressure in the ventricles caused a slowing of the heart. His most popular scientific publication was "The Physiology of Muscular Exercise" in 1919. Together with Professor Menzies from Newcastle he wrote a textbook of physiology called "Essentials of Physiology" a relatively short and concise account of physiology, much liked by medical students of the day. He was a man of small stature, not an impressive lecturer, and was dogged through his latter years by recurrent ill health.

BAIRNSDALE ULCER

v. BURULI LESIONS

A deep indolent ulcer with overhanging edges, particularly on the lower limbs. Involves subcutaneous tissue as well as skin, and is due to infection with *Mycobacterium ulcerans*.

Bairnsdale Country town in Victoria, Australia.

BAKER CYST

Enlargement of popliteal bursa or herniation of the synovial membrane of the knee joint often associated with degenerative disease of the knee.

William M. Baker (1839–1896) English surgeon, born in Andover, the son of the town's solicitor. He undertook an apprenticeship with the local surgeon, Mr. Payne, and in 1858 entered St. Bartholomew's Hospital Medical School, qualifying in 1861, when he became a midwifery assistant, and a year later entered the dissecting room. In 1867 he was elected demonstrator of anatomy. He became editor of Kirkes Handbook of Physiology, a book which had initially been designed by Kirkes and Sir James Paget in 1848. He was Sir James Paget's private assistant for some years, and became lecturer in physiology at St. Bartholomew's Hospital in 1869, a position he held until 1885. He was elected an assistant surgeon to the hospital in 1871 and a surgeon in 1882. He was surgeon to the skin department of St. Bartholomew's Hospital and wrote a number of articles on bone and joint problems. He became regarded as an expert in renal surgery, particularly nephrolithotomy.

During the last years of his life he developed locomotor ataxia and he was forced to resign his appointment in 1892. He was particularly interested in his hospital and had a superb collection of old prints and engravings of its development which he had collected over the years. He was a well built, good looking man, fond of boxing when a student, also a very keen cricketer who made a regular habit of watching the Gentlemen versus Players game at Lords. He was very attentive to his patients, and very kindly to students.

BALBIANI RINGS

Chromosome puffs.

Eduard G. Balbiani (1823–1899) French embryologist. Born in Santo Domingo, Haiti and became Professor of Comparative Embryology, College de France in 1873. He discovered schizogenesis.

BALKAN NEPHROPATHY

Interstitial nephritis of obscure etiology occurring in Rumania, Bulgaria and Yugoslavia, around the Danube basin.

BALLANCE SIGN

In a ruptured spleen, dullness in left flank does not shift whereas there is shifting dullness in the right flank.

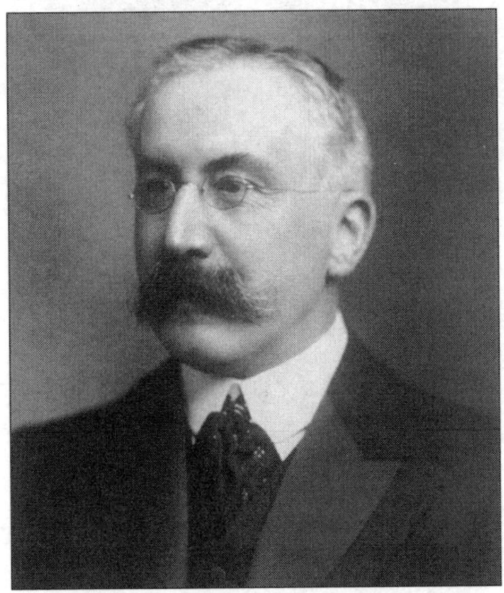

Sir Charles A. Ballance (Courtesy of the Royal Society of Medicine, London, UK)

Sir Charles A. Ballance (1865–1936) English surgeon, St. Thomas' Hospital. He entered St. Thomas' Medical School in 1876 and was a brilliant student who graduated M.B.B.S. in 1881 and interned at St. Thomas', later becoming a surgical registrar and demonstrator in anatomy. He studied bacteriology in Leipzig, attending the first course given at the University. He later worked with Horsley to remove the first spinal tumor successfully and wrote treatises on ligation of blood vessels and nerve graft of the facial nerve. He was the first President of the Society of British Neurological Surgeons and was a friend of Harvey Cushing with whom he worked in the U.S.A. Although best known for his pioneering work on nerve grafting, he did much work with Samuel Shattock on the etiology of cancer trying to implicate a protozoa with negative results. He would appear in the laboratory in the evening and often work on until midnight. He would say "at home they have yet to understand that I like my coffee cold!" He constantly preached the importance of experimental research in surgery. Following Germany's invasion of Belgium in 1914, he threw a German decoration (bestowed on him years previously) into the Thames.

BAMBERGER DISEASE

v. CONCATO DISEASE

Progressive polyserositis with effusions in the pleural and peritoneal cavities. (v. MARIE-BAMBERGER SYNDROME)

Eugen Bamberger (1858–1921) German physician.

BAMBERGER DISEASE

Palmus saltatory spasm. A tic with repeated jumping movements, achoalia (repetitive meaningless words) and abulia (inability to make decisions). This condition may be seen in schizophrenia and hysteria.

Heinrich von Bamberger (1822–1888) German physician. He first recognized Pick disease in 1872 (*v. infra*).

BANCROFT FILARIASIS

v. *WUCHERIA BANCROFTI*

Sir Joseph Bancroft (1836–1894) Born at Stretford near Manchester, he was brought up on his father's farm and apprenticed to Dr. J. Renshaw of Sale, Cheshire, "to serve in and be taught the arts, mysteries and profession of a surgeon, apothecary and man-midwife". He completed his medical studies at the Manchester Royal School of Medicine and Surgery. In 1859 he graduated M.D. at the University of St. Andrews. He practiced in Nottingham for five years, during which time he became an ardent naturalist, becoming President of the Nottingham Naturalist Society.

Ill health, probably renal in origin, since he noted "dropsy better, but still some albumin in the urine" led him to migrate to Australia as a ship's doctor on the paddle steamer "Lady Young" from

Glasgow in 1864. He was still in poor health when he arrived in Brisbane, bought land and built a house which he called "Kelvin Grove" where he established gardens and commenced his extensive plant studies. As his health became restored, he entered into active medical practice and became well known in all aspects of medical and scientific life. He investigated the properties of a number of Australian native plants and one of these he found to have potent mydriatic properties which he used in practice. This was *Duboisia myoporoides*. During the 2nd World War it was found to be rich in hyoscine, hyoscyamine and atropine and was used at that time as a source of these alkaloids for the Allies.

He made contributions to the establishment of rust-free wheat in Queensland, but his chief work for which he is remembered was his investigations on filaria. He was the first to discover the adult worm in an abscess and later live in fluid which he tapped from a hydrocele during his surgical practice. He was one of the first to suggest that disease was transmitted by mosquitoes, although it was P. Manson who reported the development of filarial embryos in the mosquito (*v. infra*). Both Manson and Bancroft thought that the method of transmission was by drinking water into which the infected mosquitoes had released the parasites.

In another capacity as Public Health Officer he had been for many years warning against drinking unboiled water in Brisbane because of the risk of typhoid and dysentery, and added filariasis to this. He thought that the fall in filarial incidence in Brisbane was due to these precautions. As Public Health Officer he often joined in public debate and apparently did not react kindly to criticism of his public health measures. In one instance he brought to the public's attention the adulteration of milk by milk vendors with roadside water which could be "proven by the naked eye evidence of small fish, tadpoles, and mosquito larvae". He said that such water should be made safe by boiling, and inspection of milk should be enforced. This led to an editorial in the local newspaper suggesting that Bancroft was begging suppliers to use clean water for adulterating milk. He thereupon attacked the newspapers and was accused by the editor of not having a sense of humor!

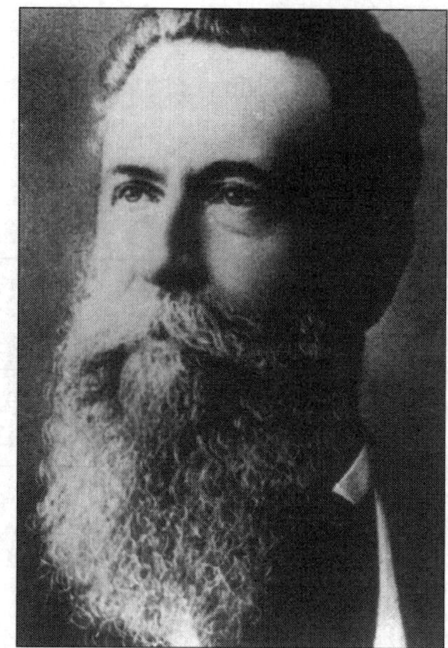

Sir Joseph Bancroft (Courtesy of Faculty of Medicine, University of Queensland, Australia)

He was a pioneer in meat preservation and commenced a factory near a property he had purchased at Deception Bay, where he not only undertook this process, but examined the possibility of tinning other foods such as fish and vegetables. He was a prominent member of the Royal Commission which examined means of control of the rabbit plague. He died suddenly of a coronary occlusion.

BANG DISEASE

Brucellosis (*v. infra Brucella abortus*), a disease in cattle which can be transmitted to man (undulant fever).

Bernhard L.F. Bang (1848–1932) Danish veterinarian and bacteriologist, who was born in Soro (Sjaelland) and studied in Copenhagen, becoming Director of the Veterinary School in Copenhagen. He cultured the bacilli of bovine tuberculosis in 1884 and isolated the organism he called *Bacillus abortus* in 1897. He was instrumental in showing that tuberculosis could be transmitted by cows' milk and in developing isolation techniques, enabling tubercle free milking herds to be established. He did this by removing all tuberculin positive cattle from the remainder.

BANTI SYNDROME OR DISEASE

Portal hypertension and congestive splenomegaly with anemia.

Guido Banti (1852–1925) Italian pathologist who was a renowned physician in Florence. Apart from his description of Banti syndrome he demonstrated that the typhoid bacillus could be found in the blood of patients with typhoid fever. He was an excellent teacher, clear in thought and expression, with a great facility for simple explanation of complicated theories. His experimental work on hemolysis led him to advocate splenectomy to treat hemolytic anemia, and its success resulted in Karnelson using splenectomy to treat idiopathic thrombocytopenic purpura.

BÁRÁNY MANEUVER

The patient is moved from a sitting position to a supine position with the head turned to one side. Nystagmus and dizziness may occur for a few seconds in patients with benign positional vertigo.

BÁRÁNY POINTING TEST

Clinical test for cerebellar function in which the patient is asked to point at a fixed object with a finger or a toe with the eyes alternately open and closed.

BÁRÁNY SYNDROME

Unilateral headache in back of the head with ipsilateral recurrent deafness, vertigo, tinnitus and abnormal pointing test, corrected by stimulating nystagmus (*v. infra*).

BÁRÁNY TEST

Caloric test of semicircular canal.

Robert Bárány (1876–1936) Austrian physician, born in Vienna, graduated from University of Vienna in 1900 and then worked with Kraepelin in Heidelberg, and also studied in Paris. In 1903 he returned to Vienna where he was a student of Sigmund Freud. A favourite story of his concerned Freud's theory that dreams were an expression of desire; Freud used to tell his students "if you can't explain your dream, come and see me". Bárány described a dream to Freud which had nothing to do with desire. Freud's retort was "That is very simple. You desire to contradict me!".

Bárány joined the Ear Clinic of Adam Politzer in Vienna in 1905 where he did his work on the effect of syringing ears to stimulate nystagmus. In 1914 he received the Nobel Prize for his work, while he was still imprisoned by the Russians, having been captured whilst serving in the Austrian Army. Prince Carl of Sweden persuaded the Czar to release him and he received his prize in Sweden and subsequently became Professor of Otology at Uppsala in 1917. He became well recognized as an able surgeon for sinus disorders, deafness and cerebellar and cerebral abscesses. He was an active pacifist and founded the International Academy of Politics and Social Science for the Promotion of World Peace in 1929. He suffered from insomnia.

BARDET-BIEDL SYNDROME

v. LAURENCE-MOON SYNDROME

Bardet-Biedl has similar features but lacks polydactyly.

BARLOW DISEASE

Infantile scurvy.

Sir Thomas Barlow (1845–1945), was the son of a Lancashire cotton manufacturer. He had a successful undergraduate career at Manchester and London, and in 1868 joined University College, London, graduating M.B. in 1873 and M.D. 1874. He became a registrar at the Hospital for Sick Children, Great Ormond Street, a physician there 10 years later, and retired to the consulting staff in 1899. He was Professor of Clinical Medicine at the University College from 1895 to 1907.

A painstaking and astute clinician, he distinguished tuberculous from meningococcal meningitis. He described a variant of Chvostek sign to detect tetany and drew attention to the relationship of tendon nodules in rheumatic fever to progressive disease and cardiac involvement. His study on infantile scurvy proved that this disease was identical to adult scurvy, an outstanding contribution at the time of introduction of artificial feeding, which led to a recognition of the disorder and reduced mortality. He became a F.R.C.P. in 1880, was elected President in 1910 and re-elected four times. He was Physician to Queen Victoria, whom he attended in her last illness; and to King Edward VII and George V.

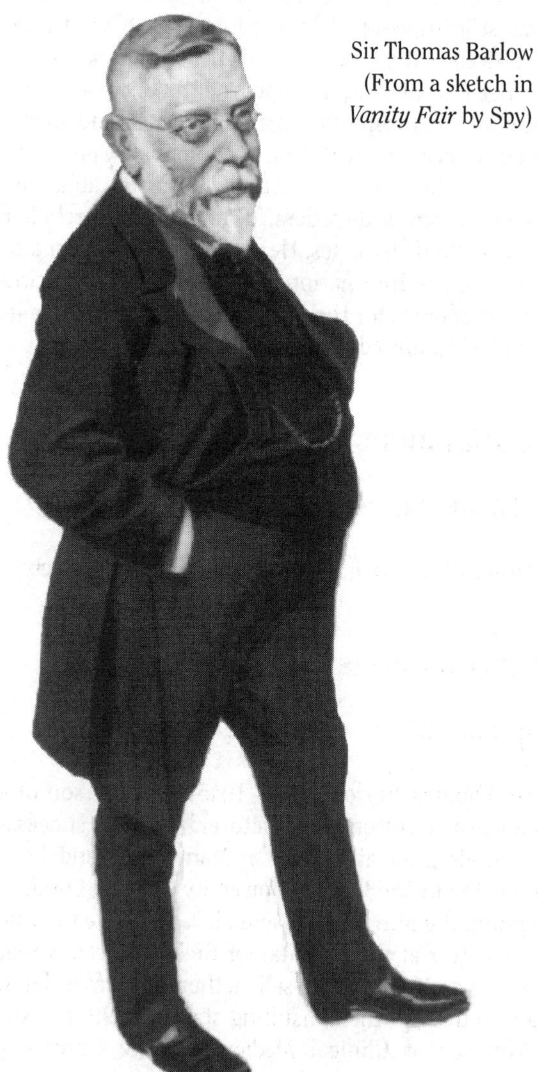

Sir Thomas Barlow (From a sketch in *Vanity Fair* by Spy)

He was created baronet in 1900 and F.R.S. in 1909. He had the North Country attributes of bluntness and honesty, but had the knack of always saying the kind thing.

BARLOW SYNDROME

Floppy posterior mitral valve cusp resulting in apical late systolic murmur preceded by an ejection click which radiates to the axilla, more commonly found in women. It may be associated with valve infection, arrhythmias and atypical chest pain. Frequently of little or no clinical significance.

John Barlow South African physician, Professor of Cardiology at University of Witwatersrand, South Africa – as a student he was nicknamed "canary" because of his references to the rare syndromes and later he kept canaries outside his office. Regarded by his colleagues as the ultimate as a clinical cardiologist in the elicitation and interpretation of cardiac signs in the classical British Paul Wood style.

BARR BODY

Condensed chromatin mass in the female cell nucleus due to the inactive X chromosome.

Murray L. Barr (1908–) Canadian physician, born in Belmont, Ontario, and graduated M.D. in 1930 from University of Western Ontario, and after 2 years in general practice returned to the Anatomy Department in 1936, intending to specialize in neurology, but World War II broke out and he joined up in 1939. After the war he returned to the University of Western Ontario and in 1949 published his work on the sex chromatin with E.G. Bertram. He became Professor of Anatomy in 1951. His initial research was neurocytology and the morphology and distribution of synaptic endings in the spinal cord – he then concentrated on anomalies of sex chromosomes in man.

BARRAQUER DISEASE

Progressive lipodystrophy.

BARRAQUER-SIMONS DISEASE

Progressive lipodystrophy.

José A.R. Barraquer (1855–1928) Spanish physician and neurologist. He was born in Barcelona and after graduation became a Faculty member of Barcelona's oldest hospital "Hospital de la Santa Creu" and in 1882 he founded its first neurology department. Here he introduced techniques of electro-diagnosis and therapy and was regarded by his colleagues as being an eccentric and given the nickname "Doctor de Pilas" (Doctor of Batteries). He described lipodystrophy in 1905 and in 1921 published the first description of the "grasp reflex". This has sometimes been called Barraquer reflex and it was his son, L. Barraquer Jnr., who connected the reflex with lesions in the frontal lobe. He was particularly interested in human behavioral problems as well as organic diseases and pioneered the Catalan School of Neurology. He enjoyed relaxing in the country and for relaxation undertook hunting and breeding carrier pigeons. He initially dissuaded his son from entering medicine, but the latter admiring his father greatly, commenced medicine in secret and ultimately the two became close collaborators.

Arthur Simons (1877–) German physician.

BARRÉ-LIÉOU SYNDROME

Occipital headache, vertigo, tinnitus and facial spasm due to irritation of sympathetic plexus around the vertebral column in rheumatoid arthritis involving the cervical spine.

Jean A. Barré (1880–1967), interned with Babinski in Paris, presented his thesis in 1912 on the osteoarthropathies of tabes, and worked with Guillain in the French Army during the 1914–18 War. He became Professor of Neurology in Strasburg in 1919, aged 39 (v. Guillain-Barré syndrome). He was particularly interested in vestibular function and disease, and founded the Revue d'Oto-Neuro-Ophthalmologie. Barré was a fine clinician who was meticulous in his examination and trained many neurologists from France and other countries who became professors.

Yong C. Liéou (1879–) French Chinese physician in Strasburg who wrote his thesis on this topic when a student of Barré.

(v. GUILLAIN-BARRÉ SYNDROME)

BARRET EPITHELIUM

Columnar esophageal epithelium which is believed to be a reparative or metaplastic response to esophageal reflux of gastric contents.

BARRET ULCER

Esophageal ulcer occurring when the normal squamous cells lining the esophagus are transformed to columnar cells resembling gastric mucosa.

Norman R. Barret (1903–1979) British surgeon. He was born in Adelaide, South Australia, educated at Eton and Trinity College Cambridge, gained 1st class honors tripos and graduated from St. Thomas' Hospital in 1928. He became surgeon at St. Thomas' and Brompton Hospitals, President of Thoracic Surgeons of Great Britain and Ireland 1962 and Editor of Thorax 1946–1971.

BART HEMOGLOBIN

Abnormal hemoglobin. Fetal equivalent of Hb H, composed of 4 α chains – first described at St. Bartholomew's Hospital, London.

BART-PUMPHREY SYNDROME

Deafness, leukonychia and knuckle pads. Autosomal dominant. Keratoderma plantaris and palmaris may also occur.

Robert S. Bart (1933–) U.S. dermatologist.

Robert E. Pumphrey (1933–) U.S. otolaryngologist.

BARTHOLIN CYST

Enlargement of Bartholin gland, situated near introitus of the vagina.

Caspar Bartholin (1655–1738) Danish anatomist and physician, born in Copenhagen. His father, Thomas (1616–80) described the intestinal lymphatics and their drainage via the thoracic duct into the venous system, edited one of the earliest medical journals, Acta Medica Hofmensia, and described an encephalitis epidemic in Denmark in 1657.

Whilst still a medical student he was appointed Professor of Philosophy, and travelled and studied extensively in Europe, and in Paris worked with the anatomist Guichard Duverney, and together they found Bartholin glands in a cow! In 1678 he commenced practice in Copenhagen.

Bartholin also discovered the sublingual glands and their ducts and later in life became interested in politics, becoming Procurator General in 1719, and Deputy of Finance in 1724.

BARTONELLA

Parasite invading red cells causing Bartonellosis – acute febrile hemolytic anemia seen in South America (v. CARRION DISEASE).

Alberto Barton (1871–1950) He was born of English parents, in Buenos Aires, Argentina, but as a child accompanied his parents to Peru and some years later acquired Peruvian nationality. He studied medicine at the Universidad Peruana de San Marcos in the Medical Faculty of San Fernando and graduated in 1900 with a thesis entitled "The bacterial pathogenesis of Carrión's disease". At the time his findings were not accepted as others isolated *Salmonella typhi* and *paratyphi* and believed these were the causative organisms. He went to London, with the support of the Peruvian government, and studied at the London School of Tropical Medicine from 1902 to 1905, when he returned to Peru. Here he continued his investigations and in 1909 published on Carrión's disease in which he again announced the discovery of the causative agent. Controversy continued until 1913 when Dr. Richard Strong from the School of Tropical Medicine at Harvard concluded that Barton had indeed discovered a new pathogenic bacillus causing Oroya Fever. Even so, Strong did not accept that the pathogenetic agent for Peruvian wart and Oroya Fever was one and the same, despite the tragic experiment of the Peruvian student Eduardo Carrión (*v. infra*) which clearly showed this to be so. In 1924 the famous Japanese bacteriologist, Hideyo Noguchi, assisted by a Peruvian scientist, Telemaco Battistini, proved that the *Bartonella* pathogen was the cause of both clinical manifestations. The first reports of this carried the authorship of both Noguchi and Battistini, but the last and more definitive article only carried Noguchi's name! Dr. Battistini, therefore, returned to Peru. Dr. Barton was the President of the National Medical Academy of Peru but was never appointed a professor in his university (the Universidad de San Marcos) in Lima, Peru.

BARTTER SYNDROME

Hypokalemic alkalosis, hyperaldosteronism with normal blood pressure and hyperplasia of the juxta glomerular apparatus.

Frederick C. Bartter (1919–1983) Physician, U.S.A., born in Manila, Philippine Islands, educated at Harvard where he graduated M.D. in 1940. He interned at the Roosevelt Hospital, New York, and worked with Fuller Albright (*v. supra*) on adrenal, parathyroid and metabolic bone disease. During this time he established the pathophysiology of the adrenogenital syndrome (1950). In 1956 he described the role of the extracellular fluid volume in the control of aldosterone secretion in man. In 1957 with W.B. Schwartz he described the syndrome of inappropriate anti-diuretic hormone (ADH) secretion in two patients with bronchogenic carcinoma with hyponatremia, inappropriate sodium loss unrelated to renal or adrenal disease, and water retention due to ADH. He moved to the National Institute for Health in Washington, D.C., in 1951 and in 1956 was appointed Chief of the Endocrinology Branch at N.I.H. He later moved to San Antonio, Texas.

BASEDOW DISEASE

Thyrotoxicosis.

BASEDOW SYNDROME

Myeloneuropathy in thyrotoxicosis not due to vitamin B_{12} deficiency.

Karl A. von Basedow (1799–1854) German physician, was a general practitioner in the town of Merseburg from 1822. In 1840 he wrote a paper on exophthalmos. Exophthalmos, goitre and palpitations were later termed the "Merseburg Triad". He also described weight loss and nervousness and suggested the use of mineral waters which contained iodide and bromide in the treatment of this condition.

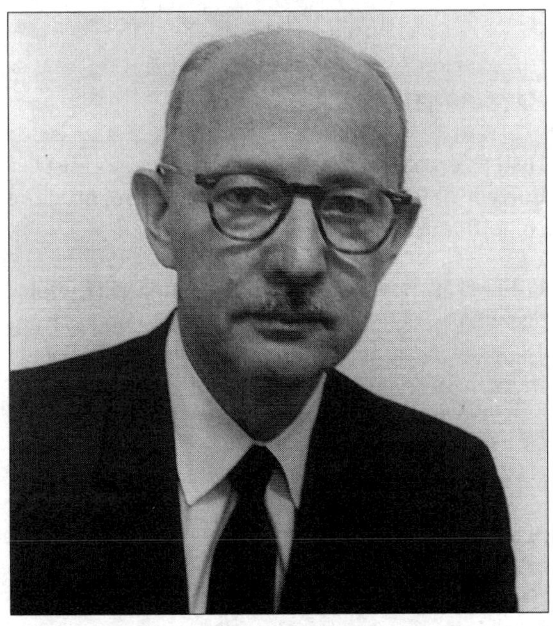

Abraham L. Kornzweig
(Courtesy of Mt. Sinai Hospital, New York, USA)

BASSEN-KORNZWEIG DISEASE OR SYNDROME

Ataxia, retinitis pigmentosa, pyramidal tract dysfunction, areflexia, anterior horn cell degeneration, burr cells in the peripheral blood, hypocholesterolemia and abetalipoproteinemia.

Frank A. Bassen (1903–) U.S. physician, Mt. Sinai Hospital, N.Y., born in St. George, Nova Scotia, Canada, and graduated from McGill in 1928. Moved to the U.S.A., practicing as a hematologist and internist in New York, 1933–1978.

Abraham L. Kornzweig (1900–) U.S. ophthalmologist, Mt. Sinai Hospital, N.Y., born in N.Y. City and graduated from N.Y. University Medical School in 1925. He trained as intern and in ophthalmology at Mt. Sinai Hospital, entering the ophthalmology service there and private practice in 1934, retiring due to ill health in 1972.

BASTIAN-BRUNS LAW OR SIGN

Complete transection of the cord above the lumbar enlargement results in a loss of deep reflexes of the lower limbs.

Henry C. Bastian (1837–1915) English neurologist, bom in Cornwall (Truro). He studied at University College and graduated from the University of London in 1861, M.D. 1866. He became Professor of Pathological Anatomy and later held the Chair of Medicine. His chief interests were in clinical neurology where he gained an international reputation and was an authority on aphasia, describing Wernicke aphasia five years earlier than Wernicke. He described word blindness and word deafness. He wrote many articles on the evolution of life, championing abiogenesis, espousing spontaneous generation and opposing Pasteur and Tyndall. He worked at the National Hospital, Queen's Square and taught one of the pioneers of neurosurgery – Victor Horsley.

Ludwig von Bruns (*v. infra*).

BATESIAN MIMICRY

A palatable species mimics an unpalatable one in appearance and thereby the prey avoids the hunter.

Henry W. Bates (1825–1892) English naturalist and explorer born in Leicester, the oldest son of a hosiery manufacturer. He was apprenticed to the trade when 13 years old but continued studying at nights and became interested in insects. In 1848 he went to the Amazon and remained there for eleven years collecting specimens and travelling. Encouraged by Charles Darwin he related his experiences in a book regarded by many as a classic, "The Naturalist on the River Amazon", in 1863. He later was appointed assistant secretary to the Royal Geographical Society and left his butterfly collection to the British Museum.

BATTEN DISEASE

v. CURSCHMANN-BATTEN-STEINHERT SYNDROME

v. SPIELMEYER-VOGT DISEASE

BATTEY BACILLUS

A strain of mycobacteria causing a lung disease like tuberculosis. First isolated at the Battey State Hospital, Georgia, U.S.A.

BATTLE SIGN

Bluish discoloration of the skin over the mastoid process suggests fracture of the base of the skull.

William H. Battle (1855–1936) English surgeon, was born in Lincoln and educated at Lincoln Grammar School, entering St. Thomas' Medical School, London, in 1873. He was an excellent student, graduating in 1877, M.R.C.S. He gained his F.R.C.S. in 1880 and became surgical registrar at St. Thomas' and in 1892 assistant surgeon. The same year he was appointed to the Lancet as general surgical advisor. He was experienced in obstetrics and had a long association with the Royal Free Hospital and taught in the Medical School for Women.

BAUMGARTEN SYNDROME

v. CRUVEILHIER-BAUMGARTEN SYNDROME

BAYES RULE OR THEOREM

A mathematical method for combining disease prevalence and characteristics of disorders to assess the likelihood of various hypotheses. This can be applied to the probabilities of diagnoses – that a given finding (e.g. malar rash or blush in systemic lupus erythematosis or mitral stenosis) may be present with a disease state or that a test may give the diagnosis (e.g. VDRL in syphilis or lupus), or the probabilities of a correct diagnosis before the performance of a test.

Thomas Bayes (1702–1761) English clergyman, mathematician and statistician. His best known work, "An Essay Towards Solving a Problem in the Doctrine of Chances", was published posthumously in 1763. It contained what has become known as Bayes Theorem of conditional probabilities which has been used in computer assisted diagnosis.

BAYLISS THEORY

Distension of a vessel results in reflex vasoconstriction which if sustained results in hypertrophy of the smooth musculature in a vessel.

William M. Bayliss (1860–1924) English physiologist who worked at University College, London from 1889 and was appointed Professor of Physiology there in 1912.

BAZEX SYNDROME

Acrokeratosis paraneoplastica. Purplish blue and erythematous lesions. Usually bilateral and symmetrical which may be hyperkeratotic. It may involve the face and extremities, pinna of the ear, bridge of the nose, hands and feet with diffuse hyperkeratosis of the palms and soles together with nail dystrophy. Predominantly occurs in males and associated with an underlying malignancy of the upper part of the respiratory and digestive systems and often precedes the appearance of the malignancy.

André Bazex (1911–1988) He was a French dermatologist who became Professor of Dermatology and Venereology at Toulouse in France.

BAZIN DISEASE

Symmetrical purple nodules due to vasculitis on the calves which break down to form indolent ulcers and leave pigmented scars, most frequently seen in adolescent girls with tuberculosis or positive tuberculin test. Erythema induratum.

Antoine P.E. Bazin (1807–1878) French dermatologist born in a small village near Paris, St. Brice-sous-Bois, the son and grandson of physicians. He was always abrasive and sarcastic in dealing with his colleagues whether senior or not and this led to movement from one hospital post to another. He finally returned to Hôpital St. Louis where as a student, he had been particularly influenced by Alibert. This was in 1847 and he remained for the rest of his professional life. In 1850 his reputation was established by his recognition with Hardy of the same fungus causing tinea capitis as well as affecting the beard and body. Liked by students and patients but had continuing running battles and sarcastic exchanges with his colleagues. Not modest, in 1860 he said "My lectures on the parasitic infections, published two years ago, have been the sensation of the medical world".

B.C.G. VACCINE

Bacillus Calmette-Guérin.

Léon C.A. Calmette (1863–1933) French bacteriologist, born in Nice; a pupil of Louis Pasteur, he introduced active immunization against tuberculosis in 1924 using a living strain of tubercle bacilli. He went to the French Naval School at Brest, graduating in medicine at the University of Paris in 1886. He entered the Colonial Service as a surgeon and founded the Pasteur Institute in Saigon and worked on snake venom and plague.

In 1895 Pasteur sent him to found the Lille Institute for Hygiene and there he commenced his work on tuberculosis. He became sub-director of the Pasteur Institute in Paris when Metchnikoff died in 1917.

Camille Guérin (1872–1961) French veterinarian born in Portiers and graduated as a vet. from Alfont. He worked with Calmette to develop the vaccine. Their investigations commenced shortly before the 1st World War and they made their first successful vaccination in 1921, but had a major set back with the Lubeck disaster when 73 of 250 infants vaccinated died of tuberculosis due to improperly prepared vaccine.

BEAU LINES

Transverse groove seen on fingernails after serious illness, e.g. myocardial infarction, or severe emotional trauma.

Joseph H.S. Beau (1806–1865) French physician, who wrote one of the early descriptions of cardiac insufficiency and asystole, sometimes termed Beau Syndrome.

BECHTEREW

v. BEKHTEREV

BECK TRIAD

Low arterial pressure, high venous pressure and absent apex beat in cardiac tamponade.

Claude S. Beck (1894–1971) U.S. surgeon, born in Shamokia, Pennsylvania. He graduated M.D. Johns Hopkins 1921, then went to Cleveland in 1924 following a period as Cabot Fellow at Harvard and associate surgeon at the Peter Bent Brigham. After some years of animal experimentation, he introduced a technique for improving vascular supply to the heart in 1936 which, after an initial wave of enthusiasm, was abandoned. Although predominantly a thoracic surgeon he made numerous contributions to vascular surgery and to neurosurgery, in particular the use of vitallium plates to close defects of the skull. He pioneered emergency surgery to re-start hearts (open cardiac massage) on patients "too good to die" and lectured widely to lay audiences on appropriate first aid techniques. He died of a stroke.

BECKER MUSCULAR DYSTROPHY

Benign X-linked recessive form of muscular dystrophy with involvement of limb girdle muscles first, and then later the pectoral muscles. Cardiac involvement is absent and the life span is often normal – as distinct from the Duchenne form of muscular dystrophy (*v. infra*). Becker also described an autosomal recessive form of myotonia congenita (cf. Thomsen Disease) which has a later onset and different inheritance.

Peter E. Becker (1908–) German human geneticist. He was born in Hamburg and worked from 1936–38 as an assistant at the Kaiser-Wilhelm Institut for anthropology and human genetics and eugenics with Professor E. Fischer. Here he was influenced by Fritz Lenz in developing his scientific approach. In 1943 he worked in the psychiatric and neurological clinic at the University of Freiberg with Professor Kay Berringer and from 1946–57 as a lecturer in that same clinic and University. He was then appointed as Professor of Human Genetics at the University of Göttingen. Over the years he has published numerous articles and books on human genetics with particular reference to the hereditary myopathies and in particular myotonia.

BECKER NAEVUS

Pigmented hairy epidermal naevus which most commonly occurs in males and is often located on the shoulder. They are often solitary and may be the size of the palm of a hand. Despite the striking appearance histological changes are slight and naevus cells are not seen in the dermis.

Samuel W. Becker (1894–) U.S. dermatologist.

BECKWITH-WIEDEMANN SYNDROME

The exophthalmos, macroglossia, gigantism (E.M.G.) syndrome. Infants are born with macroglossia and umbilical anomaly, ear lobe crease and fetal adrenal hyperplasia and other endocrine disturbances, often with hypoglycemia.

John Bruce Beckwith (1933–) Born in Spokane, Washington, graduated from the University of Washington in 1958 – he trained in pediatric pathology at the Children's Hospital in Los Angeles. In 1964 he returned to Seattle where he was on the Faculty of the University of Washington School of Medicine and Director of Laboratories at the Children's Hospital. By 1974 he was Professor of Pathology and Pediatrics at the University Washington. In 1985 he moved to Denver, Colorado where he is currently Professor of Pathology and Pediatrics of the University of Colorado School of Medicine and Chairman of Pathology at the Children's Hospital. His particular research interests include sudden death in infancy, tumor pathogenesis and classification of Wilms tumor (*v. infra*).

Hans R. Wiedemann German paediatrician, Department of Paediatrics, University of Kiel, West Germany.

BEER LAW

Transmission of light through a solution is a function of the concentration of the solution and the length of the light path.

A. Beer (1825–1863) German physicist.

BEEVOR SIGN

Upward displacement of umbilicus due to paralysis of lower rectus abdominis.

Charles E. Beevor (1854–1908) He was one of the many talented English neurologists who worked at the Brown Institute in London in research on the functions of the cerebral cortex. He collaborated with Victor Horsley, Ballance, Ferrier and a galaxy of other notables. He studied with Flechsig in Germany.

BEHÇET SYNDROME OR DISEASE

Ulcers in the mouth and urethra; thrombophlebitis; arthralgia; pyoderma; papules in eyes; uveitis. Initially described as aphthous stomatitis, genital ulcerations and iridocyclitis with hypopyon.

Hulusi Behçet (1889–1948) Turkish dermatologist. He held appointments at the University of Medicine of Gülahne, but in 1914 was appointed assistant head physician of the Kirklareli Military Hospital. He became dermatologist at the Ederne Military Hospital and in August 1918 went to Europe and worked first in Budapest and later in Berlin with Blumenthal and Cheressesky at the Charity Hospital, returning to Turkey late in 1919.

He commenced a private clinic in Cagaloglu and in 1923 was appointed assistant head physician of the Hasköy Venereal Disease Hospital. Later he transferred to the Guraba Hospital where he worked on the etiology and pathogenesis of the Eastern Boil (Baghdad Boil). During University reform in Turkey he was appointed as Professor to the Clinic of Dermatology and Syphilis in 1933, and held that position for 14 years. He became a leading figure in dermatological teaching and investigation in Turkey and also in research against syphilis and in conducting courses to train people to treat syphilis. He worked for more than 25 years on the disorder that bears his name and wrote a book on "Syphilis and Related Skin Diseases". He was a retiring, shy man who was well regarded by all of his colleagues and was well known in international circles in dermatology and described this syndrome in 1937 based on 3 patients he observed from 1924–1936. He was troubled with ill health throughout his life with chronic insomnia, spastic colitis and heart trouble. He died of myocardial infarction.

BEKHTEREV DISEASE OR SYNDROME

Ankylosing spondylitis.

BEKHTEREV NUCLEUS

Superior vestibular nucleus.

BEKHTEREV-MENDEL REFLEX

Tapping the dorsum of foot normally causes extension of 2nd–5th toes. A pyramidal lesion is characterized by flexion.

Vladimir M. Bekhterev (1857–1927) Russian neurologist. He was born in a small village, Surali, between the Volga River and the Ural Mountains. He entered the Military Medical Academy in St. Petersburg at the age of 16 and graduated in 1878. In 1884–5 he worked with Flechsig in Leipzig, visited Meynert, Westphal and Charcot, and described the superior vestibular nucleus in 1885. He was appointed Professor of Psychiatry at the University of Kazan and in 1893 succeeded his original mentor Merzhenevsky at St. Petersburg (Leningrad) (following 1917 the Institute was renamed State University of Medical Sciences). He was a faculty colleague of Pavlov and made many contributions in neuro-anatomy and clinical neurology. He and Pavlov were frequently in open conflict at meetings and there was much acrimonious debate between workers from his laboratory and those from Pavlov's. Pavlov believed work from Bekhterev's laboratory was poorly controlled and sloppy at best. Certainly Bekhterev seemed to accept his assistants' experimental findings too readily and uncritically. He died a day after chairing the All-Union Neurological Congress in Moscow.

Kurt Mendel (1874–1946) German neurologist who trained in Bielschowsky's laboratory in Berlin in 1896.

BELL PALSY

Lower motor neurone paralysis of the 7th cranial nerve.

BELL PHENOMENON

When a patient with lower motor neurone 7th nerve paralysis tries to shut his eye on the affected side it closes incompletely and the eye ball rotates upwards.

Sir Charles Bell (1774–1842) Scottish physiologist and surgeon. He was the son of an episcopal clergyman and left Edinburgh in 1801 for London, following an argument between his eldest brother, John (also a brilliant surgeon) and members of the Faculty of Medicine at the University of Edinburgh,

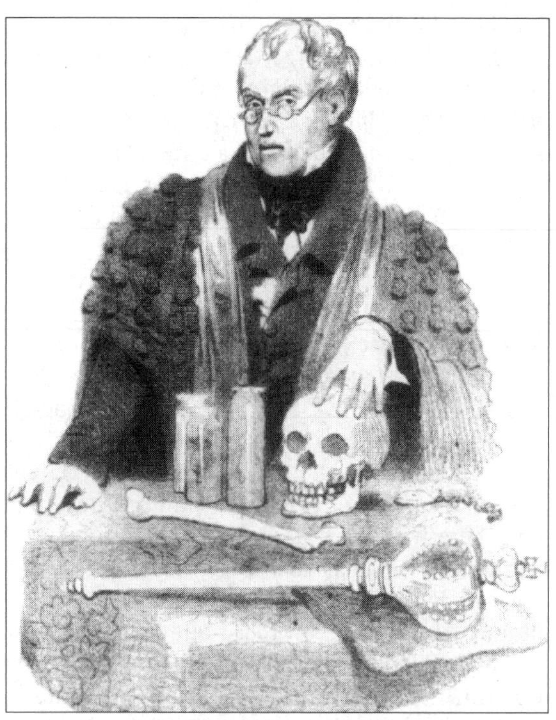

Sir Charles Bell (Courtesy of the Royal Society of Medicine, London, UK)

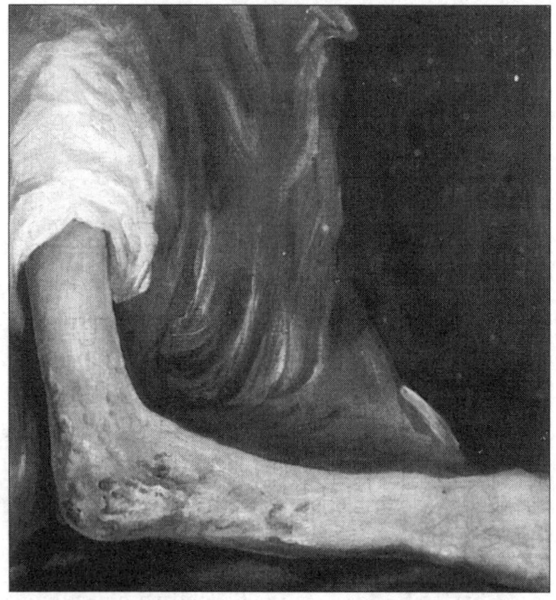

Painting by C. Bell. "Sketch in Oil of an Arm of an Officer who came to me to have his arm amputated. A musket Ball is lodged in the elbow joint, the nerves were cut, and the arm asleep, shrunk, and cold." (From the Bell Collections of the Royal College of Surgeons of Edinburgh, Scotland)

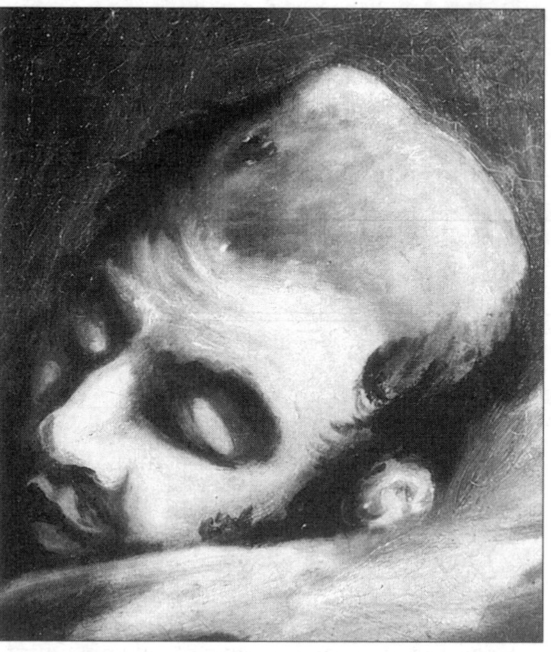

Painting by C. Bell. "Sketch of a Soldier, the ball entered in the forehead penetrated the skull, and drove up the bone, elevating the two portions at an angle. The Scalp was cut open at this part, the bone raised, and the Ball extracted, as the Dura-Mater was cut, I could expect nothing but fungus-Cerebri, I lost sight of the man and do not know his fate." (From the Bell Collections of the Royal College of Surgeons of Edinburgh, Scotland)

who denied them positions at the Royal Infirmary or the University. Bell was an accomplished artist and made his name in London initially by his publication "Essays on the Anatomy of Painting". He established that sensory and motor functions were carried by the spinal nerves and that the anterior roots carried motor fibres and the posterior roots the sensory fibres (Bell Law). It is doubtful if he recognized the significance of his finding at the time (1811), since he still held that all nerves were sensory, classifying them as sensible and insensible. He disliked vivisection and it remained for Magendie (1822) and J. Müller (1831) to establish his finding conclusively. He described proprioreceptive sensation and demonstrated that the 5th cranial nerve supplied sensation to the face and motor mastication. He was an able surgeon who attended the military hospital at Haslar to treat the wounded who had returned to England following the Battle of Corunna. In 1815 when he learnt of Waterloo he said to his brother-in-law, "Johnnie! How can we let this pass? Here is such an occasion of seeing gunshot wounds." He operated tirelessly with little sleep and made sketches and paintings of the scenes, slides of some of which are available at the Royal College of Surgeons in Edinburgh. He was a kindly man and somewhat of a dandy in dress. He founded the Middlesex Hospital and Medical School, London, and in 1836 became Professor of Surgery at Edinburgh. Viggo Christiansen of Copenhagen said, "He created modern clinical neurology in the same way his contemporary Corot created modern French landscape painting."

BENCE JONES PROTEIN

An abnormal protein found in the urine of patients with multiple myeloma, initially characterized by precipitation at 56°C and re-solution at 100°C, and now known to consist of monoclonal light chains of the gamma globulin molecules.

Henry Bence Jones (1814–1873) English physician, born in Thorington Hall, Suffolk. His mother was the daughter of Bence Bence, also of Thorington Hall and rector of Beccles, and his father was a Lieutenant-colonel in 5th Dragoon Guards. Bence Jones was educated at Harrow and Trinity College, Cambridge, graduating B.A. in 1836. He studied medicine at St. George's Hospital, and chemistry in Professor Graham's laboratory at University College under the direction of Dr. Fownes. In 1841 he went to Giessen to study in Baron Liebig's school of chemistry. He became L.R.C.P. in 1842, gained his M.B. Cambridge in 1845 and was elected that year to assistant physician to St. George's Hospital. He became a full physician and an F.R.S. in 1846 and gained his M.D. Cambridge and F.R.C.P. in 1849. In 1860 he was appointed secretary of the Royal Institution, and remained in that position for most of his life. He was an excellent physician who had a very large and wealthy practice, but he was also a highly skilled chemist who applied his knowledge to medical problems. He was a friend and great admirer of Faraday and wrote his biography. As secretary of the Royal Institution he published recent scientific discoveries for the lay public. He published on many topics, induding renal calculi, chemical analysis of the urine, and gout. His attempts to apply chemical laws to human phenomena were well ahead of his time and were not as successful as they might have been because the complexity of biochemistry and physiology were not understood. However, his insistence on the examination of the urine both chemically and with the microscope in diagnosing clinical disease, which he instilled into his students by example, not only founded an important clinical test approach but enabled scientific contributions as he showed that the sugar in diabetic urine continued to be present despite withholding sugar in the diet. His first paper on cystine calculus was in 1840, and he described the abundance of urate crystals in the urine of gouty subjects, and pioneered urinalysis as a standard step in examination. He died in congestive cardiac failure. His old teacher Liebig died in the same year and their obituaries appear alongside one another in The Lancet.

BENEDICT SOLUTION

Copper sulphate solution used to test for glycosuria.

Stanley R. Benedict (1884–1936) U.S. chemist, Professor of Chemical Pathology, Cornell University Medical College, New York, from 1912—Editor of The Journal of Biological Chemistry. He devised his solution whilst a second year student and published 9 original papers before his graduation in chemistry at the University of Cincinnati. He demonstrated that urinary ammonia was almost totally formed in the kidney and with Folin with whom he was often in debate should be credited as a major contributor to the measurement of metabolites in the blood so important in modern medicine. Apart from his development of analytical techniques he discovered new substances such as ergothioneine in the red cells. In 1920 he became editor of the Journal of Biological Chemistry and early on decided to dispense with the final "e" which terminated many biochemical compounds until he was asked by one of his colleagues whether he was going to abolish the final "e" on his favourite liqueur "Benedictine". This caused him to revise his views!

BENEDIKT SYNDROME

Ipsilateral third nerve palsy with contralateral ataxia, tremor and choreoathetoid movement of upper limb caused by a mid-brain lesion involving the 3rd nerve as it passes through the red nucleus (cf. Weber syndrome).

Moritz Benedikt (1835–1920) Austrian physician, born in Eisenstadt, Hungary, but lived all his life in Vienna. After graduation he joined the Army and fought in 1859–61 campaigns in Italy, which signalled the beginning of modern Italy. He returned to a University appointment and in 1899 became Ordinarius of Electrotherapy, a Chair just created. He was a fine teacher, an orator of wit and interested in drama. One of the founders of the General Poliklinik of Vienna, he believed the criminal was a sick person with abnormal anatomical and physiological traits. He pioneered the use of electrotherapy and made classic observations on occupational neuroses which he classified as spastic, tremulous and paralytic. He published the description of his syndrome in 1889 and his name was eponymously given to the syndrome by Charcot in 1893.

BENJAMIN SYNDROME

Hypochromic anemia with megalocephaly, small extremities and dental caries, sometimes associated with epicanthic folds, cardiac murmurs and palpable splenic tumors.

E. Benjamin German pediatrician.

BENNETT FRACTURE

Fracture of the base of the 1st metacarpal frequently following a trauma to the point of the thumb. The oblique fracture passes through the articular surface and often results in subluxation of the joint.

Edward H. Bennett (1837–1907) Irish surgeon who was born at Charlotte Quay Cork, into a family who had relatives in medicine on both sides. He graduated from Trinity College in 1859 taking a new degree M.Ch. which was given for the first time. He devoted much of his life to a collection of fractures, dislocations, diseases of the bone which he catalogued with the clinical details in the Pathology Museum at Trinity College. He became Professor of Surgery in Trinity College in 1873 and described his fracture at the British Medical Association meeting in Cork in 1880. He was one of the earliest Irish surgeons to adopt Lister's methods.

BERGER DISEASE

Glomerulonephritis with mesangial IgA deposition.

Jean Berger (1930–) He was a resident in the Paris Hospitals from 1956–60 and "Chef de Clinique" in Professor Jean Hamburger's Department of Nephrology from 1960–62. He became Professor of Pathology in 1970 at the Faculty of Medicine in the Hôpital Necker/Enfants-Malades and later Chief of the Department of Pathology at the Laennec Hospital in 1979.

BERGER RHYTHM OR WAVE

Alpha rhythm in the electroencephalogram (EEG).

Hans Berger (1873–1941) German neuropsychiatrist, was born in Neuses, near Coburg, and studied at Jena University where in 1900 he became assistant to O. Binswanger and in 1919 became his successor. He wrote numerous articles on the intracranial circulation and temperature of the brain. In 1924 he made his first electroencephalogram recording in man after some years of secret experimentation, but he did not publish his results until 1929. Apart from the EEG, he was a founder of psychophysiology. He committed suicide by hanging in 1941.

BERGERON CHOREA OR DISEASE

Sudden involuntary spasm of muscle occurring at long intervals, usually self-limited and may follow Sydenham Chorea.

Etienne J. Bergeron (1817–1900) French physician.

BERI BERI

Vitamin B_1 deficiency which can result in peripheral neuritis and/or high output cardiac failure.
Beri – a Singhalese word for weakness.

BERNARD SYNDROME

v. HORNER SYNDROME

Claude Bernard (1813–1878) French physiologist. He was born in the village of St. Julien near Ville Franche. His parents were winemakers. He was not very outstanding at school and from 1833–1834 he was apprenticed to an apothecary shop in Lyons and during that time wrote two plays which were presented, but were not greeted with much acclaim. As a result of his failure he enrolled as a medical student at the University of Paris in 1835 and soon met Magendie with whom he worked from 1839–1844 while he was doing his clinical studies at the Hôtel Dieu. He had somewhat different views to Magendie and the two split up in 1844, Bernard commenting "I consider the hospital to be a vestibule for scientific medicine; it is the first field of observation to which a physician is exposed. However the laboratory is the temple of medical science".

Bernard's initial work was in the field of digestion and he showed that gastric juice would alter sugar so that if it were injected back into the animal's veins it would no longer appear in the urine as sugar. He showed that pancreatic juice exerted a fat splitting action. In 1848 he discovered that sugar could be formed in the liver of a dog which was only eating protein and that glucose was always present in blood and in the liver and that glycogen was found in the liver. Using curare, Bernard was able to demonstrate that muscle could be excited independently of its nerve and showed that lactic acid was normally produced during muscle contraction. In 1858 he demonstrated the vasodilator action of the chorda tympani and that sectioning the cervical sympathetic nerve leads to pupillary constriction and blushing of the ear and this ultimately led to the discovery of the vasomotor nervous system. In France, Horner syndrome is referred to as Bernard-Horner syndrome. He developed the concept of the organism being an integrated whole with modulated interactions between its various units.

In his famous work "An Introduction to the Study of Experimental Medicine" he clearly outlined the scientific method of applying available methodology to prove or disprove either an established theory or a laboratory observation. He emphasized the milieu interieur (the internal environment) which the organism maintains constant in order to enable normal tissue function. He died of renal disease and a statue was erected in his honor in his birthplace, St. Julien on the Rhone.

BERNARD-SOULIER SYNDROME

Congenital bleeding diathesis associated with giant platelets with a specific membrane defect (lack of glycoprotein lb) and thrombocytopenia.

Jean Bernard (1907–) French physician, born in Paris, graduating in medicine there in 1926. He was influenced by Paul Chevallier who was the leading French hematologist of the day, and Debré. He commenced his laboratory training with Ramon at the Pasteur Institute in 1929. Active in the French resistance he was jailed during the occupation and during his incarceration composed poetry which was later published entitled "Survivance".

He is probably the most important figure in clinical medicine in France since World War II. He established a department at the Hospital Saint Louis which became an international centre for hematology and here he trained and influenced many people who later became pre-eminent in their profession in France and in other parts of Europe and the world. His renown as a physician and expertise in leukemia resulted in him acting as a consultant in the management of a leading member of the Soviet Politburo. This in turn led to a public subscription in France to establish an institute for blood disorders in Paris. He is one of the few people to be elected to the French Academy of Literature as well as the French Academy of Science.

Jean P. Soulier (1915–) French hematologist who was born in Etretat and graduated from the

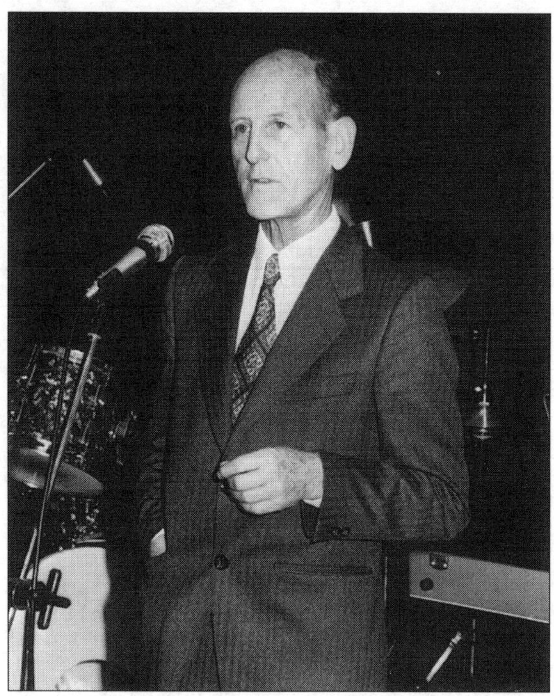

Jean P. Soulier (Courtesy of J.P. Soulier)

University of Paris in Medicine in 1944. He has been Director of the National Blood Transfusion Service in Paris since 1954. His major research interests have been in the area of blood coagulation; he has been responsible for the introduction of new techniques for investigating these problems as well as the discovery of the anticoagulant phenylindanedione and the first successful preparation of a therapeutic fraction from blood to treat factor IX and prothrombin complex deficiencies. He has written two non-medical books: "L'espace d'un matin" and "Lautreamon, genie ou maladie mentale".

BERNHARDT-ROTH PARAESTHESIA

Meralgia parasthetica. Area of pain and/or anesthesia on the antero-lateral aspects of the thigh due to compression of the lateral cutaneous nerve.

Martin Bernhardt (1844–1915) German neurologist. He was born in Potsdam and after graduating became an assistant to Leyden who was then in Königsberg. In 1869 he returned to Berlin to work in Westphal's clinic, but enlisted in the armed forces for the 1870–71 war, returning to practice as a neurologist in Berlin at its completion. His major interests were peripheral neuritis and he contributed a chapter on this to the Nothnagel "Handbook of Special Pathology and Therapy". He retired from his outpatient clinic in 1914 and died shortly after.

Vladimir K. Roth (1848–1916) Russian neurologist who was a pupil and admirer of Korsakoff (*v. infra*).

BERNHEIM SYNDROME

Right ventricle failure due to left ventricular hypertrophy causing the interventricular system to bulge into right ventricle.

Hippolyte Bernheim (1837–1919) French physician. He was appointed as Professor of Clinical Medicine in the Faculty of Medicine of Nancy in 1870. He published in many areas of medicine but in 1883 commenced his life-long interest in hypnotism and hysteria. His ideas were completely opposed to those of the Paris school led by Charcot in that he believed that hypnotism and hysteria were the results of suggestion rather than due to organic problems. This controversy raged between the years of 1885–1890 and Bernheim was proved correct. He published his major work on this in 1903, entitled "Hypnotism, Suggestion, Psychotherapy with New Considerations on Hysteria". Bernheim used the technique of trying to restore and correct emotional traumas under the influence of hypnotism and this is said to have influenced Freud who visited Nancy in 1889. Bernheim came to be known as the Chief of the "School of Nancy", a school of hypnosis.

BERNOUILLI PRINCIPLE

Fluid flowing through a tube of varying diameter travels fastest and exerts the largest lateral pressure at its narrowest point.

Jakob Bernouilli (1654–1705) Swiss mathematician who invented infinitesimal calculus and the logarithmic spiral. The family originated in Antwerp but in the 16th century moved to Frankfurt to avoid political persecution. His grandfather moved to Basel in 1622 and Bernouilli was born there. He founded the theory of probability and is said to have applied it to distribution of disease. He requested that the logarithmic spiral and the words "Eadem mutata resurgo" be carved on his headstone, but an ordinary spiral was engraved in error. Four other members of the family were famous mathematicians.

BERNSTEIN TEST

A patient's symptoms of reflux are induced by applying acid to the esophagus.

Lionel M. Bernstein U.S. gastroenterologist.

BERRY ANEURYSM

Aneurysm of the Circle of Willis which may rupture and cause subarachnoid hemorrhage. This term was introduced because the lesion looked like a berry.

BERRY LIGAMENT

Lateral fascial ligament of the thyroid gland.

Sir James Berry (1840–1946) English surgeon who was born in Canada. He pioneered thyroid surgery in England and wrote a text book on the subject which Grey Turner regarded highly. With his first wife assembled and led a medical team to Serbia in World War I and were captured by the Hungarians and repatriated through Switzerland. They returned to continue their work in Rumania.

BESNIER PRURIGO

Allergic eczema.

BESNIER-BOECK DISEASE

Sarcoidosis.

Ernest Besnier (1831–1909) French dermatologist, born in Honfleur (Calvados), son of a French customs official who moved from Givet to Marseilles then Orleans. Graduated as a doctor in 1857 and became Médecin des Hôpitaux in 1863. He studied general medicine and public health, writing on the laws which governed epidemics and the adulteration of foodstuffs as well as looking into parasitic infections and their management. In 1872 he became a physician at St. Louis Hospital and from then on specialized in dermatology. With Doyon he founded the journal "Annales de Dermatologie et de Syphiligraphie". He published a French edition of Kaposi's book "Lessons on Abnormalities of the Skin" in 1881. He was nominated for a Chair in the College of Medicine, but a sudden change in the ministry resulted in it being unsuccessful. Besnier did not protest and continued to teach at St. Louis Hospital for some years.

Caesar P. M. Boeck (1845–1917) Norwegian dermatologist. His uncle, Wilhelm Boeck, had made a considerable reputation in Norway as a research worker in syphilis. Although he was also interested in this disorder in a clinical sense, his major contributions were in the field of general dermatology, and in particular in the skin manifestations of tuberculosis which he first wrote about in 1880 and which occupied most of his research life. He particularly emphasized to his colleagues and students the importance of making such a diagnosis in the early recognition of tuberculosis and the possibility that better treatment might result in preventing severe pulmonary tuberculosis. During his study of tuberculosis of the skin, he described the formerly unknown skin disease which he called "multiple benign sarcoid". He initially looked upon it as having some connection with leukemia, but later felt it was a benign form of tuberculous infection and made the observation that the tuberculin test was usually negative. Apart from his description of sarcoid, he noted the relationship of acute rheumatic disorders with throat infections and was one of the first people to describe acne necrotica varioliformis. He was a fine, dogmatic teacher whose quick mind and fertile imagination succeeded in enthusing his students and making his teaching sessions well remembered. In 1889 he was appointed Director of Dermatology at the Rikshospitalet and teacher in dermatology at the University of Oslo. He was appointed Professor of Medicine at the University in

1896, the first dermatologist to be so appointed and this enabled the subject to become one of the major disciplines in medicine in Norway. Towards the end of his life, he was troubled by increasing attacks of angina, and died suddenly, presumably from a coronary occlusion.

BETZ CELL

Giant pyramidal cell in the 5th layer of the cerebral cortex.

Vladimir A. Betz (1834–1894) Russian anatomist and histologist. He was Professor of Anatomy at Kiev.

BEZOLD-JARISCH REFLEX

It is one of the mechanisms of bradycardia in myocardial infarction and results from the stimulation of receptors in the left ventricle conducted by the vagus nerve. This reflex promotes vasodilation, nausea, sweating, hypotension and syncope. It may contribute to vasodepressor syncope following orthostatic stress.

Albert von Bezold (1836–1868) German physiologist born in Ansbach. Son of a physician, he went to study at Munich and Würzburg and in 1857 went to work with Du Bois-Reymond in Berlin. He was appointed to the Chair of Physiology in Jena when only 23 years old and in 1865 was invited as foundation Professor of Physiology at Würzburg. His brilliant career ended there when he died of cardiac complications due to a valvular lesion following rheumatic fever as a young man.

Adolf Jarisch (*v. infra*).

BIEDL-BARDET SYNDROME

v. BARDET-BIEDL and LAURENCE–MOON

BIERMER ANEMIA

v. ADDISONIAN ANEMIA

Anton Biermer (1827–1892) Swiss Professor of Medicine at Zurich who coined the term "progressive pernicious anemia" in 1871. Although the majority and perhaps all of the patients he described did not have true pernicious anemia his paper was widely editorialised and led to a wide search for the condition and it became the popular term for the common form of B_{12} deficiency anemia.

BILHARZIA

Schistosomiasis.

Theodor M. Bilharz (1825–1862) German parasitologist who was Professor of Zoology in Cairo and discovered *Schistosoma haematobium* in 1851 and in 1853 discovered that the worm ankylostoma caused anemia and the disorder called Egyptian chlorosis.

BILLROTH GASTRECTOMY

1. Removal of lower portion of stomach with end to end anastomosis of the remaining stomach with the duodenum.
2. Gastrojejunal anastomosis with duodenal closure.

Christian A.T. Billroth (1829–1894) Professor of Surgery at the University of Vienna. Billroth performed the first successful distal partial gastrectomy in 1881. He studied with Albrecht von Gräfe in Berlin, with Hebra and Rokitansky in Vienna and with Velpau in Paris at the Charité. He became an assistant of Bernhard von Langenbeck (21 operative procedures were developed by this surgeon) in 1854. In 1855 he produced his first monograph on polyps and concluded that benign and malignant polypoid tumors of the colon were related and suggested early treatment. He published numerous works on pathology of cystoid tumors of the testis, blood vessel development and pathology and comparative anatomy of the spleen.

On Meckel's death from intestinal tuberculosis, Billroth was short-listed for the Chair of Pathologic Anatomy in Berlin with Remak and Virchow. The former had lost support because he had made

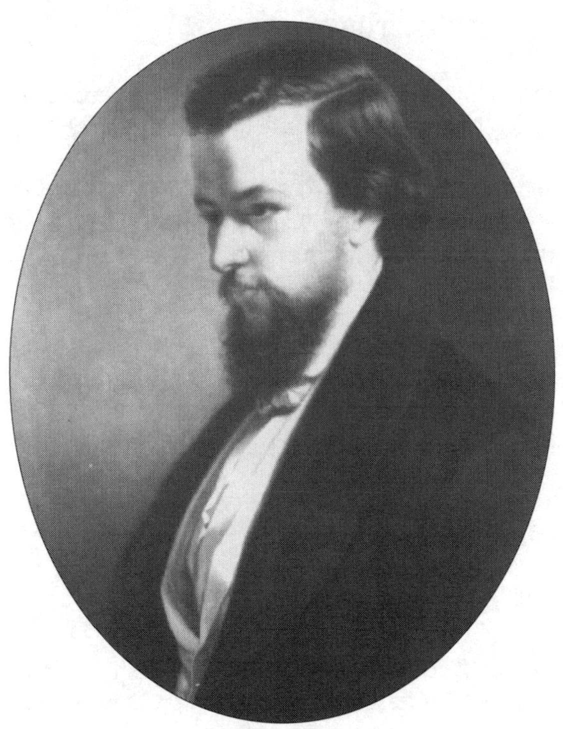

Christian A.T. Billroth (Courtesy of the Institut für Geschichte der Medizin an der Universität, Vienna)

application before Meckel's death and was Jewish, and Virchow had publicly expressed strong political beliefs favouring democracy and freedom. Following Virchow's monograph in 1848–9 "Die Medizinische Reform" which set out his strong opposition to unproven hypotheses laid down by authoritarian professors, he was dismissed from Berlin where he was a prosector. In the end Virchow was appointed with Billroth being the second candidate. Billroth next turned to teaching and writing on historical developments in surgery and was appointed Professor of Surgery in Zurich in 1860. He introduced the concept of audits, publishing all results, good and bad, which automatically resulted in honest discussion of morbidity, mortality and techniques, with resultant improvement in patient selection and care. Billroth successfully introduced laryngectomy in 1874. He wrote on modern surgical education explaining principles and not operative techniques, and his contributions in that regard were acknowledged by Flexner. He was an accomplished musician and a close friend of Johannes Brahms and was invited at times to be guest conductor of the Zurich Symphony Orchestra.

BING SIGN

Extension of the great toe following pricking of the dorsum of the toe or foot with a pin, seen in pyramidal tract lesions.

Robert Bing (1878–1956) Born in Strasburg, France, he studied medicine at the University of Basel, trained at Frankfurt/Maine, Paris, where he worked with Dejerine, in London with Sir Victor Horsley, and in Berlin. He was appointed lecturer in the University of Basel in 1907 and Professor and Head of Neurology in 1932. He wrote a book on neurology and many papers, and researched on congenital cardiomyopathy. His principal contributions to neurology were his studies on the spinocerebellar tract which he commenced with Dejerine. His textbook had 9 editions and was translated into 6 languages. He had a fondness for medical history and wrote on the history of epilepsy described by Hippocrates.

BING-NEEL SYNDROME

Tingling and light pain in the fingers and toes as an early indication of polyneuropathy which Waldenström believed to be due to a specific antibody activity of the macroglobulin but others consider may be secondary to small vessel occlusion due to hyperviscosity. Untreated progressive peripheral neuropathies may follow.

Jens Bing Danish physician who worked with immunoglobulins and was one of the first to recognize that plasma cells produce gamma-globulins.

Axel V. Neel Danish neurologist who described the syndrome in dysglobulinemia before macroglobulinemia was discovered.

BINSWANGER DEMENTIA OR DISEASE

Progressive dementia in the 5th and 6th decades, thought to be due to atherosclerosis, and characterized by memory disorders, paranoia and emotional lability.

Otto L. Binswanger (1852–1929) Professor of Psychiatry at Jena who trained H. Berger, O. Vogt and K. Brodmann.

BIOT BREATHING OR SIGN

Abrupt and irregular periods of apnoea and hyperpnea. A variant of Cheyne–Stokes respiration which may be seen in medullary compression.

Camille Biot (1878–) French physician who worked in Lyons.

BIRBECK BODIES

These are cytoplasmic inclusions seen by transmission electron microscopy which have the appearance of a tennis racquet and which are characteristically seen in epidermal Langerhans' cells. (*v. infra*)

Michael S. Birbeck British electron-microscopist.

BITOT SPOTS

Raised white patches on the bulbar conjunctivae, triangular in shape with the base near the limbus and readily dislodged. Seen in Vitamin A deficiency which may result in nyctalopia (night blindness) and keratomalacia.

Pierre A. Bitot (1822–1888) French anatomist, physiologist and surgeon. He was born in Podensac (Gie) and went to medical school in Bordeaux where he topped his class in 1846 and gained his M.D. from the Faculty of Paris in 1848 and in that year also joined the anatomy department in Bordeaux and held posts both in anatomy and physiology, becoming the titular Professor of Anatomy in 1854 and gained his Chirurgien des Hopitaux in 1856, ultimately becoming Professor of Clinical Surgery for sick children in Bordeaux in 1878. He published on a wide variety of topics ranging from hare lip to studies of the best form of ligatures to use in limb amputations and the use of quinine sulphate to prevent fever following blood transfusions as well as some aspects of cerebral anatomy and function.

BITTNER FACTOR

Factor in milk of mice with mammary carcinoma which transmits the disease to suckling mice.

John J. Bittner (1904–1961) U.S. biologist born in Meadville, Pennsylvania and graduated Ph.D. from the University of Michigan in 1930 and spent his lifetime on cancer research.

BJERRUM SCOTOMA

Arcuate scotoma seen in glaucoma.

BJERRUM SCREEN

Used to chart fields of vision accurately.

Jannik P. Bjerrum (1851–1920) Danish ophthalmologist. Professor of Ophthalmology, Copenhagen, who initially used his consulting room door to examine visual fields and from this developed his screen technique.

BJÖRK-SHILEY VALVE

Currently one of the most commonly employed prostheses in replacement of aortic or mitral valves.

Viking Olaf Björk (1918–) Swedish surgeon who was born at Sunnansgö, Sweden. He later worked in Italy, England and the U.S.A. and became Professor and Chairman of Thoracic and Cardiovascular Surgery at Uppsala University from 1958 to 1966. He later occupied a similar position from 1966 to 1983 at the Karolinska Institute, in Stockholm. He developed many methods and approaches for cardiac surgery including the first successful demonstration of a heart-lung machine with a spinning disc oxygenator in experimental animals in 1948. In 1969 he developed a new tilting disc valve prosthesis. Retiring from his chair in Stockholm he was Emeritus Professor and Director of Cardiac Research and Education at the Heart Institute, the Eisenhower Medical Center, Rancho Mirage, California, U.S.A. His interests outside medicine include sailing, golf, downhill skiing and mushroom picking, as well as looking after the family forest in Dalecarlia, Sweden.

Donald Shiley (1921–) U.S. engineer who worked originally with valves in the fuel systems of aircraft. He then worked on the Starr Edwards ball valves and developed a number of other valve prostheses. He is a keen aviator.

BLACKFAN-DIAMOND SYNDROME

v. DIAMOND-BLACKFAN SYNDROME

BLALOCK-TAUSSIG OPERATION

Palliative operation for Fallot tetralogy with anastomosis of the subclavian artery to the pulmonary artery, bypassing the pulmonary stenosis.

Alfred Blalock (1899–1964) U.S. surgeon, born in Culloden, Georgia, graduated M.D. Johns Hopkins, 1922. He was an intern and assistant resident surgeon, Johns Hopkins, 1923–25, then at Vanderbilt 1925, becoming Professor there from 1938–41, and then Professor and Director of Department of Surgery, Johns Hopkins, 1941.

Blalock had developed great expertise in vascular anastomosis in animal surgery and invited Taussig to work in his laboratory following discussions she had with him on her patients with Fallot tetralogy. After many animal experiments, Blalock performed the first Blalock-Taussig operation on a patient with Fallot tetralogy. This consisted of anastomosing the subclavian artery to the pulmonary artery at a point distal to the stenosis to enable the blood to recirculate through the lungs to become better oxygenated. The blood supply to the arm was preserved by a developing collateral circulation. The operation was most successful and opened a new era in cardiac surgery; many of the patients survived long enough to have their pulmonary stenosis and ventricular septal defect corrected by open heart surgery.

H.B. Taussig (*v. infra*)

v. TAUSSIG-BING MALFORMATION

BLAND-WHITE-GARLAND SYNDROME

Angina pectoris and myocardial infarction in young children due to anomalous origin of the left coronary artery from the pulmonary artery.

Edward F. Bland (1901–) U.S. physician who advocated pulmonary azygous vein shunt to relieve mitral stenosis.

Paul D. White (1886–1973) He was born in Boston, a son of a general practitioner. His younger sister died at the age of 12 of acute rheumatic fever and it is said that this determined his interest in cardiology. He studied medicine at Harvard, graduating in 1911, and interned at the newly established Department of Pediatrics at Massachusetts General Hospital (M.G.H.). For the next two years he was on the medical service with Dr. R.I. Lee and together they developed a technique for measuring blood coagulation, which is still commonly used, called the Lee and White method (*v. infra*). This was his first medical publication. He spent a year with Sir Thomas Lewis studying the electrocardiogram (ECG) at the University College Hospital in London. He joined up in World War I and served with the Harvard Unit with the British Expeditionary Forces near Boulogne and in 1917 helped establish the American base at Bordeaux. At the end of the war he organized an American Red Cross expedition to treat a typhus epidemic which was occurring in Macedonia and the Greek Islands, and was awarded a decoration from the Greek Government. In 1919 he returned to the M.G.H. to establish a cardiac unit. He was the author of numerous books which became standard texts in cardiology, and together with Wolff and John Parkinson, whom he had met 20 years earlier, described the Wolff Parkinson White Syndrome (*v. infra*).

In 1955 he attended President Eisenhower during his cardiac infarct and it is said that only he and the President were convinced that the President would survive. His optimistic approach to patients, mixed with common sense and a ready explanation, helped many patients who were frightened by their disease. He emphasized the importance of prevention of coronary disease and was a strong advocate of fitness and exercise in aiding its prevention. His use of the bicycle was known throughout the world and a bicycle path has been named in his honor in Boston.

Hugh Garland (1893–1973) U.S. physician. His father and grandfather both practiced medicine in Gloucester, Massachusetts, and he graduated from Harvard Medical School in 1919, and entered pediatrics. He published a number of papers including one on ectodermal dysplasia, and several papers with P.D. White and E.F. Bland on congenital heart disease. He was an interested and interesting teacher who would get students to examine his own heart to hear his patent ductus. He was always interested in literature and writing; he joined the editorial staff of the New England Journal of Medicine in 1947 with the intention of devoting only half his time to it, but the then editor, Nye, became ill, and Garland took over completely. Under his editorship, many innovations were instituted, and he contributed many fine editorials and played no small part in establishing this journal as one of the leading medical journals of the day. He was a member of the staff of the Massachusetts General Hospital from 1923–54, a member of the editorial board of the New England Journal of Medicine from 1938–1947 and editor from 1947–1967.

BLAUD PILL

Iron pill (ferrous carbonate).

Pierre Blaud (1774–1858) French physician who prescribed the pill to treat chlorosis.

BLOOM SYNDROME

Autosomal recessive disorder with sensitivity to sunlight, erythematous facial rash, short stature and increased risk of leukemia. May also have acanthosis nigricans, café au lait spots and skeletal malformation.

David Bloom (1892–) U.S. dermatologist born in Warsaw and attended school at Danzig (Gdansk) and spent one term at University of Freiburg and then when World War I broke out moved to Berne, graduating in medicine there in 1919. He migrated to the U.S.A. in 1920 and specialized in dermatology, working at the Skin and Cancer Clinic, New York University, where he first identified this group of patients as a separate form of dwarfism. At the New York University Postgraduate Medical School he taught genetic dermatology.

BLUMBERG SIGN

Rebound tenderness indicating peritoneal inflammation.

J. Moritz Blumberg (1873–1955) German surgeon and gynecologist who was initially in Berlin but moved to London. He was born in Posen and graduated from the University of Breslau (Wroclaw) in 1897 and trained with Mikulicz (*v. infra*). He investigated methods of sterilization of the surgeon's hands and invented a type of rubber glove which was widely used. In the 1st World War he fought with the German army and rapidly brought a typhus epidemic in a prisoner of war camp under control by delousing 10 000 Russian prisoners of war in a few days. At the end of the war he was presented an illuminated address by his former prisoners. After the war he returned to surgical practice and founded an X-ray and Radium Institute and organized many prenatal clinics in Berlin. With the rise of the Nazis he left Germany and resumed his medical work in England with considerable success.

BOAS SIGN

Hyperesthesia below right scapula posteriorly, 9th–11th dorsal ribs, seen in acute cholecystitis.

Ismar I. Boas (1858–1938) German physician and gastroenterologist in Berlin who wrote an authoritative textbook on "Diagnosis and Therapeutics of Disease of the Stomach". He spent a brief period in general practice before joining Prof. Ewald in Berlin as his assistant at the Augusta Hospital. Shortly after Kussmaul's (*v. infra*) introduction of the gastric tube Boas and Ewald introduced the test meal to measure gastric secretion and Boas rapidly gained an international reputation and became a world leader in gastroenterology. He was the first to recognize "occult blood" and pioneered its use in patient investigation. He founded a medical journal in 1898 and in 1920 set up the German gastroenterological society. He left Berlin for Vienna in 1936 with the rise of the Nazis and died there 2 years later as Austria too succumbed to Nazism.

BODANSKY UNIT

Measure of serum alkaline phosphatase activity.

Aaron Bodansky (1896–1941) Born in Elizabethgrad, Russia, and migrated to U.S.A. when he was 11. He graduated Ph.D. in 1923 Cornell University and M.D. University of Chicago in 1935. He was Professor of Pathological Chemistry 1930 at University of Texas and Director of Laboratories at the John Sealy Hospital. He was an excellent teacher who made numerous contributions to biochemical techniques and had a special interest in calcium metabolism. He died following complications of a mastoid operation, a pulmonary infection and acute hemorrhagic nephritis.

BOECK SARCOID

v. BESNIER-BOECK DISEASE

BOERHAAVE SYNDROME

v. MALLORY-WEISS SYNDROME

Rupture of the esophagus with spillage of gastric contents into the mediastinum.

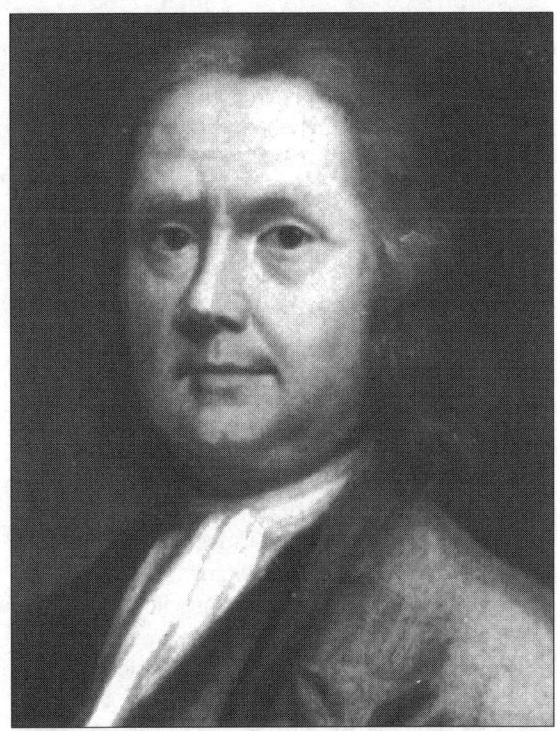

Hermann Boerhaave, (Reproduced from *"The Royal College of Physicians of London Portraits"* by G. Wolstenholm & D. Piper (Published by J & A Churchill Ltd, London, 1964)

Hermann Boerhaave (1668–1738) Dutch physician. There seems to be some dispute as to the standing of this man, but it is difficult to believe that he was not one of the "greats" since he clearly had an immense influence on medical development of his day and many would rate him with Galen, Sydenham and Hippocrates. Some writers believe that together with Sydenham he revived the Hippocratic method of clinical description and teaching at the bedside. He was the first to describe rupture of the esophagus (1724), and used the Fahrenheit thermometer in his clinic, a practice continued by his pupils van Swieten and Haen. There can be little doubt that he was a very influential teacher and probably the best known consultant physician of his time. He made Leyden the world medical center and amongst his students and pupils were Haller, Gauv, Cullen, Pringle, van Swieten and Haen, as well as Fahrenheit and Prevoost. He was consulted about the curriculum of the Edinburgh Medical School and by some is regarded as a founding father. One of his students, van Swieten, was foundation Professor of Medicine in Vienna and so his influence stretched the breadth of Europe. It is said that the only experiment Boerhaave ever performed was the effect of extreme heat on animals. His pupils, Prevoost and Fahrenheit, put a dog and a cat in an oven. They died in 28 minutes, while a sparrow died in 7 minutes in a similar experiment. Boerhaave's reputation was known in China and his works were translated in Arabic. He undoubtedly was a fine scholar himself since he knew all the European languages including Latin. During his lifetime he had his critics but he was never obviously worried by this, responding on inquiry "The sparks of calumny will be presently extinct of themselves, unless you blow on them".

He was the son of a clergyman and born at Voorhoot near Leyden and initially was going to become a clergyman. He graduated Ph.D. in 1690 at Leyden, but then decided to do medicine and graduated from the University of Harderwyk in 1693. He commenced practice at Leyden in 1701 and became a lecturer in medicine at the University and in 1709 Professor of Medicine and Botany. He was a great admirer of Sydenham, of whom he said "the light of England, the Apollo of the Art, whose name I would blush to mention without a title or of honour". He was an extremely fine lecturer and was a very pleasant man. In 1725 he developed gout which forced him, in 1729, to give up his lectures in botany and chemistry, but he continued bedside teaching until his death.

One story is that he left a book in which he had set out all the secrets of medicine. After he died it was opened and all the pages were blank except one on which was written "keep the head cool, the feet warm and the bowels open."

His description of ruptured esophagus resulted from his being called in consultation to see the Grand Admiral of the Dutch Fleet and Prefect of Rhineland Baron J. van Wassenaer who was in excruciating upper abdominal pain which failed to respond to any of the treatment of the day and the Baron succumbed undiagnosed but Boerhaave conducted an autopsy which revealed the rent in the esophagus and the contents of a previous meal and fluid in the chest.

BOGORAD SYNDROME

Unilateral lacrimation after eating or drinking following a facial nerve palsy, possibly due to misdirected nerve regeneration (crocodile tears). Loss of taste and a facial tic may also occur.

F.A. Bogorad A Russian physician, described this in 1928 although it had already been observed in 1913 by Oppenheim and Engelen.

BOHR EFFECT

The effect of carbon dioxide concentration on the dissociation of oxygen from hemoglobin.

Christian H. Bohr (1855–1911) Danish physiologist who was Professor of Physiology in Copenhagen. He made many important discoveries regarding the distribution of gases in the body.

BOMBAY BLOOD GROUP

Red cells resemble Group O but do not agglutinate with anti-H serum and their serum contains strong anti-H antibody. The first people recognized to have this group were from Bombay, India.

BONNEVIE-ULLRICH SYNDROME

Lymphedema of the hands and feet, webbing of the neck, nail dystrophy, laxity of the skin and short stature. When associated with the Klippel-Feil Syndrome (*v. infra*) it is called Nielsen Disease.

Kristine Bonnevie (1872–1950) U.S. geneticist.

Otto Ullrich (*v. infra*).

BORNHOLM DISEASE

Viral disorder with protean manifestations but characterized by attacks of severe pain, often pleural or abdominal due to Coxsackie (virus) infection.

Bornholm is an island in the Baltic Sea between Denmark and Sweden (v. Introduction).

BOSTON SIGN

v. GRAEFE SIGN

Jerking of the lagging lid in exophthalmos, seen in thyrotoxicosis.

Leonard N. Boston (1871–1931) born in Philadelphia and graduated M.D. 1896 from the Medico-Chirurgical College of Philadelphia and became Professor of Physical Diagnosis 1912–1916. He moved to the University of Pennsylvania as Associate Professor of Medicine 1919–1926 and became Professor of Principles and Practice of Medicine and Clinical Medicine, Women's Medical College of Pennsylvania in 1928. He wrote a textbook of "Clinical Diagnosis by Laboratory Methods" and co-authored "Medical Diagnosis". He died of erysipelas.

BOUCHARD NODES

Similar to, but less common than, Heberden nodes, they occur related to proximal interphalangeal joints and are seen in gout and osteoarthritis.

Charles J. Bouchard (1837–1915) French physician, who was one of the first to describe spider naevi in liver disease.

BOURNEVILLE DISEASE OR SYNDROME

Tuberous sclerosis, also termed Pringle Disease (*v. infra*).

Désiré M. Bourneville (1840–1909) French neurologist. He graduated from Paris and was awarded a gold watch for his work during a cholera epidemic in Amiens in 1866. He was a surgeon during the Franco-Prussian War and saved a number of his patients during the Commune in Paris in 1871 by his personal intervention.

He founded the Progrès Médical in 1873 and Archives de Neurologie in 1880. He established the first school for defective children. Apart from his description of tuberous sclerosis, which was separately described by Hartegin, he made observations on myxedema, cretinism and mongolism. He was physician to the pediatric service of the Bicêtre from 1879 to 1905 and when he retired remained in charge of the Foundation Vallee at the Bicêtre.

BOWDITCH EFFECT

Increase in heart rate may have a positive inotropic effect thought to be due to an increase in calcium ions made available for the contracting muscle.

Henry Pickering Bowditch (1840–1911) Hailed by many as the founding father of American physiology. He was born into a wealthy and influential Boston family with an uncle who was a prominent physician and clinical professor at Harvard (1859–1867). He entered Harvard Medical School in 1866 after being wounded in the Civil War in 1863 and resigned from the army in 1865. At Harvard he attended and was greatly influenced by the new course in physiology of the nervous system taught by Brown-Séquard (*v. infra*). He graduated in 1868 and went to Paris to work with Brown-Séquard but the latter suggested he should join Claude Bernard. He found Bernard a superb teacher but was disappointed with the laboratory facilities and in 1869 moved to Germany to work with Carl Ludwig in Leipzig at the Physiological Institute. This was the "state of the art" physiological laboratory in the world and he had an extremely productive period discovering the all-or-none principal of cardiac contraction (Bowditch Law) and the "treppe" effect. He returned to Harvard in 1871 establishing a program which brought the German laboratory approach to scientific medical research in North America.

BOWEN DISEASE

Intra-epidermal epithelioma. There is a 15-30% incidence of a malignancy with this condition.

John T. Bowen (1857–1941) U.S. dermatologist born in Boston and graduated M.D. from Harvard in 1884. He studied in Germany and Vienna spending two years there before returning as assistant physician to out-patients with diseases of the skin at the

Massachusetts General Hospital in 1889. In 1907 he was appointed Professor of Dermatology at Harvard, resigning in 1911 to become emeritus. Always rather shy, lecturing was almost torture to him. He loved "mulling" things over and investigating skin conditions by microscopy. A batchelor, he became a recluse except to his closest friends. He was afflicted with an undiagnosed form of vertigo which incapacitated him in his last years.

BOWMAN CAPSULE

Glomerular capsule of the kidney.

BOWMAN MEMBRANE

Separates corneal epithelium from the substantia propria of cornea.

Sir William Bowman (1816–1892) English surgeon and anatomist. Born in Nantwich, Cheshire. His father was a banker who was interested in botany and geology and his mother was a painter. He went to Hazelwood School, Birmingham, famous then because there was no corporal punishment. He injured his hand when he was using gunpowder and both the nature of the wound and the treatment he received from a surgeon, Mr. J. Hodgson, who gave him his first microscope, made him interested in medicine and he became apprenticed to him. He spent some time at King's College Hospital and gained his M.R.C.S in 1839 and F.R.C.S in 1844. In 1846 he was appointed surgeon to the Royal London Ophthalmic Hospital in Moorfields and was the first there to use the ophthalmoscope invented by Helmholtz. In 1856 he was appointed surgeon to King's College Hospital after a period as Assistant Surgeon. He increasingly specialized in ophthalmic surgery and succeeded Dalrymple as the leading ophthalmic surgeon. He was elected F.R.S in 1841 in recognition of his work on muscle structure. Later Bowman studied the kidney and its vasculature and was the first to appreciate that each renal tubule had a proximal dilated end with a tuft of capillaries. He received the Royal Medal of the Royal Society for his work on the microscopic anatomy of the liver and also studied the anatomy of the eye. He was granted a Baronetcy in 1884. Bowman was an intensely religious man and could recite the psalms from memory. He took the deepest interest in the welfare of his patients and with R.B. Todd (*v. infra*) established the St. John's House and Sisterhood, which trained nurses for the sick and the poor. Later he helped Florence Nightingale by sending trained nurses to the Crimea and was a life long member of the Nightingale Fund. He was a gentle, patient and thoughtful man, unrivalled in his knowledge of structure of the eye and his manual dexterity.

BRACHT-WÄCHTER BODIES

Perivascular microabscesses seen in the myocardium in acute bacterial endocarditis.

Erich F.E. Bracht (1882–) German pathologist in Berlin.

Hermann J.G. Wächter (1878–) German physician who worked in Freiburg.

BRAILSFORD MORQUIO SYNDROME

v. MORQUIO SYNDROME

BRANDT SYNDROME

(Also called DANBOLT or DANBOLT-CLOSS SYNDROME)

Steatorrhea, alopecia, paronychia, perioral and anal pustular eruptions.

Thore E. Brandt Swedish dermatologist.

Niels C. Danbolt Norwegian dermatologist.

Karl Closs Norwegian physician.

BRANHAM BRADYCARDIA OR SIGN

Compression of an arterio-venous fistula causes a slowing of the heart rate if there is a significant circulation through the fistula.

Henry H. Branham U.S. surgeon, 19th century.

BRAXTON HICKS CONTRACTION

Painless rhythmic uterine contractions occurring during pregnancy.

John Braxton Hicks (1823–1897) English obstetrician, son of a banker from Lymington, Hants, was educated as a private pupil of Rev. J.P. Zillwood of Compton Rectory near Winchester. As a boy he developed a keen interest in the natural sciences which remained with him thereafter. He was apprenticed to Dr. Fluder of Lymington, and when 18 entered Guy's Hospital Medical School. Here he was a favorite pupil of Sir William Gull, a brilliant student and a successful oarsman. He graduated M.B. in 1847 from the University of London and gained his M.D. in 1851. He entered general practice and was very successful, but in 1858 joined Guy's Hospital again as assistant obstetric physician. In 1859 he gained his M.R.C.P and became F.R.S in 1861 and full obstetric physician at Guy's Hospital from 1868–1883. He was appointed obstetric physician in 1888 to St. Mary's Hospital.

Braxton Hicks was a pioneer figure in British midwifery and published extensively both on external and internal manipulative procedures, as well as designing obstetric instruments and studying the physiology of uterine function. He presented numerous papers to the Royal Society on lichen mosses and unicellular algae and was joint author on a book on the earthworm and housefly, in which he did the engraving.

Besides his medical and scientific interests he had a superb collection of botanical specimens and Wedgewood china and was a vestryman in the Parish of St. George, Hanover Square. From his time as a student, he exhibited a classical type A personality whose mind had a number of outlets, he was a fine instructor and had a great sympathy and care for his patients' well being. He died of recurrent attacks of influenza but as he developed complete heart block terminally with glycosuria and edema it seems likely he had a myocardial infarct and diabetes.

BRENNER TUMOR

Tumor of ovary, usually benign, without known endocrine activity.

Fritz Brenner (1877–) German physician who was born in Osthofen, Germany, and graduated from medical school in Heidelberg in 1904. He then went to work in the Pathology Institute with E. Albrecht who has been termed "the kindest of all beings" because of his selfless attitude towards his assistants. In 1907 whilst working with Albrecht, he described three instances of the tumor. After this he practiced briefly in Germany, but migrated to German South West Africa in 1910 where he worked in the sea port Swakopmund. He remained there after the First War until 1922 when he moved to Windhoek, capital of West Africa and finally in 1935 he migrated to South Africa where he went into general practice in Johannesburg. It was whilst he was in Johannesburg that he was surprised to learn that his name was eponymously attached to the tumor. This tumor was in fact first described in 1899 by E.G. Orthmann.

BRESICA-CIMINO FISTULA

Arterio-venous fistula created for hemodialysis.

Michael J. Bresica (1933–) Renal physician, V.A. Hospital, New York, U.S.A.

James E. Cimino (1928–) Renal physician, V.A. Hospital, New York, U.S.A.

BREUER REFLEX

v. HERING-BREUER REFLEX

BREWER INFARCTS

Pyramidal reddened areas in the kidney seen in acute unilateral hematogenous pyelonephritis.

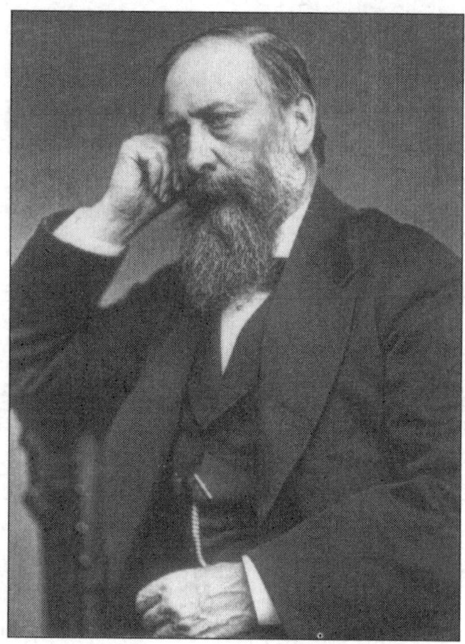

George E. Brewer (Courtesy of the Royal Society of Medicine, London, UK)

BREWER KIDNEY

Hematogenous abscess in kidney following septicemia.

George E. Brewer (1861–1939) U.S. surgeon, born Westfield, New York. He spent two years at the University of Buffalo Medical School and worked with J.F. Minor, Professor of Surgery, assisting with operations in the latter's office. He then went to Harvard, graduating in 1885. He won first place in the intern examination for Boston City Hospital and after a residency in obstetrics and gynecology at Columbia Hospital for Women, he went to Baltimore as a "Fellow by courtesy" working with W.H. Welch. He went into general practice in New York in 1887 and in 1888 became assistant to H.H. Curtis, a well known otolaryngologist. He next gained appointment as genito-urinary surgeon to F.N. Otis at the College of Physicians and Surgeons, Columbia University, and in 1892 became an assistant demonstrator in anatomy. That summer he studied anatomy in Edinburgh with Sir William Turner and Dr. Hepburn. He studied operative techniques and became junior surgeon at the Roosevelt Hospital in 1901 and with J.A. Blake founded a research laboratory of surgical pathology. In 1913 he was appointed surgical director of the Presbyterian Hospital. He wrote a successful textbook of surgery and a book on surgical diagnosis.

In 1917 he enlisted and went to France as Director of Base Hospital Unit No. 2 and served in the operating team at the Casualty Clearing Station in the Passchendale campaign and in the Argonne, and was later decorated by the Belgian Government. In 1920 he was elected President of the American Surgical Association. He returned in 1928 and went to France to renew his interest in anthropology and was made a research associate to the American Museum for National History. He developed a bladder neoplasm in 1937 which initially responded to irradiation but he died two years later in the Harkness Pavilion of Columbia Presbyterian Medical Centre.

BRIGHT DISEASE

Chronic nephritis.

Richard Bright (1789–1858) English physician, born in Bristol, son of a wealthy banker, he entered Edinburgh University to study medicine in 1808. In 1810 he went with Mackenzie's expedition to Iceland and helped with the latter's book "Travels in Iceland". He returned to commence clinical work, pathology and autopsy examination at Guy's Hospital where he was influenced by Astley Cooper. He returned to Edinburgh and in 1813 completed his thesis on erysipelis. In 1814 he travelled on the continent and learnt French and German, attending lectures in Berlin and Vienna and in 1815 he wrote a book "Travels from Vienna through Lower Hungary". He was elected assistant physician in 1820 and in 1824 became a physician at Guy's. He and Addison established an international reputation for their lecture course. Between 1827 and 1836 Bright produced three classic publications linking dropsy and coagulable urine with disease of the kidney. The chemical analyses were undertaken by a chemist, Dr. Bostock. The early publications were concerned with chronic renal disease, but later he suggested that such cases were the result of an initial, sometimes inapparent, acute episode of nephritis. Bright's

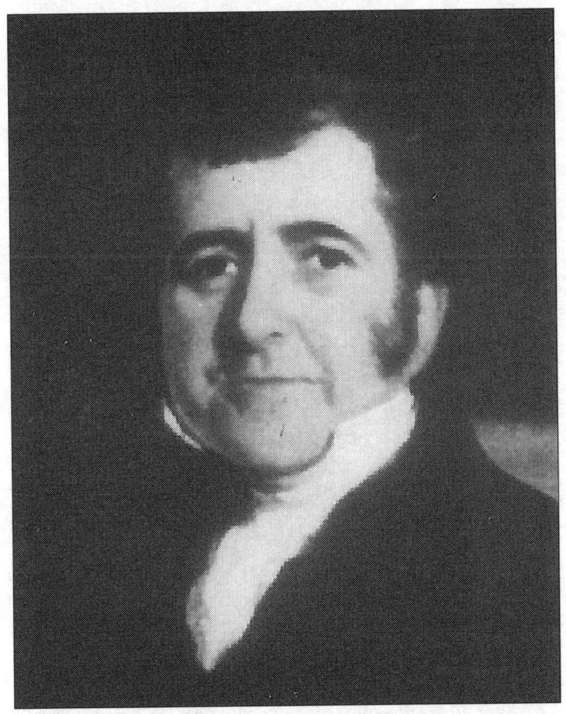

Richard Bright (Courtesy of the Gordon Museum, Guy's Hospital Medical School)

apparatus to detect protein in urine was a spoon. In his own words "one of the most ready means of detecting albumin is the application of heat by taking a small quantity of urine in a spoon and holding it over a flame of a candle. If albumin is present, you perceive before the fluid reaches the boiling point that it becomes opaque, sometimes presenting a milky appearance at the end of the spoon, which extends inwards till it meets in the centre and then breaks into a white curd". Three of his renal specimens are preserved at Guy's Hospital. Two have been reclassified as mesangiocapillary (membranoproliferative) glomerulonephritis and the other was a case of renal amyloidosis secondary to pulmonary tuberculosis. He died, not of Bright disease as had been stated (he had normal kidneys on autopsy), with an enlarged heart and aortic valve disease.

BRILL-SYMMERS DISEASE

Nodular lymphocytic lymphoma.

BRILL-ZINSSER DISEASE

Recrudescent typhus.

Nathan E. Brill (1860–1925) U.S. physician, born in New York; gained his M.D., University Medical College (New York) in 1880, interned at the Bellevue Hospital 1879–81, was appointed attending physician at Mt. Sinai Hospital in 1892 and made Professor of Clinical Medicine at the College of Physicians and Surgeons, Columbia, 1910. He translated Klemperer's book "Clinical Diagnosis" in 1898 and discovered a previously unrecognized form of typhus called "recrudescent typhus" (Brill–Zinsser Disease) in migrants from Eastern Europe without body lice. It seemed to be a recrudescence of a latent infection following primary louse-born typhus. Clinically it resembles mild typhus and may occur years after the first infection.

Douglas Symmers (1897–1957) U.S. pathologist who worked at the Bellevue Hospital, New York.

Hans Zinsser (1878–1940) U.S. bacteriologist who wrote an extremely popular book "Rats, Lice and History". He was Professor of Bacteriology at Columbia University, New York.

BRIQUET SYNDROME

Hysteria.

This eponym has been used by a group of psychiatrists who believe that hysteria is not a disease, since it may be biologically helpful, rather than unhelpful, to the patient. Some restrict this term to dyspnea and aphonia as manifestations of hysteria and Briquet ataxia to ataxia occurring in hysteria.

Paul Briquet (1796–1881) French physician who wrote a monograph on the subject in 1859.

BRISSAUD DISEASE

1. A habit spasm or tic, usually seen in children which may commence with voluntary action, but once started cannot be stopped.
2. v. GILLES DE LA TOURETTE SYNDROME.

BRISSAUD-SICARD SYNDROME

Facial hemi-spasm with contralateral paralysis of the extremities.

Edouard Brissaud (1852–1909) He was trained in neurology at the Salpêtrière by Charcot and Lasegue. He had a major interest in movement disorders and published a textbook of the anatomy of the human brain which he illustrated himself. Together with Pierre Marie he founded the French neurology journal, Revue Neurologique. He made a number of observations on psychosomatic medicine, agreeing with Babinski against the teaching of Charcot that distinction between some forms of hysteria and simulation was impossible, stating "a symptom which cannot be simulated is not a symptom of hysteria". He became Professor of Medicine in 1899 and was much liked by students because of his colorful descriptions and turn of phrase. He described one patient with Parkinsonian tremor of the tongue and lips as "he murmurs an interminable litany". He died with a brain tumor which was operated on in Paris by Victor Horsley without success. His last wish, namely that he be buried without religious observance, was denied him.

Jean A. Sicard (*v. infra*).

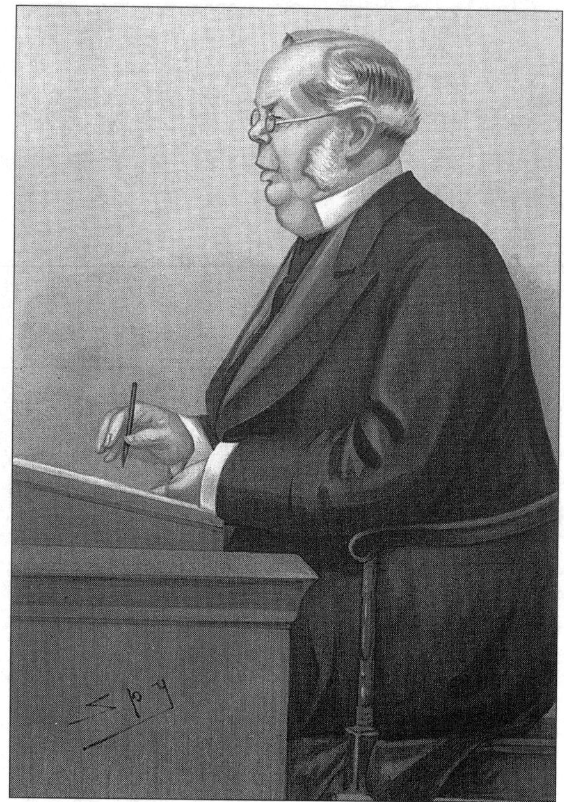

Sir William H. Broadbent (Entitled "Orthodoxy" from *Vanity Fair,* Oct 30, 1902, by Spy)

BROADBENT APOPLEXY

Intracerebral hemorrhage in which the bleeding penetrates the brain into the lateral ventricle.

BROADBENT INVERTED SIGN

Systolic pulsation seen on the posterior lateral wall of the left side of the chest which was originally thought to be due to an aneurysm of the left atrium, but more usually is a result of left ventricular hypertrophy.

BROADBENT LAW

Upper motor neurone lesions result in less paralysis in muscles concerned with bilateral contractions than those which act unilaterally.

Sir William H. Broadbent (1835–1907) An English physician who was born at Lindley, near Huddersfield in Yorkshire. He studied at the Manchester Medical School and was a brilliant undergraduate. He qualified in 1857 and went to Paris to continue his studies and returned to gain his final M.B. examination in London in 1858. In that year he joined the staff of St. Mary's Hospital and remained with that institution for the next 47 years. He was appointed in 1865 as a physician to the outpatients of the hospital and rapidly gained a reputation for being one of the finest clinical teachers of the day. His contributions to neurology were highly thought of by Hughlings Jackson and he also made a number of original contributions to cardiology and was elected F.R.S. in 1897. One of the more fashionable consultants in London he attended Prince George (later King George V) who had typhoid fever in 1891 and in 1892 he also looked after Prince Clarence whose illness, however, was fatal. Although the Spy cartoon is entitled "Orthodoxy" he was one of the early supporters for the admission of women into medical schools and with Walter Cheadle (*v. infra*) was a member of the Council of the Medical School for Women.

BROADBENT SIGN

An indrawing of the 11th and 12th left ribs with a narrowing of the space posteriorly due to pericardial adhesions to the diaphragm seen in constrictive pericarditis.

Walter Broadbent (1868–1951) English physician, son of W.H. His sign appeared in his first paper in 1895, said to be inspired by his father. He was educated at Harrow, Trinity College, Cambridge and St. Mary's Hospital, London, graduating in 1893. He served in the British Army in Italy in World War I. He was a keen rower and ice skater and had a particular love for Switzerland.

BROCA ANGLE

Parietal angle.

BROCA APHASIA

Motor aphasia.

BROCA AREA

Anterior portion of the inferior frontal gyrus. It is more developed on the left side in right handed people, and has been designated as the area of speech.

Pierre P. Broca (1824–1880) French surgeon and anthropologist, born in Sainte-Foy-la Grande near Bordeaux, son of a country practitioner with Huguenot background. He entered the Faculty of Medicine in 1841 and graduated in 1849. He was an extraordinarily prolific investigator who became Professor of Surgery in Paris having previously described muscular dystrophy (before Duchenne), rickets as a nutritional disorder (before Virchow), and venous spread of cancer (before Rokitansky). He introduced the microscope to France to diagnose cancer, wrote a classical monograph on aneurysm and introduced the use of hypnotism to surgery.

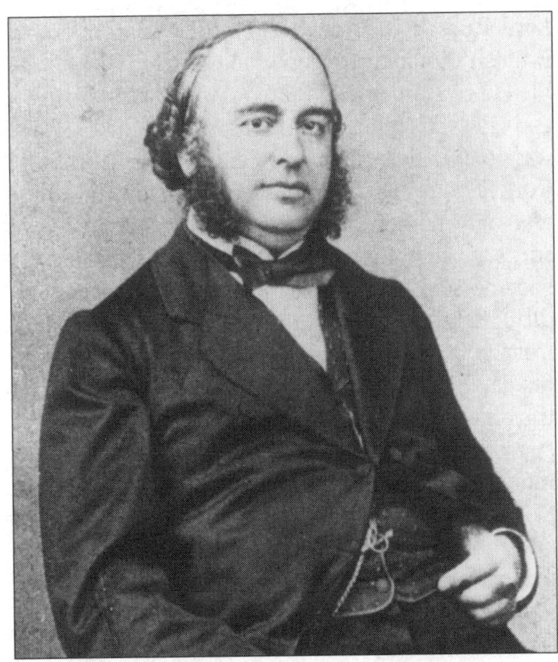

Pierre P. Broca (Courtesy of the Royal Society of Medicine, London, UK)

He shared Darwin's views in denying the immutability of race and species and founded the first Anthropological Society as well as his School and Institute of Anthropology. Broca developed the concept of left hemisphere dominance for speech from observations on brain lesions in his patients and localized it to the posterior part of the third frontal convolution. He was married to the daughter of Dr. J.G.A. Lugol (v. LUGOL IODINE), and died suddenly aged 56, possibly from a coronary occlusion.

BROCK SYNDROME

Middle lobe syndrome. Collapse and/or infective episodes secondary to compression of the right middle lobe bronchus by enlarged lymph node.

Lord Russell C. Brock (1903–1980) Baron Brock, English thoracic surgeon who operated on George VI. He was an undergraduate at Christ's Hospital and Guy's Hospital, gaining his M.B.B.S in 1927. He was Rockefeller Travelling Fellow in 1929–30 and worked with Evarts Graham (*v. infra*) in St. Louis, and here he commenced his interest in thoracic surgery. After his residency at Guy's Hospital he became surgical registrar and tutor at Guy's, and ultimately surgeon to Guy's and Brompton Hospital from 1936–1968. The leading thoracic surgeon of his day in England, he wrote important articles on the anatomy of the bronchial tree and on surgical approaches to problems of lung abscess and pulmonary stenosis. He pioneered cardiac surgery in England. A perfectionist, he was a hard task master and rather shy and reserved, but tireless in giving utmost attention to his patients and insisting on similar dedication from all associated with him.

He wrote on the life and work of Astley Cooper and had an extensive knowledge of antique furniture and prints, and the history of London. He was president of the Royal College of Surgeons 1963–66.

BRODIE ABSCESS

Chronic metaphyseal abscess in the tibia.

BRODIE SEROCYSTIC DISEASE

Usually benign, rapidly growing tumor of the breast occurring after puberty.

BRODIE-TRENDELENBURG TEST

Test for varicose veins – raise the leg until the vein is empty, then apply a tourniquet to the mid-thigh and stand the patient up and remove the tourniquet after 60 seconds. Normally the vein should fill from below within 35 seconds. Earlier filling indicates incompetence of a communicating vein; filling from above indicates saphenous vein incompetence.

Sir Benjamin C. Brodie (1783–1862) English surgeon, surgeon to St. George's Hospital, London. He was born in Wiltshire, son of a clergyman and is said to have been aided by influential friends and relatives in high places. He was a student of Sir Everard Home, lectured at Great Windmill Street (1805–1812) and became assistant surgeon and surgeon at St. George's Hospital. He was greatly influenced by Bichat and studied the effect of the brain on the heart as well as the actions of poisons from South America. He observed that respiration and cardiac function soon ceased after severing the cervical cord but could be restored by artificial respiration. His monograph "On the pathology and surgery of diseases of the joints" was a major work in its time and included a good description of Reiter Syndrome (*v. infra*) (1829). He pioneered the surgery of varicose veins. He avoided operations if possible and it was said "his vocation was more to heal limbs rather than to remove them". He became President of the Royal College of Surgeons.

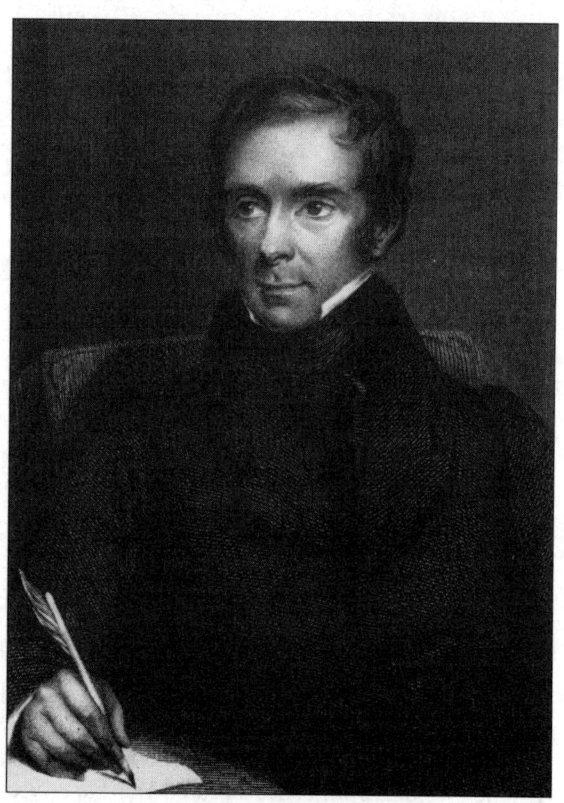

Sir Benjamin C. Brodie (Courtesy of the Royal Society of Medicine, London, UK)

Friedrich Trendelenburg (*v. infra*).

BRODMANN AREAS

Allocation of numbers to map areas of the human cerebral cortex, e.g. area 4 – motor area.

Korbinian Brodmann (1868–1918) German neurologist, born in Luggersdord Hohenzollern, and graduated in 1895. He practiced as a general practitioner and caught diphtheria and whilst recuperating he worked in a sanitorium for nervous diseases in Alexanderbad directed by O. Vogt. In 1898 he was awarded M.D. Leipzig and in 1900–01 he worked with Vogt in Berlin. During this time he developed a chart of the human cortex. There was considerable opposition to his work and he was not admitted as Privatdozent at the Medical Faculty of the University of Berlin. He died of 1918 of septicemia complicating pneumonia.

BROMPTON COCKTAIL

An analgesic mixture which is usually reserved for patients with terminal cancer, consisting of a mixture of cocaine, morphine or heroin, alcohol and some flavouring syrup.

Brompton Hospital, London Introduced first in the Brompton Hospital by H. Snow in 1896 and used around the world in various forms as an oral analgesic.

BROOKE EPITHELIOMA, SYNDROME OR TUMOR

Basal cell tumors, most commonly occurring on the face, around the eyelids and on the scalp, inherited as an autosomal dominant. They appear near puberty and become stationary after enlarging for several years.

Henry A.G. Brooke (1854–1919) English dermatologist who was renowned for his love of books and his wit. He pioneered dermatology in the English Midlands being popularly known as "Brooke of Manchester".

BROWNIAN MOVEMENT OR MOTION

Ceaseless movement of small particles in liquid or gas due to bombardment by surrounding molecules of the liquid or gas.

Robert Brown (1773–1885) Scottish botanist, who reported his discovery of the cell nucleus using a single lens microscope to the Linnaean Society in 1831.

BROWN-SÉQUARD SYNDROME OR PARALYSIS

Ipsilateral flaccid paralysis and impairment of touch, position and vibration sense with contralateral loss of pain and temperature due to a lesion sectioning one half of the spinal cord.

Charles E. Brown-Séquard (1817–1894) French physiologist and neurologist who was born in Mauritius. C.E. Brown, his father was an American sea captain from Philadelphia who disappeared at sea when Charles was a child and his mother was a French Mauritian. He took his mother's name, Séquard, after she died. He came to Paris to be a playwright but enrolled as a medical student and worked with Trousseau and Roger. He was an experimental physiologist by inclination and did much comparative work sectioning the spinal cord and examining the resultant sensory alteration which led to the description of his syndrome.

He contributed greatly to Claude Bernard's discovery of the vasomotor system by showing in the rabbit that stimulation of the cervical sympathetic caused blanching of the ear. This work took place between 1843–1852 when Brown-Séquard was living in poverty. For political reasons he went to the U.S.A. and for a short time was a Professor at the Medical College of Virginia. In 1855 he returned to Paris and practiced as a neurologist. In 1860 he was appointed Physician to the National Hospital, Queen's Square, London, the second appointment to this newly founded hospital. He spent 4½ years there and greatly influenced Hughlings Jackson. In 1864 he went to a Chair in Harvard but in 1868 returned to France, still a British citizen and politically to the left. He went to New York in 1870. In 1878 he returned to Paris and after Claude Bernard's death became a French citizen and succeeded him at the College de France. In 1889 he injected himself with testicular extract and claimed that he was greatly benefited. His reports drew much sceptical criticism but focused attention on the possibility of hormone therapy. He died from a stroke.

BRUCELLA ABORTUS

Bacteria causing infectious abortion in cattle.

Sir David Bruce (1855–1931) British physician, born in Melbourne of Scottish parents who had gone to Australia during the gold rush but returned to Scotland when he was five. He went to Edinburgh Medical School, graduating in 1881. Even as a schoolboy he was interested in natural history. He joined the army and was posted to Malta in 1886 where two years later he identified the organism causing Malta Fever from the spleen of two fatal cases (*Brucella melitensis*). His next posting was South Africa where the Governor of Natal requested the army to allow him to study a cattle disease called Nagara which he showed to be due to a trypanosome (*Trypanosoma brucei*) and that it was transmitted by the tzetse fly. This discovery led to his completing the work of Castellani (*v. infra*) who had demonstrated trypanosomes in the cerebrospinal fluid of patients with sleeping sickness. Bruce demonstrated the organism in the blood and showed that they were transmitted by the tzetse fly. He was involved in the seige of Ladysmith. Bruce was one of the great founders of the modern study of tropical medicine. He was elected F.R.S.

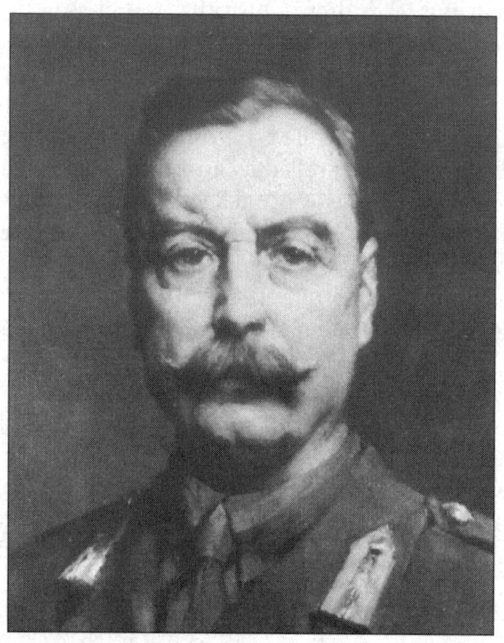

Sir David Bruce (Courtesy of the Royal Society of Medicine, London, UK)

Although Sir David was an outstanding figure, he did attract some sarcastic comments from Harvey Cushing in his book "From a Surgeon's Journal" concerning the research committee on which he and Cushing served. "General Sir David Bruce sank into a divan, stretched out his highly polished boots into the middle of the room, inserted his spurs into the rug, drew his John Bull visage deep into his clothes, turtle fashion, and slept profoundly – this was good for the General and also helped the meeting".

BRUCH MEMBRANE

The lamina vitrea – a transparent membrane next to the retina separating it from the capillaries in the choroid.

Karl W.L. Bruch (1819–1884) German anatomist. Professor of Anatomy at Giessen.

BRUDZINSKI SIGN

Sign of meningeal irritation – passive flexion of one thigh results in flexion of opposite hip and knee. When one thigh and leg are flexed and the other extended, lowering the flexed leg results in flexion of the opposite limb.

Josef Brudzinski (1874–1917) Polish physician.

BRUIT DE ROGER

v. ROGER MURMUR

BRUNNER GLANDS

Duodenal glands.

Johann C. Brunner (1653–1727) Swiss anatomist. These glands were first discovered by his father-in-law J.J. Wepfer. He was a pioneer of experimental physiology and came close to the discovery of the pancreas in dogs causing diabetes, noting excision of the pancreas caused thirst and polyuria.

BRUNS ATAXIA

Tendency to fall backwards seen in frontal lobe lesions.

BRUNS SYNDROME

Paroxysmal headache, vertigo, vomiting and sometimes falling when the head position is suddenly altered, due to lesions in the 4th ventricle.

Ludwig von Bruns (1858–1916) German neurologist in Hannover.

BRUSHFIELD SPOTS

White or light yellow pinpoint speckles seen in the iris of infants with mongolism and sometimes in normal children.

Thomas Brushfield (1858–1937) English physician.

BRUTON AGAMMAGLOBULINEMIA

Sex-linked hereditary hypogammaglobulinemia due to failure of development of B lymphocytes.

Ogden C. Bruton (1908–) American pediatrician.

BUDD-CHIARI SYNDROME

Hepatic vein occlusion resulting in hepatosplenomegaly, jaundice, ascites and portal hypertension. Characteristically the caudate lobe of the liver is spared due to direct venous channels from the inferior vena cava.

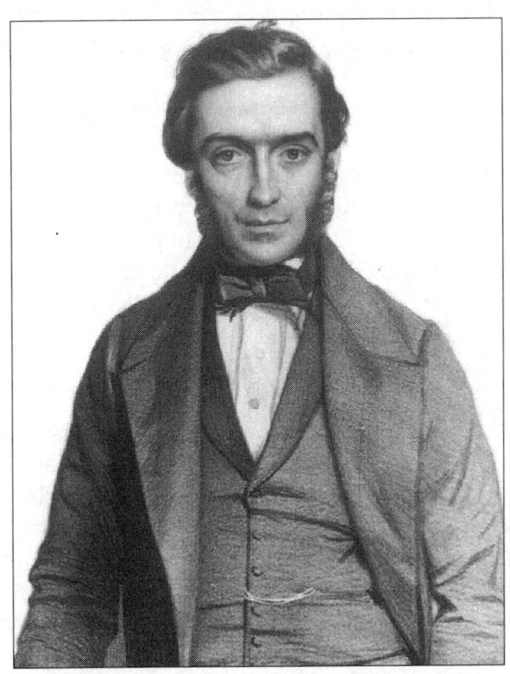

George Budd (Courtesy of the Royal Society of Medicine, London, UK)

George Budd (1808–1882) English physician. He was the son of a general practitioner at North Taunton who wrote an interesting article on an outbreak of typhoid fever in that village. Budd came from a large family of 9 sons and 1 daughter, of whom 7 sons became doctors. He received private education at his village, then went to Caius College, Cambridge, where he graduated as 3rd wrangler in 1831 and became a Fellow. He went to Paris and studied medicine and pathology before returning to London to become a student at the Middlesex Hospital. His first appointment was physician to the Dreadnought Hospital and it was here he encountered innumerable instances of liver disease in sailors returning home from the tropics which became a basis for his classical work on "Diseases of the Liver".

In 1840 he resigned to become Professor of Medicine at Kings College, succeeding Sir Thomas Watson and he and Dr. Todd were appointed physicians to the newly established Kings College Hospital where he described the syndrome in 1845. In his 23 years there he established a reputation as a clear and interesting lecturer and a fine bedside clinical undergraduate and postgraduate teacher. He was always a student's friend and was given a touching testimonial on his retirement by his students. He resigned his teaching posts in 1863 and devoted himself to private practice. In 1867 he developed glycosuria, gave up practice and went on a tour of Europe, spending the summer in Italy, and returned to the life of a country gentleman, where he enjoyed the hunt and his garden. He had recurring abdominal pain and diarrhea, became emaciated and died of pneumonia.

Hans Chiari (1851–1916) Austrian pathologist from Vienna who was Professor of Pathology at the German University in Prague. He was the son of J.B.V.L. Chiari (*v. infra*). He wrote a classical history of pathology and the first report of chorionic carcinoma of the uterus. He was a renowned histopathologist and teacher who used to rap his students over the knuckles if he caught them sectioning incorrectly. He produced a monograph on postmortem techniques in 1894 and in 1899 reviewed 13 patients with Budd-Chiari Syndrome. In 1916 he died suddenly following a throat infection.

BUERGER DISEASE

Thromboangeitis obliterans characteristically seen in smokers with a propensity for the Jewish race.

Leo Buerger (1879–1943) U.S. urologist, was born in Vienna, but his family migrated to the U.S.A. when he was one. He was educated at the College of the City of New York, Columbia University and the College of Physicians and Surgeons, where he graduated in 1901, interning on the surgical service at Lennox Hill Hospital. He studied at the Breslau Surgical Clinic in Germany for a time and then returned to private practice in New York where he had an attachment to the Mt. Sinai Hospital as a surgical pathologist. He developed a cystoscope in collaboration with F. Tilder Brown (Brown-Buerger cystoscope) and is said to have tried to change the name to that of Buerger cystoscope. He was fond of music and his first wife was a concert pianist. On his remarriage in 1929 he moved to Los Angeles to the Chair of Urology at the College of Medical Evangelists. He seems to have been a rather brash personality and was not well liked in California, and when he returned to New York in 1934 he was not reappointed to the staff of the Mt. Sinai.

BUMKE PUPIL OR SYNDROME

Transient dilatation of the pupils, which fail to respond to light and accommodation, seen in anxious or psychoneurotic patients without organic disease.

Oswald C.E. Bumke (1877–1950) German neurologist, was Kraepelin's successor in Munich. He attended Lenin's last illness, a stroke, with Foerster, Nonne and Henschen, and wrote a handbook on encephalitis. He wrote a 17 volume textbook of neurology with O. Foerster.

BUNSEN BURNER

Gas heat source.

Robert W.E. von Bunsen (1811–1899) German chemist who was Professor of Chemistry at Heidelberg – he introduced spectrum analysis.

BÜRGER-GRUTZ SYNDROME

Familial type I hyperlipidemia with eruptive xanthomata due to lipoprotein lipase deficiency, associated with pancreatitis, with onset in childhood.

Max Bürger (1885–) German Professor of Medicine and well known authority on genetics.

Otto Grutz (1886–) German dermatologist.

BURKITT LYMPHOMA

Malignant lymphoma first recognized and most commonly found in Uganda, but subsequently described in most parts of the world. It most frequently involves the mandible and retroperitoneal nodes.

Denis P. Burkitt (1907–) Contemporary British surgeon who was in the Colonial Service in Africa when he recognized this tumor. He was born in Enniskillen near Lough Erne, Northern Ireland, and graduated from Dublin University. He is well known for his work on high fiber diets in prevention and treatment of colonic disease.

BURNETT SYNDROME

Milk-alkali syndrome – hypercalcemia, azotemia and mild alkalosis.

Charles H. Burnett (1913–1967) U.S. physician. Burnett was born in Boulder, Colorado. He studied medicine in Colorado and then in New York and Boston and joined Dr. Chester Keefer at Boston University. His investigations there were interrupted by World War II when he joined the army. During his work with battle casualties, he made some important observations on shock. He returned home to study metabolic disorders and described his syndrome in 1947. He was Chairman of Medicine at Southwestern Medical School in Dallas before becoming Foundation Chairman of the Department of Medicine at the Medical School of North Carolina where he resigned because of ill health in 1965.

BURTON LINE

The lead line – a dark blue discoloration of the gums seen in patients with lead poisoning who usually have poor oral hygiene.

Henry Burton (1799–1849) Physician at St. Thomas' Hospital, London. He died of cholera.

BURULI LESIONS

v. BAIRNSDALE ULCER

Painless nodule on leg or forearm which enlarges and ulcerates due to *Mycobacterium ulcerans* infection. It is most commonly seen in children and was first noted in Buruli country near the Nile in Africa and subsequently seen in Uganda.

BYLER DISEASE

Fatal familial intrahepatic cholestasis believed to be an autosomal recessive trait seen in children of the Amish religious sect.

Byler An Amish kindred in the United States.

BYWATERS SYNDROME

Crush syndrome – lower nephron nephrosis.

Eric G.L. Bywaters (1910–) British physician, Emeritus Professor of Rheumatology, Royal Postgraduate Medical School, University of London. He was previously director of the Medical Research Council (M.R.C.) Rheumatism Research Unit at Taplow. He trained at the Middlesex Hospital, was an assistant clinical pathologist at the Bland Sutton Institute in 1935 and in 1937–39 was a Rockefeller Travelling and Harvard Research Fellow. He studied shock during World War II and observed his syndrome on air raid victims during the London blitz.

C

CABOT RINGS

Fine blue threads of nuclear remnants seen in the red cells in the peripheral blood of some patients with megaloblastic anemia.

Richard C. Cabot (1868–1939) U.S. physician born in Brookline, Mass. He was a member of the premier family of Boston which resulted in this well known limerick: "So this is good old Boston. The home of the bean and the cod. Where the Lowells talk only to the Cabots. And the Cabots talk only to God". He graduated from Harvard College in 1889 and Harvard Medical School in 1892 and remained at Harvard throughout his career, being an Instructor in 1903, Assistant Professor in 1908, Professor of Medicine in 1918, and Emeritus Professor in 1933. During the first World War he served in the Harvard Unit at Bordeaux and briefly was with the Red Cross in Paris.

He wrote a number of papers on diagnosis and was one of the early investigators to employ hypertension protocols. He introduced teaching of case histories, and wrote a book containing 702 such records. Together with his brother, Hugh, a surgeon, he initiated the clinico-pathological case conferences at Massachusetts General Hospital which provided a prototype for similar teaching exercises throughout the world. His book "Clinical Examination of the Blood" first published in 1896, in which he described his rings, went through 5 editions. He engaged in many controversies with members of his profession and established hospital social service at the M.G.H., a new departure, to be followed rapidly all over the world.

Cabot had graduated from Harvard College with honors in Classics and Philosophy and retained throughout his life an interest in ethics and philosophy. He lectured on logic at Harvard and was eventually appointed Professor of Social Ethics there in 1920, holding this position until 1934. Early in his career he attracted wide public attention by his attitudes to social aspects of medical care. In 1913 he stated that there were far too many doctors and urged re-organization of medicine into group practice. His books in the field of social welfare are still worth reading, and they include "Social Service in the Art of Healing" in 1909 and "What Men Live By" in 1914. He was widely quoted for his statement that of 400 diseases only 7 were curable by drugs and 5 by inoculations, and that the vast majority of diagnoses by doctors were wrong when compared with results of postmortem examination. In keeping with these teachings, he wrote a book "Meaning of Right and Wrong" in 1933 and one on "Christianity and Sex" in 1937. He also wrote another book entitled "Rewards and Training of a Physician" and in it

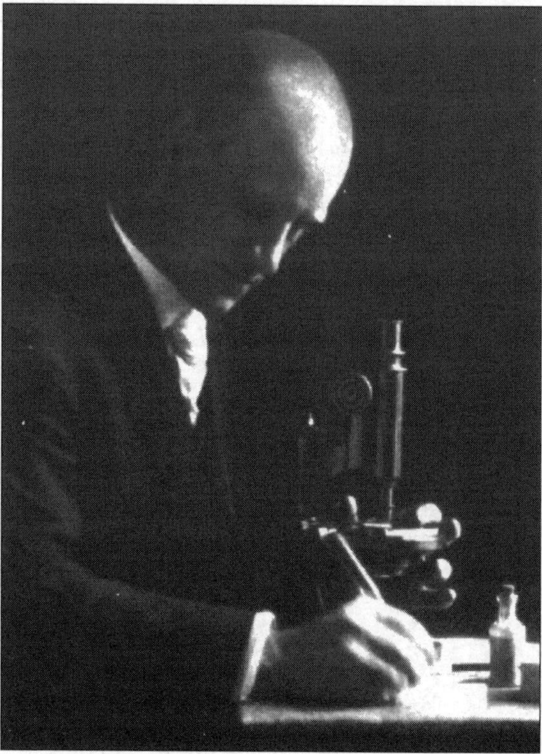

Richard C. Cabot (Courtesy of the Royal Society of Medicine, London, UK)

said "as I look over 25 years of medical work, I can remember but two patients whose lives I saved".

His clinic in Boston was conducted along classical lines in that he would read out the detail of the history and results of investigations and findings in each patient. He was very informal and would sit with his legs dangling over the edge of the table, asking his audience for suggestions as to diagnoses and slowly work up a lively discussion which at the end he would summarize, reach a diagnosis, then turn to the pathologist. In one instance it turned out that Cabot and everyone else was wrong. He said "that is the third time I have made a wrong guess" and then proceeded to go through the steps that had led him and his audience astray.

He emphasized the important role of the doctor in the care of the dying. He reputedly said that if the dying patient shared his great love of music, he would play his fiddle to him. He emphasized the importance of the correct psychological handling of a patient and the need for treating the human being as if he possessed a mind, affections, talents, vices and habits good and bad, as well as more or less diseased organs! Cabot's approach emphasizes what a physician can accomplish even when he is relatively helpless therapeutically.

A prominent Boston businessman, E. Mallinckrodt, a native of St. Louis, who went to Harvard to study chemistry, developed typhoid fever and was attended by Richard Cabot. Mallinckrodt recalled his treatment in an address at a ceremony when Ward 4 of the M.G.H. was being named the Mallinckrodt Ward. The treatment to his great discomfort had consisted of "ice sponge baths, and so thorough and conscientious were the sponsors of the baptism that to this day in troubled dreams, I think I hear the ice tinkling in the bucket and I wake up shivering". He survived the rigors of the treatment to become one of the great benefactors of American medical research.

CAFFEY DISEASE OR SYNDROME

Infantile cortical hyperostosis – self limited painful swelling of the mandible with periodic proliferation in the first 3 months of life. Other bones are sometimes affected and fever is common. It is thought to be familial, autosomal dominant.

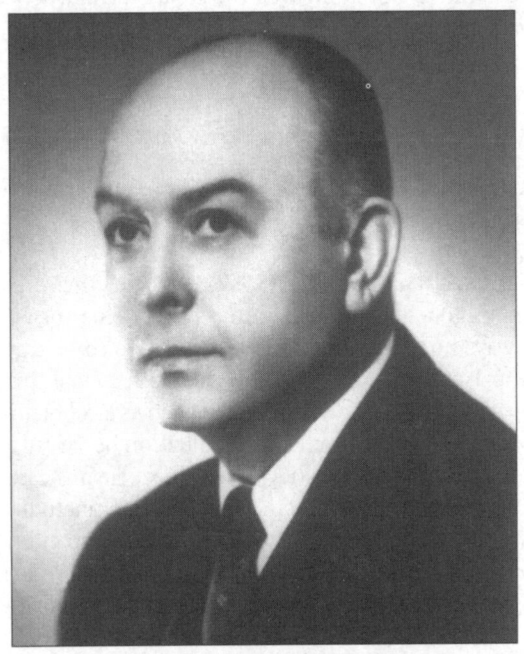

John Caffey (Courtesy of the Royal Society of Medicine, London, UK)

John Caffey (1895–1966) Emeritus Professor of Radiology, College of Physicians and Surgeons, Columbia University, New York. Born in Castle Gate, Utah, graduated in 1919 from the University of Michigan and interned at Barnes Hospital, St. Louis. In 1920 he went to Europe with the American Red Cross in Warsaw, Poland, but contracted typhus. Impressed by the lack of medical care for children in Eastern Europe he remained there after convalescence joining the Hoover Commission in Russia and stayed in Europe for 3 years. He trained in pediatrics at the Babies Hospital in New York, practiced pediatrics for a time and developed an interest in radiology and finally specialized in pediatric radiology. One of his original contributions led to the recognition of "the battered child syndrome". Always ready for argument and debate he was a born sceptic and always sure of his facts. "I wouldn't believe it even if you proved it to me!" He wrote a well known textbook on pediatric radiology. In the introduction of this book he states "Shadows are but dark holes in radiant streams, twisted rifts beyond the substance, meaningless in themselves. He who would comprehend Röntgen's pallid shades, needs always to know well the solid matrix whence they spring."

CAJAL CELLS

Astrocytes. Stellate cells which are ectodermal in origin and are present in neural tissue.

Santiago Ramon y Cajal (1852–1934) was the son of an Aragonese doctor in Spain. As a schoolboy he was always up to pranks, one of which led to three days' imprisonment. As a result, his father had him apprenticed to a hairdresser and then as a cobbler to occupy his spare time. After graduation he served as a doctor in the Spanish Army in Cuba. He protested about many of the practices of the time, including the use of the wards as stables for his commanding officer's horses. Disciplinary action was taken against him, but he was invalided out of the army, to save the authorities further embarrassment. In 1883 he was appointed to the Chair of Anatomy in Valencia and in 1887 moved to Barcelona to be Professor of Normal and Pathological Histology. Here he conducted his famous histological investigations of the nervous system and wrote a book on color photography. He said that he "worked to live, to live well and even to survive". He shared the Nobel Prize with Golgi in 1906 (*v. infra*).

CALVÉ DISEASE

Osteochondrosis of the vertebra.

Jacques Calvé (1875–1954) French orthopedic surgeon. One of the pioneers of orthopedic surgery in France, he completed his residency in Paris and worked with Menard in the Maritime Hospital at Berck. He was influenced greatly by the former, and the famous English orthopedic surgeon Robert Jones. He made many contributions to his field including the description of pseudo-coxalgia (v. LEGG-CALVÉ-PERTHES DISEASE) as well as introducing the method of treating Pott paraplegia by tapping the abscess through an intervertebral foramen. After the liberation of France he went to live in the United States (his wife was an American), but he returned to Berck in 1953 and died there in his old hospital.

CAMPBELL DE MORGAN SPOT

Cherry angioma. The incidence of this very common lesion increases with age and has no known association with disease.

Campbell G. De Morgan (1811–1876) Born at Clovelly in Devonshire he studied medicine at University College, London and then at the Middlesex Hospital where he was appointed as a surgeon in 1842. He became a Fellow of the Royal Society (F.R.S) following a contribution on bone development. He was a close friend of the sculptor John Graham Lough who was married to Sir James Paget's (*v. infra*) sister. He described the angiomas in a treatise on cancer entitled "Origin of Cancer" in 1872.

CAMURATI-ENGELMANN SYNDROME

v. ENGELMANN DISEASE; cf. RIBBING SYNDROME

CANAVAN DISEASE

Familial degenerative disease of the white matter, often called spongy degeneration of infancy. It has a predilection for families of Ashkenazi Jewish origin. Patients present at three months of age with apathy, flaccidity, an enlarging head, mental and motor retardation, progressive spasticity, blindness and optic atrophy. It is usually fatal before 3 years of age. There is macrocephaly with widespread demyelination and marked vacuolation of the deep cortical and subcortical tissue. Large protoplasmic astrocytes are present in the cerebral cortex and basal ganglion and there is a lack of myelin degradation products. It is believed to be an autosomal recessive defect.

Myrtelle M. Canavan (1879–1953) U.S. pathologist. She graduated in 1905 from the Women's Medical

College of Pennsylvania and became Curator of the Warren Anatomical Museum, Harvard University. Although Canavan reported her patient in 1931, she did not appreciate that it was a separate pathological entity, and thought her patient had a form of Schilder disease (*v. infra*).

CANNON LAW

A tissue with a deficient autonomic supply is excessively sensitive to chemical neurotransmitters.

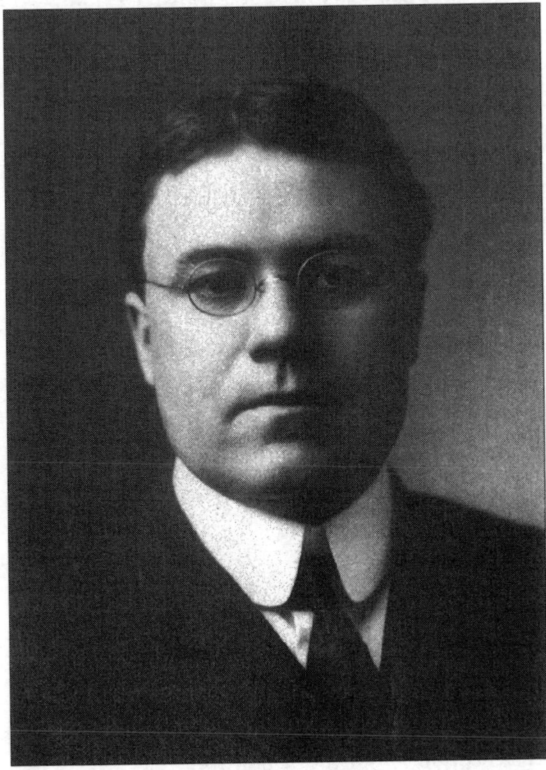

Walter B. Cannon (Courtesy of the Royal Society of Medicine, London,UK)

CANNON SYNDROME

Increase in adrenalin secretion during emotional stress resulting in palpitations and sweating.

Walter B. Cannon (1871–1945) U.S. physiologist, born in Prairie du Chien, Wisconsin, entered Harvard Medical School in 1896 and graduated 1900 to become an Instructor in Physiology. In 1906 he was appointed Professor of Physiology and stayed at Harvard until his retirement in 1942. His studies on intestinal motility, which commenced as a first year medical student, resulted in the introduction of the bismuth meal for radiological investigation of the gastro-intestinal tract. This led to his interest in the autonomic nervous system. His work contributed greatly to the concepts of chemical mediation of nerve impulses and he antedated concepts of α and β receptors with his description of sympathin E&I. Cannon served with the British Military Service in 1917, crossed the Atlantic with Harvey Cushing and Osgood (*v. infra*), worked on traumatic shock with Sir William Bayliss and was awarded the D.S.M. He wrote an interesting autobiography which outlined his philosophy "The way of an Investigator. A Scientist's Experiences in Medical Research".

CAPGRAS SYNDROME

Failure of a psychotic subject to identify an individual, despite recognition of familiarity in appearance and behavior.

Jean M. Capgras (1873–1950) French psychiatrist.

CAPLAN SYNDROME

Progressive massive necrosis of the lung in coal miners with rheumatoid arthritis.

Anthony Caplan British physician, graduated 1931, University of London. A student at St. Bartholomew's Hospital, he gained his M.R.C.P in 1935 and worked in the gold fields of South Africa as an industrial officer and subsequently in the coal mines of Wales.

CAPUT MEDUSAE (Head of Medusa)

Veins radiating around the umbilicus, seen in patients with portal hypertension.

Medusa Greek mythology. Queen of the Gorgons, who in mortal form had a head crowned with snakes and eyes which turned anyone who looked at them to stone. She was slain by Perseus who cut her head off by using his shield to look at her reflection.

CAREY COOMBS MURMUR

Short mid-diastolic mitral murmur heard in rheumatic fever and thought to be indicative of carditis.

Carey F. Coombs (1879–1932) Born in Castle Cary, Somerset. His father was a general practitioner. He trained at St. Mary's Hospital, London and in 1903 gained his M.D. He left London for Bristol initially as a medical registrar of the Children's Hospital and later was appointed to the staff of the General Hospital where he soon established himself as a fine physician and clinical investigator with a particular interest in cardiology and especially rheumatic heart disease, publishing a monograph on this in 1924. He wrote on all aspects of cardiac disease including coronary thrombosis of which he died.

CARNEY COMPLEX OR SYNDROME

Spotty pigmented lesions of the skin with myxomas of skin, breast or heart, peripheral nerve tumors (psammomatous melanotic schwannoma) (*v. infra*) and endocrine problems more commonly Cushing syndrome or sexual precocity, inherited as an autosomal dominant.

CARNEY TRIAD

Gastric epithelioid leiomyosarcoma, pulmonary chondroma and functioning extra-adrenal paragangliomas.

John A. Carney (1934–) He was born at Ballaghadereen (in English "the way of the little oak tree"), County Roscommon, Ireland. He was educated at Clongowes Wood College, Naas, County Kildare, the College of Pharmacy in Dublin, and University College, Dublin. His father had a pharmacy, and as a youngster he enjoyed being there looking at all the old remedies, pills and potions. He learned to read prescriptions (written in Latin) and to compound them. Initially he planned to be a pharmacist, but later decided to go to medical school and to return to Ballaghadereen as a general practitioner and also a pharmacist, and to continue with his father the family business. While at medical school he became interested in pathology, and on graduation M.B., B.Ch., B.A.O. in 1959, decided to abandon earlier plans and began a career in pathology. Following an internship at St. Vincent's Hospital in Dublin, he emigrated to the United States and commenced a residency in pathology at the Mayo Graduate School of Medicine in 1962. In 1966 he joined the staff of the Mayo Clinic as a consultant in the Department of Surgical Pathology. He was appointed Professor of Pathology in the Mayo Medical School in 1982.

Outside medicine, he is interested in wildlife and wild flowers. He enjoys music, grows orchids as a hobby and admits to being an excellent cook.

CAROLI DISEASE

Congenital disorder with diffusely distributed intrahepatic biliary cysts. Usually presents in the first or second decade with episodic fever, pain and sometimes jaundice. Frequently there are renal abnormalities, e.g. medullary sponge kidney. Progressive cirrhosis may lead to portal hypertension and esophageal varices.

Jacques Caroli (1902–) French physician.

CARREL FLASK

Glass container for tissue culture.

CARREL-DAKIN TREATMENT

Repeated irrigation of wounds with Dakin solution (*v. infra*).

Alexis Carrel (1873–1944) French surgeon, who was born in the village, Foy-les-lyon, near Lyons. His father died when he was four years old and to supplement his income, his mother undertook embroidering and he was very impressed by her

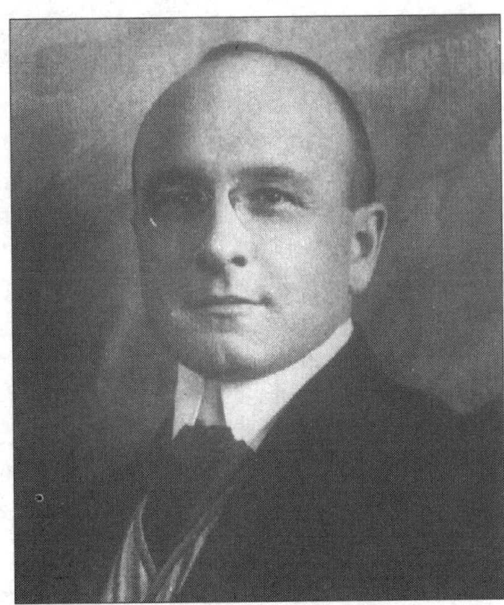

Alexis Carrel (Courtesy of the Royal Society of Medicine, London,UK)

skill with the tiny needles employed. He entered medicine at Lyons in 1890, and was already specializing in surgery when the French President Carnot was assassinated in Lyons and he was advised that the surgeons could not repair the President's portal vein which had been severed by the assassin's knife (v. Ollier). From that time on he became interested in techniques of suturing blood vessels and went to one of the finest embroiderists in Lyons, Madame Leroidier, to learn to use the tiny needles and thread which they employed and he used this in experiments on animals in vessel anastomosis. He began publishing these results in 1902, but was not popular with members of his faculty despite his undoubted clinical skills. The great French surgeon Leriche (*v. infra*) stated "He had certainly, along with Jaboulay, the best surgical hand that I ever witnessed in a career which allowed me to watch most of the greatest surgeons in the world". He had worked with Carrel when he was in Lyons. In 1903 Carrel took a pilgrimage to Lourdes and was impressed by the recovery of a young woman with tuberculous peritonitis. He strongly suggested a controlled study of the healings of Lourdes. This made him more unpopular with the Faculty and when he realized that he would not achieve any clinical advancement if he remained in Lyons, he decided to migrate to Canada and left France "to forget medicine and to raise cattle".

When he arrived in Canada he met with two physicians who encouraged him to continue his medical career in North America and he gave a paper at the French Language Congress in Montreal in 1904 which greatly impressed the Chairman of Physiology at the University of Chicago. He was offered a teaching position in Chicago and accepted, and arrived there in September 1904. Here he commenced his experimental work on vessel surgery and soon had authored publications on anastomosis of blood vessels and transplantation of a kidney.

He and his collaborator, C.C. Guthrie, performed a number of surgical heterografts and homografts with kidneys and thyroids and commenced the study of rejection problems. He rapidly gained the attention of a number of leading scientists of that time, in particular Cushing, W.S. Halstead from Johns Hopkins and Simon Flexner who was the Director of the recently established Rockefeller Institute. Both Johns Hopkins and Rockefeller offered him positions and he chose the Rockefeller which signalled the commencement of a long and happy association from 1906 to 1939. Whilst there he pioneered the development of tissue culture and with Charles Lindbergh, the aviator, developed a flask and pump for tissue culture techniques.

Carrel was a patriot and never became an American citizen. He helped a large number of French people who came to the United States for further study, one of whom was René Dubois. In 1912 he became the first person from North America to be awarded the Nobel Prize, for his work on vascular anastomosis and organ transplantation.

When the first World War broke out, he received orders to mobilize with the French Army and returned to France only to find that there was a great deal of resistance to him and his ideas; once again it was the Rockefeller Institute which came to his rescue and financed a hospital, the Rond-Royal, which was directed by him and in which, with Tuffier, he carried out experimental cardiac valvotomies; together with Henry Dakin he developed the irrigation treatment of wounds which again the French were slow to adopt. His hospital was destroyed at the end of the war by air attack and he finished the war in laboratories near Paris. He returned to the United States immediately after the war where he continued his work at the Rockefeller Institute and wrote a best selling book "Man, the Unknown".

When he retired from the Rockefeller he was planning an Institute to examine some of the social problems afflicting man, but with the outbreak of war, he returned again to France. He had a myocardial infarction in 1943 and another one immediately before the liberation. He was removed from all his offices, and he and his wife were placed under guard in Paris as collaborators. He died on November 5th, 1944, from a myocardial infarction, shortly after the French radio accused him of fleeing his guards to avoid standing trial and of being a collaborator. He had demonstrated the potential of sustaining cell lines indefinitely but these experiments were later explained by the addition of new material to the cultures by a fraudulent laboratory worker. He was the first to grow tumor tissues in vitro. He had developed techniques for preserving blood vessels in cold storage and for subsequent transplantation. He was indeed a remarkable, if rather controversial man, who made an extraordinary contribution to medical science.

Henry D. Dakin (1880–1952) (*v. infra*).

CARRIÓN DISEASE

Bartonellosis (v. BARTONELLA and OROYA FEVER). Acute hemolysis with fever and muscle pain, untreated it has high mortality.

Daniel A. Carrión (1859–1885) Peruvian medical student. Carrión inoculated himself with blood from a patient with verruga peruana (Peruvian wart), the mild form of Bartonella characterized by mild anemia and miliary nodular skin eruption varying in size from a pinshead pustule to a pea on face and limbs. He later died with symptoms of Oroya Fever, proving that it and Oroya Fever were one and the same.

CARTESIAN

Adjective referring to methods and philosophies of Descartes.

René Descartes (Cartesius) (1596–1650) Born in La Haye now La Haye-Descartes near Poitiers in France. He was educated by his maternal grandmother and nurse, and then studied at the Jesuit College in Anjou to become a scientist and philosopher who in 1662 wrote what is thought to be the first European book on physiology called "De Homine". It treated the body as a material machine directed by a soul located in the pineal. Descartes described the first experiment on reflex action – the blinking of the eyes when one pretends to strike them. He knew of Harvey's discovery of the circulation but followed Galen's teaching that cardiac movement derived from its internal fire or heat. He travelled widely throughout Europe and died in Stockholm.

CARVALLO SIGN

Murmur of tricuspid incompetence is increased in inspiration.

J.M.R. Carvallo Mexican physician, who worked at the National Cardiological Institute, Mexico City.

CASAL COLLAR OR NECKLACE

Erythematous pigmented skin lesions in pellagra.

Gaspar Casal (1681–1759) Known as the Spanish Hippocrates, he practiced in Oviedo in the Asturias from 1720–51 when he went to Madrid and was Physician to King Ferdinand. He first described pellagra (which he termed Mal de la Rosa) in a book published 3 years after his death, which recorded 30 years of observations in the Asturias on disease and epidemics, climate, fauna, minerals and flora.

CASONI TEST

Skin test for hydatid disease employing intradermal injection of sterile cyst fluid.

Tomasso Casoni (1880–1933) Italian physician who worked in Tripoli at the Victor Emanuel III Hospital.

CASTELLANI PAINT

Carbo-fuchsian solution for treatment of fungal infection.

Aldo Castellani (1877–1971) Italian tropical health expert, physician and dermatologist. He studied medicine at Florence University (1893–1899). Whilst a student he travelled with the University fencing team. The Professor who influenced him the most was Pietro Grocco (v. Grocco Triangle), who appointed him Studente Interno. Castellani was so intent on seeing patients in the ward and examining them with percussion that his fellow students nicknamed him Martellino ("little hammer"). Even as a student, dermatology attracted him, and he was taught by Professor Pellizzari, at the time the best known dermatologist in Italy. Undergraduates of the time could attend courses at different medical schools and in the summer Castellani attended various English hospitals. He was particularly impressed by Dr. Mitchell Bruce of Charing Cross Hospital. His graduating thesis was on the isolation of typhoid bacillus from the blood, and his interest in bacteriology led him to work with Professor Kruse at Bonn University. There he learned in the laboratory the technique of making broth for bacterial studies and whilst there developed a test which was used in many parts of the world to differentiate closely related bacteria. He studied at the London School of Tropical Medicine, where he was greatly impressed by the clarity and skill of Dr. Patrick Manson's lectures. Castellani was selected for an expedition to Uganda to investigate an epidemic of sleeping sickness. He discovered that the organism *Trypanosoma gambiense* was present in the cerebrospinal fluid of a majority of patients suffering from sleeping sickness and was the first person to establish its cause.

In 1903 he was appointed Professor in the Medical College of Colombo and Director of the Bacteriological Institute in Ceylon (Sri Lanka). He described this time from 1903–1915 as the happiest years of his life. He married an English woman in 1910 and his daughter subsequently married the distinguished diplomat Lord Killearn.

Castellani was a fascinating raconteur but also something of a snob and a rabid monarchist. Although an Anglophile, he never adopted English nationality, and in 1915 when Italy joined the war, he returned to the medical service of the Italian Navy. Whilst he had been in Ceylon he developed a triple vaccine (T.A.B.) and a quadruple vaccine which included cholera (T.A.B.C.) which was first used in 1916 in the Serbian Army.

Another of his accomplishments was establishing that a spirochete distinct from syphilis was the cause of yaws, and he was the first to suspect toxoplasmosis could affect man. He wrote what was probably the most authoritative text on tropical medicine of the day. Whilst one may not always have agreed with his politics, he reveals himself as a very human person in his autobiography entitled "Microbes, Men and Monarchs". During the 2nd World War his English honors were withdrawn, but later regranted by Queen Elizabeth.

CASTLE INTRINSIC FACTOR

A glycoprotein secreted in the gastric juice which binds with vitamin B_{12} and transports it across the ileum.

William B. Castle (1899–1990) American physician, born in Cambridge, Mass., he graduated M.D. cum laude in 1921 from Harvard, commenced work with Francis Peabody in the Thorndike Memorial Laboratory in 1925 and was next directed by George Minot, whom he succeeded as director in 1948. It was he who drew Pauling's attention to sickle cell anemia and this resulted in the first description of a molecular abnormality (of hemoglobin) causing a disease in man.

CASTLEMAN TUMOR

Unusual tumor which is probably a lymphoma. Usually solitary and on resection may not recur. The characteristic histologic features include an onion skin arrangement of the lymphocytes in nodules and an unusual vasculature.

Benjamin Castleman (1906-) U.S. pathologist at the Massachusetts General Hospital, Boston. For many years he edited the clinicopathological case presentations founded by R.C. Cabot (*v. supra*) in the New England Journal of Medicine.

CELSIUS

Centigrade scale of temperature.

Anders Celsius (1701–1744) Swedish astronomer born in Uppsala and became Professor of Astronomy at the University of Uppsala in 1730. He was the founder of Swedish astronomy and invented his centigrade thermometer in 1742.

CELSUS 4 CARDINAL SIGNS OF INFLAMMATION

Redness, swelling, heat and tenderness.

Aulus C. Celsus (53 B.C. to 7 A.D.) Roman physician during the time of Emperor Tiberius. He wrote numerous books on medicine in which he described the first use of a ligature. He introduced Hippocratic teaching to Rome and has been called the Roman Hippocrates. Alopecia areata is sometimes termed area celsi.

CESTAN-CHENAIS SYNDROME

Pontobulbar lesion due to tumor or occlusion of the vertebral artery below the post inferior cerebellar artery, causing ipsilateral paralysis of the soft palate and vocal cords with ocular signs, contralateral hemiplegia, sensory loss and ataxia.

cf. BABINSKI-NAGEOTTE SYNDROME; AVELLIS SYNDROME

Raymond Cestan (1872–1934) French neurologist. He was born in Gaillac, the son of a doctor who had been a student with Trousseau.

He went to medical school in Paris in 1892 and became interne des hôpitaux and student of Brissaud at the Salpêtrière in 1895. One day he spied a gong which he struck and the sound reverberated through the distant wards and one old pensioner, who had been one of Charcot's original performers on his Tuesday rounds, went into a hysterical trance.

Directed by Babinski, he was mainly interested in organic lesions such as congenital spastic paralysis which he studied with Bournville at the Bicêtre, and hemiplegia. In 1899 Raymond chose him as Chief of his Clinic and in 1902 put him in charge of the histopathology laboratory. He was the first person to describe a neurofibrosarcoma as well as the syndrome which bears his name. He was promoted agrégé in 1904, but his brother asked him to return to Toulouse. In 1913 he was appointed to a chair of psychiatry and in that capacity studied the formation of the cerebrospinal fluid and the effects of intra-ventricular injection.

Unfortunately he suffered a sudden onset of nominal aphasia and had a distressing illness for almost one year before he died peacefully in his sleep.

Louis J. Chenais (1872–1950) French physician.

CHADDOCK REFLEX

1. Noxic stimuli to the lateral malleolus may produce extension of the great toe in pyramidal lesion.
2. Noxic stimuli to the ulnar side of the forearm gives wrist flexion and finger extension in hemiplegia.

Charles G. Chaddock (1861–1936) U.S. neurologist, graduated 1885 from University of Michigan, Ann Arbor. He studied for two years in Munich (1888–1889) and four years in Paris (1896–1900) and was assistant to Babinski at La Pitié. He was appointed Professor of Nervous Diseases at the Marion-Sims-Beaumont Medical College, which became the St. Louis University School of Medicine where he succeeded C.H. Hughes (*v. infra*). He frequently returned to Paris between 1902–1921 to work with Babinski and translated some of Babinski's papers for publication in English. He translated Krafft-Ebing's "Psychopathia Sexualis" and wrote a textbook of psychiatry and a book on sexual crimes.

CHADWICK SIGN

Blue coloration of vaginovulval mucosa in early pregnancy.

James R. Chadwick (1844–1905) Born in Boston, he graduated M.D. Harvard in 1871 and spent two years in Europe visiting the major centers in Berlin, Vienna, Paris and London. He was appointed gynecologist at the Boston City Hospital and had a distinguished career becoming President of the American Gynecological Society in 1897. He was instrumental in the founding of the Boston Medical Library and was a keen proponent of cremation.

CHAGAS DISEASE

Insect vector transmitted disease due to *Trypanosoma cruzi*; the acute form causes fever, exanthemata, lymphadenopathy and meningism and chronically it can produce cardiomegaly, megaesophagus and megacolon.

Carlos J.R. Chagas (1879–1934) Brazilian physician who worked in Cruz's Institute and discovered *Trypanosoma cruzi*. He was born in Brazil and graduated in medicine from the University of Rio de Janeiro in 1903. In 1906 he was appointed director of a campaign to prevent malaria in Minas Geraes and was made an assistant at the Oswaldo Cruz Institute. He became Director of the Institute in 1917 and held this post until he died. The disease is most appropriately named after him since it is one of the few instances where the organism was found before the disease it produced was identified. Chagas first observed the crithidial stage of the flagellate in the intestine of an insect of the genus *Triatoma*. Believing it to be a stage of development of a trypanosome, he allowed infected insects to feed on marmosets and twenty days later found trypanosomes in the animal blood which he called *Trypanosoma cruzi* in honor of his mentor Oswaldo Cruz (*v. infra*). Chagas then found a disease in the region from which the infected bugs were obtained which had different characteristics to any disorder previously reported. He observed a 3 year old child with morphologically identical trypanosomes in her blood and noted Leishman-Donovan like inclusions in the brain and myocardium, thus accounting for the clinical involvement of those organs. From these surveys he suggested that the armadillo was the reservoir for the trypanosome. He made many other contributions to his country's public health and played an international role in the prophylaxis and investigation of leprosy. He was the Director General of Brazil's Department of Public Health from 1920–26 and Professor of Tropical Medicine at the University of Rio de Janeiro.

(Also called CHAGAS-CRUZ DISEASE)

Oswaldo G. Cruz (1872–1917) Brazilian physician who founded an Institute at Maguintios and became Director of Public Health at Rio de Janeiro in 1903 where he instituted dramatic reforms greatly improving the sanitary standards and providing a research milieu which gave a great boost to the study of parasitology. His institute was given his name by the government in 1908.

CHAMBERLAIN LINE

Straight line drawn from the posterior lip of foramen magnum to the posterior border of the hard palate on a lateral skull radiograph. If the dens passes through this line, platybasia exists.

W. Edward Chamberlain (1891–) U.S. radiologist whose work advanced fluroscopy and who played a major role in the American College of Radiology.

CHARCOT FEVER

Intermittent fever due to cholangitis and biliary obstruction often associated with jaundice and abdominal discomfort.

CHARCOT JOINT

Destructive joint atrophy due to neuropathology, usually secondary to syphilis but also seen with leprosy, diabetes and syringomyelia.

CHARCOT LARYNGEAL VERTIGO

Cough syncope.

CHARCOT TRIAD

Intention tremor, nystagmus and scanning speech seen in brain stem involvement in multiple sclerosis.

CHARCOT-BOUCHARD ANEURYSMS

Micro-aneurysms (≤1 mm) which are often associated with lacunae (dilatation of small arteries) in the brain. They accompany hypertension and are most commonly found in the thalamus and corpus striatum in the elderly. They are thought to be a major cause of hemorrhagic stroke.

CHARCOT-LEYDEN CRYSTALS

Colorless needle-like crystals in the sputum of patients with bronchial asthma and the feces of amebic and ulcerative colitis.

CHARCOT-MARIE-TOOTH DISEASE

Peroneal muscular atrophy. The muscle wasting usually begins in the small muscles of the feet and then the hands and remains peripheral in distribution.

CHARCOT-WILBRAND SYNDROME

Visual agnosia and inability to revisualize images once seen due to occlusion of the posterior cerebral artery of the dominant hemisphere.

Jean M. Charcot (1825–1893) French neurologist. He interned at the Salpêtrière (originally the gunpowder store for Louis XIII) in 1848 and was appointed superintendent in 1862 and became Professor of Pathology in 1872. He made clinical neurology a separate specialty and in 1882 became the first Professor of Diseases of the Nervous System. He recognized disseminated sclerosis as a distinct disease and first diagnosed it during life – previously it had been confused with Parkinsonism. His own housemaid developed the disease and he noticed that her tremor was intentional and not static. He kept her employed until she had to be admitted to the Salpêtrière where the clinical diagnosis of disseminated sclerosis was confirmed at autopsy. He depicted cortical motor centres in man, and first described syphilitic and amyotrophic lateral sclerosis and, with Vulpian, he first described ankle clonus. He studied hysteria and hypnotism and had numerous famous pupils including Marie, Babinski, Freud and Bekhterev. He introduced the study of geriatrics and recognized intermittent claudication. Charcot was a talented artist and as a lover of animals avoided animal experimentation. He had inscribed on his door "Vous ne trouverez pas une clinique des chiens chez moi". His appearance and presence apparently inspired confidence in his patients and he had an enormous practice, but he himself was said to be always rather cold and aloof.

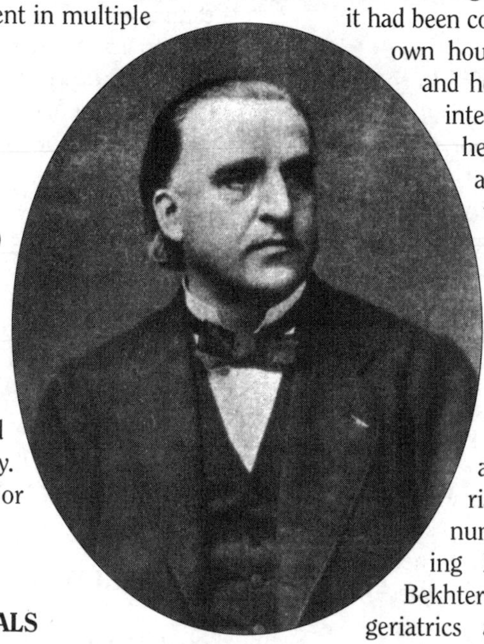

Jean M. Charcot (Courtesy of the Royal Society of Medicine, London, UK)

Charles J. Bouchard (1837–1915) (*v. supra*)

Ernst V. von Leyden (1832–1910) German physician, born in Danzig (Gdansk). He was a pupil of Schönlein and Traube and eventually followed the latter as Professor of Medicine in Berlin and took over Frerich's clinic upon his death in 1885. He founded with Frerich the journal Zeitschrift für Klinische Medizin and was coeditor of a number of other journals. He was called to treat the Czar Alexander in 1894. He was foremost in the movement for adequate hospital facilities (sanatoria) for tuberculous patients. He had a great clinical reputation and specialized in neurological problems. Northnagel was his assistant when he was in Königsberg.

Pierre Marie (1853–1940) (*v. infra*).

Henry H. Tooth (1856–1925) He was born in Brighton and educated at Rugby and then St. John's College, Cambridge, where he went in 1874. Six years later he graduated in medicine from St. Bartholomew's Hospital where he became casualty physician and following time as a demonstrator in physiology and medical tutor and demonstrator in morbid anatomy, he was appointed assistant physician in 1897, becoming a full physician in 1906 and retiring in 1921. When the Boer War broke out he joined the Army and was physician at the Portland Hospital in South Africa. He maintained his interest in army medicine, and when the Ist World War broke out he was initially placed in command of the Ist London General hospital at Camberwell and then worked overseas in Malta and at the Italian front where he was mentioned 3 times in despatches. He was a kindly teacher, well liked by students and by his medical colleagues as a consultant. He lectured at St. Bartholomew's Hospital on diseases of the nervous system and conducted weekly clinics at Queen's Square and contributed a valuable account of cerebral tumors. He was a keen musician, playing regularly in an orchestra, and was an expert carpenter. He had a cerebral hemorrhage while driving his car, and died 3 months later. Independently he described the disorder in the same year as Marie and Charcot in his Cambridge M.D. thesis (1886).

Hermann Wilbrand (1851–1935) German neuro-ophthalmologist. He worked with Laquer in Strasburg, Forster in Breslau (Wroclaw) and finally was appointed to the Chair of Ophthalmology in Hamburg in 1879. He devoted his life to the study of physiology and pathology of vision especially the visual pathway and cortical representation and projection. He showed homonomous hemianopia to be due to lesions in the optic radiations and occipital cortex as well as the optic tract and discredited Goltz's old theory of the visual centers being subcortical.

CHARNLEY PROSTHESIS

A prosthesis of the hip joint.

Sir John Charnley (1911–1982) He went to medical school at Manchester University and graduated in 1932. In World War II he undertook orthopedic surgery in Cairo and there developed a walking calliper which was officially adopted by the army. After the war he made contributions to a number of areas in orthopedic surgery and experimented in his workshop in his house on methods of fixing metal and plastics to bone and developed prostheses which were later finished by professional instrument makers, and he performed his first hip replacement in 1969. He became the first orthopedic surgeon to be elected to the Fellowship of the Royal Society in 1975. He was an enthusiastic rock climber and also fond of sports cars, especially Aston Martins.

CHASSAIGNAC TUBERCLE

Carotid tubercle on transverse process of C6.

Edouard P.M. Chassaignac (1804–1879) He was born in Nantes and became Professor of Anatomy and Surgery in Paris. He introduced modern drainage techniques to surgical practice and published a two volume textbook on this topic in 1859. He died in Versailles.

CHASTEK PARALYSIS

Fatal polyneuritis and paralysis in domestic foxes after ingestion of raw fish because thiaminase in the fish destroys thiamine.

S.J. Chastek U.S. fox breeder.

CHEADLE DISEASE

Infantile scurvy.

Walter B. Cheadle (1836–1910) English pediatrician, born in Colne, England, and educated at Caius College, Cambridge. He graduated M.B. in 1861 and joined the staff of St. Mary's Hospital in 1869–92 where he was Dean of the Medical School from 1869–73 and during his term introduced entrance scholarships and thereby enabled talented but financially embarrassed students to enter the medical school. He differentiated scurvy from rickets in 1877. He went on an exploration of Western Canada (1862–64) and wrote a book on his experiences "The Northwest Passage by Land" and in 1899 wrote another book dealing with artificial feeding of infants. He was a progressive who favoured admission of women to medical school and despite opposition from some of his colleagues was a prominent teaching member of the Medical School for Women which opened in 1874.

CHEDIAK-HIGASHI ANOMALY OR SYNDROME

Large granule in cytoplasm of neutrophils and eosinophils associated with oculocutaneous albinism, photophobia and nystagmus and recurrent pyogenic infections inherited as an autosomal recessive. The cellular defect is impairment of microtubule function. Similar giant pigment granules have been observed in other tissues, e.g. hair follicles. The disease terminates in an accelerated lymphoma-like phase with pancytopenia, hepatosplenomegaly and lymphadenopathy.

Moises Chediak (1903–) Cuban physician, born in Santiago de Cuba and went to medical school in Havana, Cuba. He was trained entirely in Cuba at the Hospital Calixto Garcia and was Professor of Clinical Pathology there when he described the anomaly.

Ototaka Higashi Japanese pediatrician, graduated from Tohoku University, Sendai, Japan. Professor of Paediatrics at Akita University.

CHEYNE-STOKES BREATHING OR RESPIRATION

Recurrent episodes of hyperpnoea followed by apnea seen in elderly patients with cerebrovascular disease and cardiac failure. Thought to be due to delay in circulation time between the lungs and respiratory centre resulting in a coarsening of the negative feedback of the blood gases.

John Cheyne (1777–1836) Scottish physician. The son of a surgeon; when 13 years old he used to help his father dress and bleed patients. He entered Edinburgh University at 15, graduated at 18, then joined the Army and served 4 years before returning to practice with his father in Leith. He was at the Battle of Vinegar Hill where the British under Sir John Moor beat the Irish. Whilst in Scotland he studied pathology and dissection with Charles Bell and wrote his first book on "Essays on the Diseases of Children" in 1801. He wrote one of the important early monographs on laryngology "Pathology of the Membrane of the Larynx and Bronchia (1809)". He first described acute hydrocephalus. In 1809 he went to Dublin and in 1812 was appointed Physician-General in Ireland. He was perhaps the founder of Irish medicine.

Ill health caused his semi-retirement and return to England in 1831. He described Cheyne-Stokes respiration in 1818. He wrote a book on apoplexy and a monograph on typhus fever.

William Stokes (1804–1878) (*v. infra*).

v. STOKES-ADAMS SYNDROME

CHIARI-FROMMEL SYNDROME

Postpartum galactorrhea with pituitary adenoma, associated with atrophy of the uterus, amenorrhea and low follicule stimulating hormone (FSH) levels in the urine.

Johann B.V.L. Chiari (1817–1854) Austrian gynecologist who was born in Salzburg and graduated in medicine from Vienna in 1841. He was appointed Professor of Obstetrics at the German University in Prague in 1853, returned to a Chair in Vienna the next year but died of cholera shortly after. He emphasized the importance of pathology in advancing gynecological practice. He trained Semmelweis in obstetrics and was the latter's ardent supporter when he first advocated asepsis in practice.

v. also ARNOLD-CHIARI SYNDROME; BUDD-CHIARI SYNDROME

Richard J.E. Frommel (*v. infra*).

CHIDO BLOOD GROUP

Present in 98% of the population and found in plasma as well as in red cells. It is closely linked to HLA and one portion of the C4 (complement) molecule.

Chido Surname of the patient in whom the antigen was first observed.

CHILAIDITI SYNDROME

Loop(s) of bowel between liver and diaphragm when the patient is upright, associated with abdominal pain, nocturnal vomiting and distension with loss of liver dullness, confirmed on X-ray.

Demetrius Chilaiditi German radiologist who described the condition in 1910.

CHINESE RESTAURANT SYNDROME

Sensation of burning pressure in the face and chest and frequently headache, produced by ingestion of monosodium glutamate used in some Chinese foods.

CHRIST-SIEMENS-TOURAINE SYNDROME

A developmental defect of the ectoderm and mesoderm structures resulting in anhidrosis, hypotrichosis and poor dental development. The facies is characteristic, with a prominent forehead, saddle nose, thick lips and fine short blonde hair. They are usually small and somewhat female in appearance. They have heat intolerance and suffer with hyperpyrexia following mild exercise due to their lack of sweat glands and this also is associated with recurrent eczema during childhood. There may be other developmental anomalies and it predominantly occurs in males and is transmitted as a recessive or dominant gene.

Josef Christ (1871–1948) German dentist.

Hermann W. Siemens (1891–1969) German dermatologist.

Albert Touraine (1883–1961) French dermatologist.

CHRISTENSEN-KRABBE DISEASE

Progressive cerebral poliodystrophy (v. ALPERS DISEASE).

Erna Christensen (1906–1961) Danish neuropathologist. She worked at the Rigshospitalet in Copenhagen and introduced neuropathology there.

Knud H. Krabbe (1885–1961) Danish neurologist at the Copenhagen Municipal Hospital and made notable contributions in comparative neuroanatomy on morphogenesis of the brains of reptiles and lower mammals.

CHRISTMAS DISEASE

Hemophilia B. Sex-linked recessive hereditary bleeding disorder identical clinically with classical hemophilia.

CHRISTMAS FACTOR

Factor IX coagulation factor.

S. Christmas Name of the patient who was recognized to be different from a classical hemophiliac.

CHURCHILL-COPE REFLEX

Increased respiratory rate due to distension of the pulmonary vascular bed.

Edward D. Churchill (1895–1972) U.S. thoracic surgeon, who described segmental pneumonectomy and bronchiectasis. Professor of Surgery at Massachusetts General Hospital, Harvard University.

O.J. Cope (1902–   ) U.S. surgeon.

CHURG-STRAUSS SYNDROME

Allergic granulomatous angiitis. There is usually a history of allergy and the main organ involvement is skin, kidney and lung with eosinophilia. Medium sized vessels are involved, with intra- and extra-vascular granulomas at varying stages of evolution.

Jacob Churg (1910–) Born in Dolhinow, Poland (now Vilnius in the Republic of Lithuania). His father was also a doctor. He graduated M.B. in 1933 and gained his M.D. in 1936. He migrated in that year to the United States and served in the Army in World War II. He joined Mt. Sinai's Department of Pathology in 1944 and was appointed Clinical Professor of Pathology in 1966. He is currently a Research Professor of Community Medicine at Mt. Sinai School of Medicine and continues to work as Chief Pathologist at Barnert Memorial Hospital Center in New Jersey. In a recent interview he commented that when he joined the hospital staff in 1943, there were 110 beds which cost $5.00 a day each. Today the hospital has 440 beds and charges nearly $500.00 a day. This remarkable man is a keen chess player and has just completed his 10th book.

Lotte Strauss (1913–1985) U.S. pathologist. She graduated from medical school at the University of Siena, Italy, in 1937 and later migrated to the United States where she undertook residency in pathology at Mt. Sinai, completing her training in 1943. She became an Associate Pathologist for pediatric pathology in 1952 and later Professor of Pathology, being awarded emeritus status on retiring in 1984.

CHVOSTEK SIGN

Tapping the face over the facial nerve in front of the tragus of the ear causes muscular twitching ipsilaterally. Seen in tetany and sometimes in anxiety states.

František Chvostek (1835–1884) Austrian surgeon, born in Mistek in Moravia, he graduated in medicine from Josef Academie in 1861. He described his sign in 1876 and investigated pathology and treatment of neurological illnesses including the use of electrotherapy.

CLARA CELL

A cell present in terminal bronchioles.

Max Clara (1899–) Austrian pathologist born at Vols and went to medical school at the University of Innsbruck and became Professor at Leipsig, Munich and Istanbul.

CLARK SIGN

Obliteration of liver dullness due to distension in peritonitis.

Alonzo Clark (1807–1887) U.S. physician from New York, who introduced opium treatment for peritonitis, replacing the popular vogue of the time, blood letting and mercurials. He was born in Chester, Vermont, and graduated M.D. from the College of Physicians and Surgeons, New York, in 1835. After visiting London and Paris he worked on principles of percussion on cadavers in the pathology department and wrote on the subject. He was a fine clinician and good bedside teacher who impressed his students with a number of aphorisms: "The medical errors of one century constitute the popular faith of the next", "Every man's disease is his personal property", "You may know the intractability of a disease by its long list of remedies", "Symptoms which cannot be readily marshalled into line must be credited to the nerves", "There is no courtesy in science". He was visiting physician to Bellevue and taught physiology and pathology with the College of Physicians and Surgeons (1848–1855), and became a Professor of Medicine (Practice) from 1855–1885. Whilst giving a lecture he had an attack of vertigo which heralded his death 6 months later, presumably due to a cerebrovascular accident. As he sank into a chair during the lecture he said, "For many years I have held this Chair, and never until this moment occupied it literally".

CLAUDE SYNDROME

Ipsilateral oculomotor palsy with contralateral ataxia and hemichorea due to a lesion in the red nucleus.

Henri C.J. Claude (1869–1945) French neuropsychiatrist and neurologist. He was assistant to Raymond (*v. infra*) and a colleague throughout his working life at the Salpêtrière with J. Lhermitte (*v. infra*). He was particularly interested in movement disorders and epilepsy and in the origin of hallucinations and the distinction between schizophrenia and hysteria. He made a number of important contributions on brain stem lesions. He pioneered the use of hyperpyrexia, electroconvulsive therapy and insulin therapy for psychiatric disturbances, in France.

CLAYBROOK SIGN

Rupture of an abdominal viscus may cause easy auscultation of heart and breath sounds in the abdomen.

Edwin B. Claybrook (1871–1931) U.S. surgeon.

CLÉRAMBAULT-KANDINSKY SYNDROME

A state in which the patient believes his mind is controlled by someone else or external forces.

(Also called KANDINSKY COMPLEX.)

Gatian de Clérambault (1872–1934) French psychiatrist, born in Bourges and gained his thesis in 1899. He became assistant physician at the special infirmary for the insane, Prefecture de Police in 1905 and became Head in 1920. Apart from his psychiatric studies he wrote on the costumes of various native tribes. He committed suicide.

Viktor C. Kandinsky (1825–1889) Russian psychiatrist.

CLUTTON JOINTS

Painless effusion into a large joint, usually bilateral, seen in congenital syphilis. The joint range is usually only limited by the effusion.

Henry Clutton (1850–1909) English surgeon, born in Sutton Walden, where his father was the Vicar. He went to school at Marlborough, had to leave because of ill health, but later went to Clare College, Cambridge, then became a student at St. Thomas' Hospital in 1872, a resident assistant surgeon in 1876, and in 1892 a full surgeon. When he died he was senior surgeon at St. Thomas' Hospital.

He was a meticulous and widely read surgeon who adopted advances rapidly, and was a very early disciple of antisepsis and became a strong supporter of aseptic techniques. He placed great emphasis on the importance of a surgeon studying and understanding pathology rather than the older school of pursuing anatomy in the pure sense. Earlier on when he was in charge of the department concerned with diseases of the ear, he was one of the first proponents for active treatment of suppuration of the middle ear and wrote a number of articles on a variety of general surgical subjects and contributed to Treves "System of Surgery" on "Diseases of bones and deformities". He also translated Von Esmarch's "Handbook for Military Surgeons". He was a very popular teacher who attracted both undergraduates and postgraduates to his rounds, but unfortunately for the last twelve years of his life his activities were somewhat limited following septicemia due to a wound infection whilst he was operating. As a result he would perform a full day's work but could not engage in any active physical activities later, and would retire to his home early and had exercise intolerance even when walking on the flat. Prior to his illness he had been a keen "bush walker" and had also enjoyed fishing. He had a great love for the visual arts and church architecture. Even though he was so exhausted at night that he would have to lie on the flat of his back unable to do anything, he still managed to be active in the College of Surgeons and died in office on the Council.

COATS DISEASE

Retinitis exudativa (circinata).

George Coats (1876–1915) Scottish ophthalmologist, born in Paisley and began his medical studies at Glasgow University in 1892 and graduated in

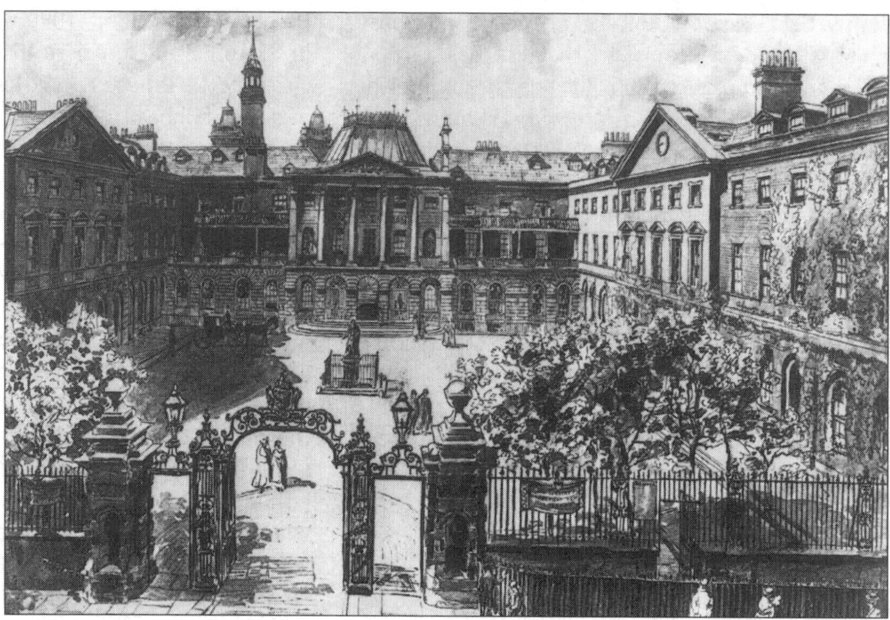

Guys Hospital, 19th century (Courtesy of the Royal Society of Medicine, London, UK)

1897. He was a resident at the Royal, Western and Eye Infirmaries in Glasgow, and continued his studies in ophthalmology in Vienna, visiting Munich, Freiburg and Zurich. He commenced work at the Royal London Ophthalmic Hospital in 1902, became a F.R.C.S in 1903 and in 1905 he was appointed pathologist at Moorfields hospital. Here he became interested in the histology and pathology of eye disease and stated that all he wanted to do was to obtain enough money to live so that he could devote most of his time to investigating these problems in the laboratory. He held numerous appointments at London teaching hospitals, but at his death was assistant surgeon to the Royal London Ophthalmic Hospital and assistant ophthalmic surgeon at St. Mary's Hospital. He wrote a number of articles on vascular diseases of the eye, one of which, on thrombosis of the central vein of the retina, was regarded as a classic. He wrote on congenital abnormalities of the eye and became very interested in comparative anatomy and pathology, spending much of his time in the zoological society gardens. One of the last papers he presented was on the retina of the fruit-eating bat. He was extremely fond of music and had an extensive musical library as well as an encyclopedic knowledge of it. He died at an early age, having already established an international reputation, and recognition in his own country as a very skilful operator and fine clinician.

COCK – PECULIAR TUMOR

Infected sebaceous cyst.

Edward Cock (1805–1892) English surgeon at Guy's Hospital who performed the first pharyngectomy in England. He was the nephew of Sir Astley Cooper and greatly revered his uncle. However, unlike him, he was an extreme conservative and was said "not to look with much favour on innovations in surgery, whether they have reference to operations or other modes of treatment". He developed a special interest in the genito-urinary tract and became well known for his treatment of stricture. He was a very successful teacher with students, although he had a marked stammer. His book "Head and Neck" was a favorite with them. Although he was a good looking man, he walked with what was described as a drooping, slouching gait and this, combined with his hesitation in speech, resulted in him being called "Old Cock" even in his younger days. He was an assistant surgeon at Guy's from 1838 to 1849 when he was promoted to surgeon. He held a number of positions in the College of Surgeons and in 1869 was elected President. He was well known to be a very kindly man. A patient of his had all his face eaten away by a rodent ulcer and lost his job as a gardener at Greenwich Hospital. Cock got him a false nose and spectacles and although his appearance was still very bizarre, hired him as his own gardener for a small plot of ground attached to his house in London. The gardener used to go through the daily routine of looking after a pocket handkerchief plot, planting seedlings that would never grow, watering, etc. and for this was paid full wages by Cock. It was related at hospital dinners that when members of the staff were toasted, Cock always got the loudest applause, and when a guest enquired why, when one considered his colleagues were all as famous or more famous teachers or clinicians, the answer given was "because he has a heart".

COCKAYNE SYNDROME

Dwarfism, microcephaly, and beak-like nose, photosensitive dermatitis, deafness, retinal atrophy, mental retardation and progressive upper motor neurone and cerebellar dysfunction, possibly due to an autosomal recessive gene.

Edward A. Cockayne (1880–1956) English physician, born in Sheffield and educated at Charterhouse and Balliol College, Oxford, doing his clinical years at St. Bartholomew's and graduating in 1907; M.R.C.P in 1909 and was elected to Fellowship in 1916. He worked at Barts and Great Ormond Street and during the Ist World War was in the Royal Navy (1915–1919). After demobilization he was appointed outpatient physician at the Middlesex Hospital and the Hospital for Sick Children, becoming a full physician in 1924 at the former and in 1934 at the latter. He combined pediatrics with general medicine and was especially interested in endocrinology and rare genetic disease in childhood. He was a younger colleague of Garrod, who undoubtedly influenced him and he became a well known entomologist and President of the Royal Entomological Society of London. He had a magnificent collection of butterflies and moths and had a unique collection of developmental anomalies, "sugaring" trees in his neighbourhood to collect specimens. He was a very modest and kindly person and a lifelong bachelor who devoted all his spare time and holidays to entomology, pursuing his prey all over the Scottish and English countryside. He published his book "Inherited Abnormalities of the Skin and Its Appendages" in 1933.

COGAN SYNDROME

1. Vertigo, tinnitus, progressive bilateral deafness, pain in the eyes and photophobia, blurred vision associated with interstitial keratitis of unknown etiology.
2. Congenital form of 3rd nerve apraxia.

David G. Cogan (1908–) U.S. neuro-ophthalmologist born in Fall River, Mass. and graduated from Harvard Medical School in 1932. Appointed Professor and Chairman of Ophthalmology in 1963.

COLEY TOXIN OR FLUID

Preparation of bacterial toxin which on injection caused febrile reaction and reduction in size of some tumor masses. The active component is now believed to be tumor necrosis factor, a cytokine.

William B. Coley (1862–1936) U.S. surgeon, born in Westport, Connecticut, graduated from Harvard in 1888, became Professor of Clinical Surgery, Cornell University Medical Center, and died following an intestinal operation. He was an honorary F.R.C.S.

COLLES FRACTURE

Fracture of the radius just above the wrist with dorsal displacement of the distal fragment.

Abraham Colles (1773–1843) Irish surgeon, born near Kilkenny, graduated in arts from Trinity College, Dublin, and obtained diploma from the College of Surgeons in the same year, 1795. That year he went to Edinburgh and gained his M.D. there in 1797. He walked from Edinburgh to London in 8 days and after a brief time there returned to start private practice in Dublin. Financially this was not very rewarding, but he was elected resident surgeon at the Steeven's Hospital. In 1804 he became Professor of Anatomy and Surgery at the College of Surgeons (Ireland) where he stayed until 1836 and built up a reputation as a surgeon and as a teacher. During that time he wrote a number of articles including one entitled "On fracture of the carpal extremity of the radius" which was published in 1814. In another he introduced mercury for the treatment of syphilis and made another original observation, "A child born of a mother who is without any obvious venereal symptoms ... and shows this disease when it is a few weeks old ... will infect the most healthy nurse ... and yet this child is never known to infect its mother." This has since been known as Colles Law, although the observation had been made earlier by Simon de Vallembert in 1565. Colles resigned his position at Steeven's Hospital in 1842 due to ill health with dyspnea and frequent attacks of gout. He died the following year and at the autopsy he had requested was found to have a fibrotic left lung and a dilated heart without valvular disease which Colles had suspected contrary to his physician Stokes (*v. infra*).

COLLET SYNDROME *or*

COLLET-SICARD SYNDROME

Fracture of the floor of posterior cranial fossa causing 9th, 10th, 11th and 12th cranial nerve palsy.

Frédéric J. Collet (1870–) French otolaryngologist – a similar patient was described by Sicard in 1917 – Collet described his patient in 1915.

Jean A. Sicard (*v. infra*).

COMBY SIGN

Buccal mucosal inflammation with whitish yellow patches seen in measles before Koplik spots appear.

Jules Comby (1853–1947) French pediatrician born in Pomadour, he went to school at Limoges and was an outstanding pupil. He studied medicine in Paris where he was a pupil of Bouchard. He trained with Hannelougue (a surgeon) with whom he wrote a paper on osteomyelitis and then worked with Grancher. He became médicin des hôpitaux in 1885 and devoted his energies to childhood illnesses founding the journal "Archives de Medicin des Enfants" in 1898 which he edited for 44 years. He wrote a popular book on pediatrics which went through several editions and was a frequent lecturer to other European countries, North Africa and Latin America.

CONCATO DISEASE

Polyserositis.

Luigi M. Concato (1825–1882) Italian physician born in Padua and became Professor of Medicine in Bologna in 1860 and in Turin in 1878 where he died. In the original description tuberculosis was the etiological agent – now the eponym is applied to all forms of polyserositis.

CONN SYNDROME

Excess secretion of aldosterone with hypertension and hypokalemic alkalosis.

Jerome W. Conn (1907–) U.S. physician who graduated from the University of Michigan in 1932. He became the Director of the Division of Endocrinology and Metabolism in 1943 and University Professor of Medicine in 1968. His major interests have been in the physiology and pathology of human metabolism and in human nutrition.

CONRADI DISEASE OR SYNDROME

Chondrodystrophia calcificans congenita. A multisystem disorder with shortening of the limbs and dwarfism as well as cataracts and sometimes icthyosis and hyperkeratosis of the palms and soles.

Erich Conradi (1882–) German physician.

COOLEY ANEMIA

Thalassemia major.

COOLEY TRAIT

Thalassemia minor.

Thomas J. Cooley (1871–1945) U.S. physician, born in Ann Arbor, Michigan, the son of a distinguished member of the Faculty of the Law School at the University of Michigan. He graduated M.D. from the University of Michigan in 1895 and then did a two year residency at Boston City Hospital following which he returned to work and teach at the medical school in Michigan. In 1900 he went abroad for a year and returned to spend a further year as a resident physician at the Boston City Hospital. In 1903 he was appointed Assistant Professor of Hygiene at the University of Michigan and remained there until 1905 when he moved to Detroit to practice pediatrics. During the Ist World War he was assistant chief of the Children's Bureau of the American Red Cross in France and the French Government awarded him a Cross of the Legion of Honour in 1924 for this work. He returned after the war to Detroit and became Head of the Pediatric Service at the Children's Hospital, Michigan, from 1921 to 1941 and Professor of Pediatrics at Wayne University from 1936 to 1941. His sub-specialty in pediatrics was hematology and he was especially interested in the anemias of childhood which resulted in the term "Cooley Anemia", an eponym he heartily disliked! He gave much of his time to community efforts to improve the standard of health care for children. He was well versed in the visual arts and music, and enjoyed fishing and golf. He died of hypertensive heart disease after being ill for some years.

COOMBS TEST

Test for detecting red cell antibodies either on the red cell (direct) or in the serum (indirect) by using rabbit anti human globulin serum (Coombs Serum).

Robin R.A. Coombs (1921–) English immunologist. Professor of Immunology at Cambridge University – graduated from Veterinary School, Edinburgh University. The test he developed is used all over the world in blood transfusion cross matching and in the investigation of anemia. He is a F.R.S and a Fellow of Corpus Christi College, and said "erythrocytes were primarily designed by God as tools for the immunologist and only secondarily as carriers of hemoglobin".

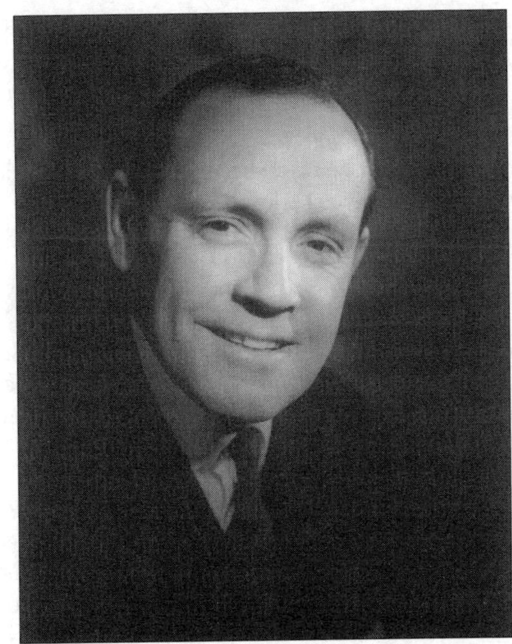

Robin R.A. Coombs
(Courtesy of the Godfrey Ardent Studios)

COONS FLUORESCENT ANTIBODY METHOD

Fluorescent antibody technique for localizing antigen in cells.

A.H. Coons (1912–) U.S. immunologist, born in New York. He went to medical school at Harvard, graduating in 1937. He commenced working on fluorescent labels for antibodies in 1941 following Marrack's demonstration that visible dyes could be linked to antibodies and act as markers. He first published on this in 1942, but the 2nd World War interrupted his studies and it was not till 1952 that he published his fluorescent antibody technique which was taken up and applied all over the world. His laboratory attracted and trained immunologists from many countries and he received many international awards in honor of his achievements including the Paul Ehrlich Prize in 1961.

COPLIN JAR

Glass vessel with vertical grooves to hold slides for staining procedure.

W.M.L. Coplin (1864–1928) U.S. physician.

CORI CYCLE

Series of enzymatic reactions converting lactic acid to glucose and glycogen in the liver.

CORI DISEASE

Amylo 1-6 glucosidase deficiency. Glycogen storage disease with hepatomegaly and sometimes splenomegaly and episodes of hypoglycemia. Glycogen storage disease Type III.

Carl F. Cori (1896–) U.S. biochemist. Professor of Biochemistry at Washington University, St. Louis, who was born in Prague and graduated from the German Medical School at the University of Prague in 1920 and migrated to the U.S.A. in 1922. He won the Nobel Prize with his wife Gerti Cori (1896–1957) for their work on glycogen debrancher deficiency, producing glycogen accumulation in liver, muscles and heart.

CORNELIA DE LANGE SYNDROME

1. Microbrachycephalia, peculiar facies, triangular mouth, hirsutism with hair to the eyebrows, limb abnormalities with mental retardation.
2. Congenitally enlarged muscles, mental retardation and sometimes spasticity and extrapyramidal disorders.

Cornelia de Lange (1871–1950) Dutch pediatrician who was born at Alkmaar in The Netherlands, studied at the University of Zurich graduating in 1897. After some time in general practice she was appointed to a children's hospital in Amsterdam and became Professor of Paediatrics at the University of Amsterdam from 1927–1938.

CORRIGAN PULSE

Collapsing pulse usually associated with aortic regurgitation and hyperkinetic circulation.

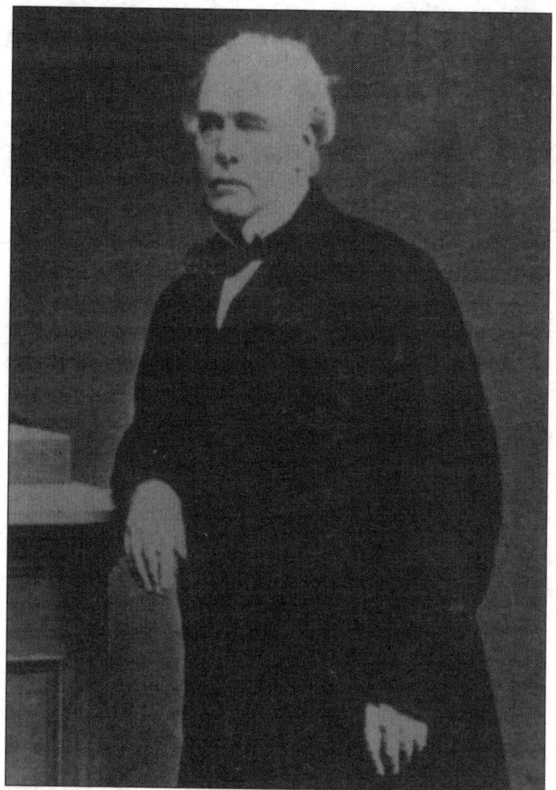

Sir Dominic J. Corrigan (Courtesy of the Royal Society of Medicine, London, UK)

Sir Dominic J. Corrigan (1802–1880) Irish physician, educated at the Catholic College at Maynooth (now a Seminary for Roman Catholic priests). His father was a dealer in hardware and fire implements. Corrigan was influenced by a general practitioner, Dr. O'Kelly, who attended the staff and students of the College and who was very impressed by Corrigan's ability and advised him to study medicine. He met a Dr. Cornelius Denver who taught him mathematics, physics and chemistry and as a result probably directed his interest into hemodynamics. He graduated from Edinburgh University, M.D., in 1825, the same year as Stokes. He returned to Ireland and practiced in Dublin, was appointed physician to the Cork Street Fever Hospital and the charitable infirmary, Jervis Street. In 1832 he published "On permanent patency of the mouth of the aorta, or inadequacy of the aortic valve", which incorporated his study of aortic regurgitation and described his pulse.

He designed an implement known as Corrigan button which is a small circular metal plate with a handle. When it is heated with a flame and touched rapidly on the skin along the course of the sciatic nerve, it acts as a counter irritant in the treatment of sciatica. In 1849 he gained an honorary M.D. degree from Trinity College, by which time he was a most successful and prosperous physician. He was elected President of the Irish College of Physicians in 1859 and retained that post until 1863, which remains the longest period anyone has held that position. Whilst he was President, he initiated a building which was completed in 1863 to give the college its first meeting place. He altered the college regulations so that it was possible to elect Fellows who graduated from any University in the United Kingdom or any foreign University. He was elected as a Member of Parliament for the City of Dublin in 1870 and was described as being a fluent speaker and in debate not given to soft words in replying to his opponents. Apart from his medical activities he promoted the Pharmaceutical Society of Ireland and was its first President and was responsible for the improvement of Dublin's water supply.

During his Presidency, the Irish College of Physicians became the first body in the British Isles to admit women to the licence examination, thus enabling them to enrol in the medical register. Five were passed in 1877 and in 1886, out of 50 women on the register, 44 were licenciates of the Irish College. It was not until 1924 that Fellowship was opened up to women! Corrigan became physician to Queen Victoria and was dubbed Sir Dominic Corrigan in 1847.

CORTI, ORGAN OF

The cochlea of the inner ear where sound is perceived by rods arranged in a spiral chamber.

Marquis A. Corti (1822–1888) Italian histologist and anatomist born in Sardinia but worked in Vienna where he was a prosector under Hyrtl. Later he worked in Berlin, Utrecht and Turin. He was never appointed to a University and worked mainly on the retina and ear. He died in Rome.

COSTEN SYNDROME

Dental malocclusion with associated neuralgic headache.

James B. Costen (1895–1962) U.S. otolaryngologist.

COUNCILMAN BODIES OR CELLS

Oxyphilic inclusion in the cytoplasm of hepatic cells seen in yellow fever—believed to represent necrosis around viral particles and may be seen in other forms of viral hepatitis and more rarely in some bacterial and even parasitic infections.

William T. Councilman (1854–1933) U.S. pathologist at Johns Hopkins and Harvard. He introduced the term amebic dysentery and distinguished the harmless *Amoeba coli* from the pathogenic *Amoeba dysenteria*. He wrote one of the early accounts confirming Laveran's discovery of the malarial parasite. He was one of the foundation editors for the section of pathology in the Journal of Experimental Medicine (1896) whose editor in chief was Welch.

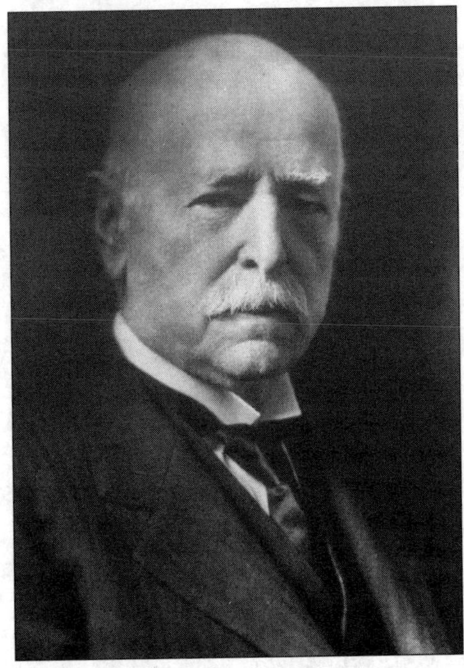

William T. Councilman (Courtesy of the Royal Society of Medicine, London, UK)

Councilman was born on a farm near Baltimore and was sent to school at St. Johns College in Annapolis, leaving aged 16. He spent the next 6 years enjoying life – but when aged 22 decided to follow his father, who was a country doctor, and entered medical school at the University of Maryland, graduating in 1878. He heard of Johns Hopkins University, which had opened in 1876, from his father, who attended Huxley's opening address. He went there on a Fellowship to work with Martin in biology and wrote his first paper "Inflammation of the cornea" and became interested in pathology. In 1880 he went to Europe where he worked in Vienna, in Strasburg with von Recklinghausen, and in Leipzig with Cohnheim and Weigert, and finally he spent some time with Hans Chiari in Prague, having first met him in Vienna.

He returned to the U.S.A. in 1883, helped John S. Billings prepare his National Medical Dictionary and performed autopsies at Bayview where for a time he was the City Coroner. In 1886 he joined Welch at Johns Hopkins and then spent another year in Europe before the opening of Johns Hopkins Hospital in 1889. In 1892 he was appointed Professor of Pathology at Harvard, the first outsider ever to be so appointed. He was a delightful, informal teacher who commented, "I think lecturing is an intellectual stimulus and comparatively harmless to the audience … it does not really matter much what the lecturer says". From his farm upbringing he was always interested in plants and planted shrubs and flowers around the Brigham Hospital and was a close friend of the Director of the Arnold Arboretum in Boston. He was one of the earliest of the conservationists and wrote a number of papers on plants, and had a bulldog called Pasco who was always at his side.

He admired tradition but was also wary of it, commenting that the reason for Johns Hopkins's initial success and enthusiasm was the total lack of it. He said, "traditions may be very important, but they can be extremely hampering as well and whether or not tradition is of very much value, I have never been certain". "It is an important thing that people be happy in their work, and if work does not bring happiness there is something wrong".

COURVOISIER LAW

In obstructive jaundice due to gallstones in the common duct, the gall bladder is impalpable and if palpable, other causes such as carcinoma of the head of the pancreas are more likely.

Ludwig G. Courvoisier (1843–1918) Professor of Surgery, Basel, born in Basel where his father was a merchant and his mother was the daughter of an English clergyman. His father developed tuberculosis and at the age of 7 he went with his parents to Malta to live with his maternal grandparents and therefore he became fluent in English. Just before entering medical school he developed typhus and spent a year recovering from that disorder. He spent some time at the University of Göttingen and then returned to Basel to graduate M.D. in 1868. Shortly after he was assistant to Professor Socien who was one of the first surgeons in Europe to sponsor Lister's antiseptic techniques.

He studied in London with Sir William Fergusson and Sir Spencer Wells and then spent a year in Vienna with Billroth and Czerny. He served in the Military Hospital in Karlsruhe during the Franco-Prussian War and then returned to Basel where he became surgeon in the small town of Riehen on the German-Swiss border. For the next 30 years this was his main post, although he opened a private clinic in Basel in 1883 which was very successful and in 1888 the University gave him the title of Professor of Surgery Extraordinary. However, it was not until the death of his old master, Socien, in 1899 that he was given beds in the hospital in Basel and became Professor of Surgery at the University of Basel. He was a pioneer in surgery of the biliary tract area and popularized cholecystectomy as an operation as well as being one of the first to remove stones from the common bile duct. Generally regarded as a safe surgeon, he had the reputation for handing over to others patients who had conditions which he considered lay outside his experience. From the time he was a small boy he took a great interest in butterflies and botany, and published over 21 papers on entomology. He gave his collection to the Natural History Museum of Basel and left his Herbarium to the Botanical Institute.

COWDEN DISEASE

Breast hypertrophy, hypoplastic jaw, papillomas of lips and mouth and scrotal or cobblestone tongue. Pectus excavatum, scoliosis and thyroid adenomata. High incidence of fibrocystic disease of the breast and also carcinoma in women. The disorder is inherited as an autosomal dominant with variable penetrance.

Rachel Cowden The praepositus of the first family described with this condition.

COWPER CYST

Retention cyst of bulbo-urethral glands.

COWPER GLAND

The bulbo-urethral glands.

William Cowper (1666–1760) Born in Petersfield, Sussex, he became apprenticed to a surgeon in London and qualified in 1691. As well as his description of the glands he wrote the first description of aortic insufficiency, one of the early operations on the maxillary sinus and a treatise on muscles. He wrote a book "Anatomy of Human Bodies" in 1698; although the text was original, most of the plates were taken from Bidloo's "Anatomia".

COXSACKIE DISEASE OR VIRUS

Coxsackie, New York U.S.A. Home town of patients in whom the virus was first isolated. The virus may cause aseptic meningitis, herpangina, myocarditis, pericarditis and pleurodynia (v. BORNHOLM DISEASE).

CRABTREE EFFECT

Inhibition of cellular respiration by high concentrations of glucose.

Herbert G. Crabtree English biochemist.

CREUTZFELDT-JAKOB DISEASE

v. JAKOB-CREUTZFELDT DISEASE

CRICHTON-BROWNE SIGN

Twitching of the outer corners of the eye and lips – an early sign of general paralysis of the insane.

Sir James Crichton-Browne (1840–1938) British physician and doyen of mental health in the United Kingdom. He was born in Edinburgh and his father was a doctor and the commissioner in lunacy in Scotland. He received his medical education at Edinburgh University where he was a pupil of Lister and later at the University of Paris.

From the start he was interested in psychiatry and as a medical student read a paper to the Royal Medical Society "Psychical diseases of early life". He graduated L.R.C. Ed. in 1861 and in 1862 gained his M.D. He then trained as a medical officer in the Derby, Devon and Warwick county asylums before becoming medical superintendent at Newcastle Asylum. He went to the West Riding Asylum at Wakefield as Medical Director, where he commenced the "West Riding Asylum Reports", the first British Journal of Neuropathology, established in 1871. He recognized the importance of and lack of facilities for research and established the first neurological research laboratory in the United Kingdom at Wakefield where Sir David Ferrier began his experiments on cerebral localization. In 1875 he was appointed Lord Chancellor's visitor in lunacy in reforms, retiring from that office in 1922. The esteem in which he was held by fellow scientists was illustrated by his proposal by Charles Darwin and his election as Fellow of the Royal Society in 1883. He was knighted in 1886.

Together with Hughlings Jackson, Sir John Buckmill and Sir David Ferrier he established a special journal for neurological research, "Brain", of which he was co-editor. He was a most imaginative speaker and impressive figure with Dundreary whiskers, who was always prominent in the public eye in debate or schooling methods, and in his intense opposition to teetotalism, maintaining "no writer has done much without alcohol". He published five volumes of autobiography and was a prominent radio broadcaster. He had an extraordinary grasp of language and knowledge of literature and was regarded as one of the best after-dinner speakers of his day.

CRI-DU-CHAT SYNDROME

Laryngeal anomaly producing a cat-like cry in infants with microcephaly and mental retardation associated with deletion of the short arm of chromosome 5.

CRIGLER-NAJJAR SYNDROME

Jaundice due to inability to conjugate bilirubin with glucuronic acid.

John F. Crigler (1919–) U.S. pediatrician who was born at Charlotte, North Carolina. He graduated from Johns Hopkins M.D. and joined the staff of the Children's Hospital in Boston in 1955. He became Chief of the Division of Endocrinology in 1965.

Victor A. Najjar (1914–) U.S. pediatrician. He was born in Zalka, Lebanon, and graduated M.D. from the American University of Beirut in 1935 and came to the U.S. in 1938 working in Pediatrics at Johns Hopkins (1949–1957) and then was appointed head of the Department of Microbiology at Vanderbilt University, Nashville in 1957. He was appointed Professor of Molecular Biology and Chief of the Division of Protein Chemistry at Tufts University, Boston in 1968.

CROCQ DISEASE

Acrocyanosis.

Jean B. Crocq (1868–1925) Belgian physician, who developed a department of neurology in Brussels. After the first World War, he became Professor of Psychiatry in Ghent. He died of encephalitis lethargica, a disease he had contracted from one of his patients.

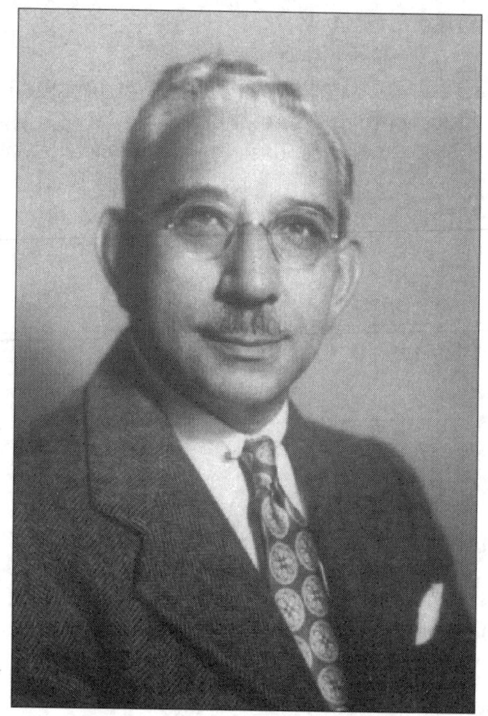

Burrill B. Crohn (Courtesy of the Royal Society of Medicine, London, UK)

CROHN DISEASE

Regional ileitis.

Burrill B. Crohn (1884–1983) U.S. physician who worked initially with Sachs (*v. infra*) at Mount Sinai Hospital, New York, screening children for cherry red spots on the retina. In 1932 when he was President of the American Gastroenterology Society he presented a paper on his new disease which consisted of abdominal pain, diarrhea and a mass often in the right lower quadrant. He was going to call the disease terminal ileitis but a friend cautioned that it may be regional, so he changed the name, and later studies proved this decision correct.

CRONKITE-CANADA SYNDROME

Alopecia, nail dystrophy, pigmentation, diffuse intestinal polyposis, protein losing enteropathy, osteomalacia, and malabsorption, which usually presents in middle or old age, etiology unknown.

Leonard W. Cronkite U.S. physician, Harvard, Massachusetts General Hospital.

Wilma J. Canada U.S. radiologist, Boston, St. Luke's Hospital, New Bedford, Mass.

CROUZON DISEASE

Cranio-facial dysostosis – hypertelorism – usually autosomal dominant.

CROUZON-APERT DISEASE

v. APERT SYNDROME

Acrocephalosyndactylia. Craniostenosis with oxycephaly and syndactyly, sometimes polysyndactyly of hands and feet, often visual failure with proptosis and ophthalmoplegia.

Octave Crouzon (1874–1938) French neurologist. Before he entered the Faculty of Medicine at the University of Paris he had already been influenced in college by Pierre Janet and had developed an interest in psychology. As a student in Paris he was very impressed by Dieulafoy as a lecturer and then by Babinski and in particular Pierre Marie. Undoubtedly this influenced him in his choice of investigation in pathology. Apart from the disorder he described he made a number of contributions to the muscular dystrophies and investigated many families from the Mendelian point of view. Graduating in 1901, he became Chef de Clinique et de Laboratoire at the Hôtel Dieu in 1906 and was promoted to Médecin des Hôpitaux in 1912. He then joined the staff of the Salpêtrière and during the war was attached to the ambulance service and then the office of the Under-Secretary of State of the service for Military Health. After the war he continued his investigations into neurological conditions, especially in hereditary dystrophies, in particular the hereditary cerebellar ataxias. Working in these areas drew his attention to the cervical and lumbar spine deformities and in turn this led to investigations on chronic rheumatic disorders with a number of his colleagues at the Salpêtrière. He maintained his interest in psychiatry and in the overall problems of the effects of disease at the personal level. He became more and more interested in the training of staff to assist patients in this regard and in the medico-legal aspects of medical problems. His deep interest in all matters pertaining to social medicine stemmed from his experiences in the war, but should also be probably dated from his student days and the influence of Pierre Janet. As a result of this, a special Chair was created for him, La Chaire d'assistance medico-sociale, to which he was appointed in 1937. A man of broad interests, he had a considerable knowledge of anthropology. He was a holder of the Croix de Guerre and a Commander of the Legion d'Honneur.

Eugène Apert (1868–1940) French pediatrician. He had an outstanding undergraduate career and was influenced by Grancher and above all Dieulafoy, with whom he became related by marriage. His graduation thesis in 1897 was on purpura. From the beginning he was interested in developmental abnormalities and published a number of instances of birth abnormalities, largely in the form of case reports. One concerned fused tower head to which his name is now attached. He wrote two books for the popular public on "Childhood Health" and "Baby Care and Welfare" which were very helpful to parents. He was greatly upset at not being promoted to Agrégé, but he continued his long interest in genetics and the study of twins. A pleasant and likeable man, he retired from L'Hôpital des Enfants Malades in 1933.

CROWE SIGN

A sign sometimes seen in lateral sinus thrombosis. Compression of the internal jugular vein on the normal side results in engorgement of the retinal vessels.

Samuel J. Crowe (1883–1955) Born in Washington and graduated from Johns Hopkins in 1903. U.S. otolaryngologist who with Cushing explored pituitary function by extirpation of the gland. He trained with Harvey Cushing, was a contemporary of Dandy and did some interesting studies of cerebro-spinal fluid physiology, showing, with A.S. Levenhart, that the drug hexemethylenamin (urotropin) is excreted into the cerebro-spinal fluid.

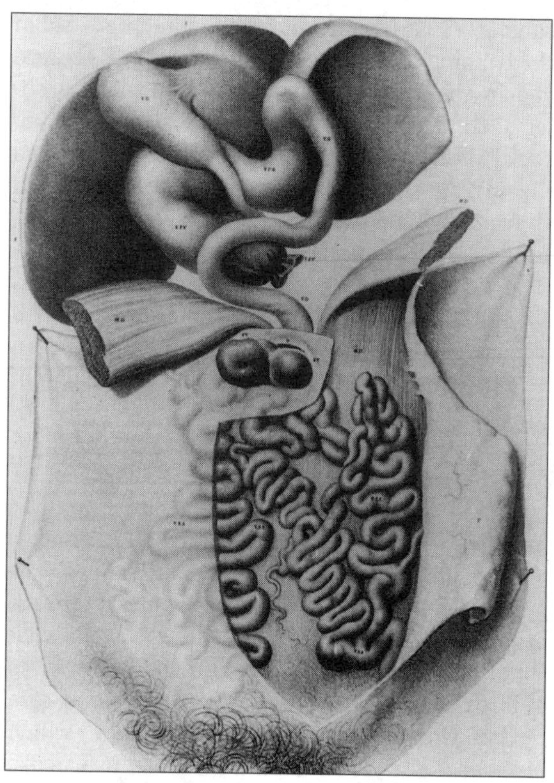

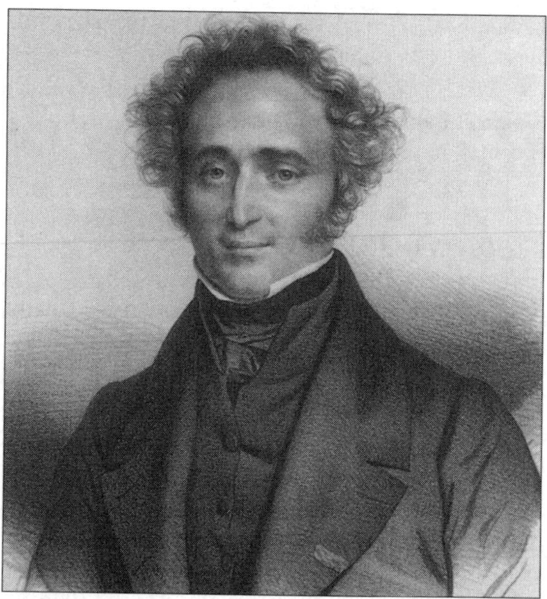

Above: Jean Cruveilhier. (Courtesy of the Royal Society of London, UK) Left: From his book *"Anatomie Pathologique du Corps Humain"*. This is the illustration of the anatomy of the veins which give rise to Cruveilhier-Baumgarten murmur. (Courtesy of the National Library of Medicine, Washington DC, USA)

He became Professor of Laryngology and Otology and Chief of Service at Johns Hopkins and died there of a myocardial infarction.

CRUVEILHIER DISEASE OR PALSY

Progressive spinal muscular atrophy (progressive muscular atrophy).

CRUVEILHIER SIGN

Impulse over the saphenous vein following coughing seen in saphenous varicosity.

CRUVEILHIER-BAUMGARTEN MURMUR OR SYNDROME

Hepatic cirrhosis with a patent umbilical vein (in fact usually varices in the falciform ligament) may cause a loud abdominal murmur and thrill over the umbilicus.

Jean Cruveilhier (1791–1874) French pathologist, born in Limoges, France, son of an army surgeon. Initially he wanted to enter the church but was compelled by his father to study medicine. After seeing his first autopsies he abandoned medical school and entered the seminary of St. Sulpice to become a priest; his father made him return to medical school where Dupuytren (a friend of his father) made him a protégé and interested him in pathology. He graduated in Paris in 1816 and practiced for 7 years in Limoges. Supported by Dupuytren he was appointed Professor of Surgery at Montpellier in 1823, in 1825 Professor of Descriptive Anatomy in Paris, and in 1836 he was appointed to the new Chair of Pathological Anatomy. He wrote many books – the best known is the "Anatomie Pathologique du Corps Humain". In this superbly illustrated work he gives an excellent description of gastric ulcer and the first pathological account of disseminated sclerosis. He reported a French soldier who in 1813 was captured by some Hungarian troops and beaten and left for dead, receiving a very powerful blow to his abdomen with a rifle butt. After 6 months stay in hospital he recovered and returned to civilian life, but some years later was troubled by abdominal swelling and a loud murmur was noted over his umbilicus. He died in 1833 and at autopsy his liver was found to be somewhat small in size, smaller than his spleen, but no cirrhosis was commented upon. There were large veins coursing from his umbilicus, connecting the systemic with his portal system. Cruveilhier speculated whether this could be congenital or acquired following the trauma.

Like John Hunter, he believed thrombosis was entirely a local event rather than a combination of local and systemic changes as proposed by Virchow. He appreciated that a cerebral lesion caused contralateral paralysis. In 1829 he saw a woman aged 45 with frontal headache, weakness of the left leg, slow speech, mental impairment and involuntary micturition and predicted a tumor of the right frontal lobe, which was confirmed at autopsy, thus anticipating Broca's demonstration by 32 years. He described pyloric stenosis secondary to pyloric hypertrophy and progressive muscular dystrophy.

Walter Baumgarten (1873–1945) U.S. physician. Born in St. Louis, Missouri, he was the son of the most outstanding physician in the Midwest who was one of the founding members of the Association of Physicians. He graduated M.D. from Washington University, St. Louis, in 1896 and was assistant in physiology at Harvard from 1897–98 and then at Johns Hopkins 1903–07. He then returned to practice in St. Louis at the Barnes Hospital and St. Luke's Hospital and retained his association with Washington University until he died when a fire destroyed his summer home at Fish Creek, Wisconsin.

CRUZ DISEASE

v. CHAGAS DISEASE

CULLEN SIGN

Bluish discoloration of the umbilicus due to blood in the peritoneal cavity (e.g. ruptured ectopic pregnancy, pancreatitis).

Thomas S. Cullen (1868–1953) U.S. gynecologist, born in Bridgewater, Ontario, Canada, a Minister's son. He graduated near the top of his class in medicine at the University of Toronto, 1890, and interned at the Toronto General Hospital; Kelly had been on a fishing holiday in Canada and performed an operation in Toronto at which Cullen was an assistant. He was so impressed by Kelly's skill that in 1891 he became junior intern on Dr. Howard Kelly's service at Johns Hopkins, and in 1893 studied for 6 months in J. Orth's laboratory in Göttingen in Europe. He returned to Johns Hopkins, first working in gynecological pathology and then going into practice as a gynecologist in 1897, retaining his association with the medical school at Johns Hopkins where he became Professor of Clinical Gynecology until 1939.

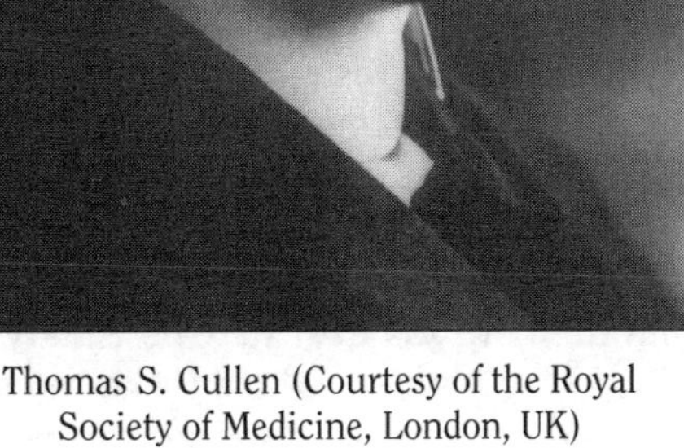

Thomas S. Cullen (Courtesy of the Royal Society of Medicine, London, UK)

He wrote the first description of pathological and clinical endometrial hyperplasia, and numerous papers. He edited textbooks on gynecology and described his sign in 1922.

CURIE, MILLICURIE, MICROCURIE

A measure of a radiation dosage or emission which pays tribute to the discoverers of radium.

Pierre Curie (1859–1906) and **Marie Curie** (1867–1934) French physicists, reported the isolation of radium from pitchblend in 1898. When it was appreciated that this element produced the same effects as X-rays it was used in the therapy of lupus and in malignant tumors. Marie was Polish and worked for years as a governess to finance her studies in Paris where she became Pierre's pupil and they married in 1895. They received the Nobel Prize in 1903. She continued their work after Pierre's death following a road accident and she was awarded the Nobel Prize again in 1911 and is still the only woman to have won it twice.

CURLING ULCER

Acute peptic ulcer associated with skin burns.

Thomas B. Curling (1811–1888) English surgeon, born in Tavistock Place, London. His father was secretary to the Commissioners of His Majesty's Customs, a post of considerable dignity and emolument. At the age of 21 when he had just become a member of the Royal College of Surgeons, Curling was appointed assistant surgeon to the London Hospital due to the influence of his uncle, Sir William Blizzard. This was deeply resented by his colleagues, as was his own rather aloof and cool manner. He was stated in one obituary to be a "man of commanding stature and though endowed with the faculty of being all things to all men, was a staunch and sincere friend whom to know was to trust and to honor".

Curling was described as not being brilliant as an operator or as a teacher, but always painstaking and accurate. He was a very strict disciplinarian and a 'terror' to the slovenly and slipshod dresser.

He was one of the first batch of 300 fellows elected under the altered Constitution of the College of Surgeons in 1843 and was made a full surgeon at London Hospital in 1849. In 1850 he was elected as a Fellow to the Royal Society. Prior to this time he had contributed frequently to the surgical literature, winning the Jacksonian Prize in 1834 for a monograph on "tetanus" and in 1842 he published his papers concerning duodenal ulcers and their association with burns, "Curling ulcers". He wrote books on diseases of the testes and of the rectum which were translated into many languages. Finally, no less a person than Jonathan Hutchison pointed to a paper of Curling's concerning two cases of the absence of the thyroid body connected with defective cerebral development which Hutchison considered anticipated the description of myxedema by Gull and others. Though he unquestionably gained the respect of his fellows, being elected to the Council of the College of Surgeons in 1864 and President in 1873, nonetheless there pervades a certain element of reservation about him – one comment made for example was that "during the early part of his life he resided in Broad Street City, but about 1858 he removed to Grosvenor Square, alleging to his professional friends that he knew where the best patients came from". Towards the end of his life he was said to be extremely pale and many people felt he was suffering from pernicious anemia. He retired to Brighton and whilst on holiday at Cannes in the South of France he developed pneumonia and died.

CURSCHMANN SPIRALS

Spiral threads of mucus expectorated by an asthmatic.

CURSCHMANN-BATTEN-STEINHERT SYNDROME

Rare hereditary syndrome with myotonia of lingual and thenar muscles, associated with atrophy of the sterno-mastoid muscles, frontal baldness, cataracts and testicular atrophy. Dystrophia myotonia.

Hans Curschmann (1846–1910) German physician, Professor of Medicine at Leipzig.

Frederick E. Batten (1865–1918) English neurologist born in Plymouth and went to Trinity College, Cambridge and then to St. Bartholomew's Hospital, graduating in 1891. He held an appointment at the Hospital for Sick Children and at the National Hospital, Queen Square, where he was Dean for 10 years and was affectionately called "Freddie" by the students. He wrote a classical description of sub-acute combined degeneration and its relation to pernicious anemia, with J.S.R. Russel and J.T. Collier, in 1900. He was a pioneer of pediatric neurology in England. He died following a hemorrhage which complicated an operation on his prostate.

Hans Steinhert 20th century German physician.

CUSHING SYNDROME OR DISEASE

1. Glucocorticoid excess syndrome with moon face, hirsutism, plethora, truncal obesity, abdominal striae, diabetes, osteoporosis, increased susceptibility to infection, cataracts, renal calculi, senile purpura, proximal myopathy and hypertension due to excess ACTH, or less commonly, an adrenal tumor.
2. Acoustic neuroma – hearing loss, ipsilateral paralysis of 6th and 7th cranial nerves, vertigo and nystagmus and cerebellar dysfunction ipsilaterally.

Harvey W. Cushing (1869–1939) U.S. neurosurgeon. He made important contributions to the physiology of the pituitary gland and/or tumors of the pituitary and hypothalamus, as well as neurosurgical techniques, reducing the mortality rate in brain surgery from 90% to approximately 8%. He also classified cerebral tumors, gliomas and meningiomas and described techniques for their removal.

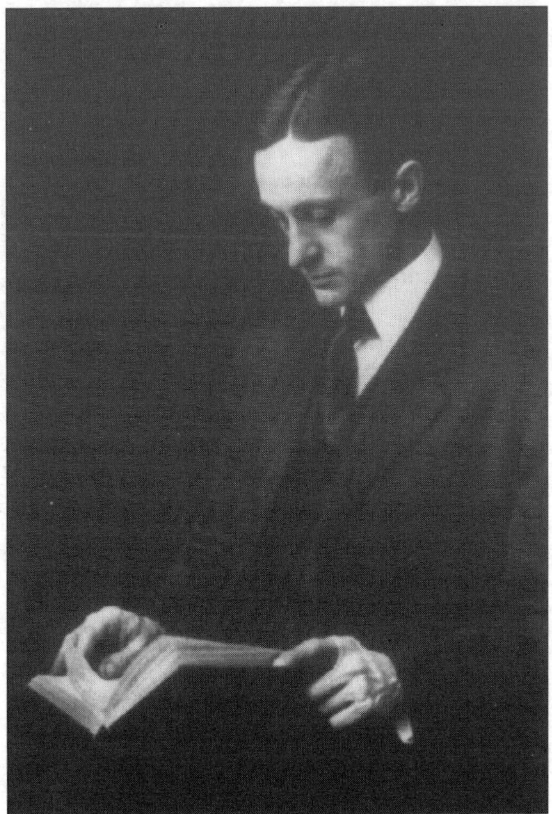

Harvey W. Cushing (Courtesy of the Royal Society of Medicine, London, UK)

He was born in Cleveland, Ohio, where his father was a stern puritanical doctor. He went to Yale College and Harvard Medical School, interned at the Massachusetts General Hopsital and then went to Johns Hopkins where for four years he worked under William Halstead. He was unimpressed both by the city of Baltimore and the hospital – "the hospital is a very sloppy place and the work of everyone most unsystematic, i.e. on the surgical side. Dr. Halstead has only operated once this month and rarely appears. Hope things clear up or I can't stand it" – an extract from an early letter he wrote home. He lived, however, next door to William Osler and a great friendship developed. After completing his time at Hopkins, he went to Europe and in Berne experimented under the direction of Theodor Kocher on the relationship between systolic blood pressure and cranial pressure. He then went to England and during a month in Liverpool took part in Sherrington's experiments on the ape motor cortex. He returned to Hopkins in 1902 and turned his attention during the next three years to patients with pituitary tumors and produced his monograph "The pituitary body and its disorders" in 1912. In 1912 he became Professor of Surgery at Harvard and Surgeon-in-Chief at the Peter Bent Brigham Hospital, where he worked for 20 years. He then moved to Yale as Sterling Professor of Neurology from 1933 to 1937 and was made Director of Studies in the History of Medicine. He died in 1939 from a myocardial infarction.

He was meticulous with his writing, it being said that every one of his publications would have been re-written 10 times. The most important contributions of his work were his development of neurosurgical skills, with particular reference to a lowering of the overall mortality rate with tumor removal such that in 1910 when he was called upon to operate on Major General Leonard Wood, Chief of Staff of the U.S. Army, to remove a large meningioma, the General returned to his official duties within a month and served throughout World War I and finally became Governor of the Philippines. He wrote a number of classics within this area including "Tumors of the Nervus Acousticus" and "Syndromes of the Cerebellar/Pontine Angle" in 1917, "Meningiomas" in 1928 and "Intracranial Tumors" in 1932, written with his assistant P. Bailey, in which he made the first serious attempt to classify gliomatous tumor based on the morphology of the central nervous system.

His investigations in endocrinological areas were not nearly as rewarding although Cushing contributed to the clinical description of the disorder to which his name is attached and believed it was a result of over-functioning adrenal cortex secondary to the basophil cells of the pituitary in every case (v. NELSON SYNDROME). Cushing could be an extremely exasperating and hard task master. His sarcasm and stormy outbursts occurred most frequently in the operating theater when he would reduce student nurses to tears (sometimes he apologized), but to his patients he was always a man with great charm, very gentle and sympathetic and never in any form of hurry. Cushing had a brush with the military hierarchy during World War I. As a Colonel with a Harvard Unit serving with the British Expeditionary Forces, he made some harsh criticism of a British surgeon (in a letter to his wife which was intercepted by French censors, who handed it on to the British government). He was even threatened with a court martial. The matter was smoothed over eventually by him being transferred to an American command. In 1936 he published "From a Surgeon's Journal, 1915–18" of his experiences in World War I which gives poignant descriptions of the wounded and a sad account of the death of Osler's only child Revere, at whose side he stayed until he died. He comments on the irony of a grandchild of the famous American patriot (Paul Revere) being buried wrapped in a Union Jack.

One frequently told story about Cushing is that during his Johns Hopkins days when exchanging stories on Paris with William McCallum, Cushing casually remarked "let us meet at the top of the Eiffel Tower 10 years from now on July 4th at 2.00 in the afternoon, and continue this conversation". The incident was not mentioned again. McCallum went to Paris and went to the top of the Eiffel Tower but could not find Cushing; he then noticed an iron staircase which went up to the very top; on clambering up, he was greeted from a small lookout with "Well, Willy, I had almost despaired of you getting here". One of Cushing's accomplishments was his two volumes "A Life of Sir William Osler" which won him the Pulitzer Prize.

CUVIER DUCTS

The two cardinal veins.

Georges L.C. Cuvier (1769–1832) French scientist, and a Baron. He was born in Montbeliard. He was one of the founders of modern morphology as well as paleontology and comparative anatomy. He was the discoverer of the pterodactyl and believed that fossil species disappeared with natural sudden catastrophes and opposed Darwinian theories. He published his magnum opus, a 20 volume study on fossils and living animals in 1817. He established the first University Professor of Pathology at Strasburg in 1819 to which J.F. Lobstein (*v. infra*) was appointed.

D

DA COSTA SYNDROME

Circulatory neurasthenia – cardiac neurasthenia – effort syndrome; cardiac neurosis.

Jacob M. Da Costa (1833–1900) Born on St. Thomas in the West Indies of Spanish and Portuguese extraction, he left with his parents when only four years old for Europe, and went to school in Dresden where he studied modern languages and became multilingual. He entered Jefferson Medical College (Philadelphia) in 1845 and graduated 3 years later. He spent one and a half years in Paris where he was a favorite pupil of Trousseau and then went to Vienna where he worked with Hyrtl. He returned to Philadelphia in 1853 where he practiced and taught students and postgraduates as lecturer in medicine at Jefferson Medical College, and wrote a very popular textbook "Medical Diagnosis". He became Professor of the Theory and Practice of Medicine in 1872 and resigned in 1891. During the Civil War he served at the Military Hospital in Philadelphia and gathered much of the evidence for his syndrome which he described in an article in the American Journal of Medical Science in 1871.

DAGNINI REFLEX

Percussion of the radial aspect of the back of the hand causes adduction and extension where there is hyper-reflexia or pyramidal tract lesion.

Guido Dagnini (1905–) Italian physician, born in Bologna, and graduated from the University of Bologna in 1931, becoming assistant in the Department of Pathology and Professor of Medical Pathology in 1938. He became Head of the Ospedale Maggiore (Major Hospital) of Bologna in 1953, retiring in 1975. Initially his major research interests were neurology but later he turned to cardiology.

DAKIN SOLUTION

Antiseptic solution containing sodium hypochlorite, used in cleansing wounds.

v. CARREL-DAKIN TREATMENT

Henry D. Dakin (1880–1952) Born in London, England, son of a Leeds iron and steel merchant, he worked in the U.S.A. at the Rockefeller Centre where he contributed to studies of carbohydrate metabolism, oxidation and the reduction reaction, and introduced dichloramine T (now used commonly in isotopic labelling techniques) as a substrate for sodium hydrochlorite to release chlorine locally at wound sites.

He was brought up in Leeds where he studied organic chemistry and after graduating he went to London in 1901 and worked at the Lister Institute of Preventive Medicine (then the Jenner Institute). It was here that he first became interested in enzymes and studied the mode of action of lipase. At this time he collaborated with A. Kossel in Heidelberg where they discovered arginase and Dakin proposed the concept that the primary action of an enzyme consists in its labile attachment to the substrate.

In 1905 he was invited by Christian A. Herter, the founder of the Journal of Biological Chemistry, to work in his private laboratory in New York. When Herter died in 1910, Mrs. Herter requested that he continue to direct the laboratory in New York and they later married. Dakin examined beta (β) oxidation of fatty acids and extended the previous observations reported by Knoop. He investigated the aromatic amino acids and examined alcaptonuria. He studied the metabolic fate of amino acids and in particular examined their glucogenic and ketogenic functions. He examined the structure of certain proteins and showed that crystalline albumins of eggs from hens and ducks differed greatly in their immunological specificities although their overall amino acid composition was very similar, and from his studies suggested a different distribution of the constituent amino acids in different proteins. In this he worked in collaboration with Sir Henry Dale and used to comment that "Dale and he proved that a hen was not a duck".

In 1914 he went to Europe after the outbreak of World War I and there collaborated with Alexis Carrel at a French military hospital and developed his solution for treating wounds. One of these involved the use of chloramine-T, and he went on to employ this substance for sterilization of drinking water and organized and directed its use in the hospital ship Aquatania during the Gallipoli campaign. Following the war, he continued his work on the amino acid content of proteins and also the oxidative metabolism of fatty acids. Around this time he expended much energy and effort, together with a young clinician, attempting to isolate the antianemic factor in liver which had been demonstrated by Minot and Murphy.

Dakin was elected Fellow of the Royal Society when he was aged 37, and was awarded the Davy Medal by that Society. Although he collaborated with a number of people, he preferred to work on his own and had his own private laboratory in a house with beautiful grounds overlooking the Hudson River. There he would take a daily constitutional walk with his Alsatian dogs, whom he adored, and there despite Prohibition he made wines! He was an extremely honest and modest man who refused to speak in public, and in 1926, after he had submitted a paper about thyroxine to the Journal of Biological Chemistry, discovered that a former associate had independently reached similar conclusions, and so withdrew the paper! His nickname was "Zyme".

DALLDORF TEST

Capillary fragility test employing a suction cup.

Gilbert J. Dalldorf (1900–) U.S. pathologist who first isolated the Coxsackie virus from feces of children. Born in Davenport, lowa, he graduated M.D. from New York University in 1924 and studied pathology at the Pathologisches Institut, Freiburg 1925–6 and became Professor of Pathology, Sloan Kettering Division, Cornell University in 1960.

DALRYMPLE DISEASE

Inflammation of the cornea and ciliary body.

DALRYMPLE SIGN

Widened palpebral fissure or lid spasm seen in thyrotoxicosis.

John Dalrymple (1804–1852) English ophthalmologist. He was the son of a surgeon, William, who had trained with Astley Cooper. John was initially apprenticed to his father at the Norfolk and Norwich Hospital and later studied at Edinburgh University. He then went to London, gained his M.R.C.S. in 1827 and worked at Moorfields Eye Hospital as a demonstrator. He was appointed assistant surgeon in 1832 and published his book "Anatomy of the Human Eye" in 1834. He retired due to ill health in 1849 and became F.R.S. in 1850. His magnum opus was an atlas "Pathology of the Eye" which was published in 1852 and he died shortly thereafter, bequeathing the paintings in the atlas to the library of the Royal London Ophthalmic Hospital. He was widely regarded for his skill as a surgeon and attached little importance to his sign. He was a member of the Microscopical Society and undertook the histological examination of the bone tumors found in the first patient described with multiple myeloma and who was reported on by Bence Jones (*v. supra*). He also took part in the autopsy of the celebrated surgeon Robert Liston.

DANA SYNDROME

v. PUTNAM-DANA SYNDROME

DANBOLT SYNDROME *or*

DANBOLDT-CLOSS SYNDROME

v. BRANDT SYNDROME

DANCE – SIGNE DE DANCE

Empty right iliac fossa found in children with intussusception.

Jean B.H. Dance (1797–1832) Born in St. Pol he obtained his M.D. in Paris in 1818 and became Head of the Cochin Clinic in 1830. He wrote a book "Guide pour l'Étude de Clinique Médicale', described tetany and worked on uterine phlebitis and cholera. He died of cholera.

DANDY-WALKER SYNDROME

Failure of development or obstruction of the foramen of Luschka and Magendie giving internal hydrocephalus.

Walter E. Dandy (1886–1946) U.S. neurosurgeon. He was born in Sedalia, Missouri, two years after his parents had migrated to the U.S.A. from Barrow-in-Furness, Lancashire, England. His father was a train driver, a socialist and a Plymouth Brethren. Dandy went to the University of Missouri where he became interested in science through the Professor of Zoology, W.C. Curtis. He was an outstanding student and a fine athlete, and was offered a Rhodes scholarship, but since at the time he could not continue medicine at Oxford, he declined and entered Johns Hopkins Medical School, where he graduated M.D. in 1910. Whilst a student he had impressed Halstead, who suggested to him that he spend his first year in the surgical Hunterian laboratory. Here he came in contact with Harvey Cushing and undertook his first laboratory work which was a study of the blood supply to the pituitary. In 1911 to 1912 he was Cushing's clinical assistant, but both men possessed somewhat similar temperaments and they had numerous clashes during the year. Although all the other positions on the staff had been filled, the Director of the hospital decided Dandy should stay, with K.D. Blackfan, a resident in pediatrics, and they studied the pathogenesis of hydrocephalus and the physiology of the cerebrospinal fluid. This original work impressed Halstead so that he had no hesitation in finding Dandy a place on his staff and in 1916 he was appointed Chief Resident.

In 1917 he commenced a search for a method of localizing brain tumors. Initially he studied the X-ray changes in 100 patients with intracranial symptoms suggestive of a new growth and showed this technique on its own to be of limited value, destruction of the sella turcica due to increased pressure being a late phenomenon. He then investigated the possibility of using radio-opaque dyes in animals and found that this gave excellent delineation, but the substances were too irritating for the nervous tissue. It is said his idea of air encephalography originated when he was operating on a patient with an X-ray showing gas under the diaphragm following a perforated typhoid ulcer. Another anecdote is that of his attending a boy who had fractured his skull and X-ray showed air in the ventricles and this gave him the idea. In 1918 he introduced the technique of pneumoencephalography and ventriculography in patients with hydrocephalus. In 1934 he drew attention to the compression of the trigeminal nerve in the cerebellopontine angle by vessels or tumor as a cause of trigeminal neuralgia.

Dandy was an extremely skilful surgeon who introduced many techniques to deal with cerebral aneurysm and acoustic neuromas. He organized the first postoperative recovery room which was the forerunner of intensive care areas.

Arthur E. Walker (1907–) U.S. neurosurgeon, Johns Hopkins, who wrote a monograph "The Primate Thalamus" in 1938 and also edited "A History of Neurological Surgery" (1951).

DANE PARTICLES

40–45 nm particles found in Australia antigen +ve sera and thought to be hepatitis B virus.

David S. Dane English pathologist, Bland Sutton Institute, Middlesex Hospital.

DANLOS SYNDROME

v. EHLERS-DANLOS SYNDROME

DANYSZ PHENOMENON

A decrease in antitoxin neutralizing capacity when toxin is added incrementally rather than all at once.

Jean Danysz (1860–1928) Polish pathologist who lived in Paris, studied rat plague and applied radium to malignant tumors (1903).

He was born in Chylin, Poland, and came to France at the age of 19 years. He was always very conscious of his Polish origin and associated with many of the Polish expatriots in France. Graduating in natural science, he worked first in the anatomy laboratory of the Museum of Natural Science on the worm *Taenia fenestrata* and he became interested in parasitic infestations in agriculture. He joined the Pasteur Institute in 1893 and worked on diseases which might control animal pests such as mice and rats and this enabled him to study and make contributions to the understanding of epidemics of disease.

Later he devoted his attention to control of insect agricultural pests, particularly in relation to the sugar beet, and silk worm disease. He gave advice to a number of governments concerning similar problems – in Portugal, oak tree parasites – in Transvaal, South Africa, a cattle disorder, and in Australia, destruction of rabbits. In 1902 he published his observations on neutralization of toxins by antitoxins. He was always original and inquisitive in his endeavours, never fearing to follow his own inner feelings and intuitions as evidenced by a book he wrote on the origin of 'psychic energy'.

DARIER DISEASE

1. Pseudoxanthoma elasticum.
2. Erythema annulare centrifugum.
3. v. HAILEY-HAILEY DISEASE.
4. Keratosis folliculosis, dominant inheritance.

DARIER SIGN

Stroking of the skin results in erythema and edema in mastocytosis (urticaria pigmentosa).

Jean F. Darier (1856–1938) French dermatologist who was born in Budapest of a French Huguenot family who had emigrated after the revocation of the Edict of Nantes. Although he commenced medical studies at the early age of 15, he decided to leave for Paris and in 1878 to 1880 he was firstly extern and then intern at Parisian hospitals. He became a naturalized Frenchman and settled in Paris. Following his graduate thesis in 1885, he Joined Ranvier's laboratory in the College de France. He was the last surviving member of the celebrated "Big Five" – Besnier, Brocq, Darier, Sabouraud, all dermatologists, and Fournier, whose prime interest was in venereal disease. This group made the Paris School of Dermatology one of the most famous of its time. Following his training in Ranvier's laboratory in histology he became Médecin des Hôpitaux and worked at La Roche Foucauld, La Pitié, Broca and finally St. Louis.

He was an extremely cultivated and charming person who collected objets d'art and had a very keen sense of humor. He was fluent in German and Italian but although he could read English well (his favourite author was Rudyard Kipling), he would rarely be persuaded to speak English. He wrote a textbook called "Practice of Dermatology" which went through many editions and was translated into German and French.

DARLING DISEASE

Histoplasmosis.

Samuel T. Darling (1872–1925) U.S. pathologist, described histoplasmosis in 1906 whilst at Ancon in the Canal Zone in Panama.

DARROW SOLUTION

Electrolyte solution containing potassium.

Daniel C. Darrow (1895–1965) U.S. pediatrician. Professor of Pediatrics, Duke University, North Carolina.

DARWIN TUBERCLE

A small prominence which occurs in some ears about ⅔ up from the bottom of the helix.

Charles R. Darwin (1809–1882) English biologist whose theory of evolution revolutionized scientific thinking. He was born in Shrewsbury, the son of a doctor and the grandson of a famous physician, Erasmus Darwin. On his mother's side his grandfather was the potter, Josiah Wedgewood. He began to study medicine in Edinburgh but, perhaps because he was so bored by the lectures of the professor of anatomy, Munro Tertius, who used to read verbatim the lectures that his father had prepared, he changed his interest to botany. Later he undertook the famous voyage on the H.M.S. Beagle as its naturalist. On his return he lived an extraordinarily reclusive life at Down House in Kent. There has been much speculation on his medical problems ranging from depression to Chagas disease with which some believe he was infected during his field trips in South America. During this time he wrote his famous book "The Origin of Species" and in it proposed his theory of natural selection as the explanation of evolution with much subsequent controversy and debate. He became an F.R.S. in 1839.

DAVSON-DANIELLI MODEL

Cell membrane model postulating bimolecular lipid layers.

H. Davson English physiologist.

J.F. Danielli (1911–) English biologist born in Wembley and gained his Ph.D. at the University of London. Fellow St. John's College, Cambridge, and appointed Professor of Zoology, King's College London (1949–61).

DEBRÉ-DE TONI-FANCONI SYNDROME

v. FANCONI SYNDROME

DEBRÉ-FIBIGER SYNDROME
(also called PIRIE SYNDROME, FIBIGER-DEBRE-VON GIERKE SYNDROME)

Variant of Wilkins Syndrome with pseudospasm of the pylorus, causing vomiting, dehydration and death.

DEBRÉ-MARIE SYNDROME

1. Infectious edematous polyneuritis – fever is followed by edema of the hands and feet with hand and foot drop and a normal cerebrospinal fluid.
2. Dwarfism and disordered water metabolism with sexual infantism.

DEBRÉ-SEMALAIGNE SYNDROME (also called KOCHER-DEBRÉ-SEMALAIGNE SYNDROME)

Muscle hypertrophy in association with weakness and slowness of movement seen mainly in cretins.

Robert Debré (1882–1978) French pediatrician who wrote on many aspects of pediatrics including an excellent book on measles in 1926. His son became Prime Minister of France.

J. Fibiger (*v. infra*).

E. von Gierke (*v. infra*).

Julien Marie (1899–) French pediatrician.

Georges Semalaigne French pediatrician.

DEGOS DISEASE

Also called fatal cutaneo-intestinal syndrome; characterized by the association of skin papules due to vasculitis, multiple infarcts of the gastrointestinal tract, sometimes with involvement of the nervous system and avascular patches in the conjunctivae.

Robert Degos (1904–) French dermatologist at the Hospital St. Louis.

DEITERS CELLS

Cells on the basilar membrane of the internal ear.

DEITERS NUCLEUS

The lateral vestibular nucleus.

Otto F.K. Deiters (1834–1863) German physician and histologist who made a number of contributions in neuro-auditory anatomy and in the structure of the internal ear. He was a pupil of Virchow in Berlin and later Professor of Anatomy and Histology at Bonn. He discovered astrocytes in 1863. He published an account of the neurone which was an important contribution to the neuronal theory, showing that each cell has an axis cylinder and from it branches a series of dendrons which form aborisations linking other nerve cells.

DEJERINE-KLUMPKE SYNDROME OR PARALYSIS

Lower brachial plexus palsy (Waiter's Tip).

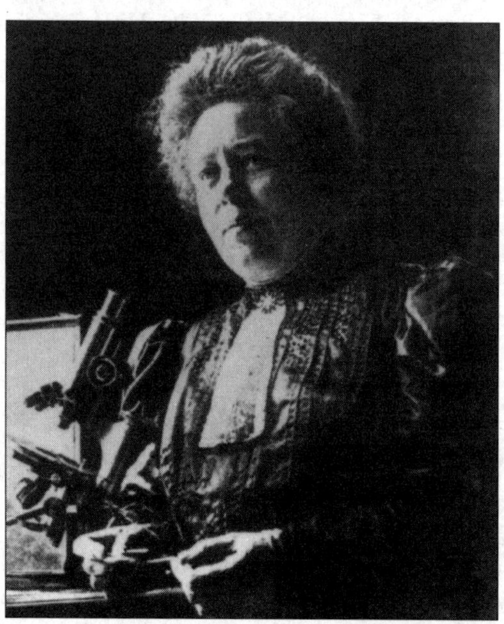

Augusta Dejerine-Klumpke (Courtesy Bibliothèque Interuniversitaire de Médecine, Service Photographique)

Augusta Dejerine-Klumpke (1859–1927) French neurologist and wife of J.J. Dejerine. She was born in San Francisco but studied medicine in Paris and in 1887 was the first woman to receive the title "interne des hôpitaux" against great opposition. She carried on her husband's research and practice when he died in 1917, and wrote an important treatise on the neurological features of lead poisoning.

DEJERINE ANTERIOR BULBAR SYNDROME

Occlusion of the anterior spinal arteries resulting in involvement of the cortical spinal tracts, medial lemnisci and hypoglossal nerves. Eye movement may be impaired and also bladder and bowel function if the medial fasciculus is also involved.

DEJERINE CORTICAL SENSORY SYNDROME

Loss of proprioception, stereognosis with retention of touch, pain, temperature and vibration seen in parietal lobe lesions.

DEJERINE-LANDOUZY DYSTROPHY OR MYOPATHY

Facioscapulohumeral muscular dystrophy.

DEJERINE-ROUSSY SYNDROME

v. LEVY-ROUSSY SYNDROME

Thalamic syndrome.

DEJERINE-SOTTAS DISEASE OR NEUROPATHY

Hypertrophic interstitial neuropathy resulting in palpable nerve trunks with weakness and muscle atrophy, motor and sensory involvement. Onset in early childhood with autosomal recessive inheritance.

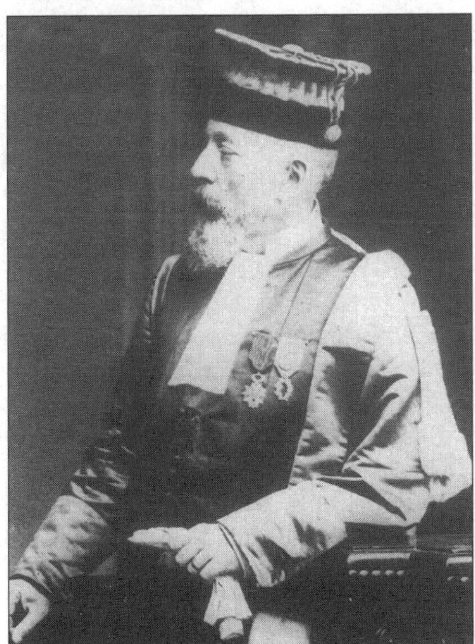

Jules J. Dejerine (Courtesy Bibliothèque Interuniversitaire de Médecine, Service Photographique)

DEJERINE-THOMAS ATROPHY

Olivopontocerebellar atrophy.

Jules J. Dejerine (1849–1917) French neurologist who was born in Geneva, Switzerland. He was an enthusiast about outdoors sports, fishing, boxing and swimming. In 1871 he went to Paris to continue clinical studies and joined Vulpian to become his most famous pupil. He held appointments at the Bicêtre and Salpêtrière.

One of the pioneers of localization of function in the brain, he ascribed word blindness to lesions of the superior marginal and angular gyri. He made contributions to functional disorders.

He was an outstanding clinician in every way and was especially sympathetic and thoughtful with his patients. His approach to psychiatric problems was basically that of reassurance, sympathy and vigorous persuasion, enthusiasm and encouragement. This was often successful. He used to say to his students, "It is rare that you will be able to use subtle logic; it is your heart that carries you along – if I may express myself thus – and much more than your reason. In man, emotion is almost everything and reason very little".

Louis T.J. Landouzy (1845–1917). French physician. He was born in Rheims, the son and grandson of doctors. He commenced his medical studies in Rheims, but moved to Paris in 1867 and became the hospital resident there in 1870. In 1890 he was appointed physician to the Hopital Laennec and three years later became Professor of Therapeutics in the Faculty of Medicine in Paris and the Dean of the Faculty.

Although he is best remembered for his description of facioscapulohumeral muscular dystrophy, his major research was in the area of tuberculosis and he showed that lesions from erythema nodosum in patients with tuberculosis would produce the disease when injected into guinea pigs. He championed the idea that laryngeal tuberculosis was due to direct surface infection in opposition to Calmette. He was one of the foremost workers in recognizing that tuberculosis was a social disease and campaigned vigorously for its eradication by education of the lay public. He had a great facility in physical examination and expressed himself clearly which made him an outstanding student teacher. He was interested in hands and disease, and made the comment concerning the little finger of a patient "tells his past, shows his temperament and foretells his future". He coined the term camptodactyly to describe flexure contracture of the finger(s) at the proximal interphalangeal joint. He was a keen supporter of spas, fond of travel, and appreciative of the visual arts as well as a keen collector of books. He died following surgery with uremia.

Gustave Roussy (1874–1948) French pathologist (*v. infra*).

Jules Sottas (1866–1943) French neurologist.

André Thomas (1867–) French neurologist.

DE LANGE SYNDROME

v. CORNELIA DE LANGE SYNDROME

DEL CASTILLO SYNDROME

Small testes and sterility in otherwise normal looking males. The germinal epithelium is absent although Sertoli and Leydig cells are normal (*v. infra*). Testicular dysgenesis syndrome.

E.B. Del Castillo Argentinian physician and endocrinologist.

DE MORGAN SPOTS

v. CAMPBELL-DE-MORGAN SPOT

DE MUSSET SIGN

The visible nodding of the head in time with arterial pulsation in patients with aortic insufficiency. It is a rare association and can be seen in other situations such as massive left pleural effusion.

Alfred De Musset (1810–1857) French poet. George Sand became his mistress but left him for Chopin. It was first described by his brother Paul in the biography he wrote of Alfred. Paul and his mother observed it whilst they were having breakfast in 1842. When told of this Alfred put his thumb and forefinger on his neck and the head stopped bobbing. He said "You see, this dreadful malady is cured by a method which is not only simple but inexpensive as well".

DE MUSSY POINT

Intersection of a line drawn along the left sternal edge and lower border of 10th rib in the epigastrium – diaphragmatic pleurisy may give referred pain and tenderness there.

N.F.O. Guineau de Mussy (1813–1885) French physician.

DENNIE-MARFAN SYNDROME

Spastic paraplegia and mental retardation in children with congenital syphilis which usually commences in early childhood.

Charles C. Dennie (1883–1971) U.S. dermatologist. He wrote a book on the history of syphilis.

Antoine B.J. Marfan (1858–1942) French pediatrician (*v. infra*).

DENNY-BROWN SYNDROME

Bronchogenic carcinoma associated with degeneration of the dorsal ganglion cells and myopathy.

Derek Denny-Brown (1901–1981) Boston neurologist. He was born in New Zealand and later trained as a neurologist in England at Oxford and London, before migrating to the U.S. to work at Harvard.

DENVER CLASSIFICATION

A classification of chromosomes numbering 1-22 from the largest to the smallest, including other characteristics e.g. length of arms, site of centromere. Agreed upon at a meeting in Denver, Colorado.

DE QUERVAIN DISEASE

1. Subacute thyroiditis.
2. Inflammation of the styloid process of the radius.

Fritz de Quervain (1868–1940) Swiss surgeon who came of Huguenot stock and trained with Langhan (*v. infra*) in pathology and spent three years with Kocher (*v. infra*) in Berne.

He published over 300 papers, many of which were devoted to thyroid disease, ranging from technical procedures on thyroidectomy to the epidemiology of thyroid disease. He wrote one of the leading surgical textbooks of the day "Special Surgical Diagnosis". He was a strong proponent of a general approach to the patient and teaching rather than an artificial division into specialist areas and brooked no opposition on this point. He was one of the earliest clinicians to appreciate that post operative pneumonia was often really a pulmonary infarct due to embolism. He died of acute pancreatitis.

DERCUM DISEASE

Adiposis dolorosa – symmetrically distributed tender subcutaneous lipomas, associated with peripheral neuropathy.

Francis X. Dercum (1856–1931) U.S. neurologist, born in Philadelphia and together with Osler, Pepper and others founded the Anthropological Society and agreed to leave their brains for study! He edited a textbook of neurology and investigated a number of neurological and psychological conditions. He was the first to photograph people having fits and was among the earliest to photograph and classify abnormal gaits. He was particularly interested in hysteria and its manifestations as well as the use of suggestion in its treatment.

D'ESPINE SIGN

Mediastinal lymph node enlargement may cause whispering pectoriloquy over the spinous processes of 4th, 5th and 6th thoracic spines.

Adolph d'Espine (1844–1930) D'Espine was a Swiss pediatrician who studied medicine in Paris, becoming an intern des hôpitaux de Paris in 1867.

He returned to his native Geneva and soon became interested in pediatrics, and by 1877 published with his classmate C. Picot a book entitled "The Manual of Diseases in Childhood". This was an immediate success and D'Espine became Professor of Paediatrics at the University of Geneva and held this position for some 40 years, training innumerable students. One of these, P. Gautier, succeeded him to his position when he retired in 1921.

During the Ist World War, D'Espine played a leading role in the operations of the Red Cross and in particular he helped in campaigns to care for children of refugees and those who had been abandoned, or injured, during the Ist World War. He wrote numerous articles in the French, German and Swiss literature.

DE TONI-FANCONI SYNDROME

v. FANCONI SYNDROME

DEVIC DISEASE

Optic neuritis.

Eugene Devic (1858–1930) French physician who practised in Lyons.

DEVIL GRIP

Epidemic pleurodynia.

v. BORNHOLM DISEASE

DIAMOND-BLACKFAN SYNDROME

Congenital hypoplastic anemia characterized by progressive anemia with sparing of white cells and platelets.

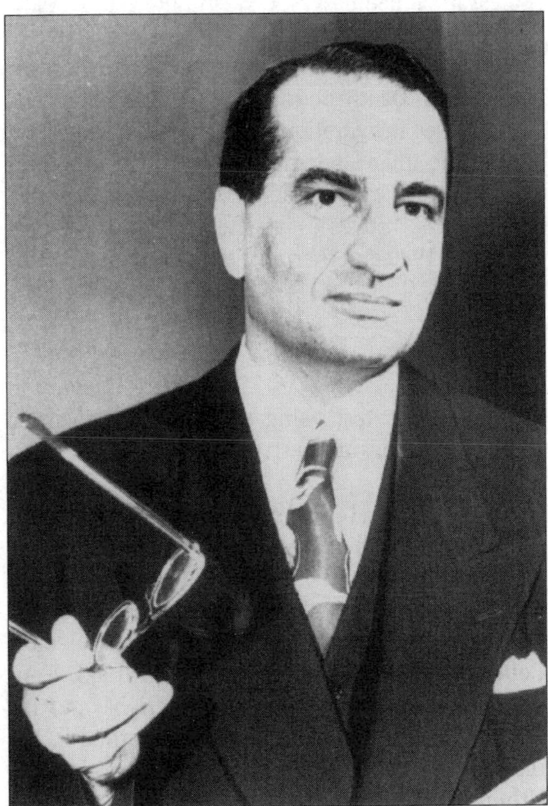

Louis K. Diamond (Courtesy of the Royal Society of Medicine, London, UK)

Louis K. Diamond (1902–) Born in New York City, he graduated M.D. Harvard in 1927, then interned and was chief resident at the Children's Hospital, Boston. He became Chief of Hematology there from 1951–1968 and Professor of Pediatrics 1963–68. With Sidney Farber (*v. infra*) he instigated modern chemotherapeutic techniques in the treatment of childhood leukemia and made a number of studies on rhesus disorders. His department became a focal point for hematological pediatric training in the U.S.

Kenneth D. Blackfan (1883–1941) Went to the Albany Medical School of Union University, New York. He was influenced by working with Richard Pearce, Professor of Pathology, during the summer vacation. He graduated aged 22, and went back to his home town to be a general practitioner. Encouraged by Pearce in 1909, he went to the Foundling Hospital in Philadelphia to commence his career as a pediatrician. In 1911 John Howland, Professor of Pediatrics at Washington University, St. Louis, offered him a residency and in 1913 he followed Howland to Johns Hopkins where he worked with Dandy on internal hydrocephalus, and later showed dehydration to be the most important problem in infant diarrhea. He was a superb clinician and dedicated teacher. He was appointed Professor of Pediatrics at the University of Cincinnati in 1920 and then in 1923 at Harvard.

DICK TEST

Intracutaneous test using streptococcus toxin to detect prior exposure to streptococcus.

George F. Dick (1881–1957) U.S. physician, born Fort Wayne, Indiana, and graduated M.D. Rush Medical College in 1905, held a number of pathology appointments in Chicago and was appointed Professor of Clinical Medicine, Rush Medical College in 1918 and Chairman 1933–1945. Considerable controversy occurred when he and his wife Dr. Gladys Dick patented their method in the U.S.A. and applied for a patent in England in 1927 although they derived no personal remuneration since an independent charitable body had been established.

DIEGO ANTIGEN

A blood group antigen which is extremely rare in European and West Africans, found in Chinese, Japanese and South American Indians and presumed to be of Mongolian origin and inherited as a dominant. It was initially found in a Venezuelan patient of that name with erythroblastosis fetalis.

DIETL CRISIS

Recurrent pain in the costovertebral angle with vomiting, nausea, tachycardia and hypotension due to ureteral obstruction.

Joseph Dietl (1804–1878) A Polish physician born in Cracow, he was one of the members of the New Vienna School (which included Skoda), which endorsed views of therapeutic nihilism. In 1851 he said that a physician should not be judged by the success of his treatment but by the extent of his knowledge. "As long as medicine is an art, it will not become a science. As long as there are successful physicians there will be no scientific physicians". This type of attitude died hard but the arrival of Virchow and his demolition of Rokitansky's first book and philosophies like those espoused by Dietl brought a new era.

DIEULAFOY DISEASE

Gastric erosion or ulcer complicating pneumonia.

Georges Dieulafoy (1839–1911) French physician who influenced many graduates. Born in Toulouse he graduated in Paris in 1869 – he became Professor of Medicine and Chief of the medical service at the Hôtel Dieu in 1869. He invented a suction pump to evacuate body fluids and worked on numerous topics including typhoid, Bright disease and appendicitis. He wrote a manual on pathology and was elected President of the French Academy of Medicine in 1910. He died in Paris.

DIGEORGE SYNDROME

Thymic aplasia, associated with absence of the parathyroid glands and frequent infections due to lack of T cell lymphocytes. B cell lymphocytes are present in normal numbers and immunoglobulin levels may be normal.

Angelo M. DiGeorge (1921–) U.S. pediatrician. He was born in Philadelphia and went to Temple University School of Medicine graduating in 1946. From 1947–49 he was stationed at Linz, Austria with the U.S. Army Medical Corps. He returned to train in pediatrics at St. Christopher's Hospital for Children and is currently Professor of Pediatrics, and Chief of the Endocrine and Metabolic Service there.

DIGHTON SYNDROME

Osteogenesis imperfecta with deafness.

C.A.C. Dighton (1885–) English otolaryngologist.

DI GUGLIELMO ANEMIA OR DISEASE

Acute or chronic erythroleukemia. A variant of acute leukemia, it is a term used to encompass a number of entities whose relationship is still uncertain, including refractory sideroblastic anemia, refractory anemia with excess blast cells and preleukemia. Some authorities demand the presence of PAS-positive erythroblasts and/or morphological abnormalities in red cell proliferation to make the diagnosis.

Giovanni Di Guglielmo (1886–1962) Italian hematologist and physician, born in Sao Paolo, Brazil, of Italian parents. At the age of 6 he went to Italy to complete his education and after graduating in medicine returned to Sao Paolo to practice. However, he yearned to return to Italy and six months later was back in Naples where he worked with A. Ferrata who interested him in research and hematology. In 1929 he was appointed Professor of Medical Pathology at Pavia and later Professor of Medicine at Catania. He held similar posts at Naples and finally in Rome.

DIOGENES SYNDROME

Gross neglect in old age

Diogenes (412–323B.C.) Greek philosopher who abandoned all his creature comforts and worldly goods.

DISSE SPACE

Peri-sinusoidal space in the liver.

J. Disse (1852–1912) German anatomist.

DIVRY-VAN BOGAERT DISEASE

Angiomatosis of skin and cerebral meninges with progressive demyelinization of white matter, clinically characterized by familial dementia, epilepsy, pyramidal and extrapyramidal disturbances, visual field defects and a progressive course.

Paul Divry (1889–) Belgian neurologist.

Ludo Van Bogaert (1897–) Belgian neuropathologist who founded a large department in Antwerp during the first half of this century.

DOEHLE BODIES (DÖHLE)

Light blue cytoplasmic inclusions in polymorphs up to 1–2 in diameter, seen in burns, infection and the May-Hegglin anomaly (*v. infra*).

Karl G.P. Doehle (Döhle) (1855–1928). He was born in Muhlahausen in Thuringen. He graduated in medicine in 1881 in Kiel and became an assistant at the Kiel Pathological Institute in 1883 where he remained until his retirement in 1924. For many years he was Heller's assistant and was promoted to Professor in 1896 and became Head of the Department at the Pathological Institute in 1908, and a full Professor in 1921.

Döhle was one of the first, if not the first, to differentiate syphilitic inflammation of the aorta from atherosclerosis. Looking for parasitic lesions causing disease, he noted the inclusion bodies of leukocytes in blood in patients with scarlet fever and he initially believed these to be specific, and to represent spirochetes. He found that he could differentiate inclusion bodies in the leukocytes in scarlet fever from those occurring in other illnesses. These suggestions were not confirmed. Although a very good histopathologist, he published relatively little and being somewhat of an introvert avoided medical congresses and therefore he was relatively unknown outside his Institute. It was only through the efforts of Heller that his work on syphilitic aortitis eventually achieved recognition. He was, however, a very successful teacher of students and postgraduates.

DONAHUE SYNDROME

Leprechaunism. Autosomal recessive lipodystrophy with motor and mental retardation, progeria and a grotesque facies.

William L. Donahue (1906–) Canadian pathologist.

DONATH-LANDSTEINER TEST OR PHENOMENON

Serum produces hemolysis after incubation with red cells at 4°C and subsequent re-warming to 37°C.

Julius Donath (1870–1950) German physician.

Karl Landsteiner (1868–1943) (*v. infra*).

DONNAN EQUILIBRIUM

(Also called GIBBS-DONNAN EQUILIBRIUM)

If a solution of permeable electrolytes, e.g. NaCl, is separated by a semi-permeable membrane and on one side a non-permeable substance, e.g. a protein, is introduced, there will be a re-distribution of permeable electrolytes so that overall electrolyte concentrations will be equal on both sides of the membrane.

Frederick G. Donnan (1870–1956) English physical chemist. He studied at Queen's University, Belfast and then at Leipzig, Berlin and London. He was appointed Professor of Chemistry at University College, London, in 1913 and retired from there in 1937. Invented a drop pipette to study oil dispersion and studied detergent action of soap.

J.W. Gibbs (*v. infra*).

DONNÉ CORPUSCLES

Fat cells in colostrum.

Alfred Donné (1801–1878) French physician, born in Noyon, he studied in Paris and became Chef de Clinique at the Charité Hospital where he gave courses in microscopy. He became Inspector General of the University of Paris. He noted the third cellular element in blood viz. the platelet, in 1842, but mistook them for fat globules of chyle. He published an atlas with the first engraving from a photomicrograph and first described *Trichomonas vaginalis*, initially believing that it caused gonorrhea but later established that it was often found in the female genital tract. He died in Paris.

DONOVAN BODIES

Chromatin masses which look like a closed safety pin in bacteria called *Calymmatobacterium granulomatis*. This bacterium is responsible for granuloma inguinale characterized by cutaneous and mucocutaneous ulceration in the inguinal region.

Charles Donovan

(*v. infra*) LEISHMAN-DONOVAN BODIES.

DOPPLER EFFECT, PHENOMENON, PRINCIPLE

When a source of light or sound is moving rapidly the wave-lengths appear to decrease or the pitch of the sound increases as the object gets closer, e.g. an approaching train and vice versa.

Christian J. Doppler (1803–1853) Austrian physicist and mathematician. This effect is used in the ultrasound diagnostic techniques to delineate body organs.

He was born in Salzburg. Initially taught mathematics at a high school in Prague and then joined the Technical Institute in Prague becoming a Professor of Mathematics and Geometry there from 1841–7. He held other appointments in Germany, but finally was appointed Professor of Experimental Physics at the University of Vienna and the Director of the Physics Institute. He investigated the colors of double stars and suggested a technique of measuring their distance from earth and the diameters of fixed stars.

DOROTHY REED CELL

v. REED-STERNBERG CELL

DOUGLAS BAG

A bag for collecting expired air for respiratory function studies.

Claude G. Douglas (1882–1963) English physiologist who graduated in medicine from Oxford and Guy's Hospital in 1908. He was appointed as Fellow at St. John's College and worked with and was greatly influenced by J.B.S. Haldane, with whom he investigated the effects of altitude on respiration and the blood gases in expeditions to the Peak of Teneriffe in 1910 and Pikes Peak, Colorado in 1911.

He joined the Royal Army Medical Corps (RAMC) in 1914 and in 1915 when the Germans used gas, he played an important role in developing gas masks and was mentioned in despatches four times and awarded the Military Cross. In 1918 he returned to Oxford and became renowned as an investigator with a flair for developing instruments and as a kindly and enthusiastic teacher with a keen sense of humor.

Apart from the bag (1911), he developed with F.H. Courtice, gas analysis and blood gas analysis apparatuses and with these techniques studied many aspects of respiratory physiology, and fat and carbohydrate metabolism. He and Haldane discovered the reverse Bohr effect (raising O_2 pressure in the blood increases CO_2 dissociation). He first reported ketones in the urine after prolonged exercise (sometimes called Courtice-Douglas effect).

In the 2nd World War he again worked on defence against gas attack and chemical warfare, and after the war returned to his teaching in physiology at Oxford, collaborating with R.G. Bannister (the first man to run a mile under four minutes) on the effects of exercise on respiratory control.

DOUGLAS POUCH

Anatomical space between uterus and rectum.

James Douglas (1675–1742) Scottish physician and anatomist. He obtained his M.D. at Rheims and returned to London and practiced midwifery and became physician to Queen Caroline. Became F.R.S. in 1706. He described the Guernsey Lily and was the first to compile a comprehensive bibliography of medical literature. He encouraged William and John Hunter in their anatomical school. He did public dissections at his home and died in London.

DOVER POWDER

Analgesic mixture of 10% opium, 10% ipecacuanha and 80% lactose.

Thomas Dover (1660–1742) Born in Warwickshire, he studied medicine at Oxford and Cambridge, graduating in 1687 and then worked with Thomas Sydenham in London who treated him for smallpox and later he advocated inoculation of smallpox as a method of controlling and preventing the disease. He practiced in Bristol and later, perhaps influenced by his rich adventurer and slave-trading patients, abandoned medicine. He led a successful buccaneer expedition against Spain in South America. In 1709 he rescued the ship-wrecked Scottish sailor, Alexander Selkirk, upon whom Defoe based his novel Robinson Crusoe. Dover returned to England in 1711 extremely rich and practiced medicine again in London.

DOWN SYNDROME

Mongolism. Sometimes called LANGDON-DOWN SYNDROME.

John L.H. Langdon-Down (1828–1896) English

physician. Down was his father's Irish family name, where his great-grandfather was the Protestant Bishop of Derry, whilst his mother's family (Langdon) migrated from Cornwall to Devon 200 years earlier. He was born at Tor Point, Cornwall, and left school at the age of 13½ to assist his father who was a pharmacist. In 1847 he enrolled as a student at the pharmaceutical society of London and in 1849 became assistant to Professor Redwood and subsequently assisted Faraday in some of his experiments on gases. He became ill and spent the next three years recuperating in Dartmoor, walking and riding. He lectured at Tor Point in chemistry and wanted to continue in science, but when his father died in 1853 he entered medical school at the age of 25 at the London Hospital, largely for financial reasons. He graduated M.B. University of London in 1858, coming second to Sir William Broadbent (*v. supra*). He then became resident physician and superintendent of the Earlswood Asylum and was elected assistant physician to the London Hospital in 1859 shortly after Mr. Jonathan Hutchison (*v. infra*) had been elected assistant surgeon. He became lecturer on materia medica and therapeutics at the London Hospital Medical College and afterwards lecturer in the principles and practice of medicine. For the first 9 years following this appointment he continued to live at the Earlswood Asylum and to work there and superintend the asylum's organization and development. This resulted in a model for the care of the mentally ill in the United Kingdom. Many of Down's publications related to mental ill health. He published on edema and its management and on the classification of mental disease. He was an early protagonist for training the mentally retarded and when he moved to set up consultant practice in London in 1868 he established a home for training feeble-minded children of the well-to-do, this being the first of its kind. He described mongolism in his Letsom lectures entitled "On some of the mental afflictions of childhood and youth" delivered in 1887. He passed on to medical students a piece of advice given to him by an old man when he left his village, "My lad, you take your aim; be sure you aim high enough. That's the thing – aim high enough" and he added some advice of his own. "The formula to solve problems, the secret that will command success, the talismanic charm which turns everything to gold, the potent spell at which all difficulties vanish. It is earnest and persistent work. Let it be supplemented by a gentle Christian life, terminated by a peaceful, hopeful death". He had what was called a severe bout of influenza in 1890 and never recovered completely. One morning he collapsed at his breakfast and was dead 10 minutes later at his home in Hampton Wick.

DOWNEY CELLS

Atypical lymphocytes seen in infectious mononucleosis.

Hal Downey (1877–1959) U.S. hematologist. He was born in State College, Pennsylvania, where his father was a mathematician. As a child he spent 6 years in Hannover, Germany, where he went to school, and completed his schooling in Minneapolis. He enlisted for the Spanish-American War and served in the Philippines from 1898–1899. He returned to the University of Minnesota where he gained his Masters Degree in Zoology in 1904. He was a keen cyclist and was once arrested by a Minneapolis policeman for "having pedalled his racing bike too fast in town, with head down"!

His first research concerned the urogenital organs of a Mississippi river fish. His interest in hematology was aroused when he found that the kidney was the chief hemopoietic organ in the species he was studying. He lived in Germany for two years when he worked in Pappenheim's laboratory at the University of Berlin and with Weidenreich at the Anatomical Institute in Strasbourg in 1911. Apart from this time, he was a member of the University of Minnesota from 1903–1946. He was Professor of Zoology until 1929 when he became Professor of Anatomy. Following his early work on comparative hematology, he turned increasingly to studies of mammalian species and man, studying the origin of the blood platelet and the use of supravital stains in examining hemopoietic tissue and its origin and function.

By 1923 he was beginning to examine the pathological disorders of man and made a number of important morphological contributions to such disorders as leukemia, Gaucher disease and the lymphomas. In 1936 he published the first of his articles on infectious mononucleosis which were to prove classics of morphological description and illustration which distinguished this benign disorder from the leukemias. He was described as an inspiring teacher – his lectures were always philosophical and enquiring. A story he would tell all his doctoral students on the eve of their exams was about his own examination when he was asked to name the cells of the blood. He had to be asked to name them several times before he "got around to remembering the red cells". From 1913–1959, except for the World Wars, he was the American editor of Folia Haematologica and was the first English-speaking investigator to have this honor.

DOYNE CHOROIDITIS

Familial involvement of macula with retinal degeneration and yellow white drusen (*v. infra*) deposits in a mosaic pattern giving a honeycomb appearance.

DOYNE IRITIS

Small gray precipitate on the anterior surface of the iris.

Robert W. Doyne (1857–1916) British ophthalmologist. He was born in Wexford, the son of the Reverend P.W. Doyne, and educated at Marlborough and Keble College, Oxford. He entered the Bristol Medical School and then St. George's Hospital, London, gained his M.R.C.S. and practiced briefly in Bristol. He joined the Navy in 1883 and left the service in 1885 when he married and settled in Oxford. He gained his F.R.C.S. in 1892, became interested in ophthalmology and commenced an eye dispensary in a builder's yard at Oxford. From this meagre beginning, through his energy and the help of a number of friends, the Oxford Eye Hospital developed. Doyne gave his services tirelessly to this institution until he retired after 25 years of continuous service in 1912. He was consulting ophthalmic surgeon at the Radcliffe Infirmary and the first reader in ophthalmology at the University of Oxford, a post which he held for 11 years. He was a skilful ophthalmological surgeon and became well known in England and internationally through his writings on a number of subjects including a book on "The More Common Diseases of the Eye". He wrote on retinitis pigmentosa, visual sensation, perception, appreciation and judgement, and conjunctivitis. He instituted regular ophthalmological congresses in Oxford. He was a kindly and generous host and was a very keen fencer, who founded the Oxford Fencing Club.

DRAGSTEDT OPERATION

Complete vagotomy and gastrojejunostomy for duodenal ulcer.

Lester R. Dragstedt (1893–1975) U.S. surgeon born in Anaconda, Montana. He gained his M.D. from Rush Medical College in 1921 and studied at the University of Vienna 1925–26 and became Professor and Chairman of the Department of Surgery, University of Chicago from 1925–1959.

DRESSLER BEAT

Fusion beat. This is usually ventricular in origin and results from impulses occurring from two different sites with resultant changes in the QRS in the electrocardiogram.

DRESSLER SYNDROME

v. HARLEY DISEASE

Chest pain, pericardial in nature, occurring 2–3 weeks post myocardial infarction. It tends to recur, often associated with fever and pleural effusion, and occasionally arthralgia.

William Dressler (1890–1969) U.S. physician, educated in Vienna and practiced there until 1938 but left Europe for the United States with the Nazi takeover of Austria. He was born in Budzanow, Poland, graduated M.D. Vienna in 1915 and was associate chief of the heart hospital in Vienna from 1924–1938. He became chief of the cardiac clinic at

Maimonides Hospital, Brooklyn, N.Y. and was co-author of a book on cardiology.

DRIESCH LAW OF CONSTANT VOLUME

The differences in total mass of an organ are due to the number and not the volume of cells, e.g. the nerve cells of man or woman are approximately equal in size; the renal cells of a man or mouse are also similar in size.

H.A.E. Driesch (1867–1941) German biologist, studied zoology at Freiburg, Jura and Munich and became Professor at Heidelberg University. An experimental embryologist, he championed the importance of protoplasm in the control and development of tissue vis à vis the nucleus.

DRINKER RESPIRATOR

"Iron lung". A machine to maintain respiration in patients who have muscular paralysis.

Philip Drinker (1894–) U.S. public health engineer.

DRUSEN BODIES

Glial tissue in the retina which may resemble papilledema when it is close to the optic disc – hereditary, often bilateral and symmetrical. Sometimes associated with hereditary forms of choroiditis

v. DOYNE CHOROIDITIS.

DRUZA

Bohemian word for crystals embedded in a rock.

DUANE SYNDROME

Congenital fibrosis of the external rectus. On attempted adduction of the affected eye, there is contraction of the globe and narrowing of the palpebral fissure. It is more common in females than males, and often familial, resembling 6th nerve palsy.

Alexander Duane (1858–1926) U.S. ophthalmologist, one of the early American investigators in ophthalmology who was especially interested in accommodation and strabismus.

He was born in Malone, New York, the son of General James Duane, and entered the Union College where he graduated M.D. in 1881. He interned at New York Hospital and began practice in New York City in 1884. He became an authority on the physiology of optics and also movements of the eyes and their motor anomalies. He contributed numerous papers as well as devising a successful student's medical dictionary and making contributions to various American ophthalmological textbooks, but perhaps he was most noted for his translation of the textbook by the Viennese authority Fuchs (*v. infra*).

He served in the Spanish-American War as a lieutenant in the American Navy and in the Great War as a signal officer on the American ship "Granite State". He was also the author of a monograph entitled "Rules for signalling on land and sea" which was first published in 1899.

DUBIN-JOHNSON SYNDROME

Liver anomaly with jaundice and hepatic pigmentation due to retention of conjugated bilirubin. (cf. ROTOR SYNDROME.) The liver shows melanin deposition in the centrilobular zone. The bromosulphthalein excretion test shows a secondary rise and the gallbladder is not visualized with oral cholecystogram. Estrogen and the oral contraceptive pill may increase bilirubin levels and precipitate jaundice. Thought to be autosomal recessive form of inheritance.

Isadore N. Dubin (1913–1980) U.S. pathologist. Professor of Pathology, Medical College of Pennsylvania, Philadelphia.

Frank B. Johnson (1919–) He was born in Washington D.C. and graduated from Howard University, Washington D.C. in 1944. Initially interned at the Medical Center, Jersey City, and became a resident in pathology there in 1945 and stayed on as a resident in pathology for one year. He then spent two years as Acting Pathologist and Director of Clinical Laboratories at the Howard University College of Medicine, becoming a Certified Pathologist in 1949. He trained in histochemistry with Dr. Isidore Gersh at the Anatomy Department in the University of Chicago and returned to become Chief of Laboratories Methods Section at the Armed Forces Institute of Pathology in Washington D.C. in 1952. He has remained there in various positions, being appointed in 1990 as Chief, Division of Chemical Pathology, Department of Environment and Toxicology.

DUBOWITZ SYNDROME

Congenital dwarfism with hypoplasia of the mandible, zygoma and malar bones, hypoplasia of the supraorbital ridges and large ears, giving a characteristic facies. The skin is thickened and eczematous and the patient is sometimes mentally retarded.

Victor Dubowitz (1931–) English pediatrician born in Beaufort West, South Africa and graduated M.B., Ch.B. University of Capetown in 1954 gaining his M.D. in 1960 and migrating to England to the University of Sheffield where he gained his Ph.D. in 1964 and became consultant pediatrician at the United Sheffield Hospitals. His research interests are largely in the diseases of muscles.

DUCHENNE ATTITUDE

Lowering of the shoulder with external rotation due to paralysis of the trapezius.

DUCHENNE DISEASE

1. Tabes dorsalis.
2. Progressive bulbar palsy.

DUCHENNE PARALYSIS

Progressive bulbar palsy.

DUCHENNE-ARAN DISEASE

Progressive muscular atrophy, with symmetrical involvement of the hands, forearms and shoulder girdle muscles with muscular atrophy and fasciculation.

DUCHENNE-ERB PALSY, PARALYSIS OR SYNDROME

v. ERB-DUCHENNE PARALYSIS

DUCHENNE-GRIESINGER DISEASE

(Also called DUCHENNE MUSCULAR ATROPHY OR DYSTROPHY)

Pseudo-hypertrophic infantile muscular dystrophy, an X-linked recessive disorder which usually commences before 5 years of age and involves pelvic muscles. Muscle enzymes are very high and progression is usually rapid so that patients are incapacitated by adolescent age. Abnormalities have been noted in the red cell membrane.

Guillaume B.A. Duchenne (1807–1875) He was born in Boulogne, where he attended college at Douai and despite his father's efforts to induce him to follow the family seafaring tradition, his love of science drove him to Paris where he studied medicine in 1827 under the direction of Laennec, Dupuytren, Magendie and Cruveilhier, graduating in 1831. He practiced in Boulogne for five years, but after his wife died in childbirth, he was separated from his only son by his wife's family, and he returned penniless to Paris. There he went into private practice and pursued his clinical neurological studies in a very unorthodox but effective fashion. He has been described perhaps somewhat romantically as a strange mariner-like figure who used to haunt the major Parisian teaching hospitals, particularly in the morning, seeking out patients and studying their neurological problems.

He examined each patient very carefully and at great length and would hold informal discussions with the ward residents or physicians who initially held him somewhat in contempt and whom he called "monarchs" of the ward. He never held an appointment at a Paris teaching hospital or at the University, nor did he seek one. However, his

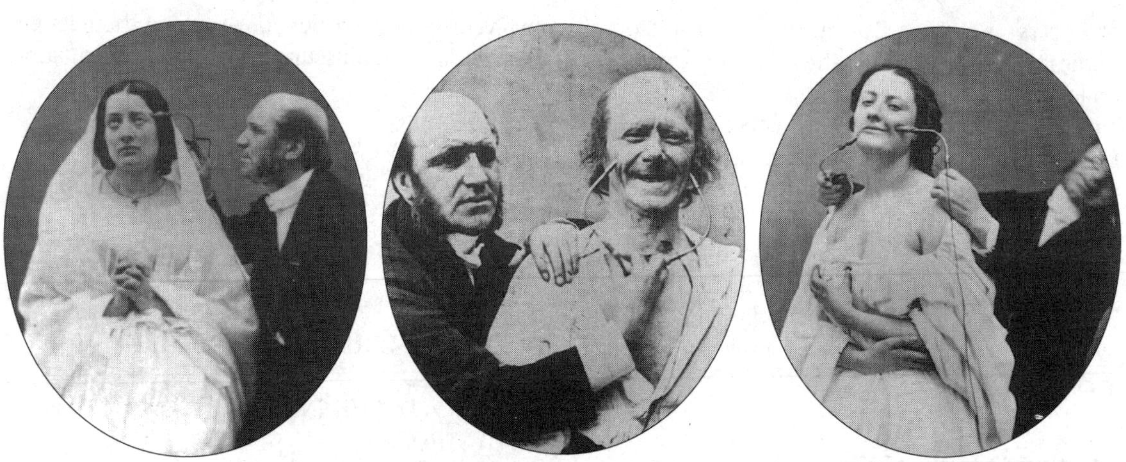

Guillaume B.A. Duchenne (From *"Mechanisme de la Physionomie Humaine, un Analyse Electro-Physiologique de L'Expression des Passions, Avec Atlas"* by G.E.A. Duchenne [Courtesy of the National Library of Medicine, Washington D.C., USA])

extraordinary abilities soon became well known around the Paris hospitals. He discovered that external electrical stimulation could cause muscle movement and initially employed this as a form of therapy, but then appreciated its possibilities as a diagnostic method. He employed this technique to analyse the mechanism of facial expression which was published and illustrated by many striking photographs. It was largely Duchenne who introduced the painstaking and at times flamboyant physical examination and interrogation which have become the stamp of all modern neurologists. He would cap a satisfactory answer to one of his queries or performance of a neurological maneuvre with an explosive "bon"! His clinical ability was such that Charcot dubbed him "The Master" and Trousseau held him in the highest esteem.

Duchenne was possibly the first person to use a biopsy procedure to obtain tissue from a living patient for microscopic examination. This aroused a deal of controversial discussion in the lay press concerning the morality of examining living tissues. Apart from Duchenne's description of the disorders to which his name is attached, he also was the first to distinguish upper and lower motor neurone causes of 7th nerve paralysis.

He made important contributions to our understanding of lead palsy and pointed out that the profound paralysis of poliomyelitis must be due to a lesion which he located in the anterior horn cells of the spinal cord. This extraordinary man had a touching reunion with his estranged son in 1862 when the latter took up neurology in Paris, but the son died in 1871 from typhoid fever. Following this, Duchenne apparently deteriorated rapidly with cerebral atherosclerosis (? depression) and he died in 1875 from a cerebral hemorrhage. He had set the stage for what was to become one of the most exciting eras of clinical neurology anywhere in the world.

François A. Aran (1817–1861) French physician at Hôpital St. Antoine who published the first account of progressive muscular atrophy, freely acknowledging Duchenne.

Wilhelm Griesinger (1817–1868) German neurologist who described splenic anemia in children in 1866. He was the first German to advocate humane treatment for insanity and in 1854 he concluded that the worm ankylostoma caused Egyptian anemia, independently of Bilharz (*v. supra*).

DUCREY BACILLUS

Hemophilus ducreyii.

Augusto Ducrey (1860–1940) Italian dermatologist who became Professor of Dermatology in Pisa and

Rome. He isolated the bacillus causing chancroid lesions or soft chancre in 1888.

DUFFY SYSTEM – BLOOD GROUP

Erythrocyte antigen found in a patient named Duffy who had received multiple transfusions. This system may be important in malarial infectivity. Duffy –ve cells are resistant to the invasion by some forms of malarial parasites.

DUGAS TEST

Test for dislocated shoulder. When the hand of the affected side is placed on the opposite shoulder the elbow cannot touch the chest.

Louis A. Dugas (1806–1884) U.S. surgeon, born in Washington, Georgia, and went to medical school in Philadelphia and Baltimore, graduating from the medical department of the University of Maryland in 1827. He spent some years training in Europe and in 1832 helped to establish the Medical College of Georgia, where he became Professor of Surgery. He became editor of the Southern Medical and Surgical Journal from 1851–1858 and during that time published a paper on "New Diagnosis in Shoulder Dislocations" in which he described his sign. He was also interested in geology and in 1834 was elected to the Geological Society of France.

DUHRING DISEASE

Dermatitis herpetiformis – an itchy eruption which occurs in attacks with symmetrically distributed vesicles, pustules or bullae, variable eosinophilia is usually present, together with fever.

Louis A. Duhring (1845–1913) Born in Philadelphia and gained M.D. in 1867 at the University of Pennsylvania. He studied dermatology in Paris, London and Vienna and returned to open a dispensary for skin diseases in Philadelphia in 1870 and became Professor of Diseases of the Skin at the University of Pennsylvania in 1876. He described the condition in 1884, and wrote the first American textbook of dermatology.

DUKE BLEEDING TIME OR TEST

A platelet function test performed by puncturing the ear lobe and determining the time taken for bleeding to cease.

William W. Duke (1883–1945) U.S. physician, born Lexington, Missouri, and graduated M.D. Johns Hopkins in 1908. He worked with W.H. Howell at Johns Hopkins and with him showed that stimulation of the vagal supply of the mammalian heart caused secretion of potassium. He worked at the Massachusetts General Hospital, the University of Virginia and the University of Berlin before commencing practice in Kansas City, Missouri. He was Professor of Experimental Medicine there from 1914–1918. He made a number of important studies of platelet physiology including their rate of regeneration and the part played by platelets in preventing hemorrhage. He was prominent in the field of allergy.

DUKES DISEASE

v. FILATOV SPOTS

Roseola infantum or exanthem subitum.

Clement Dukes (1845–1925) English physician. Born in London, the son of a clergyman, he studied medicine at St. Thomas Hospital, where he was a brilliant undergraduate. He gained his M.R.C.S. in 1867 and graduated M.B.B.S. London in 1869 with honours. He interned at St. Thomas and then at the Hospital for Sick Children, Great Ormond Street. He also worked at the City of London Hospital for Diseases of the Chest and the Royal Ophthalmic Hospital, Moorfields and in 1871 was appointed medical officer at Rugby school, a position he held until 1908. He gained his M.D. London in 1876 and later became F.R.C.P. At Rugby he gained worldwide renown for his books and articles on schoolboy health and health care.

In 1900 he published an article entitled "On the confusion of two diseases under the name of

Rubella (Rose Rash)". In this he distinguished the two disorders rubella and roseola infantum, and concluded that they were two similar, but etiologically and pathologically distinct, infections. In 1901 he reported an epidemic in school children which he differentiated from scarlet fever, common measles and rubella, and called the fourth disease. Although this "4th disease" was much debated and questioned during his day, history has vindicated his view.

DUNCAN DISEASE OR SYNDROME

X-linked recessive combined immunodeficiency disease with a propensity to malignant lymphoproliferative disease of the B cell type and fatal outcome following exposure to the Epstein-Barr virus.

Duncan was one of the early kindred described.

DUPUYS-DUTEMPS PHENOMENON

Paradoxical lid retraction present in Bell palsy.

Louis Dupuys-Dutemps (1871–) French ophthalmologist who worked with Cestan on the pupillary reflexes.

DUPUYTREN CONTRACTURE

Thickening and eventual contracture of palmar fascia resulting in flexure of 4th and 5th fingers predominantly. There is an association with alcoholic cirrhosis and manual work, but in many instances the etiology is uncertain.

Baron Guillaume Dupuytren (1777–1835) He was born in Pierre-Buffiere in 1777, the son of an impoverished advocate. He was an extremely attractive and intelligent child and was kidnapped at the age of 4 by a rich lady from Toulouse but returned to his family. He attracted the attention of an Army Officer in the town, who took him into Paris at the age of 12 where he attended school. After finishing his course there he returned home wanting to join the Army, but his father insisted that he become a surgeon. He returned to Paris and entered medical school, but went through an extremely difficult period because of his poverty. When 18 he obtained a post as prosector at the École de Santé (School of Health) where he was placed in charge of all the autopsies at the medical school, and this laid a foundation for his future interest. When he was 24 he was appointed Chef des Travaux Anatomiques and soon had written a monograph on pathological anatomy based on his autopsy findings. Here he also gave a course in pathology with Bayle and Laennec as assistants. He and Laennec parted on very bad terms since Laennec felt Dupuytren was endeavoring to gain credit for Bayle's work.

Dupuytren was first appointed to the Hôtel Dieu in 1802 and became a full staff member in 1808. In 1812 he became elected to the Chair of Operative Surgery after much opposition and in 1814 became Surgeon in Chief and in this position performed an incredible amount of work and was regarded even by those who had disliked him as one of the outstanding surgeons of his day. Percy, a lifelong friend of Larrey, said of him "first of surgeons and last of men". He was also called Le Brigand d'Hotel Dieu by Lisfranc, a surgical colleague at La Pitié, a gentleman renowned for his many asides about his colleagues.

It seems certain that Dupuytren himself pursued all of those who were against him, such as Velpau, throughout his life. He is said to have seen 10 000 patients annually outside of his hospital work, and certainly amassed a fortune and died a millionaire. His lectures were obviously first rate, since he attracted students from countries all over the world, and although he was renowned for his parsimony, he offered Charles X, after his dethronement, a million francs, or one third of his fortune, an offer which the King declined. Dupuytren had been created a Baron by Louis XVIII and was appointed first surgeon to Charles X. In 1833 he had a stroke whilst lecturing but persisted and finished the lecture, but from that time on he was an invalid and died a little more than a year later.

Dupuytren never operated if an operation could be avoided, but he was the first person to successfully remove the lower jaw. He not only described

Dupuytren contracture, but devised an operation to cure it, and also the operation for correction of wry neck by sectioning the sternomastoid muscle. He developed an enterotome and his instrument or a modification of it was used by surgeons such as Astley Cooper and Mikulicz. In fact, as is the wont of eponyms, it is often called the Mikulicz enterotome.

One of Dupuytren's sayings was "rien n'est pas tante redouter pour un homme que la mediocrité (nothing should be feared so much for a man as mediocrity"). Whilst he was nobody's friend in Paris, he certainly was well liked and honored in countries such as England and Italy.

DUROZIEZ DISEASE

Mitral stenosis.

DUROZIEZ MURMUR

Systolic and diastolic murmur heard over the femoral artery on compression with the bell of the stethoscope, in aortic regurgitation or other disorders with a wide pulse pressure.

Paul L. Duroziez (1826–1897) French physician. He was born in Paris in 1826 and graduated in 1853. As a student he won the Corvisart Prize for his discussion on digitalis. In 1856 he became Chief of Clinic with Charcot and in 1870 served as a surgeon in the Franco-Prussian War. He was in general practice and held no official hospital appointment, but was widely acclaimed because of his articles on mitral stenosis as well as other cardiac disorders. He was highly respected by his physician colleagues and was elected President de Societé de Medicine in 1882 and Chevalier of the Legion of Honour in 1895.

DUSARD SYNDROME

Congenital dysfibrinogenemia with deficient lysis of fibrin and probably associated with a thrombotic tendency.

Dusard is the surname of a family with this syndrome.

E

EAGLE MEDIA

Tissue culture media.

Harry Eagle (1905–) Born in New York and graduated M.D. from Johns Hopkins in 1927. U.S. pathologist and bacteriologist who developed the media whilst working at the National Institutes of Health, Washington, D.C. He developed a test for syphilis and became Professor of Bacteriology at the Albert Einstein University, New York.

EAGLE SYNDROME

Symptoms may include hemifacial pain or a constant pain or nagging dull ache in the pharynx, ear pain, difficulty in swallowing and a sensation of a foreign body, in the pharynx. Palpation of the tonsillar fossa on the side involved usually reproduces the pain. It is due to an elongated styloid process and the symptoms are relieved by operation and shortening of the elongated styloid process.

Watt W. Eagle (1898–) American otolaryngologist.

EALES DISEASE

Recurrent retinal and vitreous hemorrhage of unknown etiology, occurring in young adults, usually males, giving sudden visual impairment.

Henry Eales (1852–1913) English physician, born at Newton Abbot, the son of the Vicar of Yealmpton in Devonshire. He became apprenticed to the village doctor and following an outbreak of scarlet fever which led him to test patients' urine for the presence of protein, he incidentally examined his own and found himself to have heavy proteinuria. As a result, he had a year's convalescence before he enrolled in medicine at the University College, London. He had a fine undergraduate record and graduated M.R.C.S. in 1873 and then interned at the Birmingham and Midland Eye Hospital. He was demonstrator in anatomy and medical tutor at Queens College, and in 1878 was appointed honorary surgeon to the Eye Hospital, where he remained for 35 years. He was well known for his abilities with the ophthalmoscope and built up a very big consulting practice. He wrote a number of papers, amongst which was a review of the appearance of the retina in patients with renal disease. Apart from occasional migraine he enjoyed good health and the proteinuria did not return. Shortly before his death he developed pain in his left calf which waxed and waned for 10 days, forcing him to go to bed, and he died sometime thereafter following a syncopal attack, possibly due to a pulmonary embolus.

EATON AGENT OR VIRUS

Mycoplasma pneumoniae. Eaton agent pneumonia. Primary atypical pneumonia. Cold agglutinins are present in 50% of instances.

Monroe D. Eaton (1904–) Born in Stockton, California, graduated M.D. Harvard 1930 – U.S. bacteriologist who first reported his finding in 1944, becoming Associate Professor of Bacteriology and Immunology at Harvard in 1947.

EATON-LAMBERT SYNDROME

v. LAMBERT-EATON SYNDROME

EBERS PAPYRUS

16th century B.C. Egyptian papyrus on many aspects of medicine.

Georg M. Ebers (1837–1898) German Egyptologist. He discovered the papyrus (of 110 pages) in Luxor, Thebes, in 1872. It refers to diabetes mellitus (1502 B.C.), trachoma, hook worm and filariasis as well as forms of arthritis and offers a large number of remedies. There was also a short psychiatric section. He initially studied law and then hieroglyphics and became Professor of Egyptology in Leipzig in 1875. He wrote numerous scientific books on Egypt and a number of novels.

EBSTEIN ANOMALY OR MALFORMATION

Congenital anomaly of tricuspid valve obstructing right ventricular filling and producing cyanotic heart disease.

EBSTEIN DISEASE

1. Armani-Ebstein nephropathy (*v. supra*).
2. Ebstein anomaly – a congenital defect of the tricuspid valve.

Wilhelm Ebstein (1836–1912) German physician, a pupil of Frerichs, Virchow and Romberg who worked and taught at Breslau (Wroclaw). In 1874 he was appointed to the Medical Clinic at Göttingen and became Director (1877), replacing Hasse, who was forced to resign because of his political views. He made many contributions to the study of metabolic disease, produced urinary calculi experimentally and noted cylinduria in diabetic coma. Among his important works was a review of kidney disease in one of the standard medical texts. In 1892 he published his article "The Diagnosis of Incipient Pericardial Effusions" and wrote a section on renal disease in the book "Senile Diseases" which was published by Schwalbe. His other contributions of importance were a book "Obesity and Its Treatment" which went through 7 editions and another on "Diabetes Dietetic Management". He wrote on the medical illness of prominent Germans in history, e.g. Luther, Schopenhauer, and medicine in the Talmud and Bible. Ebstein was reputed to be a superb clinician with a wide circle of friends and a keen interest in literature and the visual arts.

ECK FISTULA

Anastomosis of the portal vein to the inferior vena cava, thus bypassing the liver.

Nicolai V. Eck (1847–1908) Russian physiologist who introduced the technique to study liver function in 1877.

ECONOMO DISEASE

Encephalitis lethargica.

Konstantin von Economo (1876–1931) Austrian neurologist. Born in Braila (Rumania) of wealthy Greek parents, he was brought up in Trieste and forced by his father to study engineering. After two years in Vienna he changed over to medicine and after graduation spent one year at the University clinic, under Nothnagel, then went to Paris where he worked for a year in psychiatry with Magnan and in neurology with Pierre Marie. He visited Bethe in Strasburg and Kraepelin in Munich and wrote a paper on the anatomy of normal nerve cells. In 1906 he returned to the Psychiatric Clinic of Wagner von Jauregg. He was interested in ballooning, became one of the first pilots in Austria (1908) and served as a pilot in the 1st World War in the Tyrol. In 1916 he was ordered back to Vienna to treat brain injuries and commenced his studies on encephalitis. He wrote extensively on Wilson Disease, the nature of sleep and an authoritative text on the histology of the cerebral cortex. In 1931, after declining an invitation to replace von Jauregg, he became director of a Brain Research Institute. He died suddenly of heart disease – presumably a coronary.

EDDOWES DISEASE OR SYNDROME

Osteogenesis imperfecta.

Alfred Eddowes (1850–1946) British dermatologist. He was the son of a doctor, born in Pontesbury, Salop. He entered medical school in the University of Edinburgh where he graduated in 1873, gaining his M.D. three years later, then worked at St. Bartholomew's Hospital and studied in Vienna, Hamburg and Paris. He worked as a resident officer at the Royal Salop Hospital for 4 years and then in general practice in his native county for 11 years before coming to London, where he gained his M.R.C.P. in 1897 and specialized in dermatology, working in skin departments in a number of hospitals including St. John's Hospital for Diseases of the Skin in Leicester Square. He was appointed Honorary Dermatologist to the Artists' Section of the Stage Guild.

EDINGER-WESTPHAL NUCLEUS

Autonomic nucleus of the 3rd nerve.

Ludwig Edinger (1855–1918) German neurologist who was the founder of comparative neuro-anatomy. Born in Worms, on the Rhine, the son of a wealthy textile manufacturer, he was given a microscope by his mother when he was 14. He was fascinated by it and learned the technique of embedding and mounting. He was a poor student at school and on finishing, threw his books over his garden wall, only to retrieve Homer, Horace and Sophocles!

At Heidelberg he was bored by famous names like Friedrich Arnold in anatomy, whose theories he despised, and Bunsen the physicist and Theodor Schwann, but was very influenced by the clinical neurology lectures by E. Leyden, read his book on comparative anatomy and in 1877 worked with Wilhelm Waldeyer in Strasburg and published his first paper. He was assistant to A. Kussmaul the same year and saw the pathologist von Recklinghausen at work. In 1879 he commenced academic work in Giessen with Franz Riegel and in 1881 spent a year in travelling, visiting Berlin (Westphal, Wernicke and Ehrlich), Leipzig (Erb, Strümpell, Möbius, Kraeplin and Flechsig) and Paris (Charcot). He regarded Leyden, Kussmaul and Erb as his teachers in neurology. In 1883 he came to Frankfurt to practice neurology but he soon turned to the laboratory and in 1885 published a classical text on the structure of the nervous system, which related structure with function and clinical neurology.

In 1885 he became closely associated with Carl Weigert who had just perfected his stain for the myelin sheath and built up and financed a neurological institute. He was made Ordinarius in neurology in 1914 at the recently founded Goethe University in Frankfurt and his institute was funded by "Ludwig Edinger Stiftung".

Throughout his career he pursued the relationship of structure with function as "to investigate brain anatomy alone is to pursue a sterile science". He wrote a book on the clinical application of neuro-anatomy in 1909. He was the first to describe the vertebral and dorsal spinocerebellar tract and to distinguish the paleo-encephalon from the neoencephalon and the paleo-cerebellum and neo-cerebellum. Although Roussy and Dejerine are usually mentioned when thalamic pain is discussed, Edinger was the first to describe it and verify it at autopsy some 15 years earlier. He was also a hypnotist, a fine artist and a collector of objets d'art. He died of a coronary thrombosis post-operatively.

Karl F.O. Westphal (1833–1890) German neurologist. Born in Berlin the son of a prominent physician. He studied medicine at Berlin, Heidelberg and Zurich. In 1857 he was an assistant in the smallpox section of the Charité Hospital in Berlin and a year later moved to the psychiatric division working with Griesinger, van Horn and Ideler. In 1891 he became Privatdozent in psychiatry and in 1874 Professor. He described the nucleus in the adult two years after Edinger had demonstrated it in the fetus. He made many contributions, in particular identification of pseudosclerosis (Wilson disease), demonstrated the relationship of general paralysis of the insane with tabes dorsalis, described periodic paralysis and first described agoraphobia (fear of open places). He trained a number of world famous neurologists, including Arnold Pick and Hermann Oppenheim, and Wernicke was his assistant. Together with Erb he was the first to describe the deep tendon reflex. He was the first Professor of Neurology appointed in Berlin.

EDWARDS SYNDROME

Trisomy 18 – a severe and usually fatal dysmorphic condition with death occurring in the first few weeks of life. The characteristic 'pinched' facial appearance, the small size at birth, the clenched fingers, the short big toe, all usually coupled with a major lethal malformation involving the heart and/or the esophagus, prompt an early diagnosis. The spectrum of defects externally and internally, as recognized at post mortem, is wide. A few, without lethal malformations, survive but are severely retarded both intellectually and physically.

Jack H. Edwards (1928–) English medical geneticist who followed an unorthodox medical career. While at Cambridge to study medicine, he devoted much of his time to the intricacies of algebra and gliding, the latter providing a necessary practical application of his mathematical knowledge. After qualification he held posts in neurology and psychiatry, became a Medical Officer on the Falkland Islands and after that joined the Population Research Unit at Oxford. He then moved to Birmingham as a clinical geneticist at the time that chromosomal analysis had become feasible in man. Later he was the first Professor of Clinical Genetics in the University. Election to the Fellowship of the Royal Society of London and a move to the Chair of Genetics at Oxford followed but before these events had occurred he had continued with his interests in chromosomal defects in man, carried out collaborative studies on the zygosity of new-born twins and their placentation, as well as pursuing a mathematical interest in a population genetic study in Iceland. In retrospect, his genetic interests and publications have followed three main paths. The first has been in biometrics, a field of great complexity that deals with the fundamental sums of genetics. The second has been a devotion to the construction of computer programs to map the human genome and, lastly, the application of logic to existing genetic theory and biological processes. His ability to recognize and exploit the crucial but anomalous result and successfully challenge accepted truths have also led to wide recognition. The heterogeneity of genetic disease, the mechanisms of somatic and gonadal mosaicism, uniparental disomy and the resurrection of the phenomenon of anticipation were topics that he devoted himself to in the late 1980s.

EHLERS-DANLOS SYNDROME

Hyperelasticity of the skin, easy bruising and joint extensibility usually due to faulty collagen synthesis. Mitral valve prolapse (v. BARLOW SYNDROME) is usual and congenital cardiac defects, e.g. atrial septal defect, are common. Most forms have an autosomal dominant inheritance but some are autosomal recessive.

Edward Ehlers (1863–1937) Danish dermatologist. His description appeared in 1901. Professor of Clinical Dermatology at Copenhagen and made contributions on leprosy. He was Danish President of the Alliance Francaise.

Henri A. Danlos (1844–1912) French physician and dermatologist, who was born in Paris. His father wished his son to enter a family business and his initial education was aimed in that direction, but he himself decided he wanted to do medicine and without his parents' knowledge changed to a medical course and graduated in 1869. Initially he was most interested in laboratory work, although his doctorate in 1847 concerned the effects of menstruation on skin problems. When 37 years old he was promoted to Médecin des Hôpitaux and worked with Vulpian, giving him a well rounded clinical training. He was Chef de Service in 1885 at Hôpital Tenon, but it was not until 1895 that he finally realized his ambition of being appointed to the Hôpital Saint-Louis. Shortly after his health became delicate and after four years he had to withdraw from the hospital laboratory and clinical work and from that day he became depressed. He was the first person to use radium to treat lupus erythematosus of the skin, applied radium to the treatment of breast cancer and in the treatment of keloid. He described numerous therapeutic approaches to psoriasis and syphilis and compared the various procedures for treatment of skin tuberculosis.

EHRLICH REAGENT

Dimethylaminobenzaldehyde.

EHRLICH TEST

Test for urobilinogen using Ehrlich reagent

EHRLICH TUMOR

Transplantable tumor originally derived from breast carcinoma in mice – it grows in solid and ascitic forms.

Paul Ehrlich (1854–1915) German physician and scientist. He was born in Strehlen, Silesia, went to medical school at Breslau and studied in Strasburg, Freiburg and Leipzig where he graduated in 1878. He had been an indifferent student, but had devoted much of his time to studying staining techniques and whilst at Strasburg he had studied lead poisoning and developed a Fuchsin stain which identified lead in the tissues. This led to his thesis that certain tissues had a particular affinity for specific chemicals:

In 1878 he became Frerich's assistant in Berlin and commenced his studies of staining techniques. Here he developed the idea of spreading blood thinly on a glass slide and fixing it prior to staining with his dyes which he noted had a selective affinity for certain cells. This enabled him to classify the granulocyte series as well as to study the morphological changes in the bone marrow in anemic states. Using these techniques he was the first to describe the megaloblast and to discover the mast cells, as well as reporting the first patient with aplastic anemia and writing a classic textbook on hematology in which he described such phenomena as thrombocytosis associated with blood loss. During this time he introduced his diazoreaction for urobilinogen and greatly improved the staining methods for tubercle, showing that it was acid fast. He is said to have shown little interest in clinical medicine and spent most of his time in his small laboratory with its array of stains and various techniques for purifying and filtering them, and he used a form of paper chromatography to study some of the properties of these stains. Ehrlich remained with Frerich until 1885 and then became Gerhardt's (*v. infra*) assistant until 1890 when he moved to Koch's Institute for Infectious Diseases with a title equivalent to Associate Professor. He published a monograph entitled "The oxygen requirements of the organism" in 1885 and here he promoted a side chain hypothesis with a lock and key model for antibody formation which is now accepted as one of the ways antigens can select the appropriate lymphocyte to transform and produce clones of lymphocytes producing specific antibodies. At the time his hypothesis was vigorously debated and attacked, although Wassermann has stated that without this theory he would never have developed his Wassermann Test (*v. infra*). Whilst at Koch's Institute Ehrlich developed a technique to measure diphtheria toxin and later accused von Behring of stealing his ideas. When the latter came to develop diphtheria

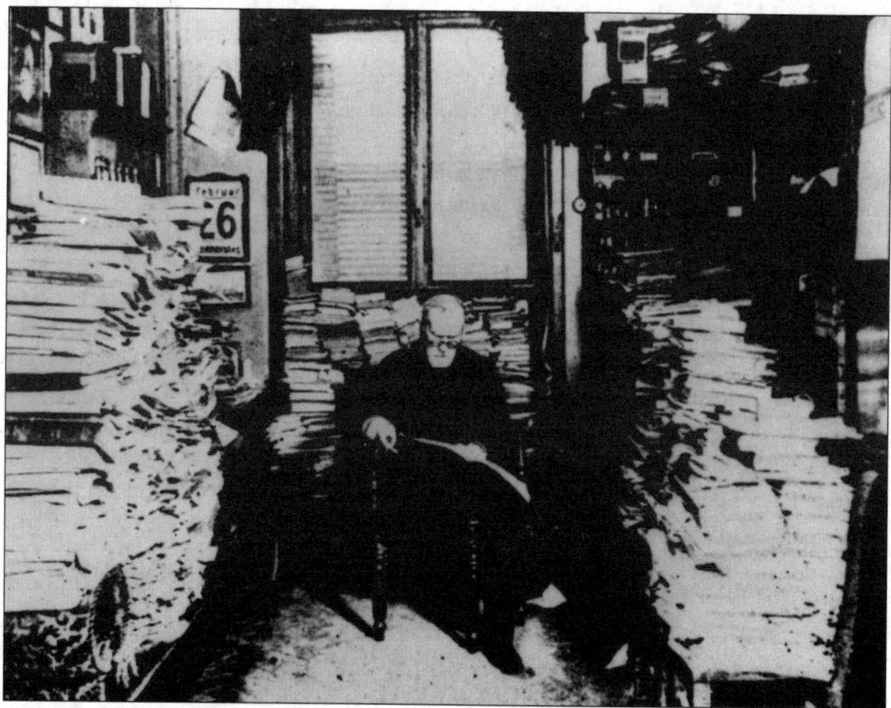

Paul Ehrlich in his study.
Reproduced from *"Paul Ehrlich"* by Martha Marquardt (Published by William Heineman Medical Ltd. 1949)

antitoxin in a quantity sufficient to be used in the treatment of diphtheria, he required a quantitative technique to measure its efficacy and there seems little doubt that he did use Ehrlich's method to do this and there was considerable bitterness and debate.

In 1899 Ehrlich went to Frankfurt-am-Main as Director of the Royal Institute of Experimental Therapy. Here he continued his studies on antibody formation, and proceeded to investigate the use of experimental animals in the study of cancer as well as employing animals infected with organisms such as the trypanosome and using these animals as a screen to select useful drugs against infection and tumors. It was by the use of this technique that he discovered the arsenical compound Salvarsan which he termed 606 (since he had investigated 605 previous compounds) and this compound proved to be effective against syphilis. Ehrlich's persistence, method and meticulousness is shown by the way in which he personally vetted the initial material and the initial studies on his compound in patients with disease. It was a considerable time before he allowed the preparation to be prepared commercially. He was perhaps made even more cautious by the relatively recent failure of tuberculin to affect tuberculosis (v. Koch). Ehrlich's treatment was effective against trypanosomiasis as well as syphilis and undoubtedly was one of the major advances of the time.

There was considerable opposition in some instances on moral grounds; the Orthodox Church of Russia for example held that venereal disease was a punishment imposed by God for an immoral action. The German police objected to it on the grounds that every common prostitute must sooner or later become infected with syphilis, and if Ehrlich's preparation 606 was as active as claimed, then she could be cured and become infected repeatedly and so remain a permanent danger. Despite all the controversies, Ehrlich won the Nobel Prize in 1908.

Ehrlich was a patient and kindly man and had the habit of jotting down ideas and instructions to his assistant in a notebook interleaved with carbon paper. The recipient would have to sign and take away the written instructions while the copy remained in Ehrlich's book, a practice some of his colleagues found disagreeable. He was always an extremely modest person who enjoyed the simple pleasures of life and apparently was a good raconteur and listener to broad stories, as well as an avid reader of thrillers. One of his proudest moments was the receipt of a postcard from a patient thanking him for being cured with Salvarsan. He carried that in his wallet all the time. When asked what he considered was the guiding idea of his scientific life he mentioned that when he was 20 years old he was waiting in his uncle's laboratory (Weigert) and he looked down the microscope at a prepared slide which was colored blue and red and although at the time he had no histological knowledge, it struck him that some parts of the cells were colored red and others blue. He realized at once that certain parts of the cell had an affinity for the acid red dye stuff while the other parts had the same affinity for the basic blue and therefore was able to take up the color. That meant different parts of the cell could be differentiated by different dye stuffs. This led on to all of his studies of drug affinity. One of Ehrlich's maxims was that good research required "Geduld, Geschick, Gluck und Geld (Patience, Ability, Luck and Money)".

Ehrlich's name was a household word in Germany until the Nazis came to power when they persecuted his widow and confiscated his property. Professor Sir Almroth Wright, a pupil of Ehrlich's, arranged for Burroughs Wellcome to provide an income for her to live comfortably until her death.

Ehrlich was undoubtedly one of the greatest geniuses of his time. He could well be regarded as the father of hematology, immunology, chemotherapy and pharmacology. He was the first to relate chemical structure with function successfully.

EINTHOVEN LAW

The potential difference in lead II is equal to the algebraic sum of the potential differences of leads I and III of the electrocardiogram.

EINTHOVEN TRIANGLE

An equilateral triangle with apices at the left and right wrists and left hip which are assumed to be equidistant from the heart.

Willem Einthoven (1860–1927) Dutch physiologist. He was born in Semarang, Java (Indonesia), where his father was in medical practice, but after his father died in 1870, his mother took her six children back to Holland and settled in Utrecht. There he went to school and eventually to University where he was particularly influenced by the physicists, Buys and Ballot, and then the anatomist Koster and the ophthalmologist Snellen, and finally the Professor of Physiology, Donders. He succeeded Heynsius as Professor of Physiology at Leyden University, receiving his invitation before he had actually passed the final State examination in medicine, 1886. With his sound knowledge of physics, he developed instruments for recording minute electrical changes which had not been previously available and as a result was able to record electrical traces of the heart and founded the modern science of electrocardiography. Although others had demonstrated that electrical impulses from the heart could be detected, his instrument was the first practical and accurate electrocardiograph. This led to clinical application, both in diagnosis and physiology. He developed instrumentation for recording heart sounds, was awarded the Nobel Prize for his work in 1924 and in 1925 was elected as a foreign member of the Royal Society.

He is remembered by most of his physiological colleagues and clinical peers as a very modest person who was profoundly courteous and very hospitable. He could speak three languages fluently as well as his native Dutch and this no doubt helped his influence in international scientific circles. However, one incident which shows that Einthoven may not have been above criticism concerned a paper presented by Craib, then a relatively recent medical graduate who was working at Johns Hopkins on electrocardiography at an International Congress in Stockholm, which was chaired by Einthoven. At the end of Craib's paper Einthoven stopped the session and refused to allow any questions, went over to Craib whose paper had challenged some of the basic tenets upon which electrocardiography had been based, and roundly abused him as being a disgrace for presenting such obviously false information. Craib's work proved to be correct!

EISENMENGER COMPLEX (TETRALOGY)

Congenital cyanotic heart lesion consisting of a ventricular septal defect, dextraposition of the aorta and resultant pulmonary hypertension.

EISENMENGER SYNDROME

Any left to right shunt which develops pulmonary hypertension with consequent reversal of the shunt and cyanosis, e.g. patent ductus arteriosus.

Victor Eisenmenger (1864–1932) German physician.

EKBOM SYNDROME

Restless legs syndrome – unpleasant sensation in the lower limbs when the patient is at rest, often associated with an intolerable restlessness, cramps which may interfere with sleep. It is associated with iron deficiency, drugs (phenothiazine), barbiturate withdrawal, diabetes, uremia, neuropathy and chronic respiratory illness as well as following a cerebrovascular accident.

Karl-Axel Ekbom (1907–) Swedish neurologist, University of Uppsala who became Professor of Neurology there in 1958.

ELLIS-VAN CREVELD SYNDROME

Chondroectodermal dysplasia. Polydactyly, chondrodysplasia with dwarfism, hidrotic ectodermal dysplasia and congenital heart defects; short, thick digits (six fingered dwarfism). The extra digit is usually on the ulnar side, sparse hair, dystrophic nails, defective dentition, cryptorchidism and epi- or hypospadias may occur. It is thought to be autosomal recessive.

Richard W.B. Ellis (1902–1966) English pediatrician who came from a Quaker family. He commenced his medical studies at King's College, Cambridge where his particular heroes were Barcroft and Adrian. He then went to St. Thomas' Hospital where he qualified in 1926. His training was somewhat unusual in that he did not stay with the one hospital as was then the custom, but undertook registrar posts at St. Thomas' and then the London and later the Hospital for Sick Children, Great Ormond Street. He spent a year in Blackfan's Department (*v. supra*) at the Boston Children's Hospital. He was appointed physician for children's diseases at Guy's Hospital in 1936 and shortly after went to Spain to help with the 4,000 Basque children who were refugees from the Spanish Civil War and he adopted two children whom he brought back to England. There he met his future wife who he married in 1941.

When World War II broke out he went to Hungary and Romania to take care of Polish refugees and then joined the Royal Air Force. After the war he returned to Guy's Hospital to develop the pediatric department but when a chair of pediatrics failed to be established he left to become Professor of Child Life and Health in Edinburgh. There he wrote a popular text book "Diseases of Infancy and Childhood" and became increasingly interested and involved in child development and the social interactions which influence it.

He was diagnosed with cancer when he was 56 years old and 6 years later continued his work despite bone secondaries with resultant pathological fractures. He was a keen oil painter and had a great interest in antique furniture.

S. van Creveld (1894–1971) Dutch pediatrician.

v. VAN CREVELD-VON GIERKE SYNDROME.

ELLSWORTH-HOWARD TEST

Failure of parathormone to induce phosphate diuresis in pseudohypoparathyroidism.

Reed E. Ellsworth U.S. physician, Johns Hopkins. He made many contributions to calcium metabolism but perhaps his best known was the solution of the controversy between Albright and Collip as to whether the parathormone acted directly on bone (Collip) or indirectly by causing phosphaturia (Albright). Ellsworth and Futcher tied off the ureters in an animal and showed parathormone injection still caused calcium increase, thus proving Albright wrong.

John E. Howard (1904–1985) U.S. physician, Johns Hopkins. He went to college at Princetown and entered Johns Hopkins Medical School in 1924. After graduating in 1928 he spent two years at the Massachusetts General Hospital and then two further years as Assistant Resident at Johns Hopkins. In 1934 he was appointed as Instructor in Medicine and became Physician to the Johns Hopkins Hospital. He became Director of the Division of Endocrinology and Metabolism and in 1960 became a full Professor. A quote from Howard is that "Serendipity hovered around my door due to an aberrant gene from my great-great-grandfather. At the Battle of Cowpens a retreat was ordered but General Howard had charged and the first defeat of Tarleton's British regulars resulted". Howard has felt that serendipity has been with him throughout his research career. Whilst investigating pheochromocytoma, he was asked to see a patient who recently had a normal appendix removed following an acute episode of abdominal pain. Hypertension had developed rapidly after the operation and continued for two months. An X-ray suggested the possibility of adrenal tumor and although they did not expect to find a pheochromocytoma, an abdominal exploration was undertaken. At the operation the surgeon noticed a curious area in the kidney and removed it in the belief that it could be cancerous. The patient's condition improved and after the operation the patient became normotensive. The renal lesion was an infarct. Fifteen years later Howard was asked to see a patient with identical problems with exactly the same result following nephrectomy. A subsequent patient was diagnosed pre-operatively by aortography. This led Howard, together with a member of his department, to investigate techniques for differentiating these problems and led to the development of tests designed to study the differential renal function in renovascular hypertension. Howard's group over the years made numerous contributions to the area of renal stone formation and in particular to the thesis that some urines in patients who form renal stones lack an inhibitor which normally prevents calcification. Studies using phytic acid in the management of renal stones led to the serendipitous finding that increased phosphorus excretion by the urine could be useful in preventing oxalate stone formation. During the Second World War, Howard made important observations on potassium metabolism which led to the introduction of potassium in the recovery phase of diabetic acidosis.

ELY SIGN

Patient lies prone with feet over the end of the table. The heel is placed towards the buttock with the thigh hyper-extended. Discomfort indicates a hip lesion or psoas irritation ipsilaterally.

Leonard W. Ely (1868–1944) U.S. orthopedic surgeon. He graduated M.D. from the College of Physicians and Surgeons, New York in 1895 and served as a captain in the U.S. Army medical corps in World War I. He was on the staff at the Presbyterian Hospital in New York but moved to California where he became Professor of Surgery (orthopedic) at the Stanford University School of Medicine from 1924–1934.

ENGELMANN DISEASE

(cf. RIBBING SYNDROME), sometimes called **Camurati-Engelmann Syndrome**.

Progressive diaphyseal dysplasia. Results in hyperostoses of the long bones, osteosclerosis and muscular dystrophy going on to cause anemia and hematological complications due to increasing thickening of bone cortex.

Guido Engelmann (1876–1959) Austrian orthopedic surgeon who worked in Kienböck's department in Vienna. He was born in Olmütz (Mähren) and studied medicine in Vienna where he worked in Albert's surgical clinic before becoming an assistant to von Hoffa in Berlin. He returned to Vienna to practice orthopedic surgery and wrote a book "Genetic Lesions in Orthopaedic Surgery" with Bertha Aschner in 1928. He left Austria in 1938 and settled in the U.S.A., dying in California.

Mario Camurati (1896–1948) Italian orthopedic surgeon, Bologna.

EPSTEIN SYNDROME

The nephrotic syndrome: edema, proteinuria, hypoalbuminemia and hyperlipidemia.

Albert A. Epstein (1880–1965) U.S. physician. He was a student of Emanuel Libman (v. LIBMAN-SACHS ENDOCARDITIS) and was on the house staff of Mt. Sinai Hospital in 1908 and continued his association, becoming an associate physician in 1923, resigning in 1928 to become attending physician at the Beth Israel Hospital and the Hospital for Joint Diseases in New York. He made a number of contributions to diabetes and renal disease including a microchemical method for estimating sugar in the blood which he developed in 1914.

EPSTEIN-BARR VIRUS (EBV)

Herpes-like virus associated with infectious mononucleosis and Burkitt lymphoma.

Michael A. Epstein (1921–) He was born in London and studied medicine at Cambridge University and the Middlesex Hospital Medical School. He moved from the Middlesex to become Professor of Pathology at the University of Bristol in 1968. Following a presentation in 1961 by Denis Burkitt of his epidemiological studies at the Middlesex Hospital he investigated Burkitt lymphoma for causative viruses and established a Burkitt lymphoma cell line which on examination with the electron microscope revealed particles morphologically similar to herpes virus. Biological tests demonstrated that this was a new human herpes virus and it became known as the Epstein-Barr virus. The virus is the cause of infectious mononucleosis or glandular fever, and is associated with nasopharyngeal carcinoma as well as Burkitt lymphoma.

Yvonne Barr (1932–) She was born in London and obtained her Ph.D. from the University of London in 1966. She joined Epstein's laboratories to work on this project. She married an Australian and is currently in residence there.

ERB PARALYSIS

v. ERB-DUCHENNE PARALYSIS.

ERB POINT

2–3 cm above clavicle in front of the transverse process of 6th cervical vertebra.

ERB SCAPULOHUMERAL MUSCULAR DYSTROPHY

Autosomal recessive. Muscular dystrophy occurring in adolescents.

ERB SIGN

1. Loss of the knee jerk as an early sign of tabes dorsalis.
2. Use of galvanic current to diagnose tetany.

ERB-DUCHENNE PARALYSIS

Upper brachial plexus paralysis

ERB-GOLDFLAM DISEASE

Myasthenia gravis.

Wilhelm H. Erb (1840–1921) German neurologist. He was the first clinician to use the reflex hammer as a routine in physical examination. Born in Winweiler, the son of a forester, he studied medicine at Heidelberg, Erlargen and Munich. In 1865 he was appointed Privatdozent for medicine at Heidelberg and Associate Professor in 1869. In 1880 he went to Leipzig as Professor of Medicine, but returned to Heidelberg where he spent most of his life – he succeeded his teacher N. Friedrich in 1883. He made early observations relating to syphilis and tabes dorsalis, popularized electrodiagnosis in neurology and demonstrated increased motor nerve irritability in tetany (Erb phenomenon). He was an excellent teacher although something of a martinet with a short temper – one of his sayings to his students, who included E. Remak and Nonne, was "Pray every morning before you get out of bed – O Lord let me not idle away my life today". He occupied the same position in German neurology as Charcot in France and Gowers in England.

G.B.A. Duchenne (*v. supra*).

S.V. Goldflam (*v. infra*).

ERBEN PHENOMENON, REFLEX OR SIGN

Slowing of the pulse when the head and trunk are flexed due to vagal stimulation.

Siegmund Erben (1863–) Austrian neurologist who worked in Vienna.

ERDHEIM SYNDROME *or*

SCAGLIETTI-DAGNINI SYNDROME

Cervical spondylosis secondary to acromegaly often with clavicular hypertrophy.

Jakob Erdheim (1874–1937) German pathologist. He wrote a classical paper on aortic medionecrosis and made many contributions on pituitary disorders including pituitary dwarfism. He influenced Fuller Albright (*v. supra*) during his time in Germany.

O. Scaglietti (*v. infra*).

G. Dagnini (*v. supra*).

ERLENMEYER FLASK

Conical flask.

E. Erlenmeyer (1825–1909) German chemist born in Wehen. He was a pharmacist in Heidelberg and became a Professor of Chemistry at the Polytechnikum Munich in 1868. He introduced the term hydroxyl and made important contributions to the chemistry of aliphatic components and alcohols.

ESCHERICHIA COLI

Gram negative bacteria.

Theodor Escherich (1857–1911) German pediatrician and bacteriologist, born in Ansbach, who wrote the first account of *Bacillus coli* infections in children (1885) when he was Docent in Children's Diseases in Munich. He became a professor in Graz 1894 and finally Vienna in 1902 and wrote on childhood tetany, diphtheria and croup.

EUSOL

Antiseptic solution for wound irrigation – chlorinated lime and boric acid in water.

Edinburgh University Solution.

EUSTACHIAN TUBE

Duct connecting the middle ear with the pharynx.

Bartolomeo Eustachios (1524–1574) He was Professor of Anatomy at the Collegio delle Sapienze in Rome (1555–1568). He was physician to the Pope and Professor of Anatomy in Rome until his death. In 1552 he completed a set of anatomical plates which remained unprinted in the Papal library for 162 years. Pope Clement XI gave them to his physician Lancisi, who on the advice of Morgani published them in 1714. Apart from the Eustachian tube he discovered the adrenal gland, the thoracic duct and the 6th nerve. He described the cochlea, the pulmonary veins and gave the first accurate description of the uterus and placenta and wrote about the structure and nerve and blood supply of the teeth.

EVANS BLUE

Diazo dye which combines with albumin and may be used to estimate blood volume and cardiac output.

Herbert M. Evans (1882–) U.S. anatomist and physiologist. Born in Modesto, California, graduated M.D. Johns Hopkins in 1908. He was appointed Professor of Anatomy, University of California, Berkeley, in 1915. He studied human chromosomes and reported them to number 48 in 1918. He discovered vitamin E and linolenic acid and investigated the effects of growth hormone and isolated a number of the pituitary hormones.

EVANS SYNDROME

Coomb positive acquired hemolytic anemia and idiopathic thrombocytopenic purpura.

Robert S. Evans (1912–1974) U.S. physician, Seattle. He graduated from Harvard in 1938 and was a resident at the Massachusetts General Hospital for the next three years, after which he became a resident at the Thorndike Research Laboratory of Harvard. He first moved to Stanford Medical School but shortly afterwards went to Seattle as head of medicine at the Seattle Veterans' Hospital until his death, in a motor car accident. "Bud" was first of all a general physician with research interests in immuno-hematology, but especially in hemolytic anemia. He was, however, best known to those around him for his humanity and an annual award to the most caring physician is given in his name.

EWART SIGN

Dullness to percussion, increased fremitus and bronchial breathing beneath the angle of the left scapula in pericardial effusion.

William Ewart (1848–1929) English physician. He was born in London, but his mother was French and he was educated partly in England and at the University of Paris. He joined the medical school at St. George's Hospital in 1869 and whilst still a student worked in a field hospital during the

Franco-Prussian War where he described how the German surgeons showed great reluctance to operate. "They were always anxious to give unaided nature her last chance, by which they often seemed to deprive the patient of his." (The French performed 14,000 amputations during this war and 10,000 of these died of sepsis so the Germans' reluctance to operate was well founded.)

He qualified L.R.C.S. in 1871 and L.R.C.P. in 1872, then went to Gonville and Caius College, Cambridge, where he graduated in 1876 with a first class of the natural science tripos and gained his M.B. degree in 1877. After working in Berlin he returned to London to St. George's Hospital where he lectured on physiology and also was a Curator of the Museum. At the same time he became assistant physician at the Brompton Hospital, and he undertook the pathology examinations at both hospitals. In 1882 he was elected assistant physician at St. George's Hospital and resigned his Brompton appointment. In 1887 he became a full physician and retired in 1907.

His major work stemmed from his extensive knowledge of the chest and resulted in an atlas of the anatomy of the bronchi and pulmonary blood vessels, and a number of small publications on physical examination. In view of his interest in tuberculosis and its relation to climate he examined the climatic conditions of a number of the southern counties. He was a devout Catholic and something of an eccentric, and students and patients alike appeared to find him somewhat confusing during his clinical rounds. He was constantly on the look-out for rare cases, but it sometimes appeared that his elaborate examination and knowledge often led him to lengthy conclusions which could be readily explained more simply. The comment was made in one of his obituaries that "apart from his excellence in his hospital work, he did not possess the qualities that appealed to the public, nor was he able to render the prompt and straight-forward assistance to family practitioners that they and their patients expected at consultations". It therefore seems that although this man had commendable attributes, he was not a success as a consultant physician. In his later years he developed severe rheumatic disease and (still a bachelor) lived at his club, the Atheneum, and died in St. Mary's Hospital.

EWING SARCOMA

Malignant bone tumor occurring in children or young adults.

James Ewing (1866–1943) U.S. pathologist, born in Pittsburgh, he graduated from Amherst College and obtained his medical degree from Columbia University in 1891. After interning there he went to the Pathology Department of Columbia where he worked until 1899, when he was appointed Professor of Pathology at Cornell University. There he taught for the next 33 years and made a number of contributions to clinical pathology of blood and neoplastic diseases, was a founder of the "Journal of Cancer Research" and wrote an important textbook "Neoplastic Disease".

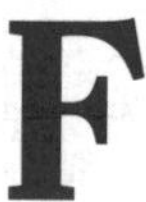

FABRICIUS – BURSA OF

Lymphoid structure in birds' intestine which is the origin of B lymphocytes, i.e. cells concerned with antibody production. Removal of the bursa in embryo results in an animal unable to produce antibodies.

Hieronymous Fabricius ab Aquapendente (1553–1619) Professor of Anatomy at Padua, he taught students from Poland, Germany and England, one of whom was Harvey. He demonstrated valves in veins and Harvey told Robert Boyle that it was this observation of his former teacher which made him embark on his study of the circulation. Fabricius was the founder of comparative embryology but followed Galen's view in most areas, even using his actual words.

FABRY DISEASE

v. ANDERSON-FABRY DISEASE

Angiokeratoma corporis diffusum universale. Transmitted by X-linked gene; it results in a progressive accumulation of the glycolipid ceramide trihexoside in glomeruli due to absence of α-galactosyl hydrolase. Patients present with the skin lesions, small red spots seen on the lower abdomen, thighs and scrotum, corneal opacities, episodes of fever, primary parasthesia of the extremities and peripheral edema and renal failure. The disorder was described in 1898 by Fabry in Germany and Anderson in England.

Johannes Fabry (1860–1930) German dermatologist who first described the condition as "purpura hemorrhagica nodularis".

FAHR DISEASE

Intracerebral vascular calcification which characteristically involves the small vessels of the deep cortical layers, and the lenticular and dentate nuclei and is unrelated to atherosclerosis. It can be familial.

Theodor Fahr (1877–1945) German pathologist who worked with Volhard (*v. infra*).

FAHRENHEIT

Fahrenheit temperature scale – freezing point is 32°F and boiling point is 212°F. Normal body temperature is 98.6°F. Now largely replaced by Centigrade, but was the most common temperature scale in the U.K., U.S.A. and Australia before World War II.

Gabriel D. Fahrenheit (1668–1736) German instrument maker who invented the mercury thermometer (1714) and was elected F.R.S. for his achievement. He worked with H. Boerhaave (*v. supra*) who suggested that he multiply the scale he had intitally adopted, 8 divisions for freezing and 53 for boiling water by four, giving the range of 32 to 212. Two years later Celsius proposed 0–100 but it was too late to gain universal agreement.

FAIRBANK DISEASE

Hyperostosis generalisata with striation. A disorder of bone with obliteration of the medullary cavity and irregularity of the ossification of epiphyses resulting in enlargement and X-ray appearance of striations in the vertebrae.

Sir Thomas Fairbank (1876–1961) English orthopedic surgeon who qualified M.B. from Charing Cross Hospital in 1898 and the following year took his dental degree. He volunteered for the South African War and was with Lord Robert's contingent at Paardeverg, the surrender of General Cronje.

At the end of the Boer War he returned to London and was appointed orthopedic surgeon to Charing Cross and also to the Children's Hospital, Great Ormond Street, the first appointment of this kind in London. He made a number of investigations on congenital dislocation of the hip and in 1914 visited centers on the east coast of America. At the outbreak of World War I he went to Belgium and France and later to Salonika with the Royal Army Medical Corps. He was decorated on numerous occasions. At the end of the war he was placed in charge of the orthopedic department at King's College Hospital where he made a number of significant contributions. He received his knighthood for services given to the Ministry of Health during World War II as well as the many contributions he had made to the orthopedic literature. He wrote an important textbook on skeletal abnormalities "An Atlas of General Affections of the Skeleton".

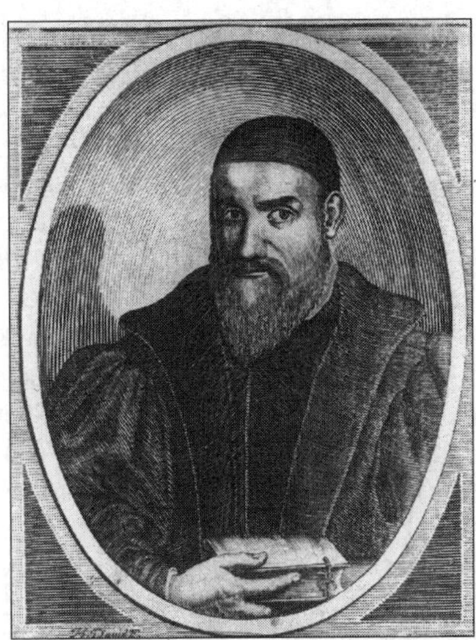

Gabriele Fallopio (Courtesy of the Royal Society of Medicine, London, UK)

FAIRLEY TEST

Bladder washout test to determine the site of urinary infection.

Kenneth F. Fairley (1927–) Australian physician, Royal Melbourne Hospital, Victoria, Australia.

FALLOPIAN TUBE

Oviduct.

Gabriele Fallopio (1523–1562) Italian anatomist who made many original observations including the description of the inguinal ligament, the ileocecal valve and the hard and soft palate. He extensively studied the anatomy of the ear and discovered the aqueduct of the vestibule, the osseous labrynth and the chorda tympani and the canal of the facial nerve. He was a pupil of Vesalius and in turn had Fabricius as one of his students who succeeded him to his chair of anatomy and surgery in Padua when he died of pleurisy. He was a keen botanist and the plant genus *Fallopia* is named after him.

FALLOT TETRALOGY OR TETRAD

Congenital cyanotic heart disease due to ventriculoseptal defect, pulmonary stenosis, right ventricular hypertrophy and dextraposition or over-riding of the aorta.

Etienne-Louis A. Fallot (1850–1911) French physician, born in Cette (Sete) which is on the Mediterranean. He went to medical school at Montpellier in 1867, was a resident in Marseilles where he wrote a thesis on pneumothorax. In 1888 he was appointed Professor of Hygiene and Legal Medicine in Marseilles. At his request no obituary was written. The tetrad was first described by Stensen (*v. infra*).

FANCONI ANEMIA

Congenital hypoplastic anemia often associated with skeletal abnormalities, e.g. extra phalanges as well as non-specific chromosome changes, sometimes terminating with leukemia.

FANCONI SYNDROME

(Also called DEBRÉ-DE TONI-FANCONI SYNDROME and LIGNAC-DE TONI-FANCONI SYNDROME)

Hereditary disorder of renal tubular function with renal rickets resistant to vitamin D; glycosuria, aminoaciduria, and hyperphosphaturia. A similar syndrome can be seen in adults, with osteomalacia – usually acquired, e.g. multiple myeloma, drugs.

Guido Fanconi (1882–1979) Swiss pediatrician. In 1930 he gave a paper to the 2nd International Conference of Paediatrics in Stockholm in which he advocated the use of raw fruit in the treatment of acute diarrhea. One discussant told him he was crazy, but this led to the development of pectin as an antidiarrheal agent. He was one of the first pediatricians to recognize and employ intravenous fluid and electrolytes to treat dehydration in children. He undertook clinical investigations on rickets and calcium metabolism and was the first to describe a pneumonia with a positive Wassermann reaction in nonsyphilitic subjects (? lupus). He was one of Europe's foremost pediatricians and in the later years of his life did much to sustain the International Paediatric Association, being Secretary-General until 1965.

Robert Debré (*v. supra*).

Giovanni de Toni (1896–1973) Italian pediatrician from Bologna.

FARBER DISEASE

Disseminated lipogranulomatosis giving nodular plaques in the skin, recognizable at birth or shortly after; the substance accumulated is mainly chondroitin sulphate B.

Sidney Farber (1903–1973) He was born in Buffalo and at school was tackle on the football team and additionally gave violin lessons and taught calculus at the Buffalo Technical High School in the evenings. He learned about the strengths of German medicine from his older brother, Marvin, who was studying philosophy in Germany and in 1923 he studied medicine at Heidelberg and Freiburg where he was particularly influenced by Pick, Benda and Aschoff. He returned to complete his medical training at Harvard and he graduated M.D. in 1927. He was particularly attracted by Professor S. Burt Wolbach who was chairman of pathology and became a full time pathologist at the Boston Children's Hospital in 1929. He spent his whole working career there, apart from spending a year at the Pathological Institute in the University of Munich (1928–1929) and at Professor C. Heyman's laboratory of pharmacodynamics at the University of Ghent. He was appointed Professor of Pathology in Harvard Medical School in 1948 and was involved in a number of histopathological descriptions including the disorder to which his name is attached. It is, however, in the development of chemotherapy that he made his most important contribution and initiated the first studies on actinomycin D on Wilm's tumor of the kidney, completely changing the outlook of this disorder. He and his co-workers pioneered the use of folic acid antagonists in the treatment of acute childhood leukemia and developed effective chemotherapy protocols for treatment of other childhood hematological malignancies. He became a national figure in community fund-raising for cancer and was a central figure to the fund-raising efforts for the Cancer Research Foundation and the Jimmy Fund in Boston. His many contributions have been recognized by the establishment of the Sidney Farber Cancer Institute. His firm belief in his objectives led him at times to be rather aggressive in criticism and it was commented that "the wrath of contradiction of his beliefs was incredible".

FAVRE DISEASE

1. Lymphogranuloma venereum.
2. Acroangiodermatitis – angiodermatitis of the lower limbs due to venous insufficiency.

Maurice Favre (1876–1954) French dermatologist and physician, born near Lake Leman in the locality of Rousses, Jura, he went to Lyons and was a pupil of Renault from whom he learned the techniques of histopathology and of Gailleton who taught him dermatology. He became Médecin des Hôpitaux in 1909 and was promoted to Agrégé de Médecine Generale in 1920. He was Professor of Anatomical Pathology for 10 years from 1927–1937, and during this time made numerous contributions, particularly to disorders of the connective tissue and disorders involving the lymphatics and blood vessels. He became Professor of Clinical Dermatology, retiring in 1943. Like most dermatologists of his day he was involved in the management and treatment of patients with venereal disease and published on syphilis. In 1913 he described the disorder lymphogranuloma venereum which he separated from other forms of venereal disease, calling it lymphogranuloma inguinale. He deplored the many names which later became attached to this disorder, of which he used to say "it had a good father, but bad sponsors". He described accurately both the clinical picture and the pathology of this condition and suggested that it was due to a virus. Later the introduction of the Frei (*v. infra*) reaction made the disorder easier to diagnose. Favre was one of the first to describe the pathology of a viral illness and in France to propose a classification for the lymphomas.

FAZIO-LONDE ATROPHY OR DISEASE

Hereditary bulbofacial progressive muscular atrophy.

E. Fazio (1849–1902) Italian physician who also wrote a monograph on public hygiene.

P.F.L. Londe (1865–1944) French neurologist.

FEDE-RIGA DISEASE

Ulcer on the under-surface of the tongue caused by the lower teeth when infants are still suckling.

Francesco Fede (1832–1913) Italian pediatrician.

Antonio Riga (1832–1919) Italian physician.

FEER DISEASE

Acrodynia – Pink disease.

SWIFT DISEASE (*v. infra*).

Emil Feer (1864–1955) Swiss pediatrician. His full name was E. Feer-Sulzer. One of the leading pediatricians of his day, he was Professor of Pediatrics in Heidelberg, Germany, from 1907–1911 and in Zurich from 1911–1929. He wrote a textbook of pediatrics which was internationally acclaimed and of which there were 18 editions with translations into many languages. He wrote another book entitled "Diagnosis of Diseases of Children" which ran for six editions. He was an excellent clinical observer who spent 15 years as a general practitioner prior to his specialization in pediatrics. He published over 105 papers in all fields of pediatrics ranging from nutrition to diphtheria and tuberculosis and eczema, but his most famous paper was that on "vegetative neurosis" which became known as Feer illness, in a paper which appeared in a volume dedicated to Heubner in a Festschrift for his 80th birthday. He trained innumerable pediatricians, many of whom went on to higher academic honors and held chairs in countries such as Germany and Poland. He devoted much of his life to development of the Children's Hospital at Zurich.

FEGELER SYNDROME

Capillary naevus preceded by sharply defined erythema and slight edema of the forehead and cheek following trauma to the neck. It is in the distribution of the Vth nerve and may be associated with ipsilateral weakness and hyperesthesia in the arm and leg.

Ferdinand Fegeler German dermatologist.

FEHLING TEST

Test for reducing substances (e.g. glucose) in the urine using Fehling solution, a mixture of copper sulphate, potassium hydroxide and potassium sodium tartrate.

Hermann von Fehling (1812–1855) German chemist whose test for sugar enabled the first quantitation of glycosuria in 1848.

FEIL-KLIPPEL SYNDROME

v. KLIPPEL-FEIL SYNDROME

FELTY SYNDROME

Pancytopenia, especially neutropenia and splenomegaly in rheumatoid arthritis.

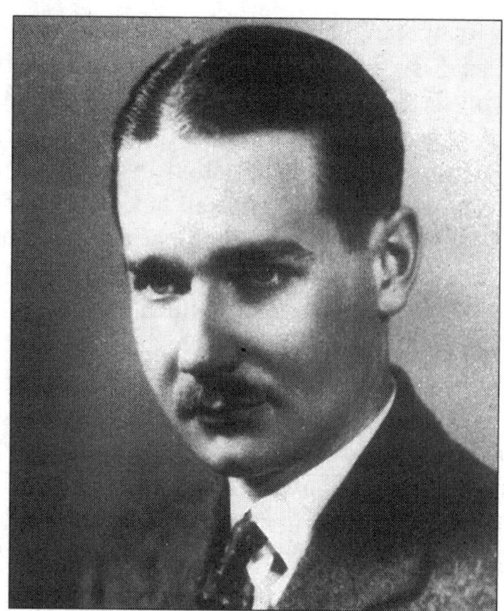

Augustus R. Felty (Courtesy of the Royal Society of Medicine, London, UK)

Augustus R. Felty (1895–1964) U.S. physician, Johns Hopkins Medical School. He was born in Abilene, Kansas, where his father, J.W. Felty, and his uncle were in general practice. His father moved to Hartford, Connecticut, and there he went to school and entered Yale College in 1912, intending to become an academic in the classical languages. He heard Sir William Osler lecture and decided to enter medical school. Graduating from Yale in 1916, he went to Johns Hopkins Medical School and graduated M.D. in 1920. After an internship on the Osler service from 1920–1921 he went to Columbia Presbyterian Hospital in New York as research fellow and there studied water and electrolyte acid base problems in dogs in which pyloric obstruction had been induced. He returned as an assistant resident to Johns Hopkins from 1922 to 1924 and it was during this period that he described Felty Syndrome. He published some papers on infectious diseases and epidemiology and although interested in a career in academic medicine felt obliged to take over his father's practice at Hartford where he remained until he retired in 1958. He died suddenly from a stroke.

FENWICK DISEASE

Gastric atrophy associated with pernicious anemia.

Samuel Fenwick (1821–1902) English physician. He was born in Northumberland at Earston House into a family which played a part in the history of the country for more than seven centuries (De Fenwyke was selected by William I to guard the border against the Scots), but his father lost his money and Fenwick was obliged to enter a professional career and he was apprenticed at the age of 14 to the Royal Infirmary at Newcastle. After 7 years he gained his M.R.C.S. (England) and in 1846 M.D. from the University of St. Andrews. He practiced in North Shields and soon built up a clinical reputation and published research on digestion and absorption in lower animals. His interest in histology led to his appointment as a lecturer in the Durham School of Medicine. He established a consulting practice in Newcastle, but in 1862 he moved to London and commenced practice in Harley Street, which at the time had only one other medical man in practice there. He was initially appointed as Assistant Physician to the Hospital for Diseases of the Chest, Victoria Park, and a few years later gained a similar post at the London Hospital. Apart from his busy consultant practice, he collected pathological specimens and conducted clinical investigations concerning mainly the diseases of the digestive system, and in 1865 published a book entitled "The Morbid States of the Stomach and Duodenum". He also released a book for medical students which resulted from his teaching, both at Newcastle and London Hospitals entitled "The Student's Guide to Medical Diagnosis". In it he instructs, "Remember to commit all your observations to writing. The number of well-recorded cases is invaluable and forms the best practice of physic for your future reference and guidance. Describe only what you see and hear, do it in the simplest language and do not allow your expressions to be influenced by any pre-conceived opinion as to the nature of the disease you are investigating. Be exact in your description of physical signs and as much as possible employ your pencil in marking on diagrams of the body the precise spots at which you discover any signs of disease. In this way, with ordinary industry in collecting cases and perfect honesty in recording your observations, you cannot fail quickly to surmount the difficulties of medical diagnosis". This was an extremely successful book which went through nine editions and was published in many languages. In 1879 he published a companion volume "Outlines of Medical Treatment". He wrote numerous papers, but his most important contribution was the description and discovery of atrophy of the stomach associated with pernicious anemia. He also made some excellent observations on perforation of the appendix and abscess formation. He was extremely popular with patients who gained great comfort from his presence at their bedside, "his presence was invariably attended by mental, if not physical, relief". He was an excellent teacher and consultant who still had a busy practice until a few weeks before his final illness. He died from cardiac failure due to aortic atheroma which was said to have involved his aortic valves.

FÉRÉOL NODE

Periarticular subcutaneous nodes in acute rheumatism.

L.H.F. Féréol (1825–1891) French physician.

FEULGEN REACTION

Staining reaction for DNA.

Robert Feulgen (1884–1955) German chemist who developed the technique and worked in Giessen.

FIBIGER TUMOR

Squamous cell carcinoma of the stomach in the rat caused by larvae of the nematode *Spiroptera neoplastica.*

Johannes A.G. Fibiger (1867–1928) Danish pathologist who was Professor of Pathology at the University of Copenhagen. One of the pioneers of experimental carcinogenesis he won the Nobel Prize in 1926 for his discovery of the spiroptera carcinoma, but this work has never been reproduced.

v. DEBRÉ-FIBIGER SYNDROME

FICK PRINCIPLE

$$\text{Cardiac output} = \frac{\text{oxygen consumption}}{\text{arteriovenous oxygen difference}} \times 100$$

Adolf E. Fick (1829–1901) German physiologist who was born in Kassel and went to medical school at the University of Marburg. Here he became a friend and pupil of Carl Ludwig who at the time was a Prosector to Fick's elder brother. He studied for a while in Berlin with Müller and Du Bois-Reymond and returned to Marburg to graduate. He worked briefly with his elder brother and then went to Zurich to renew his relationship with Ludwig who by then had become Professor of Physiology. When Ludwig left to take up an appointment in Vienna, he stayed on working under Professor Moleschott until 1862 when his former chief moved to the University of Turin, and he was appointed Professor of Physiology at Zurich. Whilst here he worked on diffusion and also the thermodynamics of muscular contraction with which he was helped by R. Clausius. In 1865, together with Wislicenus, he climbed one of the mountains to test Liebig's theory that albumin was the source of muscular energy. He was always interested in mathematics and physics, and applied these to the study of electrical stimulation in muscle work. In 1867 he discovered that muscle contraction and carbohydrate metabolism were linked. In 1868 he was appointed to the University of Würzburg where he remained until he retired in 1899. He developed and described his "Fick principle" here and published it in 1870. It was also here that he developed plethysmography to study blood flow through the arm. In 1882 he correlated mechanical conditions with heat production in muscle and produced evidence that muscle energy is transferred directly into work without heat being an intermediary. He was concerned with many social aspects including alcoholic consumption, education and even dress, and wrote several articles on political and other questions. He died suddenly on vacation.

FIEDLER MYOCARDITIS

Viral myocarditis.

Carl L.A. Fiedler (1835–1921) German physician who worked in Dresden.

FILATOV DISEASE

Infectious mononucleosis.

FILATOV SPOTS

v. KOPLIK SPOTS

FILATOV-DUKES DISEASE

v. DUKES DISEASE

Nil F. Filatov (1846–1902) Russian pediatrician, who came from an aristocratic family and was born at Pensa and received his initial schooling there in an institute for nobility. He entered medical school when 17 years old and graduated from the University of Moscow to go back to his district to practice as a country doctor. He did not find this intellectually rewarding, however, and undertook further training in Vienna, Paris, Berlin and in particular with Professor Steiner in Prague. After 2 years he returned to Moscow and began working and teaching in the old Children's Hospital in 1876. On the death of Professor Tolsky he was appointed as Professor of Paediatrics and also Director of a new Children's Hospital which was opened at that time. In 1892 the Moscow Paediatric Society was founded and Filatov was appointed as its president, to which position he was re-elected annually till he died. For the 3 years prior to his death he suffered from angina pectoris, but died suddenly of a stroke.

He first described glandular fever, which he called idiopathic adenitis, in his 2 volume textbook "Lectures on Acute Infectious Diseases of Children" which was published in Moscow in 1885–7. He described rubella in the same book.

FINKELDEY CELLS

v. WARTHIN-FINKELDEY GIANT CELLS

FISHER SYNDROME

Ophthalmoplegia, ataxia and loss of tendon reflexes – possibly a variant of Guillain-Barré Syndrome. Complete recovery is usual.

Miller Fisher U.S. neurologist at Massachusetts General Hospital and Harvard Medical School.

FITZGERALD TRAIT

Also called Flaujeauc and Williams trait or kallikrein deficiency, resulting in prolongation of clotting tests employing contact activation but rarely causing hemostatic problems or symptomatology. These were the names of patients in whom the defect was first appreciated.

FITZGERALD-GARDNER SYNDROME

v. GARDNER SYNDROME

FITZHUGH-CURTIS SYNDROME

Pain in the right upper quadrant of abdomen due to gonococcal peritonitis.

Thomas Fitzhugh (1894–1963) U.S. physician who was born in Baltimore, Maryland, but spent his early life in Charlottesville, Virginia, where his father was Professor of Latin. He gained his M.A. from the University of Virginia and enlisted in the U.S. army, serving as a private at the Base Hospital at St. Denis, France, in 1914–18. On his return he commenced medicine at the University of Virginia but graduated M.D. from the University of Pennsylvania where he remained for the rest of his professional career as chief of the hematological section of the University Hospital from 1929 until he retired in 1955. He was an outstanding teacher at the bedside who despite his busy practice made a number of contributions including the introduction of the term maturation arrest which he proposed in a patient with agranulocytosis, drawing analogy with red cell changes in pernicious anemia. He wrote a number of papers on the spleen, splenectomy and purpura and drew attention to the possible relationship of gall bladder disease and angina. He served with the U.S. army again in the 2nd World War being in charge of the 20th General Hospital in Assam, India and later being promoted to the rank of Colonel. He died of a bronchogenic carcinoma.

Arthur H. Curtis (1881–1955) U.S. obstetrician. He was born in Portage, Wisconsin, and went to medical school at Rush Medical College, Chicago, graduating in 1905 and interning at the Cook County Hospital. He undertook postgraduate work overseas and served with the American Forces overseas in World War I. He became Professor of Obstetrics and Gynecology at the Northwestern Medical School and was author of a textbook on "Gynaecology" and "Gynaecological Diagnosis" as well as editor of "Obstetrics and Gynaecology". He had a passionate interest in American football and was head football coach both at the University of Kansas in Lawrence and the University of Wisconsin in Madison. He died of a myocardial infarction.

FLATEAU (FLATAU) SYNDROME

Torsion dystonia, an autosomal recessive disorder with bizarre movements which may only be brought on by physical activity. Several reports have suggested that these patients often require less than normal time for sleep. The mean age of onset is around 11 years with movements of the trunk and neck being the most commonly involved.

FLATEAU-SCHILDER DISEASE

v. SCHILDER DISEASE

Edward Flateau (Flatau) (1869–1932) Polish neurologist. He was born in Plock and went to medical school at the University of Moscow where he graduated M.D. in 1892, being greatly influenced by the psychiatrist Korsakoff and the neurologist Kozhevnikof. He then went to work in Berlin with K. Mendel with whom he published a large atlas which was translated into many different languages. He worked with Waldeyer and J.K. Goldscheider (*v. infra*), and with him studied the influence of heat and chemicals as well as mechanical injuries to nerves. This work aroused much discussion and was emphasized by Nissl who was an opponent of the neurone theory. In 1896 he enunciated the Flatau law "the greater the length of the fibres in the spinal cord, the closer they are situated to the periphery". This followed his re-examination of Bastian's work on the results of section of the spinal cord.

In Waldeyer's laboratory he worked on comparative anatomy and by 1899 had established a name for himself both in Germany and abroad, but at that stage decided to return to Poland, where he went into private practice, but developed a private laboratory and eventually obtained an appointment in 1907 to the Jewish Hospital in Warsaw and in 1912 founded the Neurobiological Institute of Poland.

He wrote on almost every aspect of neurology, but in particular he made fine contributions on disseminated encephalomyelitis which in some circles is termed the Flatau-Redlich disease. He also made classical descriptions and studies on tumors of the spinal cord, migraine and tuberculous meningitis. Together with E.J. Remak he wrote a section on neuritis and polyneuritis for Nothnagel's textbook, and was very fond of quoting the latter "Only a good man can be a good physician". He died of a brain tumor.

FLECHSIG TRACT

Dorsal spinocerebellar tract.

Paul E. Flechsig (1847–1929) German neurologist. The son of a Protestant clergyman, he was born in Zurckav, Saxony, and studied medicine at Leipzig. He graduated in 1870 and served as a surgeon in the Franco-Prussian War, then returned to Leipzig and commenced his work on myelogenesis which led to his studies on the spinocerebellar and pyramidal tracts, and his conclusion that the function of the tracts required myelination. He mapped out various areas of the brain and assigned functions to them, and was the first to describe the auditory radiation. He had many famous students, including O. Vogt and Bekhterev. He was rather a stern figure who said it is the duty of a Professor to think "other than others". He intensely disliked socialism.

FLETCHER FACTOR

Prekallikrein. Fletcher factor was noted in coagulation studies which revealed a slow contact activation. It is not associated with abnormal bleeding.

Fletcher was the name of the patient in whom the defect was first recognized.

FLINDT SPOTS

v. KOPLIK SPOTS

Nicholaj Flindt (1843–1913) Danish physician.

FOIX SYNDROME

Paralysis of the 3rd, 4th, 5th and 6th cranial nerves together with proptosis and edema of the eyelids. There may also be trigeminal neuralgia.

FOIX-ALAJOUANINE SYNDROME

Subacute necrotizing myelopathy. This is often associated with thrombophlebitis or vascular malformation of the spinal cord. This results in spasticity of the lower limbs, sensory changes and sometimes loss of sphincter control.

Charles Foix (1882–1927) French neurologist who was born at Salies-de-Bearn near Bayonne, France. He studied medicine at the University of Paris and was a pupil of Pierre Marie. He was an intern in 1906, Médecin des Hôpitaux in 1919 and Agrégé in 1923. He taught at Guillain's Clinic at the Salpêtrière and at Achard's at the Hôpital Beaujon. His main approach was to relate thrombosis of specific arteries at autopsy with symptoms and signs that he had established in his patients and he wrote a book on the blood supply of the brain. He simultaneously described Schilder Disease so that this disorder is sometimes known as Schilder-Foix Disease.

A most impressive teacher and clinician, he was almost as much at home with general medicine as he was with neurology, and during the 1st World War was put in charge of a tuberculosis service. He was an accomplished poet, but even a better lyricist.

Théophile Alajouanine (1890–) French neurologist who was a pupil of Dejerine and worked with Guillain and Foix. He wrote prolifically on many neurological topics but was especially interested in aphasia.

FOLEY CATHETER

Urethral catheter which is retained by inflating a balloon.

Frederic E.B. Foley (1891–1966) U.S. urologist who worked in St. Paul, Minnesota. He also pioneered a new procedure for relieving stricture at the uretero-pelvic junction.

FONG LESION OR SYNDROME

Nail-Patella Syndrome. Transmitted as autosomal dominant. Nails of thumbs and great toes most commonly involved, ranging from longitudinal ridging to anonychia and there may be abnormalities with the iliac bones (symmetrical), e.g. horns, a cloverleaf area of pigmentation around inner margin of iris, sometimes mental defectiveness and renal abnormalities.

Edward E. Fong (1912–) U.S. radiologist who described the iliac horns as a chance radiological finding in a woman on whom intravenous pyelography was performed. He was at the time a Captain in the U.S. Army Medical Corps (1945).

FORBES DISEASE

Excessive glycogen storage is due to a deficiency of amylo-1-6, glucosidase (debrancher enzyme) resulting in hepatomegaly, cardiomegaly and muscle weakness.

Also termed Type 11 of Cori.

Gilbert B. Forbes (1915–) U.S. pediatrician born in Rochester, N.Y. and graduated M.D. from University of Rochester in 1940. Interned in pediatrics at Strong Memorial Hospital, Rochester, and then went to the St. Louis Children's Hospital in 1941, eventually becoming Associate Professor

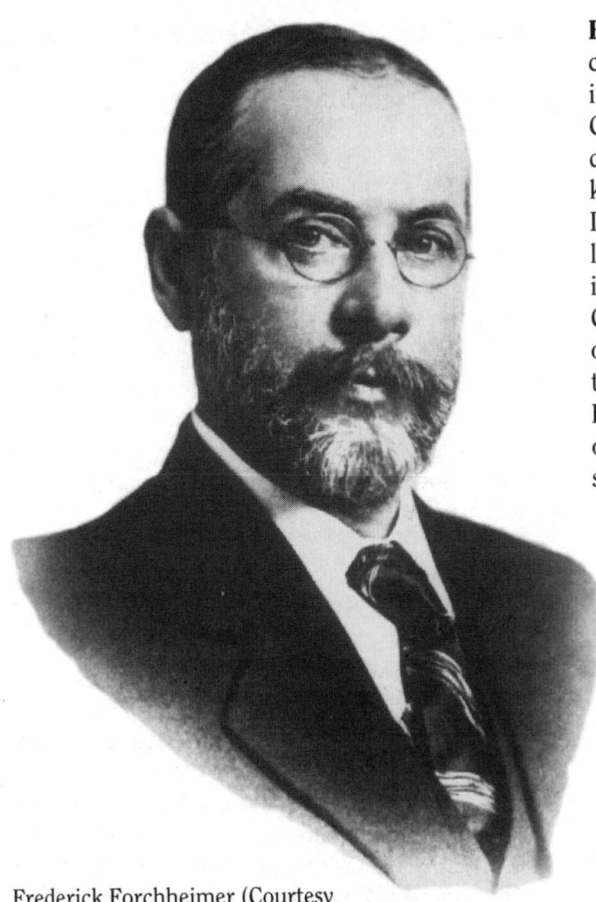

Frederick Forchheimer (Courtesy of the Royal Society of Medicine, London. UK)

there. In 1953 he returned to Rochester University, becoming Professor of Pediatrics in 1957.

FORBES-ALBRIGHT SYNDROME

Galactorrhea with intrasellar tumor.

Anne Forbes U.S. physician, Professor of Medicine, Massachusetts General Hospital.

Fuller Albright (*v. supra*).

FORCHHEIMER SIGN

Rose red maculopapular eruption of the soft palate preceding skin eruption of rubella (cf. KOPLIK SPOTS).

Frederick Forchheimer (1853–1913) U.S. pediatrician. His early reputation was established when in 1875 he became an instructor in the Medical College of Ohio and soon after founded a clinic for diseases of children, which was one of the first of its kind in the United States. He became Professor of Diseases of Children in the same College and published extensively on pediatrics and in particular, in 1892, a book entitled "Diseases of the Mouth in Children" where he described his sign. He was one of the medical leaders in Cincinatti and at the time of his death was Professor of Medicine and Head of the Department of Medicine in the College of Medicine in the University of Cincinatti. His standing in the United States is shown by the fact that he was elected President of the Association of American Physicians in 1911 and received an Honorary Doctor of Science degree from Harvard University in 1912. He died following an operation on his prostate gland to relieve acute retention.

FORDYCE LESION

Angiomas of the scrotum. Commonly seen in the elderly, these are venous in origin and appear as small blue lesions 1–2 mm in diameter usually following the course of a vein. They are of no significance.

FORDYCE SPOTS

White or yellow spots 1 mm in diameter on the mucosal surface of lips, cheeks or tongue – mucosal sebaceous cysts.

John Fordyce (1858–1925) U.S. dermatologist. He described the lesions in 1896 and practiced in New York.

FORSSMAN ANTIGENS

Heterophile antibodies – antibodies directed against antigens which occur naturally in other species.

M.J. Forssman (1868–1947) Swedish pathologist who became Professor of General Pathology and

Bacteriology at Lund University, Sweden. He made important observations on nerve regeneration as well as discovering and investigating the Forssman antigens.

FOSTER KENNEDY SYNDROME

Unilateral optic atrophy with contralateral papilledema and anosmia usually due to a frontal lobe tumor.

Robert Foster Kennedy (1884–1952) Born in Belfast, Ireland, he graduated in medicine in 1906 from the Royal University of Ireland. He then worked at the National Hospital, Queen's Square, and in particular was influenced by Sir William Gowers, Hughlings Jackson, Sir Victor Horsley and Sir Henry Head. After four years there he was invited in 1910 to come to the recently established New York Neurological Institute. When the Ist World War broke out in 1914 he went to France and worked in a French Military Hospital and subsequently with a British unit. He worked close to and in the front line and having a number of narrow escapes himself understood some of the problems better than most. He was the first to point out that shell shock was hysteria and he believed that this rose from an insoluble conflict between the soldier's instinct for self-preservation and his herd instinct. He outlined this in a paper he published in 1918 entitled "The nature of nervousness in soldiers" and in this he crossed swords with Freud's views on the application of psychoanalysis to psychosomatic illness. He pointed out that in the Ist World War there were more neuroses, but no more psychoses. When he returned to the U.S. there was an encephalitis epidemic and his wards at the Bellevue Hospital, New York, were full of these patients. In 1923 he published a paper "Epilepsy and the convulsive state" in which he described the "Foster Kennedy Syndrome". He wrote extensively on tumors involving the brain and the resultant symptomatology produced and was one of the first to use electroconvulsive treatment in the management of psychosis. He became Professor of Neurology at Cornell University and in 1940 was elected President of the American Neurological Association. He contributed to many areas of neurology and neuropsychiatry, but perhaps is best remembered for his work on tumors, lesions of the hypothalamus and functional psychosomatic disorders, especially those related to war service.

He was a kindly man who had a ready turn of phrase and was well known for his cutting remarks and aphorisms. He was not unknown to unobtrusively slip a few dollars to a poverty stricken patient from the Lower East Side of New York as the best method of treatment for a problem. He was awarded the Chevalier of the Legion of Honour by France and he died in his own ward in Bellevue Hospital following an intestinal hemorrhage which was a complication of periarteritis nodosa which developed 12 months earlier.

FOTHERGILL DISEASE

Trigeminal neuralgia or tic doloreaux.

John Fothergill (1712–1780) English physician, who was born in Carr End, Yorkshire. He was a Quaker who studied medicine at Edinburgh university – being a dissenter he could not enter an English University. Although initially enrolled as an apothecary, he was noticed by Monro (*v. infra*) who influenced him to change to medicine. He graduated in 1736 and went to St. Thomas's Hospital, London, and there developed a reputation for kindness and help to the poor which led him to remark later "I climbed on the backs of the poor to the pockets of the rich". He described both diphtheria and streptococcal throat but did not differentiate the two. He worked extraordinarily long hours and gained one of the most lucrative practices in London, and was the first Edinburgh graduate to become a Fellow of the Royal College of Physicians. J. Wakley Lettsom was a protégé of his. Benjamin Franklin wrote to him "By the way, where do you intend to live?", when he collaborated with Franklin in a plan for reconciliation between the U.S.A. and England in 1774. Lord North proposed that he become Physician to the King but he declined. He had many Quaker relationships with Americans in Philadelphia and aided many Americans who came to London to study medicine after the Revolution. He also donated money and anatomical papers, models and skeletons to the Pennsylvania Hospital. He was very active in prison reform and the abolition of slavery. Apart from tic doloreaux, he first described the association of coronary sclerosis with angina pectoris. He had a magnificent botanical garden and collection of insects, shells and drawings, which he left to his friend William Hunter after he died.

FOURNIER DISEASE OR GANGRENE SYNDROME

Fulminating infection of the scrotum leading to gangrene and commonly associated with diabetes. The infective agents are anaerobic *Bacteroides fragilis* and the aerobic *E. coli*.

Jean A. Fournier (1832–1914). French venereologist who described the condition in 1883. He wrote a book on the effects of congenital syphilis and in it first described the anterior bowing of the tibia.

FOVILLE PARALYSIS OR SYNDROME

Conjugate ocular paralysis with or without peripheral 7th nerve palsy and contralateral spastic paralysis due to lesion in the pons.

Achille L.F. Foville (1799–1878) French neurologist who wrote on comparative neuroanatomy. Whilst an intern at the Salpêtrière worked with a number of famous Parisian physicians including Esquirol, and commenced his work on anatomy and physiology of the nervous system and was especially intrigued by cerebral localization. He published clinical observations on insanity, and in 1825 he was appointed Medical Superintendent at the Saint-You Asylum in Rouen which had just been opened. He soon became well known, publishing papers on disorders of the nervous system and developing an outstanding reputation as a Director of Asylums and became Professor of Physiology at the Medical School at Rouen. Ill health forced him to resign from Saint-You in 1833 and he spent some time in travelling, including a trip to Africa and America. He returned to Paris and re-commenced his studies on the brain, and when Esquirol died he was appointed successor at Sharenton in 1840. Four years later he published an important work on the anatomy of the nervous system of the spinal cord which was one of the best works prior to the introduction of the microscope. He lost his post at Sharenton during the Revolution in 1848 and commenced private practice. For the next 20 years he was regarded as one of the best physicians treating mental disorders in Paris. He retired to Toulouse where he continued in a role as a consultant physician. He described his syndrome in 1848.

FOWLER POSITION

Semi-reclining position in bed which was used as part of the treatment of peritonitis.

George R. Fowler (1848–1906) U.S. surgeon. Professor of Surgery, New York Polyclinic School, who performed the first thoracoplasty in 1893. He was born in New York City and later moved to Jamaica, Long Island, where his father was the master mechanic in charge of the repair shops of the Long Island railroad. When he was 12 the Civil War broke out and he ran away to join up, but was found by the police and returned safely to his parents. He was working as an apprentice in the railway repair shop when he went to the assistance of a worker who had had an accident. This commenced his interest in medicine and he enrolled in the Bellevue Hospital Medical College, graduating in 1871. He was too poor to undertake internships and he immediately went into practice where he worked as a general practi-

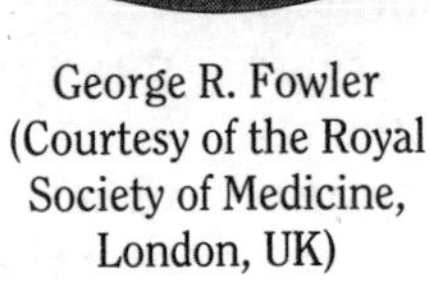

George R. Fowler (Courtesy of the Royal Society of Medicine, London, UK)

tioner for 15 years, but became increasingly interested in surgery. He was one of the first to adopt Lister's ideas concerning antisepsis, but it was some time before he could gain a hospital appointment.

In 1883, he finally gained an appointment to a newly opened hospital, St. Mary's Hospital. During the Spanish-American War he was commissioned a Chief Surgeon of Division and Chief of the Operating Staff of the 7th Army Corps, a role he fulfilled throughout the war. In 1890 the State of New York instituted a State Board of Medical Examiners and he was appointed as one of its organizers and a Chair of Surgery was given to him, a position he retained whilst he lived. He was an extremely energetic man who appeared to be tireless both day and night and his most important contributions were on the subjects of the early operative treatment of appendicitis and his method of positioning the patient for the treatment of general peritonitis, "Fowler Position", and also his innovation of decortication of the lung in chronic emphysema. He was one of the first to advocate early radical surgical interference in appendicitis (1894). In 1906 he had just finished his book on surgery, and whilst travelling to a medical meeting he had acute abdominal pain and on operation was found to have a gangrenous appendix, developed paralytic ileus and on the 6th post-operative day had a heart attack and died.

FOWLER SOLUTION

Potassium arsenate solution used to administer arsenic therapeutically, e.g. in treatment of leukemia.

Thomas Fowler (1736–1801) English physician. He introduced his solution in 1786. He was an acquaintance of William Withering whom he first met when Fowler was an apothecary in York. Later he studied medicine at Edinburgh, graduating in 1778 and introduced his arsenical solution as a treatment for fevers and subsequently he took over Withering's practice in Stafford, and with the apothecary Hughes produced a quack remedy of liquor arsenalis called "Tasteless ague and fever drops".

FRANCIS TRIAD

Asthma, nasal polyps and aspirin sensitivity.

Clement A. Francis (1898–1951) English otolaryngologist. He was born in Queensland, Australia, son of a well known Brisbane ear, nose and throat surgeon, who had suggested the theory that asthma was often due to vasomotor abnormalities. His father returned to London to practice as an asthma specialist. He served in the Royal Field Ambulance as a lieutenant in Palestine and following the war studied medicine at Cambridge and St. Bartholomew's Hospital, London, graduating in 1925. He specialized in otolaryngology, studying in London and Vienna, and was appointed surgeon to the Metropolitan Ear, Nose and Throat Hospital. Here he developed a fine reputation as a dexterous surgeon and continued his father's treatment of asthma using light cauterization of the nasal septum. He published numerous papers on allergy and asthma and was the first to lay emphasis on the group of asthmatics who were aspirin sensitive. A keen sportsman, he was a member of the Marylebone Cricket Club (MCC) and a good cricketer as well as golfer.

FRANÇOIS SYNDROME

v. HALLERMAN-STREIF-FRANÇOIS SYNDROME

Jules François Belgian ophthalmologist. He was Professor of Ophthalmology in Ghent from around 1950 to 1980 and was renowned for his surgical ability as well as his diagnostic acumen.

FRANK CAPILLARY TOXICOSIS

Non-thrombocytopenic purpura.

Alfred E. Frank (1884–1957) German physician. He identified diabetes insipidus as being due to a lesion of the posterior pituitary.

FRANK SIGN

Oblique fissure of the ear lobe associated with coronary disease, hypertension and diabetes. This is an

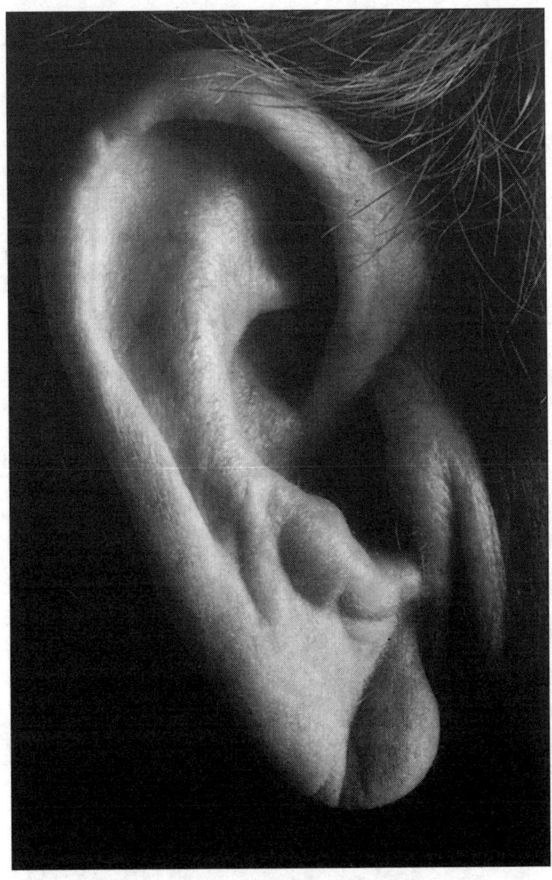

Frank sign

acquired sign and must be distinguished from the congenital crease seen in newborn infants, a feature of Beckwith Syndrome (*v. supra*) which may also be present in normal children.

Sanders T. Frank (1938–) U.S. chest physician. He was born in Middletown, Connecticut and graduated M.D. from the New York Medical College in 1943. He is the Director of Respiratory Care at the Garfield Medical Center, Monterey Park, California and an Associate Clinical Professor of Medicine.

FRANKLIN DISEASE

Heavy chain disease. Dysproteinemia where the paraprotein is a dimer of the heavy γ chain of the γ globulin molecule.

Edward C. Franklin (1929–1982) U.S. investigator, New York School of Medicine, New York. He was born in Berlin and migrated to the U.S.A. in 1939. He graduated M.D. from the New York University (NYU) School of Medicine in 1950 and worked at the Rockefeller and then at NYU where he became a Professor in 1968.

FREEMAN RULE

cf. McNAGHTON RULE

Mental disease or circumstance preventing a person having knowledge of what he is doing makes him not responsible for crimes committed.

U.S. vs. Charles Freeman, 1966.

FREI DISEASE

Lymphogranuloma venereum.

FREI TEST

Intracutaneous injection of material from the infected gland.

Wilhelm S. Frei (1885–1943) German dermatologist, born in Neustadt (Prudnik), Upper Silesia, and studied at the Robert Koch Institute in Berlin, University of Göttingen and Breslau, and was appointed Privatdozent in Dermatology in 1923 and Professor in 1926 at the Berlin-Spandau Municipal Hospital. He migrated to the U.S. and was resident physician in dermatology in the Montefiore Hospital in New York, 1937 and 1938. Apart from his research on venereal disease he published on allergic skin diseases.

FREIBERG DISEASE

v. KÖHLER DISEASE

Albert H. Freiberg (1868–1940) U.S. surgeon. He was born in Cincinnatti, Ohio, and studied medicine at the Medical College of Ohio and later the

Medical Department of the University of Cincinnati in 1890. After graduation he studied in Würzburg, Berlin, Strasburg and Vienna, and returned to the U.S.A. to commence practice in Cincinnati in 1893. From 1902 to 1938 he was Professor of Orthopedic Surgery at the University of Cincinnati College of Medicine. He was an accomplished violinist and a keen amateur botanist and photographer who was particularly active in trying to improve the lot of crippled children and had a keen social conscience.

FREY SYNDROME

Auriculo-temporal syndrome. Sweating, flushing and warm feeling in the distribution of the auriculo-temporal nerve which may be triggered by eating and may follow surgery, or injury to parotid, 7th nerve palsy or diabetes.

Lucie Frey (1889–1944) Polish physician who practiced in Warsaw. She was killed by the Nazis.

FREUDIAN

Refers to theories of Freud.

Sigmund Freud (1856–1939) Austrian psychiatrist who was born in Freiberg in Moravia and came to Vienna aged 4, where he studied medicine. He worked in Bruche's physiology laboratory from 1876–1881, gaining his doctor's degree. He then worked in the Institute of Cerebral Anatomy, under Meynert, and became Privatdozent in Neuroanatomy in 1885. With Kolles he studied the treatment of morphine addicts with cocaine. He revolutionized psychiatric theory and management, emphasizing the importance of repressed and suppressed sexuality, and introduced questioning under hypnosis, interpretation of dreams and the psychoanalytic approach to therapy. He was a pupil of Charcot and became a Professor of Neurology in Vienna where he developed an internationally famous school with students such as Jung and Adler.

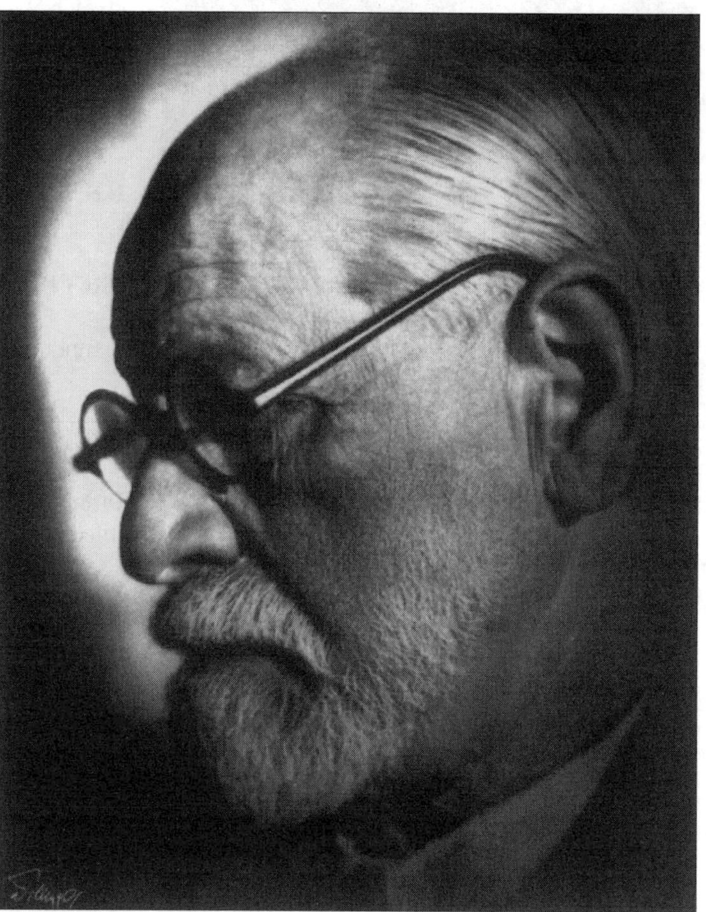

Sigmund Freud (Courtesy of the Royal Society of Medicine, London, UK)

FREUND ADJUVANT

Emulsion added to antigen which greatly increases an animal's response to the antigen following injection.

J.T. Freund (1891–1960) Hungarian bacteriologist who lived in the U.S.A.

FRIDERICHSEN SYNDROME

v. WATERHOUSE-FRIDERICHSEN SYNDROME

FRIEDLANDER BACILLUS

Klebsiella pneumoniae.

FRIEDLANDER CELLS

Cells of uterine deciduis.

FRIEDLANDER PNEUMONIA

Pneumonia caused by the bacillus.

Carl Friedlander (1847–1887) German pathologist and bacteriologist. He was born at Brieg (Silesia) and studied medicine at Breslau, Würzburg, Zurich and Berlin.

He was assistant firstly to Heidenhain and later worked with von Recklinghausen. Apart from discovering the bacillus which bears his name, he also edited a journal and undoubtedly would have made many more contributions to medicine but developed pulmonary tuberculosis and died five years later.

FRIEDMAN TEST

Modification of Asheim-Zondek pregnancy test, using rabbits instead of mice.

Maurice H. Friedman (1903–) U.S. physiologist and physician. He was born in East Chicago, Indiana, and graduated M.D. from the University of Chicago in 1932 after gaining a Ph.D. in physiology in 1928. After interning at the Michael Rees Hospital he joined the physiology department at the University of Pennsylvania becoming assistant professor. During World War II he investigated the circulatory effects of dive bombing. At the end of the war he became involved in clinical medicine and later went into private practice.

FRIEDREICH ATAXIA

Hereditary spinocerebellar degenerative disease. Clinical manifestations are ataxia, diminished deep tendon reflexes, upgoing plantars, high plantar arch and nystagmus. 30–50% have clinical cardiac manifestations and up to 90% have ECG anomalies relating to an associated cardiomyopathy.

FRIEDREICH DISEASE OR SPASMS

Paramyoclonus multiplex.

FRIEDREICH SIGN

Inspiration causes a lowering in pitch of the percussion note of a cavity in the lung.

Nikolaus Friedreich (1825–1882) German neurologist. He was born in Würzburg and succeeded Virchow as Extraordinarius in the Chair of Pathology there. A year later he went to Heidelberg (1857) as Professor Ordinaire of Pathology and Treatment. He was a fine clinician and teacher, and his pupils included A. Kussmaul, Fr. Schultze and W. Erb. He wrote a significant treatise on progressive muscular atrophy which he dedicated to his teacher Virchow: "To me as a clinician the principles of cellular pathology have become the cynosure in the labrynth of pathological process".

FROEHLICH SYNDROME

Adiposogenital dystrophy. Pituitary tumor with obesity and sexual infantilism.

Alfred Froehlich (1871–1953) Austrian physician who described his syndrome in 1901. He was born in Vienna and went to medical school there, graduating from the University of Vienna in 1895 when he joined the medical department of Professor Nothnagel as well as having an attachment to the Institute of Pathology with Professor S. Basch. In 1901 he described "a case of tumor of the hypophysis cerebri without acromegaly" with an emphasis on the obesity and infantilism associated with pituitary tumors.

In 1901 he visited Liverpool and worked with Sir Charles Sherrington and whilst he was there met Harvey Cushing (*v. supra*) and a life-long friendship developed. He became very interested in the physiology and pharmacology of the nervous system, and joined Langley in Cambridge in 1904 where he studied the autonomic nervous system.

He became a full time member of the Department of Pharmacology at the University of Vienna in 1905, initially under the direction of H. Meyer and then D.P. Pick. He investigated the pharmacology of cocaine with Otto Loewi and he also examined the effects of the pituitary on the autonomic nervous system. He had a long interest in comparative pharmacology and physiology and spent time in marine laboratories in Naples and Helgoland, Germany, as well as Woods Hole, Massachusetts. From 1919 to 1939 he was a full Professor of Pharmacology and Toxicology but following Hitler's invasion of Austria, he migrated to the United States where he joined the May Institute of Medical Research of the Jewish Hospital of Cincinnati. Here he had an association initially with I.A. Mirsky, and later Dr. Sol Sherry, who were Directors of the Institute, and there he continued his experimental studies on the central nervous system.

An extremely cultured man, he had wide interests. In 1908 he met Rudyard Kipling in Switzerland and until World War I there was a lively correspondence between the two, and an annual rendezvous in Switzerland. He was a superb conversationalist and had a deep understanding of both science and the arts. He loved music and was an accomplished pianist, having studied harmony with the Austrian composer Anton Bruckner.

FROIN SYNDROME

High protein in the CSF associated with xanthochromia and coagulation due to obstruction of the spinal subarachnoid space.

Georges Froin (1874–) French physician who described the above in 1903.

FROMENT SIGN

Ulnar palsy results in paralysis of adductor pollicis, so that if a patient holds a piece of paper between the index finger and thumb the thumb flexes.

Jules Froment (1878–1946) A French physician who graduated in 1906 and in World War I was with the front line troops in an ambulance, but in 1915 was recalled to the neurology service at Rennes where he found many cases of peripheral nerve injuries which became one of his major interests. Shortly after, he was sent to Paris to work with Babinski, who had a major influence on him. After the war returned to Lyon and studied the epidemic of encephalitis which occurred between 1918 and 1922 and its resultant complications of Parkinsonism. He developed a long standing interest in aphasia and language difficulties in general. In 1938 he was appointed Professor of Clinical Medicine succeeding Professor Paviot and held the chair until 1945 when he resigned due to ill health.

FROMMEL DISEASE

Involution of the uterus following prolonged lactation.

Richard J.E. Frommel (1854–1912) German gynecologist who was born in Augsburg and studied medicine at Munich and Göttingen finally graduating from the University of Würzburg. He worked in Vienna and Berlin where he was Schroder's assistant, spent some time in private practice and was appointed Professor of Obstetrics in Erlangen where he gained a reputation as a teacher and published widely on clinical aspects of his discipline as well as an investigation of the placenta of the bat. He retired to private practice in 1901 and died of appendicitis.

FRORIEP INDURATION

Fibrous myositis following inflammation.

Robert Froriep (1804–1861) German anatomist and surgeon with whom Virchow (*v. infra*) worked as an assistant. He worked in Berlin.

FUCHS ATROPHY

Peripheral atrophy of the optic nerve.

FUCHS DYSTROPHY

Familial degenerative condition of the eye seen more commonly in women, with clouding of the cornea and often complicated by glaucoma.

FUCHS PHENOMENON

Paradoxical lid retraction associated with eye movements during 3rd nerve regeneration.

Ernst Fuchs (1851–1930) Austrian ophthalmologist who practiced in Vienna. He studied medicine in Vienna where he was a pupil of Billroth and following graduation became an assistant to Arlt who was then Professor of Ophthalmology in Vienna, and for whom throughout his life Fuchs had the greatest admiration and respect. His earliest work consisted of an examination of the pathology of conditions of the eye and this approach enabled him to publish in 1881 an analysis of sarcoma of the uveal tract based on 259 patients. In the same year he was appointed to the Chair of Ophthalmology in the University of Liege. It had been pointed out earlier that myopia was often associated with crescents observed with the ophthalmoscope on the outer margin of the optic disc due to choroidal atrophy. In 1882 Fuchs emphasized the difference between the acquired atrophic crescents and congenital crescents due to a defect in the development of the choroid which usually occurs at the lower margin of the optic disc and which is small and oval horizontally – a condition often referred to now as Fuchs Colomboma. In 1885 he returned to Vienna, publishing an important paper on the anatomy of the iris, and in 1889 the first edition of his textbook of ophthalmology "Lehrbuch der Augenheilkunde". This book was taken from his lectures in an endeavor to ensure that his students listened to his lectures rather than distract themselves by taking notes. It was a classic in its time and published in all European languages as well as Japanese and Chinese (v. DUANE). He employed the then new technique of using large print for material suitable for students and small print for that which he felt was important for people who were continuing to study ophthalmology as a postgraduate exercise. Beer was the first Professor of Ophthalmology in Vienna, appointed in 1812, and he was succeeded by Fuchs' teacher, Arlt, who rapidly made Vienna the centre of the world for this speciality. Fuchs added to this renown and an idea of the number of patients he saw may be gauged from an article in 1897 on "retinitis circinata" where he states that of 70,000 patients he had seen during the 7½ years in his clinic, he had only seen 11 patients with this rare condition.

The Shah of Persia, Nasr-ed-Din, sent his favourite wife, who had been diagnosed as having a cataract, together with several other women with cataracts, to Fuchs for his treatment. When Fuchs examined her he found that she had glaucoma and there was nothing he could do, but he was able to remove the cataracts from the women who accompanied her. The Shah could never comprehend how Fuchs could restore the sight of servants and could do nothing for his favorite concubine.

Fuchs was a great traveller and also enjoyed walking on his vacations in out-of-the-way places. Besides his clinical descriptions of diseases of the eye and his accurate recording of the various afflictions of the retina, as well as his interest in histopathology, he also was an innovator in surgery. Largely through his efforts the age-old custom of a patient after a cataract operation being kept in bed with both eyes covered in a dark room for a week before the dressings were changed, was abandoned and he introduced early ophthalmoscopic examination after these operations which enabled him to discover that choroidal detachment was far more common than had previously been imagined. He visited most European countries and in 1911 undertook a lecture tour of the United States.

At the outbreak of the 1st World War he was a very wealthy man as one might imagine from the size of his practice, and he lived accordingly, but after the war, due to the inflation that ensued, he became quite hard up, and in view of his age could do little about it, although he was helped greatly by his friends and admirers, who enabled him to undertake a lecture tour to the United States; subsequently he visited Spain, Egypt and Asia Minor.

A tall man with a slight stoop, he apparently embodied all Osler's ideals of equinamitas, maintaining a calm and unruffled exterior and never being angry or impatient. He spoke excellent English and maintained his investigatory curiosity right to the very end, when he died with angina pectoris.

G

GAISBÖCK (GEISBÖCK) DISEASE OR SYNDROME

Stress polycythemia or relative polycythemia. A somewhat controversial syndrome where the patient presents with headache, neurasthenia and elevated hematocrit and hemoglobin, but the red cell mass is found to be normal and the plasma volume is reduced.

Felix Gaisböck (Geisböck) (1868–1955) Austrian physician.

GALENICAL

Any medicine prepared from plants in contradistinction to chemicals.

Claudius Galen (130–200 A.D.) Born in Pergamum, now Bergama in Turkey. He was the son of an architect and studied at a number of the leading medical schools of the time (Smyrna, Corinth and Alexandria). At 28 he returned to Pergamum where he was surgeon to the gladiators for the next 4 years and then went to Rome where he commenced practice and gave lectures on anatomy. He rapidly became a well known physician and treated the Emperor Marcus Aurelius when reputedly he had intestinal colic following the consumption of a large amount of cheese. He became the Emperor's personal physician and accompanied him on a military expedition to Germany. After the Emperor's death he was appointed personal physician to the succeeding Emperors, Commodus and Septimus Severus. When he retired he ceased practice and travelled extensively. He was the first person to prove that arteries carried blood and to describe the cranial nerves and sympathetic system and showed that section of the spinal cord caused paraplegia. He was also the first to describe arterial aneurysm and distinguish between pneumonia and pleurisy. He added loss of function to the 4 classical signs of inflammation already described by Celsus, namely redness, heat, pain and swelling. Unlike Hippocrates, he had a great faith in drugs and had a plant collection from all corners of the globe. He wrote an incredible volume of work and always seemed to have an answer or cure for everything, again unlike Hippocrates. Although he seems never to have dissected a human body, his principles of physiology and anatomy were blindly accepted for almost 15 centuries and indeed they were regarded by the medical establishment of most countries in Europe as an infallible dogma which it was a sin to contravene.

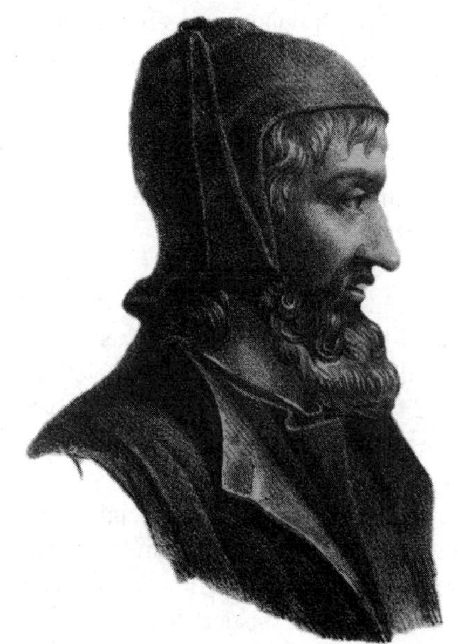

Claudius Galen (Courtesy of the Royal Society of Medicine, London, UK)

GALVANIC CURRENT

Continuous electric current in one direction.

Luigi Galvani (1737–1798) Born in Bologna, where he studied medicine, and graduated in 1759. He was Professor of Operative Surgery and Anatomy (1766).

He demonstrated that two dissimilar metals on contact with frog's muscle caused it to contract, generating an electric current, and that animal tissue could generate electricity. Shortly before his death he was dismissed from his position because he refused to swear allegiance to the new Cisalpine Republic.

GAMNA-FAVRE BODIES

Cytoplasmic inclusions seen in lymphogranuloma venereum.

GAMNA-GANDY BODIES

Brown nodules in the spleen due to deposition of hemosiderin and calcium seen in congestive splenomegaly.

Carlos Gamna (1886–1950) Italian physician.

M. Favre (1876–1954) French physician (*v. supra*).

Charles Gandy (1872–) French physician.

GAMPER BOWING REFLEX

Reflex seen in children with severe brain damage and occasionally in normal premature infants, due to release of the pons from cortical impulses. With the sacrum held, the hips are extended and the baby's head and trunk elevate from the supine position as in a bow.

Eduard Gamper (1887–1938) Austrian neurologist. Born in Kappl (Tirol) and went to university at Innsbruck graduating in 1911. He was appointed Professor of Psychiatry and Neuropathology at Innsbruck in 1930, then went to the German University at Prague and finally joined Spielmeyer in Munich.

GAMSTORP DISEASE

Periodic paralysis, usually with hyperkalemia. It has an autosomal dominant inheritance and in its mildest form expresses itself as asymptomatic myotonia.

Ingrid Gamstorp (1907–) Swedish pediatric neurologist who also described another unusual muscle disorder characterized by myokynesia (persistent quivering in a few muscle fibres, live flesh), cramps, hyperhydrosis and sometimes muscle wasting. She was Professor of Child Neurology at Uppsala but described the periodic paralysis whilst working in Lund.

GANSER SYNDROME

Nonsensical or wrong answers to questions, seen especially in prisoners awaiting trial, and believed to be a form of hysteria.

Sigbert J.M. Ganser (1853–1931) German psychiatrist, born in Dresden. Worked in Munich as von Gudden's assistant and suggested to Nissl (*v. infra*) that he examine the pathology of cortical cells. He became Professor and Head of Neurology at Dresden and here taught and trained Quekenstedt (*v. infra*).

GARDNER SYNDROME

Autosomal dominant. Variant of congenital polyposis of the colon – adenomatous polyposis of the large bowel with multiple osteomata of the skull and mandible and multiple epidermoid cysts and soft tissue tumors of the skin.

Eldon J. Gardner (1909–) U.S. geneticist born in Logan, Utah, and gained his Ph.D. at the University of California in 1939 in zoology. He was teaching a course in genetics at the University of Utah and mentioned in one of his lectures a study which was being commenced there on inheritance of various types of cancer. At the end of the talk a pre-medical student came up to him and told him that he knew of a family from his home town who had a high incidence of cancer. It was the study of this family which resulted in the description of the syndrome. He was appointed Professor of Zoology at Utah State University from 1949–1974 and is now emeritus Professor of Zoology at the University. He has written a textbook on genetics and another book on the history of biology, and over the years his research interests have been in drosophila and human genetics.

GARLAND TRIANGLE

An area of relative resonance found near the spine posteroinferiorly in the presence of a pleural effusion.

George Minot Garland (1848–1926) U.S. physician who graduated from Harvard in 1874, was assistant in physiology (1877–1881) and then Instructor in Clinical Medicine 1881–1892 at Harvard and finally physician at Massachusetts General Hospital, Boston.

GARROD HYPOTHESIS

One gene, one enzyme defect.

GARROD PADS

Pads present on the dorsal aspect of the proximal interphalangeal joints, which may be painful on flexion.

Sir Archibald Garrod (1857–1936) English physician at St. Bartholomew's Hospital. He wrote a treatise on gout and devised a test for uric acid and porphyrins. He was the son of another distinguished physician, Sir Alfred Garrod. Garrod graduated from Oxford University and St. Bartholomew's Hospital and succeeded Osler on the latter's death, as Regius Professor at Oxford. He discussed inborn errors of metabolism in his Croonian Lecture which was published as a book in 1909 and was a milestone in medical genetics. He was elected F.R.S. in 1910. He first clearly distinguished rheumatoid arthritis from rheumatism and gout, in 1890, and made many contributions to the chemistry of urine and urinary pigments, especially in the fields of porphyria and cystinuria. He was a co-editor of the Quarterly Journal of Medicine for 20 years. His three sons died in the 1st World War. His daughter became a well known archeologist and anthropologist at Cambridge University, where he and his wife went to live after he retired from Oxford in 1927.

GARTNER CYST

Benign cyst in the antero-lateral wall of the vagina. A remnant of Gartner Duct.

GARTNER DUCT

Ductus epoophri longitudinalis. It may persist in the mesosalpinx near the ovary or the lateral wall of the vagina.

Hermann T. Gartner (1785–1827) Danish surgeon who was born in St. Thomas, then a Danish possession in the West Indies. When he was 10 years old he returned to Copenhagen. He studied medicine in Copenhagen graduating in 1807 and worked in London and Edinburgh. He served in the army in Norway and later entered practice. In 1824 he was appointed as a surgeon in the Danish army.

GASSER CELLS

Inclusions in lymphocyte or monocyte cytoplasm which stain dark red-purple with Romanowsky stains are seen in mucopolysaccharide syndromes, e.g. Hurler, Hunter, but not in Morquio Syndrome.

GASSER SYNDROME

1. Acute transient aplasia of erythropoietic tissue in young children, cause unknown but probably related to infections, e.g. parvovirus.
2. Acute hemolytic uremic (HUR) syndrome in children.

Conrad Gasser (1912–) Swiss pediatrician who was born in Chur and studied medicine in Rome, Vienna and Berlin before graduating in Zurich (1937) where he joined Professor G. Fanconi's department in 1941. Whilst performing reticulocyte counts on newly admitted children he noted some with a reticulocytopenia, and marrow examination revealed a dramatic reduction in erythropoiesis which he reported in 1949. He described the Gasser cells in 1950 and reported the HUR syndrome in 1955. He was appointed Professor at the University of Zurich in 1962. He has made numerous contributions in pediatric hematology including ABO incompatibility causing hemolysis in the newborn (1948).

GASTAUT SYNDROME

Hemi-convulsion hemiplegic epilepsy in young children who may have an associated aura of fear and display sucking movements. The signs are ipsilateral.

Henri Gastaut (1915–) French neurologist.

v. LENNOX-GASTAUT SYNDROME

GAUCHER CELLS

Large histiocytes (20–80 μm) with an eccentrically placed nucleus and fibrillar looking cytoplasm (onion skin).

GAUCHER DISEASE

Familial disorder due to deficiency of β glucocerebrosidase resulting in accumulation of glucocerebroside in cells. Features include hepatosplenomegaly, skin pigmentation, pingueculae of the sclera, bone lesions and later anemia and thrombocytopenia.

Phillipe C.E. Gaucher (1854–1918) French physician and dermatologist. As a student he was greatly influenced by Hillairet and this determined his direction into dermatology and together they wrote a book on the "Theory and Practice of Skin Disease" which was published in 1881. He trained with Potain and Bouchard and so had a thorough grounding in clinical medicine as well as in the laboratory approach to research. He was appointed Chef de Clinique Médicale in 1882 and Médecin des Hôpitaux in 1886, gaining his agrégé in 1892. He worked with Professor Fournier and when Fournier retired in 1902 he was appointed to the chair of Dermatology at the Hôpital Saint-Louis where he remained for 15 years. In 1882 he described Gaucher Disease and wrote on many aspects of medicine, but in particular dermatology and syphilis.

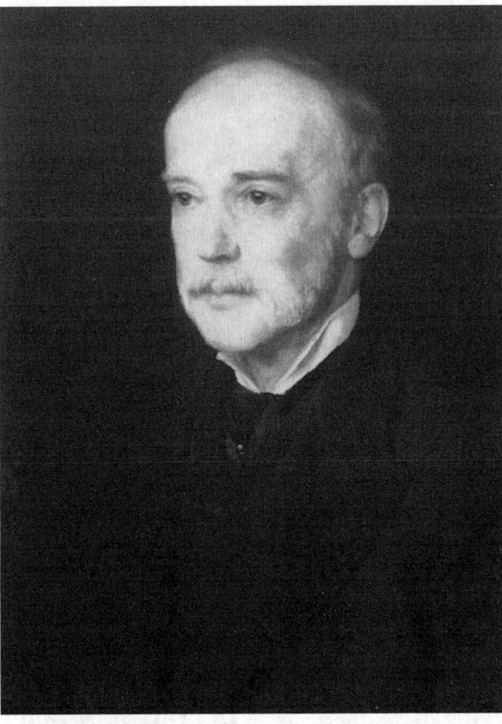

Samuel J. Gee, (Reproduced from *"The Royal College of Physicians of London Portraits"* by G. Wolstenholme & D. Piper (Published by J & A Churchill Ltd, London, 1964)

During the 1st World War he was placed in charge of the Military Hospitals in Paris and he was said to be a little distant and reserved, and to have always carried himself as if he had a uniform on.

GEE DISEASE

(Also called GEE-HERTER DISEASE, GEE-HESS-THAYSEN DISEASE, HEUBNER-HERTER DISEASE)

Infantile celiac disease.

Samuel J. Gee (1839–1911) English pediatrician and physician. He entered University College Hospital as a medical student in 1857 and graduated M.D. University of London in 1861. He served as a house surgeon at the University College Hospital and subsequently at Great Ormond Street Hospital for Sick Children. He became a member of the Royal College of Physicians in 1865 and a Fellow in 1870, and in 1871 gave the Goulstonian Lectures, his lecture title being "Heat of the Body". In 1866 he was an assistant physician of St. Bartholomew's Hospital. This was one of the rare occasions where St. Bartholomew's Hospital had appointed someone from outside their own hospital. Initially he was in charge of the skin department, but in 1870 became demonstrator in morbid anatomy and from 1872–1878 he was lecturer in pathological anatomy. He became a physician at St. Bartholomew's in 1878 and from that year until 1893 he lectured in medicine. In 1901 he was appointed physician to the Prince of Wales and he retired in 1904.

His family was not well to do, and he had no influential relatives to help him, but he rapidly made his mark and by 25 he had already contributed articles to one of the leading textbooks "Reynolds Systems of Medicine". A few years following his election as assistant physician to St. Bartholomew's Hospital he published a book entitled "Auscultation and Percussion together with Other Methods of Physical Examination of the Chest" which rapidly became extremely popular, and which had six editions, the first appearing in 1870.

Although shy and somewhat withdrawn he was an excellent teacher who would frequently drive home a point with an aphorism and these sayings became very well known amongst the student population, together with attempts at imititating a mannerism of speech which he had. It is not surprising that his other book entitled "Medical Lectures and Aphorisms" was also popular and reached a third edition in 1907. He died suddenly from a coronary occlusion, and at the autopsy, which he had requested, was shown to have extensive atheromatous changes in the aorta and its valves.

Christian A. Herter (1865–1901) U.S. physician (*v. infra* HUEBNER-HERTER DISEASE)

Thorvald E. Hess-Thaysen (1883–1936) Danish physician.

GEHRIG DISEASE

Amyotrophic lateral sclerosis.

Lou Gehrig (1903–1941) U.S. baseball player. He studied for two years at Columbia University before joining the New York Yankees in 1923 playing with them until 1939. He was nicknamed "Iron Horse" since he rarely missed a game in his career, playing 2,130 consecutive major league fixtures. He was a member of the famous "Murderers Row" which included the legendary Babe Ruth. Unlike Ruth, he was a rather retiring and shy person and died in 1941 of amyotrophic lateral sclerosis. He was the hero of an emotional movie picture and was played by Gary Cooper. He was the American League's most valuable player four times and elected to the National Baseball Hall of Fame in 1939 with a lifetime batting average of .340 including 493 home runs.

GEIGER COUNTER

Geiger-Müller counter.

Instrument for detecting radioactivity.

Hans W. Geiger (1882–1945) German physicist who worked with Rutherford at Manchester University before the Ist World War and returned to Germany when war broke out. He was involved in a German effort to develop the Atom bomb in World War II. He devised his instrument whilst working in Rutherford's laboratory and later (1928) collaborated with Müller in an improved design.

W. Müller German physicist.

GÉLINEAU DISEASE

Narcolepsy–involuntary periods of sleep.

GÉLINEAU-REDLICH SYNDROME

Narcolepsy.

Jean B.E. Gelineau (1859–) French physician.

Emil Redlich (1866–1930) Austrian neurologist who worked with H. Obsteiner while the latter was the Director of the Neurologisches Institut of the University of Vienna and proposed with him that tabetic degeneration of the posterior columns begins in the posterior roots.

GELLÉ TEST

In deafness due to a conduction defect pressure over the external auditory canal does not change the loudness of bone conduction.

Marie E. Gellé (1834–1923) French surgeon and otologist.

GEODE CYST

Bone cyst seen in rheumatoid arthritis due to the intraosseous inclusion of synovial membrane.

Geode is a geological term referring to a stone containing a cavity lined with crystals or mineral matter.

GERHARDT DISEASE

Erythromelalgia.

Idiopathic paroxysmal vasodilation of peripheral vasculature especially in the feet, causing a burning sensation – occurs equally in both sexes and hands are less commonly also involved. It is sometimes completely relieved by aspirin.

GERHARDT SIGN

Change of percussion note over a lung cavity when the patient stands or lies flat.

GERHARDT SYNDROME

Bilateral abductor paralysis of the larynx.

Carl A.C.J. Gerhardt (1833–1902) German physician, from Spega, and Professor of Medicine at Jena (1861), Würzburg (1872) and Berlin (1885), where Paul Ehrlich worked with him as an assistant, but Ehrlich became unhappy because Gerhardt wanted him to become more clinically involved. He was interested in laryngology and wrote on croup and vocal cord paralysis and tests of percussion and auscultation. A founder of pediatrics, he edited an authoritative book of the time. Weir-Mitchell described erythromelalgia also in 1872 (*v. infra*).

GERLACH TONSIL

Lymphoid tissue around the internal auditory meatus.

GERLACH VALVE

Mucosal fold near the orifice of the appendix.

Joseph von Gerlach (1820–1896) German histologist, born in Mainz. He was one of the pioneers in the introduction of staining techniques in histopathology. In 1847 he injected capillaries with a mixture of carmine, ammonia and gelatine and in 1855 he was employing carmine as a nuclear stain. He experimented with aniline and gold chloride and as result of his work differential staining advanced rapidly.

GERLIER DISEASE OR SYNDROME

Paralytic vertigo, endemic in Switzerland, occurring in cattle workers, and often with associated severe headache, photophobia and bilateral ptosis.

E. Felix Gerlier (1840–1914) Swiss physician, described the disorder in 1886.

GERSTMANN SYNDROME

Right-left apraxia, acalculia, agraphia, finger agnosia and often alexia, constructional apraxia and homonomous hemianopia due to a lesion in the (L) parietal angular gyrus.

GERSTMANN-STRÄUSSLER-SCHEINKER DISEASE

Progressive cerebellar ataxia, pyramidal and sometimes extra pyramidal signs with dementia. First described in a Viennese family, it is usually autosomal dominant but in some instances a slow virus has been suggested. Amyloid plaques are present throughout cerebrum and cerebellum. Its onset occurs in the 5th decade.

Josef Gerstmann (1887–1969) U.S. neuropsychiatrist who studied with Wagner von Jauregg in Vienna.

E. Sträussler Austrian physician.

I. Scheinker Austrian physician.

GHON LESION OR TUBERCLE

Calcified area in the chest X-ray due to healed primary tuberculosis.

Anton Ghon (1866–1936) Austrian pathologist. He was born in the town of Villach and went to medical school in Graz where he graduated in 1890. He worked for a while in Vienna in the dermatology department, but was unhappy in this area and moved to pathology where he was an assistant to Weichselbaum and in 1897 he was a member of the Austrian commision which studied the plague in Bombay. In 1902 he was appointed an Associate Professor in Vienna, becoming a full Professor in 1910 when he moved to the German University of Prague to replace von Kretz. Working with a number of collaborators he undertook many original studies in the area of bacteriology, particularly that in relation to meningitis and gonorrhea. When relatively young he developed tuberculosis of the larynx, but fortunately recovered from this. In 1928 he had his first myocardial infarction and another a year later, but he recovered well from this and worked at the German University in Prague until his retirement. A few months later he died with tuberculous pericarditis.

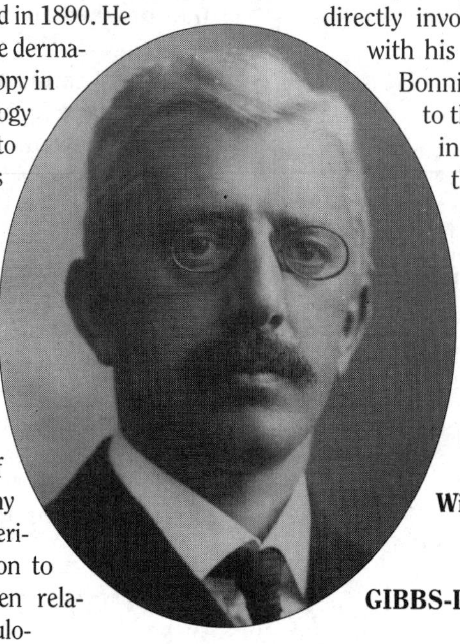

Anton Ghon (Courtesy of the Institut für Geschichte de Medezin an der Universität, Vienna)

GIARDIA LAMBLIA

Flagellated protozoan which may infect man and cause abdominal discomfort and diarrhea.

Alfred Giard (1846–1908) French biologist, born in Valenciennes and educated in Paris where he obtained his D.Sc. in 1873 at the Sorbonne. He became Professor of Natural History at the University of Lille and in 1874 established a marine zoological station at Wimereux, near Boulogne. He was elected to Parliament in 1882, but lost his seat at the next election in 1885. He made many contributions to cytology, and was the author of over 600 scientific papers in the field of biology and zoology. He was especially concerned with the interrelationships between host and parasite and introduced the term "parasitic castration" in animals and plants to denote changes in the secondary sexual characteristic of the host caused by the parasite, even when it does not directly involve the host gonads. Together with his student and collaborator, Jules Bonnier, he made many contributions to the study of parasitic infestations in marine animals, particularly the crustacea. In 1888 the town council of Paris endowed a lectureship of evolution for him at the Sorbonne which became a chair. Through his students and works he exerted a great influence on the development of biological sciences in France.

Wilhelm D. Lambl (*v. infra*).

GIBBS-DONNAN EQUILIBRIUM

v. DONNAN EQUILIBRIUM

Josiah W. Gibbs (1839–1903) U.S. physicist (Professor at Yale 1872–79) who studied with Clausius (at Zurich) and Helmholtz (who also taught Röntgen). Clausius and Kelvin proposed the second law of thermodynamics and Gibbs applied it to chemical reactions. His work resulted in the founding of physical chemistry.

GIEMSA STAIN

Stain for blood film and bone marrow.

Gustav Giemsa (1867–1948) German chemist, born in Blechhammer, Upper Silesia. He studied pharmacy, chemistry, bacteriology and mineralogy at Leipzig University. He worked for some years in Tanzania (then German East Africa) and in 1900 was appointed Director of the Department of Chemistry at the Institute for Naval and Tropical Medicine in Hamburg. He developed his stain for various cytological preparations to investigate protozoal infestations. He was a pioneer in chemotherapy and became a Privatdozent in Chemotherapy at the University of Hamburg in 1919.

GIERKE CORPUSCLES

Thymic corpuscles.

Hans P.B. Gierke (1847–1886) German anatomist who described the tractus solitarius (Gierke respiratory bundle).

GIERKE DISEASE (Type I of Cori).

Glycogen storage disease with hypoglycemia and cirrhosis and hepatomegaly, due to a reduction or absence of glucose-6-phosphatase. This was the first recessively inherited disorder shown to be due to deficient activity of a specific intracellular enzyme.

Edgar von Gierke (1877–1945) German pathologist born in Breslau (Wroclaw) and went to University of Heidelberg and Freiburg in Germany, joining the faculty of University of Heidelberg in 1905 and spent some time at the Cancer Institute, London, 1907 and returned to become head of the Department of Pathology at the Charité Hospital, Berlin. Served in the Medical Corps in World War I and described the disorder and its pathology in 1931. He also researched bone tumors and thyroid gland structure.

GIESON

v. VAN GIESON

GIFFORD REFLEX

Constriction of the pupil when the orbicularis oculi is contracted with the eyelids held open.

GIFFORD SIGN

Lid lag in hyperthyroidism.

Harold Gifford (1858–1929) U.S. ophthalmologist. Born in Milwaukee he graduated M.D. from the University of Michigan in 1882. He studied abroad and was appointed Ist assistant to Horner (*v. infra*) in Zurich. He returned to America and commenced practice in Omaha in 1886. He was an ardent socialist and conservationist. He was nonetheless well liked and respected by his conservative colleagues as is emphasized by the orthodox newspaper the "Omaha Post of the American Legion" declaring him "The city's most valuable citizen" in 1928.

GIGLI SAW

Flexible wire saw used in cranial and other bone operations.

Leonardo Gigli (1863–1908) Italian gynecologist who developed his instrument to perform pubiotomies (1894) and then adapted it for craniotomies (1898).

GILBERT SIGN

Patients with cirrhosis of the liver pass more urine when fasting than following a meal.

GILBERT SYNDROME OR DISEASE

Fluctuating benign jaundice secondary to glucuronyltransferase deficiency. This results in an increase in unconjugated bilirubin which is accentuated by infectious illness or fasting. Its incidence varies from 1–2% in females and 3–7% in males and is most commonly diagnosed by chance investigation.

Nicholas A. Gilbert (1858–1927) French physician. He was born in Buzanchy in the Ardennes, and graduated from the University of Paris with a gold medal in 1885. He was particularly influenced by Bouchard, Hanot, Fournier, Grancher and Hayem. His principal work was in liver disease, particularly cirrhosis, and its classification, portal hypertension, and familial jaundice. With numerous other workers, he published papers on a range of subjects from tuberculosis of birds and mammals and the pneumonia caused by psittacosis, to blood diseases, which he studied when a student of Hayem. He was author and co-author of a number of books in medicine. In 1901 he became Professor of Therapeutics to the Faculty and in 1907 a member of the Academy of Medicine, and in 1910 Professor of Clinical Medicine at l'Hôtel Dieu. Although outwardly cold and rather distant, he developed very close relationships with people, had numerous friends and was highly respected and liked by his students.

GILCHRIST DISEASE

North American blastomycosis.

Thomas C. Gilchrist (1862–1927) U.S. physician. He was born in Crewe, England, and studied medicine at the Manchester Royal Infirmary, qualifying M.R.C.S. Eng. and L.S.A., London, 1887. He did not sit his final M.B. London because of a serious illness. He went to Baltimore where he became assistant to the Professor of Dermatology. He was an enthusiastic research worker and teacher and became interested in blastomycosis. He became Professor of Dermatology at Johns Hopkins in 1898 and in 1907 the University of Maryland conferred on him an honorary M.D. He was President of the American Dermatology Association in 1909 and died of cirrhosis of the liver.

GILFORD-HUTCHINSON DISEASE

v. HUTCHINSON-GILFORD SYNDROME

GILLES DE LA TOURETTE DISEASE OR SYNDROME

Violent muscular jerks of the face, shoulders and extremities beginning in childhood with spasmodic grunting, explosive noises or coprolalia. Samuel Johnson is thought to have had this problem.

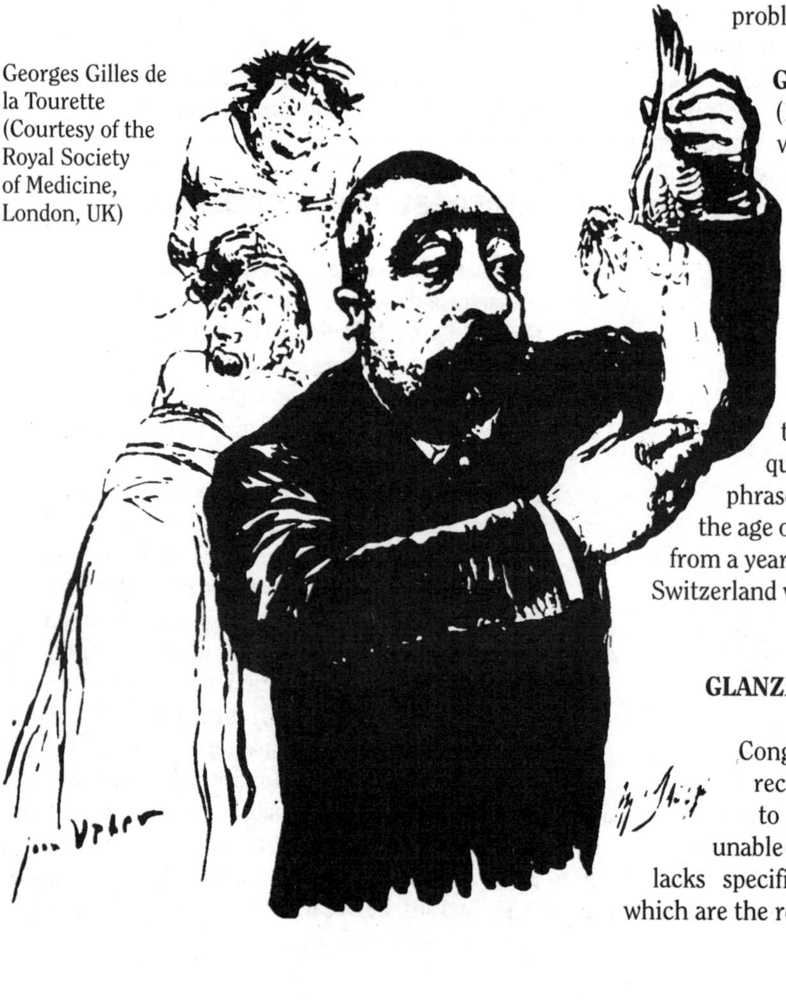

Georges Gilles de la Tourette (Courtesy of the Royal Society of Medicine, London, UK)

Georges Gilles de la Tourette (1857–1904) French neurologist who wrote extensively on hypnotism and hysteria and was a student of Charcot at the Salpêtrière. He emphasized the character of the gait in neurological disorders as well as his more famous description of tics. The patient he initially described died aged 85 years and the obituaries in the Paris papers quoted some of her more colorful phrases. Her disorder commenced at the age of 7 and remained with her apart from a year long remission during a trip to Switzerland when she married.

GLANZMANN DISEASE

Congenital thrombasthenia with a recurrent bleeding diathesis due to defective platelets which are unable to aggregate. Their membrane lacks specific glycoproteins IIb and IIIa which are the receptor for fibrinogen.

GLANZMANN AND RINIKER LYMPHOCYTOPHTHISIS

Swiss type agammaglobulinemia with absence of the thymus, severe cytopenia, recurrent infections and failure to form antibodies.

Edward Glanzmann (1887–1959) Swiss pediatrician who wrote on nutritional aspects of childhood anemias and first described goat's milk anemia (1916) and Glanzmann disease in 1918. He was born in Lucerne and went to medical school in Zurich, Berlin and Berne, graduating M.D. in 1914 and was assistant to Prof. Czerny at the Pediatric Clinic in 1932.

P. Riniker Swiss pediatrician.

GLAUBER SALT

Sodium sulphate.

Johann R. Glauber (1604–1668) German chemist who had no formal training. He was born in Carlstadt and became the greatest analytical chemist of his time and published a book on chemical methods. He was secretive and was said to have sold some of his secrets to manufacturers several times over!

GLÉNARD DISEASE

Generalized ptosis of intra-abdominal organs.

Frantz Glénard (1848–1920) French physician who left Paris to live at Vichy because of ill health.

GLEY CELLS

Interstitial cells of the testis.

GLEY GLANDS

v. SANDSTRÖM BODIES

Parathyroid glands.

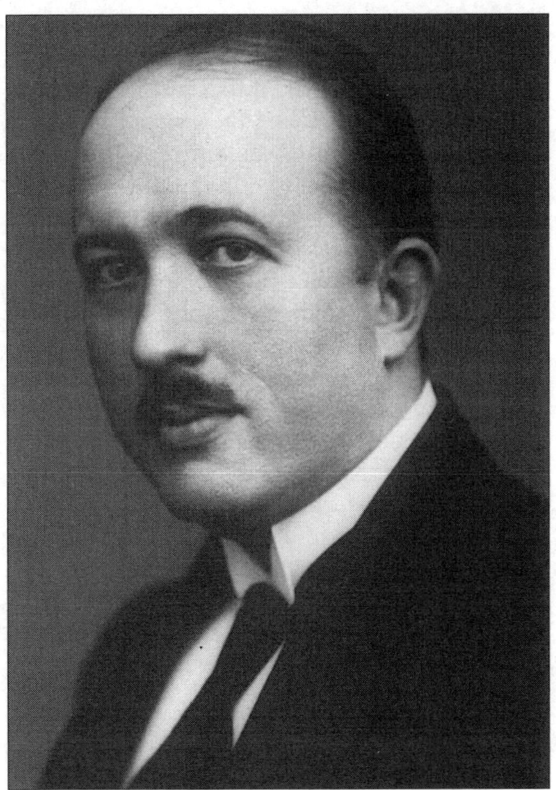

Edward Glanzmann
(Courtesy of Madam Kaiser-Glanzmann)

Marcel E.E. Gley (1857–1930) French physiologist. He was first influenced to take up physiology by Beaunis in Nancy. When 23 years old he went to Paris to work with Marey at the College of France, and in 1883 was appointed Prosector in Physiology in the Faculty of Medicine there and Professor Agrégé in 1889, Assistant to the Museum of Natural History in 1893 and finally in 1908 he was appointed to a chair of General Biology in the College of France. Although he had been taught in classical physiology by Beaunis and Marey, in the stimulation of nerves and the use of kymograph preparations and vivisection, he turned his attention to the study of internal secretions and chemicals which directly influence cells and tissue function. In 1890 he was studying the function of the thyroid gland and in the course of experiments on thyroidectomy in rabbits, he noted that there were two small glands beneath the thyroid and it was not long before he realized that he had re-found the glands first described by Sandström in 1880 and reported in a work which had been completely ignored. He had called them the para-thymic glands. He investigated the function of these glands further by removing the thyroid and leaving the glands behind and finding that the animals would survive this operation but that if he removed the parathyroid glands they died shortly after. In 1894 with the Italian Dr. Vassale, he demonstrated the importance of extracts of the thyroid glands in treating animals which had had their thyroids removed and was therefore one of the first people to demonstrate the effectiveness of such replacement in myxedema. Although Claude Bernard had shown that the liver was capable of internal secretion (blood glucose) and external secretion (bile in 1855), it was not until 1890 that Brown-Séquard widened this concept. Following work he undertook with D'Arsonval using testicular extractions he suggested that cells could produce an internal secretion which was capable of influencing other cells more distantly placed, through the circulation rather than by some mechanism requiring the function of the nervous system. From 1897 Gley stressed the importance of this function and he conducted numerous experiments with his student Pezard to show how such products in the blood could react harmoniously in controlling cell function. Together with L. Camus he worked on experimental production of antibodies and showed that there was both a natural as well as an acquired immunity in the production of hemolysis in animals. He made numerous communications on many topics ranging from the two types of pancreatic secretion to the property of normal serum in inhibiting proteolytic enzyme action and the presence and importance of calcium and iodine in the blood.

Besides his research, Gley was a superb lecturer and teacher of students, and was able to communicate his convictions and enthusiasms to all who made contact with him.

GLISSON CAPSULE

Capsule of the liver.

Francis Glisson (1597–1667) English physician who was born in Rampisham, Dorsetshire, but spent most of his life in London. He introduced the idea of irritability and showed that muscle did not increase in bulk during contraction by immersing an arm in water and showing no volume change during contraction.

He went to Gonville and Caius College, Cambridge, and took his M.D. in 1634. In 1635 he became a member of the Royal College of Physicians and became Regius Professor of Physic at Cambridge until his death. Apart from his anatomical study of the liver, he also described scurvy and gallstones and published a treatise on rickets in 1668 and in this described splints and orthopedic measures for the management of the bony deformities. He was one of the founders of the Royal Society and President of the Royal College of Physicians (1667–1669).

GMELIN TEST

Urine is layered over nitric acid and if bilirubin is present, various coloured rings are seen at the junctions.

Leopold Gmelin (1788–1853) German chemist from Göttingen who confirmed the presence of hydrochloric acid in gastric juice and studied the constituents of bile. In 1817 he became Professor of Chemistry and Medicine at the University of Heidelberg and together with F. Tiedemann, another chemist, published a book on digestion which included microscopic and chemical observations on this.

GODTFREDSEN SYNDROME

Ipsilateral blindness, trigeminal neuralgia, XIIth nerve paralysis and ophthalmoplegia due to invasion of the cavernous sinus by a tumor. Also called the cavernous sinus-nasopharyngeal syndrome.

Erik Godtfredsen Danish radiologist.

GOLDBLATT HYPERTENSION

Experimental renal hypertension, produced by clamping the renal artery.

Harry Goldblatt (1891–) U.S. pathologist, born in Muscerine, lowa, and graduated M.D. from McGill University in 1916, and after training in pathology in Canada and the U.S. went to the Lister Institute, London, as a Beit Fellow (1921– 24). He returned to Case Western Reserve in 1924 where he became Professor of Experimental Pathology from 1935–46. He moved to the University of Southern California, becoming Professor of Experimental Pathology there in 1955. His other research interests were experimental cancer, rickets and the effects of light.

GOLDENHAR SYNDROME

Oculo-auriculo-vertebral dysplasia.

The features include conjunctival dermoid cysts, auricular appendices with pretragal blind fistulae. The skull may be asymmetrical with micrognathia, with other skeletal abnormalities being accessory ribs and abnormal vertebrae.

Maurice Goldenhar French physician. A pupil of Professor Klein (*v. infra*). He described his syndrome in a doctoral thesis under the direction of Professor Klein at the ophthalmological clinic in Geneva.

GOLDFLAM DISEASE OR SYMPTOM COMPLEX

Myasthenia gravis.

Samuel V. Goldflam (1852–1932) Polish neurologist. He was born in Warsaw and went to school and university there graduating from the Faculty of Medicine in 1875 and then working in Professor Lambl's clinic (*v. infra*). In 1882 he studied with the famous neurologists Westphal and Charcot and then returned to Warsaw to teach neurology in the manner of the Grand Masters. He published in many areas of neurology, having particular interest in the significance of reflexes, neurological aspects of syphilis and eye reflexes, as well as a monograph that he published with S. Meyerson "On the Sounds in the Ear and Head". During the Ist World War he worked as a volunteer at the Jewish Hospital with his great friend, the director, E. Flateau (*v. supra*). He died of a mediastinal tumor. T. Willis first described myasthenia in 1685 and Erb in 1878.

GOLDSCHEIDER DISEASE

Epidermolysis bullosa.

Alfred Goldscheider (1858–1935) German Professsor of Medicine. He was born in Sommerfield, the son of a doctor and entered the Royal Friedrich Wilhelm Institute in Berlin as a student in 1876. He passed his state medical exams in 1881 and after a few years of military service he returned to the Friedrich Wilhelm Institute in Berlin. In 1891 he was ordered as Surgeon Major to the clinic of Ernst von Leyden. In 1894 he became the director of the Municipal Hospital of Moabit and in 1906 the Director of the Rudolf Virchow Hospital. In 1910 he was appointed as Senator's successor to the Outpatient Department of the Royal University of Berlin, and in 1919 this became the III Medical University Clinic which he continued to direct, even after his retirement in 1926, until 1933.

He served in the Ist World War and was particularly prominent in the adoption of anti-typhoid techniques and in the early diagnosis of typhoid fever and tetanus, and was one of the sanitary experts of the German Army. His initial research revolved around the physiology of the senses, and the structure of reference of skin senses to the spinal cord, as well as the problems of pain. He wrote a monograph with Ernst von Leyden on disorders of the spinal cord and the medulla oblongata and was a prominent exponent of the art of percussion and physical examination, which made him an excellent teacher of students. He promoted the importance of physical and dietary care in helping a patient combat illness. He firmly believed that students should be trained in reliable work and in thinking scientifically, and not in ingenuity! Because of the relative lack of effective therapy, he proposed that "an entirely scientifically regulated and determined therapy was unthinkable" (v. Skoda), and was also suspicious of the beginning of intrusion of techniques and laboratory studies in arriving at a diagnosis. He died in Berlin following cardiac arrhythmia which led to a stroke.

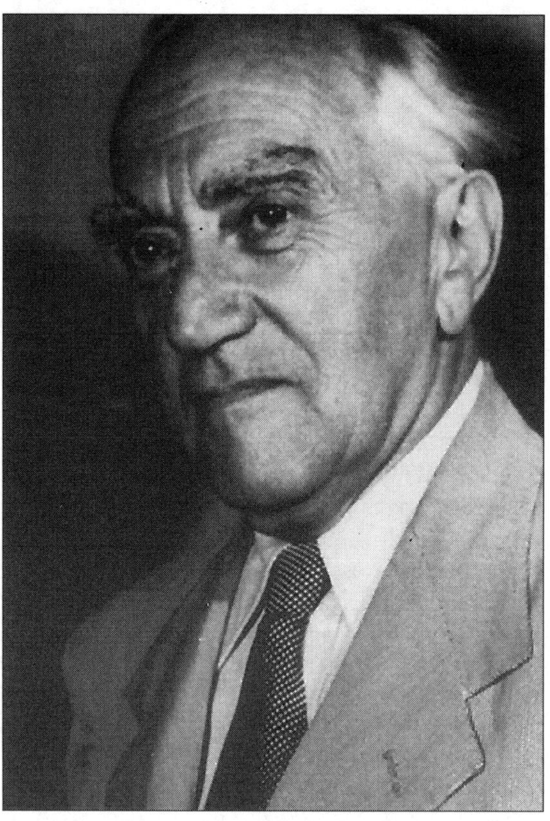

Kurt Goldstein (Courtesy of the Royal Society of Medicine, London, UK)

GOLDSTEIN CATASTROPHIC REACTION

Extreme agitation and anger observed in patients with acute loss of cognitive skills, provoked when the lost skill is attempted. Behavior is composed when doing tasks of which they are capable.

Kurt Goldstein (1878–1965) U.S. neurologist. Worked with L. Edinger on the diencephalon and lateral spinothalamic tract. He studied in Paris with G. Marinesco and C. von Monakow.

GOLGI APPARATUS

Specialized portion of the endoplasmic reticulum which is the site of synthesis of some of the intracellular granules and is important in the processing of some intracellular proteins.

GOLGI CELLS

Motor and sensory nerve cells.

Camillo Golgi (1844–1926) Italian histologist, born in Conteno, Lombardy, in the Alps (now called Conteno Golgi); his father was the local doctor. Golgi graduated from Pavia in 1865, did his medical training in Ospedale di San Matteo in Pavia and worked and trained in the laboratories of G. Bizzozero (the discoverer of the platelet), who became a close friend. His first publication was on pellagra, the next on smallpox and he made the first major publication on the pathology of the bone marrow. Following this he turned to the nervous system and studied psammomas and neuroglia of the grey and white matter. For financial reasons he became chief physician in a small town, Ospizio-Cronici in Abbiategrasso, and here in his kitchen, working mainly at night by candlelight, he discovered a silver chromate method for staining nerve tissue. In 1875 at the age of 32 he was appointed Extraordinarius in Histology at the University of Pavia, and remained there for the rest of his career. He described his Type I (motor and long axons) and Type II cells (sensory and short axons) in the

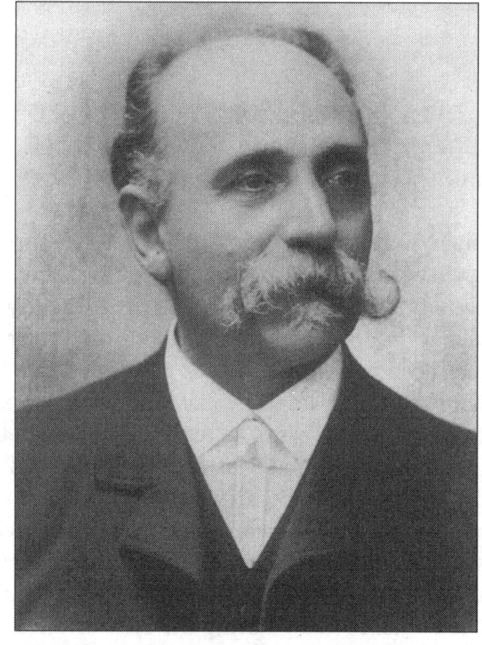

Camillo Golgi (Courtesy of the Royal Society of Medicine, London, UK)

cerebral cortex, and the intracellular organelle, the Golgi apparatus in 1858, although it had earlier been described by Von La Valette St. George in the sexual cells of snails. In 1890 his interest turned to research in malaria and he demonstrated that in relapsing malaria the organism develops in the organs whilst in the attack it cycles in the red cell. He recognized that the severity of an attack of malaria was proportional to the number of parasites in the blood, and reported the distinguishing morphological features of the parasite of quartan and tertian malaria, and that the fever corresponds to the release of merozoites.

His neurological discoveries had paved the way for the acceptance of the neurone, although his theories concerning the "nerve net" were wrong. Cajal described the two of them as "two Siamese brothers attached at the back" and the two certainly never saw "eye to eye" as is seen by Golgi's attack on Cajal at Stockholm when they were jointly awarded the Nobel Prize in 1906.

GOLL COLUMN OR TRACT

Fasiculus gracilis medullae spiralis.

GOLL NUCLEUS

Gracilis nucleus

Friedrich Goll (1829–1903) Swiss physician and anatomist. Goll was born in Zofingen in the Canton Aarga but moved to Zurich with his parents when he was quite young and graduated there in medicine in 1847. He was particularly influenced by the botanists Heer and Naegli, and the physiologist Ludwig, as well as the clinicians Hasse, Lebert and Billroth. He graduated in medicine in 1851 and then went to Paris and worked with Claude Bernard for 2 years. He returned to Zurich and established himself as a general practitioner from 1854 to 1862, when he joined the Faculty of Medicine. In 1863 he was placed in charge of the University's outpatient department and when a vacancy occurred in the Pharmacology Institute he was made Director. Goll published very little following his initial work on the anatomy of the spinal cord, and he was not made an Associate Professor until 1885, but this was in part due to a very limited number of appointments.

In 1871 he joined a number of other Swiss doctors on the battlefields of the German-French war to help the wounded. He was a very friendly person who was extraordinarily kind, and it was said that he never failed a candidate. He was particularly fond of the Swiss Alps and spent all of his vacations in the high mountain region, away from the tourist areas. During a vacation trip in Nice he had a stroke which left him aphasic. He lived for 3 years following this episode but was never able to participate actively because of his physical disabilities.

GOLTZ SYNDROME

Focal dermal hypoplasia syndrome, syndactyly and teeth abnormalities. Inherited as an autosomal dominant.

Robert W. Goltz (1923–) American dermatologist.

GOMBAULT DEGENERATION OR DEMYELINATION OR NEURITIS

Segmental demyelination.

François A.A. Gombault (1844–1904) French neurologist.

GONZALES BLOOD GROUP

Antigen GOa found in a Mrs. Gonzales which has been reported only in the blood of black people.

GOOD SYNDROME

Agammaglobulinemia associated with thymoma with deficiences in both humoral and cellular immunity with resultant recurrent fungal, viral and pyogenic infections.

Robert A. Good (1922–) For many years Professor of Pediatrics at the University of Minnesota and then Director of the Sloan-Kettering Institute, New York (1973–1980). He graduated M.D. from the State Medical School in 1947. His studies on "Experiments of Nature" in children with problems in their immune system greatly advanced knowledge of the interaction of cellular and humoral immune responses. His investigations helped establish the importance of the thymus and his recognition of the role of the Bursa of Fabricius in the chicken contributed greatly to the recognition of B and T cell lymphocytes and their functions.

GOODELL SIGN

Softening of the cervix uteri as a sign of pregnancy.

William Goodell (1829–1894) U.S. gynecologist, born in Malta, the son of a missionary who had been stationed in Beirut, but who had temporarily moved to Malta because of the Battle of Navarino. He graduated from Williams College in 1851 and studied medicine at the Jefferson Medical College, graduating in 1854. He then returned to Constantinople and three years later married at Smyrna. Becoming dissatisfied with medical practice in Turkey, he returned to the United States in 1861. In 1870 he was appointed lecturer in the diseases of women at the University of Pennsylvania and became Clinical Professor of Gynecology in which post his lectures attracted people, not only from the medical profession, but also lay people and lawyers. He wrote a popular book at the time "Lessons in Gynaecology" which was first published in 1879. He was conservative in his approach to operative procedures, but nonetheless had a very wealthy practice which was said to have returned him $50,000 per year, and was a leading teacher of obstetrics and gynecology in Philadelphia, publishing over 100 papers. He suffered throughout his life with gout and two years before his death developed insomnia which could not be relieved by the hypnotics of the day. He resigned from his Chair in 1893 and died following a stroke.

GOODMAN CAMPTODACTYLY B

Scoliosis, arachnodactyly, hammer toes, fibrous tissue hyperplasia with flared nostrils and camptodactyly (flexion of fingers at one or both interphalangeal joints).

Richard M. Goodman Israeli geneticist.

GOODPASTURE SYNDROME

Acute glomerulonephritis with hemoptysis, intrapulmonary hemorrhage and anemia.

Ernest W. Goodpasture (1886–1960) U.S. pathologist who was born in Montgomery County, Tennessee. Graduated from Johns Hopkins University in 1912 and was the Rockefeller Fellow in Pathology at Johns Hopkins from 1912–1914 when he moved to Harvard. In 1924 he was appointed Professor of Pathology at Vanderbilt University and remained in that position until 1955. In 1934, with C.D. Johnson he first showed that mumps was due to a filterable virus. He was one of the early workers to establish chick embryo techniques in the study of viruses.

GORDIACEA

Nematomorpha (horse hair worms) which are parasites of arthropods but have been found in the intestinal and urinary tracts of man and in orbital and external ear inflammations.

Gordius Greek mythology. The complicated Gordian knot was tied by Gordius, King of Gordion in Phrygia. It was said that whoever untied it would rule Asia. Alexander the Great cut it with his sword.

GORDON REFLEX OR SIGN

1. Compression of the calf muscles may result in dorsiflexion of the great toe or all toes in pyramidal tract disease.
2. Compression of the forearm muscles or pisiform bone may result in flexion of all fingers or the thumb and forefinger in pyramidal tract disease.

Alfred Gordon (1874–1953) U.S. neurologist and psychiatrist. Born in Paris, France, and graduated from the University of Paris in 1895. He worked in Paris, Berne and Munich before migrating to the U.S.A. in 1899. He was best known for his book "On the Study of Reflexes". A regular participant and member of the Philadelphia Neurological Society at which he was a discussant after most presentations. He never achieved prominence in academic appointments although at one time an associate in nervous and mental disease and an instructor in neuropathology at the Jefferson Medical College.

GORDON SYNDROME

A congenital, often familial renal tubular disorder resulting in hyperkalemia with hyperchloremic acidosis despite normal glomerular filtration rate. When familial the inheritance is dominant. The biochemical features are the mirror image of those in another congenital but rarely familial renal tubular syndrome with renal salt wasting (v. Bartter syndrome). The hypertension and biochemical abnormalities are corrected by strict dietary salt restriction or by potassium wasting diuretics.

Richard D. Gordon (1934–) Australian endocrinologist born in Brisbane and graduating from the University of Queensland Medical School. He later trained with Grant W. Liddle (*v. infra*). Currently he is Professor of Medicine at the University of Queensland and Head of the Endocrine Hypertension Research Unit, Greenslopes Hospital, Brisbane.

GORDON TEST

Test once used for Hodgkin disease by intracerebral inoculation of a suspension of Hodgkin's lymph node into a laboratory animal, resulting in eosinophilia.

Mervyn H. Gordon (1872–1953) English bacteriologist. He was born in Harting, Sussex, and spent his childhood in the village which overlooked Chichester Harbour. His father was a local vicar who had an interest in archeology and history which his son soon shared. From Marlborough he went to Keble College, Oxford, and then to St. Bartholomew's Hospital where he qualified in 1898 and commenced work in bacteriology. He became the Head of Bacteriology at St. Bartholomew's Hospital. Whilst at the hospital, Lord Horder was one of his assistants and aided him in some of his initial work on classification of meningococci and streptococci. Gordon was a leading authority on this subject and he developed a flocculation technique for the diagnosis of smallpox. This technique was a great advance in its time, being reliable, rapid, and sensitive. In the 1914–18 war he made a major contribution in the epidemiology, diagnosis and serotherapy of meningitis, the material for this study largely coming from epidemics from the army barracks. This work led to the detection of distinct serological types of meningococcus. In 1923 he resigned his appointment to the hospital and teaching staff at St. Bartholomew's Hospital to become a full time research worker, changing his field from that of bacteria to that of viruses.

He transmitted mumps to monkeys for the first time and made contributions to psittacosis. In 1929 he commenced studying the etiology of Hodgkin Disease, endeavoring to prove that this was a viral disorder. Whilst his work in this area has not stood the test of time, there is no question that he was one of the United Kingdom's leading bacteriologists who was a great enthusiast and a very keen raconteur, with a fine sense of humor. His experiments on air-borne transmission led to him being invited to examine the environment of the House of Commons and its ventilation. In descriptions of his experiments in the House of Commons, he used to recount that a characteristic streptococcus in the mouth of a Cabinet Minister was recovered in plates exposed in the ladies' gallery.

He was a man with wide interests who was a very ardent archeologist, and in recognition for his achievements was elected as F.R.S. in 1924. He was a nephew of the naturalist F.T. Buckland and gave an interesting account of this man who discovered John Hunter's body in the vaults of St. Martin-in-the-Fields in 1859.

He wrote "It is the glory of a good bit of work, that it opens the way for still better, and thus rapidly leads to its own eclipse. The object of research is the advancement, not of the investigator, but of knowledge."

GORLIN SIGN

Ability to touch the tip of the nose with the tongue in patients with Ehlers-Danlos syndrome (*v. supra*).

GORLIN SYNDROME

Multiple basal cell carcinomas and cysts of the jaw with palmar and plantar pits, bifid ribs, mesenteric cysts and scoliosis, often autosomal dominant.

Robert J. Gorlin (1923–) U.S. dental pathologist. Professor of Oral Pathology, University of Minnesota.

GOTTRON SIGN

Symmetrical violaceous to erythematous scaly patches or papules which may progress to atrophic areas with telangiectasia and are said to be present in one third of patients with dermatomyositis. Most frequently present on the dorsum of the hand over the heads of the 2nd and 3rd metacarpals.

Heinrich Gottron (1890–1974) German dermatologist who published a wide range of articles on contact dermatitis, amyloid and leukemic infiltrates and skin manifestations.

GOUGEROT-BLUM DISEASE

Pigmented purpuric lichenoid dermatitis.

Henri Gougerot (1881–1955) French physician. He was born at Ouen–sur–Seine and went to medical school at the University of Paris where he qualified in 1908. In 1910 he became Professor Agrégé in the Faculty of Medicine and served in the French Army in the Ist World War, being awarded the Croix de Guerre. In 1909 he first described hemisporosis and with de Beurmann he delineated sporotrichosis in 1912. In 1928 he was appointed to the Chair of Dermatology and Syphilology at Paris University and became Chief Physician at the Hôpital St. Louis, posts he held until he died. He wrote on numerous other aspects of dermatology including sarcoidosis, lupus and cutaneous papillomatosis, edited one of the French journals of dermatology and with Darier and Sabouraud edited the text of dermatology "Nouvelle Pratique Dermatologique" which was published in 8 volumes in 1936. In 1936 he was made an honorary foreign member of the British Association of Dermatology. He had a prodigious output of papers, which numbered 2500!

Paul Blum (1887–1933) French dermatologist who graduated from the University of Paris and worked for a while at the Pasteur Institute. He became an assistant to Gougerot at L'Hôpital St. Louis and Physician in Chief L'Hôpital St. Lazare and L'Hôpital de Saint-Denis.

GOWERS MYOPATHY

Distal muscular dystrophy.

GOWERS PHENOMENON

Passive dorsiflexion of the foot produces pain along the course of the sciatic nerve when the former is compressed.

GOWERS SIGN

1. Irregular contraction of pupil as an early sign of tabes.
2. Inability of a patient with proximal myopathy to stand from a sitting position with the arms outstretched.

GOWERS SOLUTION

Diluent of sodium sulphate and acetic acid for red cell counting.

GOWERS TRACT

Anterior spinocerebellar tract.

Sir William Gowers (1845–1915) He was educated at Christchurch School, Oxford, and was an apprentice to Dr. Simpson, a medical practitioner in Essex. He then went to University College Hospital, London, qualified M.R.C.S. in 1867 and took his M.B. degree in 1869. He became a Fellow of the Royal College of Physicians in 1879 and Fellow of the Royal Society. He was knighted in 1897. At University College Hospital he was a student and protege of Sir William Jenner whom he greatly admired. He was initially appointed as Assistant Physician at the National Hospital for the Paralyzed and Epileptic, and to a similar post at University College Hospital, where he ultimately became Professor of Clinical Medicine. In 1878 he invented a hemoglobinometer and designed a blood cell counting chamber in which the slide on which the cells were counted had micrometric squares etched, rather than being placed on the eye piece as had been originally evolved by Hayem. He wrote and personally illustrated an atlas of ophthalmology entitled "Medical Ophthalmology" which was published in 1897. He epitomized the strengths of British neurology and was one of its foremost practitioners, synthesizing the concepts and ideas of people such as Hughlings Jackson, Ferrier and Horsley. He was an inspiring teacher who attracted many students and postgraduates, but was extremely dogmatic and aggressive. His writings were concise and always to the point and he followed his own dictum "words have a strong tendency to cause opacity if they be numerous". In 1880 he published "Diagnosis of Diseases of the Spinal Cord" which was an elegant demonstration of the relationship between anatomy, physiology and the patient's symptoms. This book contained a description of a tract in the spinal column, now called the anterolateral fasciculus which was subsequently described by Bekhterev, who named it Gowers Tract. In 1886–1888 he published his book "A Manual of the Diseases of the Nervous System" in two volumes which is still a masterpiece and which he illustrated himself. He was a painter and etcher of considerable ability whose paintings were shown by the Royal Academy of Arts. He was a forceful proponent of the use of shorthand and he himself was an excellent stenographer using shorthand for all his notes of his patients and he founded a Society of Medical Stenography. One story told of him later in his life was that he grabbed hold of a perfect stranger in the street and said "Young man, do you write shorthand" to which the shocked man answered, "No, I don't" whereupon Gower dropped his arm, saying "You are a fool and will fail in life". He had a great interest in nature and was particularly fond of Ruskin's work and had an extensive interest and knowledge of mosses, and was interested in wild flowers, archeology and architecture. He personally studied the remains of some of the old Suffolk churches and wrote about them and their history. Perhaps his greatest contribution was his systematic classification of nervous diseases and his ability to relate clinical facts with pathological change. In teaching he would emphasize the patient's symptoms, the clinical signs that were associated, and finally, definitely and clearly outline the changes in the nervous system which would be associated with these symptoms and signs.

GRAAFIAN FOLLICLE

This is the term used for the oocyte in the ovary.

Reiner de Graaf (1641–1673) He was born in Schoonhaven in Holland. His father was a well known architect and engineer who invented a number of water-driven machines. De Graaf entered medicine at Utrecht and transferred to the University of Leyden where he was taught by Sylvius de la Boë (*v. infra*) and one of his fellow students was N. Stensen (*v. infra*). He carried out early experiments on the functions of the pancreas employing an external fistula in a dog using a goose quill. For this work he was awarded an M.D. In 1665 he went to Paris and his work was published in French where it remained the authoritative text on the pancreas until Claude Bernard disproved his conclusions some 200 years later. In 1666 he returned to Holland and practiced in Delft and studied the male and female generative organs and in studies on rabbits, goats and other animals he showed that in the female the ovary contained structures which he identified as the equivalent to eggs in the ovaries of birds and he traced the passage of these ova down the oviducts into the uterus. He wrote an excellent description of the human testes. He published these findings in 1672 but did not succeed his former teacher Sylvius to the Chair of Anatomy at Leyden when it was vacated in 1672, perhaps because he was a Catholic. In 1673 he sent Leeuwenhoek's letters to the Royal Society. He died of the plague.

GRADENIGO SIGN OR SYNDROME

Paresis of the lateral rectus with pain in the temporo-parietal region, resulting from an abscess of the apex of the petrous bone secondary to otitis media and mastoiditis.

Giuseppe Gradenigo (1859–1926) Italian otolaryngologist. He described the sign in 1904 and was founder of the "Archivi Italiani di otologia e laringologia".

GRAEFE SIGN

Lid lag in exophthalmos.

PSEUDO GRAEFE PHENOMENON OR SIGN

Elevation of upper eyelid looking down, due to aberrant regeneration of the 3rd nerve after injury.

GRAEFE-SJÖGREN SYNDROME

Autosomal recessive disorder with spinocerebellar ataxia, retinitis pigmentosa and deafness which may be associated with congenital cataracts and mental retardation.

Friedrich W.E.A. von Graefe (1828–1870) Was the founder of scientific ophthalmology. The son of the Prussian Surgeon-general and a brilliant student, he received his medical degree in Berlin in 1847 and then studied in Prague and, influenced by F. Arlt, went into ophthalmology, studying in Paris, Vienna and London. He was the first clinician to use Helmholz's recent discovery, the ophthalmoscope, routinely, and he diagnosed sudden visual loss due to retinal artery embolism, optic retinitis and was one of the first to treat glaucoma successfully. He introduced several operations, wrote a textbook and founded a journal, Arch. für Ophthalmologie. He became Associate Professor of Ophthalmology in Berlin in 1857 and Professor in 1866. Students flocked to him from all over the world, including Argyll Robertson and Theodor Billroth, who was impressed by "his great personal kindness and his great humility. He was very rich and used to treat all poor patients with eye disease for nothing". He died of tuberculosis.

T. Sjögren (*v. infra*).

GRAHAM LAW

The rates of diffusion of any two gases are inversely proportional to the square roots of their densities.

Thomas Graham (1805–1869) Scottish chemist, Glasgow. Professor of Chemistry, Andersonian University, Glasgow (1830–37), then at University College, London (1837–55), then became master of the mint (1855–1869). He pioneered physical chemistry. He made important investigations on osmotic pressure "the conversion of chemical efficiency into mechanical power" and introduced the distinction between crystalloid and colloid.

GRAHAM STEELL MURMUR

Pulmonary diastolic murmur associated with pulmonary hypertension.

Graham Steell (1851–1942) Scottish physician. He was the younger son of Sir John Steell, a Scottish sculptor, who made the statue of Sir Walter Scott in Princes Street, Edinburgh. Steell was educated in the Edinburgh Academy, and initially wanted to join the Army, but was persuaded by his brother to enter medicine. He qualified in Edinburgh in 1872 and following a short time in Berlin he became house physician at the Edinburgh Royal Infirmary, working with G. Balfour who stimulated his interest in cardiology. For several years he worked in fever hospitals in Edinburgh, London and Leeds, and his M.D. thesis was on scarlet fever. In 1878 he was appointed as resident medical officer to the Manchester Infirmary following a prior appointment in the Department of Materia Medica in therapeutics in Edinburgh as assistant to Professor T. Fraser. In 1883 he became assistant physician to the Manchester Royal Infirmary and remained at that hospital until he retired in 1931. He wrote a textbook on cardiology in 1906 which was praised by the then doyen of cardiology, McKenzie, and he described the murmur that bears his name in 1888 in the Medical Chronicle. He wrote a number of small monographs concerning physical signs of cardiac disease. He always used a monaural stethoscope made of box wood with a bell shaped ear piece. He was a great lover of animals and one of the first advocates in modern times of the importance of physical exercise in the treatment and prevention of heart problems.

After he retired he went to live with his son, who was in practice in Derbyshire, who to his horror one day found his old father embarking on some research on the color sense of some young bullocks, by waving a red handkerchief at them.

GRAHAM TEST

Oral cholecystogram.

Evarts A. Graham (1883–1957) U.S. surgeon, Professor of Surgery, Washington University, St. Louis. His original work book can be seen on display at the Washington University library, St. Louis. He was a pioneer in lung surgery and was the first to remove a lung for cancer. He was a heavy smoker but on becoming convinced of the relationship of tobacco and carcinoma of the lung reduced his cigarette consumption. After he and an associate demonstrated the carcinogenic effects of cigarette tar in animals, he stopped smoking altogether, only to die of lung cancer.

GRAM STAIN

Microbiological stain using crystal violet. Bacteria taking up the stain are called Gram +ve (e.g. *Streptococcus, Staphylococcus*), and those not, Gram –ve (e.g. *Salmonella*).

Christian Gram (1853–1938) Danish physician. His stain demonstrated structural variation in bacterial cell walls and enabled a ready classification of bacteria.

He studied botany at the University of Copenhagen and was assistant to Japetus Stenstrup. Throughout his life he had a great interest in plants and this introduced him to the basis of pharmacology of the day and the use of the microscope. He entered medical school in 1878 and in 1883 became a doctor and then resident physician at Kommune Hospital. For some years he was the district physician in Copenhagen. In 1891 he became lecturer in pharmacology and that same year was appointed Professor. In 1892 he became physician and chief at the Frederiks Hospital and in 1900 resigned his Chair of Pharmacology to take up that of Medicine. His initial work concerned the study of the red blood cells in man with particular reference to their size in health and disease. He was one of the first to recognize that macrocytes were characteristic of pernicious anemia and that there was often an increase in red cell size in jaundice. The work that gained him international reputation was his development of a method for staining bacteria. This appeared in a small paper in Friedlander's Archives. Gram did not initially attempt to use his technique for separating bacteria into two groups, although he had noted that pneumococci, in particular, stained intensely whilst other bacteria such as typhoid did not. Later the stain played a major role in classification of bacteria and demonstration of the structural variation in bacteria cell walls led to their ready classification.

Gram was a very modest man and in this initial publication he stated, "I have therefore published the method, although I am aware that as yet it is very defective and imperfect; but it is hoped that also in the hands of other investigators it will turn out to be useful". After his appointment as Professor of Internal Medicine, he published four volumes of clinical lectures which became standard reading in Denmark. He was a fine clinician whose thorough and meticulous examinations were sometimes found to be too extensive for his students' and assistants' liking, but the thorough clinical grounding he gave them was appreciated later in their practice. Following his retirement in 1923 he lived inconspicuously until his death.

GRASSET-GAUSSEL PHENOMENON OR SIGN

A sign of upper motor neurone involvement in which the patient with hemiparesis lying on his back can raise either leg separately but cannot raise them together. If the paralyzed leg is raised it will fall when the unaffected leg is passively raised.

Joseph Grasset (1849–1918) French physician who practised in Montpellier.

A. Gaussel (19th C.) French physician.

GRAVES DISEASE

Hyperthyroidism.

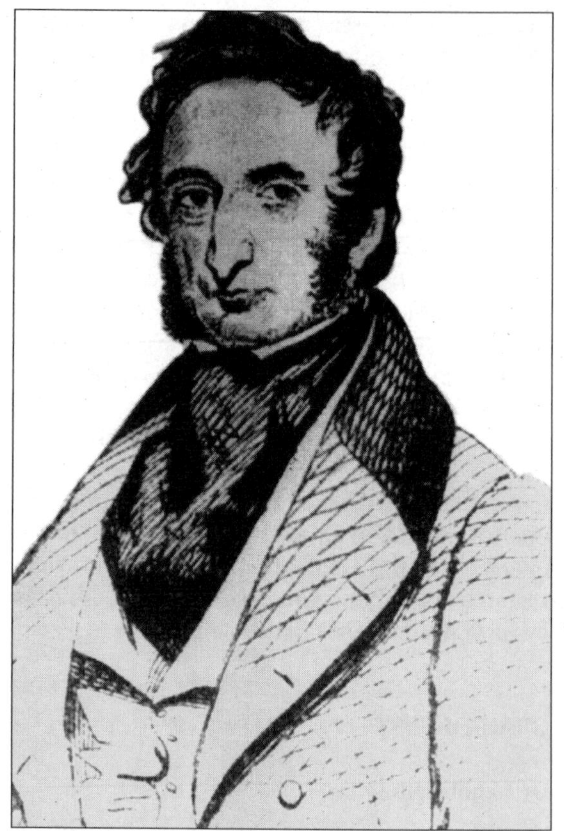

Robert J. Graves (Courtesy of the Royal Society of Medicine, London, UK)

Robert J. Graves (1797–1853) Irish physician, born in Dublin, he was the son of a clergyman. He graduated after a brilliant undergraduate career at Dublin in 1818 and studied in London and Edinburgh and on the continent. He had a great talent for languages and was once imprisoned for 10 days in Austria whilst travelling on foot without a passport as a German spy, since no one believed an Englishman could speak German so well. On another journey he saved a ship and its mutinous crew by assuming command during a storm in the Mediterranean. During a gale the ship sprang a leak, pumps failed and the crew attempted to abandon ship but Graves holed the one lifeboat with an axe and repaired the pumps with leather from his own shoes and all aboard survived. Whilst travelling in the Alps he became acquainted with the famous painter J.M.W. Turner and they travelled and painted together for several months eventually parting company in Rome. He returned to Dublin in 1821 to be Chief Physician at the Meath Hospital. He introduced bedside teaching and student clerking to medicine in England and Ireland and apart from hyperthyroidism also described angioneurotic edema, scleroderma, erythromelalgia, the pin hole pupil in pontine hemorrhage and cough fracture.

Graves showed the qualities which would ensure a great teacher. He was tall, somewhat swarthy with a vivacious manner and taught in English not in Latin or Dog Latin as was still the case in most classes in the 1830s. In his introductory lecture he said, "From the very commencement the student should set out to witness the progress and effects of sickness and ought to persevere in the daily observation of disease during the whole period of his studies". As well as the practical importance of bedside learning to ensure that a graduate was not "a practitioner who has never practiced" he emphasized the importance of research, "learn the duty as well as taste the pleasure of original work". He was sometimes sarcastic and in dealing with a colleague's attack on the use of the stethoscope which was advocated by himself and Stokes he wrote "We suspect Dr Clutterbuck's sense of hearing must be injured: for to him the 'ear trumpet' magnifies but distorts sound, rendering it less distinct than before". His published "Clinical Lectures" were a model for the day and highly recommended by none other than Trousseau (*v. infra*). He light-heartedly suggested to W. Stokes (*v. infra*) on a ward round that his epitaph be "he fed fevers".

GRAWITZ TUMOR

Hypernephroma – renal cell carcinoma.

Paul S. Grawitz (1850–1932) German pathologist born in Zerrin bei Butow in Pomerania on the Baltic Sea. He studied in Halle and Berlin, and when a student was assistant at the Pathological Institute of Berlin University where he helped Rudolf Virchow with his collection of pathology bottles. He became assistant at the Institute and was highly thought of by Virchow so that when Professor Ponfick went on leave for one semester from the University of Rostock he recommended Grawitz as a temporary replacement. He then remained with Virchow until 1886 when Professor Grohe in Greifswald became ill and Grawitz was appointed Senior Lecturer. When Professor Grohe died in 1887 Grawitz was appointed Professor of Pathology and Director of the Pathological Institute and remained in those positions until he retired in 1921. His initial work with Virchow concerned the possible movement of malignant cells. He then became interested in bacteriology and before the day of Koch's culture methods he succeeded in growing a fungus and a pathogen of favus and in infecting man with them from culture. While he was still in Berlin he wrote his papers on "The origins of kidney tumours of the suprarenal gland tissue" from which the name Grawitz tumors has arisen, although he mistook their true origin. After he moved to Greifswald he continued his interest in skin inflammation and tissue reaction to different stimuli. In a paper in 1892 "On the sleeping cells of the connective tissue and their behavior during progressive nutritional disturbances" he developed his theory of sleeping cells and the idea that mesenchymal cells can degenerate so that they lose their nucleus and become tissue fibrils and elastic fibres but on certain stimuli re-acquire nuclei and cell bodies, detach themselves from the union in fixed cells and become wandering cells again. This was the manner in which he thought tissue leukocytes arose. These views have been proven incorrect, and they were indeed challenged even in his day. Nonetheless these techniques were the beginnings of the ideas of tissue culture, and some of Grawitz's experiments on transplantation and implantation of cornea and cardiac valve tissue show how in some ways he was ahead of his time. Nonetheless he seems to have been unfortunate in that most of his theories, for which he fought so hard, were totally incorrect, and in 1902 he proposed the idea that thymus death was the cause of the demise of otherwise healthy children, these days known as "cot deaths".

Grawitz shunned scientific meetings, for example he never once went to a meeting of the German Pathological Society, but he promulgated and advocated and persecuted his ideas fearlessly through the literature. Although he had a sarcastic sense of humor, he was well liked by the students and his Faculty colleagues both as a person and a teacher. Apart from his initiation of the use of tissue culture, he will probably be best remembered for the very fine pathological collection that he established at his University and Institute. His careful cataloging grew into a book which he liked to call "The Manual for the Self Study of Pathological Anatomy". Virtually all of the pathological specimens were labelled by him personally, and he is said to have stated "if you want to have a good collection, you must devote about 2 hours a day to it".

GREENFIELD DISEASE

Metachromatic leukodystrophy

v. HENNEBERG DISEASE and SCHOLTZ DISEASE.

Joseph G. Greenfield (1884–1958) English neuropathologist. His father was Professor of Pathology and Clinical Medicine in Edinburgh. He graduated from Edinburgh and was house physician to Sir Byron Bramwell, one of the great clinicians and neurologists of the time at the Edinburgh Royal Infirmary. In 1910 he went to Queen Square, first as a house physician, after which he worked in Stewart's Pathology Department in Leeds, returning to become pathologist at Queen Square, succeeding Kinnier Wilson in 1914. He remained there for 35 years and made many contributions to pathological classification, especially in encephalitis and diffuse sclerosis. He was not an experimental pathologist but encouraged others and wrote important texts of the time on staining techniques and the cerebrospinal fluid.

GREGG TRIAD

Cataracts, heart defects and deafness occurring in children whose mothers have had rubella during the pregnancy.

Sir Norman Gregg (1892–1966) Australian ophthalmologist. A keen sportsman he represented New South Wales at cricket and toured Tasmania in a team captained by Victor Trumper. He graduated in medicine from the University of Sydney in 1915 and spent three years with the Australian Army in France winning the Military Cross for gallantry in action. He returned to Sydney in 1919 as a resident medical officer and then went to England and worked at Moorfields Eye Hospital returning to Sydney in 1923 to private practice with appointments at the Royal Alexandra Hospital for Children and the Royal Prince Alfred Hospital. He described the association of rubella in pregnancy with congenital malformations in 1941 and by sound clinical observation opened a new field of obstetric and pediatric research.

GREIG HYPERTELORISM

Ocular hypertelorism resulting in widely spaced eyes and mental retardation. The vertex is high and there is a low forehead. It is sometimes associated with osteogenesis imperfecta, Sprengel deformity (*v. infra*) and some other anomalies of the skull.

David M. Greig (1864–1936) Scottish surgeon. He was born in Dundee, and studied medicine at the Universities of St. Andrew's and Edinburgh and graduated from the latter in 1885. Following this he served in the Army, both at home and in India, and in 1900–1901 he was with General Buller's army in the Boer War. He returned to Dundee where he was a surgeon at the Royal Dundee Infirmary and a lecturer in clinical surgery and spent much time supervizing the Baldovan Institution for mentally defective children. In 1921 he was appointed conservator of the Museum of the Royal College of Surgeons in Edinburgh. This was a particularly appropriate appointment because he had diverse interests, but a particular penchant for rare disorders and peculiar manifestations of disease in general, and gathered specimens rather like a philatelist collects stamps. He had over 300 skulls, for example, and he incorporated them into the College Museum after his appointment. His interest in the skull which was pursued throughout his life may have commenced with his first publication in 1891 "A case of gunshot injury in which a piece of lead remained embedded in the skull for 31 years" in the Edinburgh Medical Journal. He described many types of congenital deformities of the skull and even discussed the cephalic features of Sir Walter Scott. He wrote on all aspects of surgery, including new methods for sterilizing and storing glass, modifications of instruments, and new surgical approaches. He published on the organization of army medical services and a number of aspects of medical problems arising in the army. He was a thoughtful reader, interested in music, and even published his own book of verse "The Rhymes of D.R.I." which looked at some of his colleagues of the Royal Dundee Infirmary in a light-hearted manner and records reminiscences of his medical student days. His publications were extremely varied, ranging from intussusception and Henoch-Schönlein purpura to a recovered stab wound of the heart, congenital edema, a number of publications on lymphomas involving various parts of the anatomy including the skin, all varieties of anatomical congenital abnormalities, hydrophobia, syringomyelia, a case of vicarious menstruation, and a case of hypertrophy of the labia minora. He had a continuing interest in abnormalities of the scapula and torticollis. He was a particularly careful and lucid writer who paid particular attention to the use of illustrations in his contributions to surgical pathology.

GREY TURNER SIGN

v. TURNER SIGN

GRIESINGER DISEASE

1. Pseudohypertrophic infantile muscular dystrophy.
2. Ankylostomiasis causing anemia.

GRIESINGER SIGN

Swelling over the mastoid process due to thrombosis of the transverse sinus.

Wilhelm Griesinger (1817–1868) German neurologist from Stuttgart. He was a pupil of Schönlein and assistant to Wunderlich before he succeeded Romberg in 1865 at the Charité and founded a psychiatric journal in Berlin. He favored the no restraint system in the treatment of the insane – apart from his many contributions to psychiatry he described hookworm infection "tropical chlorosis" (1826) and wrote important descriptions of infectious diseases. He introduced the idea of a psychiatric clinic for patients before admission and on discharge from asylums.

GROCCO SIGN

Triangular area of paravertebral dullness on the opposite side to a pleural effusion.

GROCCO TRIANGLE

Paravertebral triangle.

Pietro Grocco (1856–1916) Italian physician, Professor of Medicine at Perugia and Florence, who made a number of studies of respiratory disease and described his sign in 1902. He was an interesting and inspiring teacher with a knack for simple explanations of complex problems.

GROENBLAD-STRANDBERG SYNDROME

Pseudoxanthoma elasticum with angioid streaks in the retina. The skin abnormality has been likened to the appearance of the skin of a plucked chicken and is most marked in the neck, axilla and flexures. There is an association with vascular disease.

Ester E. Groenblad (1898–) Swedish ophthalmologist.

James Strandberg (1883–) Swedish dermatologist. Professor of Dermatology in Stockholm.

GRUBER SYNDROME

v. MECKEL SYNDROME

Autosomal recessive disorder characterized by microcephaly, occipital encephalocoele, abnormal facies, polycystic kidney and other somatic abnormalities – also termed dysencephalia splanchnocystica.

Georg B. Gruber (1884–1977) German physician.

GRUBER TEST

Auditory test using a tuning fork.

Josef Gruber (1827–1900) Austrian otolaryngologist. He was born at Kosolup in Bohemia, went to school in Budapest and studied medicine in Vienna, where he was highly thought of by both Hyrtl and Rokitansky. He graduated in 1855 and spent the next 5 years as an assistant at the Allegemeine Krankenhaus. During this time he published articles on both dermatological and surgical topics, but became most interested in diseases of the ear, and acting as his own teacher studied the anatomy and pathology of the auditory system. He was made Privatdozent in Otology in 1863 as a result of his publications in his field. He wrote a book on the topic in 1870 and at this period also, together with Voltilini, Rudinger and Beber-Liel, he founded a journal on the subject.

In 1873 he was made Extraordinary Professor, and together with Politzer was appointed Director of the new clinic for Ear Disease at the University of Vienna. He was the first to discover the benefits of early operation in middle ear infection in order to prevent deafness and involvement of the mastoid and central nervous systems. His clinics attracted people from all over the world and in 1889 he was given the rank of Ordinary Professor which he had to resign in 1898 because of age, at which time the Emperor of Austria awarded him the Order of the Iron Crown (3rd class).

GUILLAIN SIGN

In meningism pinching the skin over or squeezing the quadriceps femoris on one side results in flexion of the contralateral hip and knee.

GUILLAIN-BARRÉ SYNDROME

Acute symmetrical lower motor neurone paralysis which commences distally but spreads proximally and may involve the bulbar region and the diaphragm. It is believed to be viral in origin and is usually self-limiting, the patient often recovering completely. Characteristically the lumbar puncture shows a high protein concentration but few cells.

(Also called LANDRY-GUILLAIN-BARRÉ SYNDROME v. Introduction)

Georges Guillain (1876–1961) French neurologist, born in Rouen. He wrote a book on Charcot, "J.M. Charcot, His Life, His Work". He studied the cerebrospinal fluid and described the syndrome in two French soldiers. He was Professor of Neurology, Paris Faculty of Medicine, 1923–1944.

Jean A. Barré (*v. supra*).

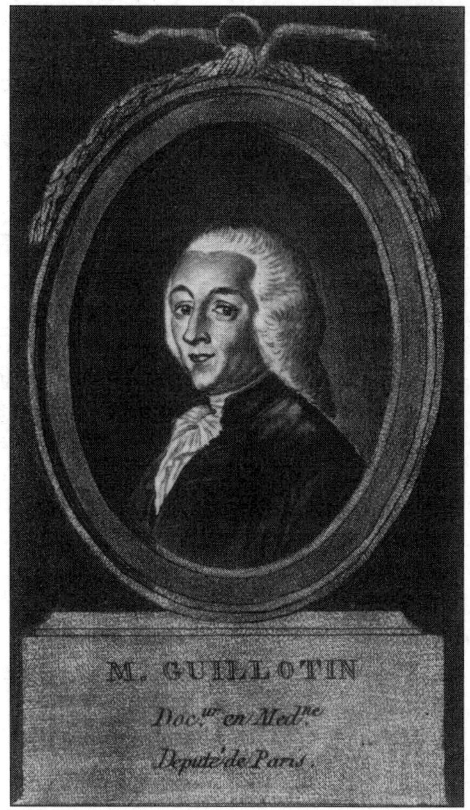

Joseph I. Guillotin (Courtesy of the Royal Society of Medicine, London, UK)

GUILLOTINE

French instrument for execution by decapitation. A term applied to some surgical instruments which work on a similar principle.

Joseph I. Guillotin (1738–1814) He was born in Saintes and initially was interested in the Arts and became Professor of Literature at the Irish College at Bordeaux, but later studied medicine at Rheims where he graduated in 1768 and two years later graduated from the University of Paris. He was appointed to the government committee to examine the exhibitions then being undertaken by Mesmer and became one of the 10 Deputies of Paris in the Assemblée Constituante. In 1789 he proposed that there should be a uniform method of executing by decapitation in place of the inhumane methods such as burning, mutilation, drowning and hanging. His colleagues, however, laughed when he claimed that a machine that he had designed could cause immediate and painless separation of the head from the trunk. It was not until 1791 that a law was passed that everyone condemned to death in France should be decapitated.

Dr Antoine Louis who was the secretary of the surgical academy, together with Schmidt, a German piano maker and Sanson, the executioner, made the machine without any reference to Guillotin. Initially the machine was called "la Louisette" or "la petite Louisson" before it finally became the "guillotine".

Guillotin was one of the first French doctors to support Jenner's (*v. infra*) discovery and in 1805 was the President of the Committee for vaccination in Paris. Guillotin was imprisoned because a letter from Count Méré, who was about to be executed, commended his wife and children to the doctor's care. When Robespierre fell from power, he was released and died with a carbuncle on the left shoulder.

GULL DISEASE

Myxedema (hypothyroidism).

Sir William Gull (1816–1890) English physician, born in Colchester, England. His father was a barge owner and died of cholera, leaving his family poor. Gull was helped by Mr. Harrison, secretary of Guy's Hospital, who made him his protégé. He studied at Guy's Hospital, graduating M.B. in 1841, University of London, and M.D. in 1846. He became lecturer in medicine there in 1856, F.R.S. 1858 and was created a Baronet in 1872 when he treated the Prince of Wales who had typhoid. He was physician to Queen Victoria. His description of myxedema (1873) was not the first but he was one of the first to attribute the clinical picture to the thyroid. He noted the involvement of the posterior column in tabes, described intermittent hemoglobulinemia (1866) and with Sutton the pathological changes in chronic nephritis. He wrote on anorexia nervosa, was one of the pioneers of the use of ricinis in the treatment of tenia, and wrote the first description of syringomyelia and steatorrhea due to intestinal lymphoma. He was an attractive teacher and famous for his epigrams: "Savages explain, science investigates"; "The road to a medical education is through the Hunterian Museum and not an apothecary's shop"; "We have no system to satisfy, no dogmatic opinions to enforce. We have no ignorance to cloak, we confess it"; "I do not say no drugs are useful, but there is not enough discrimination in their use".

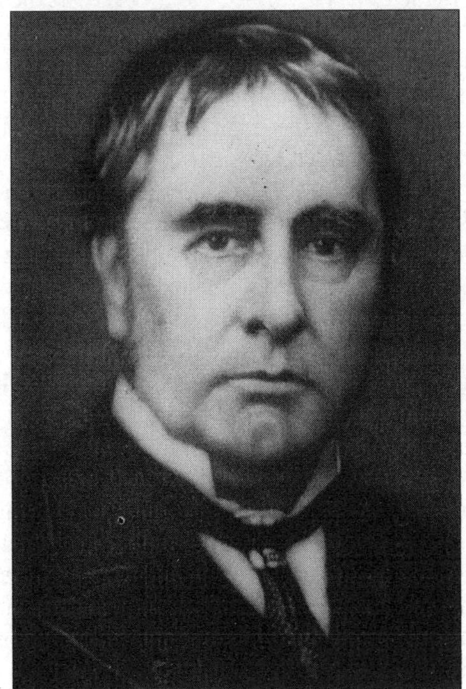

Sir William Gull (Courtesy of the Royal Society of Medicine, London, UK)

He died a very wealthy man, being especially able at handling neurotics and his immense success in practice was shown at his death when he left a fortune of 344 000 pounds. To one such hypochondriac he said "You are a healthy man out of health". This satisfied the patient so much he wanted to know why the other doctors had not told him.

GUMPRECHT SHADOWS

Degenerated nuclei (naked nuclei) seen in the peripheral blood films of patients with leukemia.

Ferdinand Gumprecht (1863–) German physician.

GUNN

v. MARCUS GUNN

GUTTMANN SIGN

Bruit heard over the thyroid gland in thyrotoxicosis.

Paul Guttmann (1834–1893) German physician who was director of the Moabit Hospital, Berlin. He graduated from medical school in Berlin in 1858 and was particularly influenced by Griesinger and J. Meyer with whom he worked as an assistant and by Traube who guided his clinical career. He wrote a book on diagnostic techniques and physicial examination and investigated the mode of action of antipyretic drugs as well as the structure and function of the sympathetic nervous system. He played a major role in treating and controlling an outbreak of cholera in Berlin.

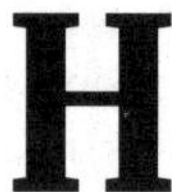

HAENEL SIGN

Analgesia to pressure on the eyeball in tabes dorsalis.

HAENEL VARIANT

Progressive muscular atrophy affecting only the upper limbs.

Hans Haenel (1874–1942) German neurologist.

HAFF DISEASE

Myositis and myoglobinuria due to eating fish that have ingested industrial wastes.

Königsberg or Kurische Haff (inlet or harbour) where the first cases were reported in 1924 and thought due to arsenical preparations used in cellulose factories and dumped into the water, accumulating in eels living in the water and in turn eaten by the fishermen.

HAGEMAN FACTOR

Factor XII – (a contact factor) – is a plasma protein which on activation by surface contact sets off chain reactions activating the clotting, kinin, fibrinolytic and complement pathways.

Mr. Hageman A railroad engineer (train driver), who was noted to have a grossly prolonged clotting time yet had no bleeding manifestations and died of pulmonary embolism.

HAILEY-HAILEY DISEASE

Familial benign pemphigus, an autosomal dominant lesion which most frequently involves the nape, or lateral aspects of the neck and axillae (sometimes called DARIER DISEASE).

William H. Hailey (1898–1967) American dermatologist in Atlanta, Georgia.

Hugh E. Hailey (1909–) American dermatologist.

HAJDU-CHENEY SYNDROME

Loss of the terminal phalanges of the hands and feet sometimes giving the appearance of clubbing with osteoporosis, scoliosis, loss of the teeth and coarse hair. The face is characterized by bushy eyebrows, broad nose, receding and pointed chin. It is an autosomal dominant in some families.

Nicholas Hajdu (1908–) Graduated in medicine at Prague University in 1934 and worked at the first university clinic for medical diseases there until 1939. It was here that he first became interested in radiology, since he had the task of screening schizophrenics who were being checked for tuberculosis before treatment with hypoglycemic shock. He was unsupervized and he recalls the eerie sensation of being surrounded by a dozen of such patients in a room filled with unguarded high tension cables which when the pilot light failed would be plunged into complete darkness. He migrated to England and requalified in medicine there and spent a year in general practice before enrolling in the British Government scheme to train radiologists for the armed forces. He undertook this at St. George's Hospital. He was appointed as an Assistant Radiologist in 1947 and it was during this time that he noted the then unrecorded combination of skeletal changes which has subsequently been named after him. He was appointed Consultant Radiologist at St. George's Hospital in 1949 and remained there for 25 years until his retirement.

William D. Cheney (1918–) U.S. radiologist. He was born at Tekonsha, Michigan, and graduated

M.D. from the University of Michigan in 1943 to undertake his residency at Wisconsin General Hospital in Madison, Wisconsin. He commenced his training in radiology at the St. Joseph's Mercy Hospital in Ann Arbor, Michigan, and on completion of this in 1950, he practiced at the Edward Sparrow Hospital in Lansing, Michigan.

HALBERSTAETER BODIES

v. PROWAZEK-HALBERSTAETER BODIES

HALLERMAN-STREIFF-FRANÇOIS SYNDROME

Congenital short stature, bird-like facies, atrophy of the skin, cataract, micro-ophthalmia and mental retardation.

Wilhelm Hallerman (1901–) German ophthalmologist.

Enrico B. Streiff (1908–) Swiss ophthalmologist. Born in Genoa, Italy, and graduated from the University of Genoa in 1933. He became Privatdozent in ophthalmology in Geneva in 1933 until 1944 when he was appointed professor in Lausanne.

Jules François Belgian ophthalmologist.

HALLERVORDEN-SPATZ DISEASE OR SYNDROME

Progressive pallidal degeneration or adult amaurotic idiocy, a heredo-familial condition commencing in childhood with progressive rigidity, speech difficulties, dementia, optic atrophy and hyperkinesis with deposition of iron in the substantia nigra and globus pallidus.

Julius Hallervorden (1882–1965) German neurologist, born in East Prussia. He came to Kraepelin's clinic in Munich to spend sabbatical leave and brought with him the brain of a girl who had suffered with the syndrome. He met Spatz there and together they described the syndrome. Hallervorden worked with Spatz from then on. He loved symphonic music.

Hugo Spatz (1888–1969) German neurologist and son of the editor of München medizinische Wochenschrift. He entered medical school in Munich and proceeded to Heidelberg, graduating in 1914 and going straight to the Western Front for the duration of the war. He joined Kraepelin's Forschungsanstalt für Psychiatrie in Munich and was influenced there by Nissl, Brodmann and especially Spielmeyer. He was a morphologist who could both elaborate and stimulate thought, and made numerous contributions especially in the field of extrapyramidal neuropathology. He was appointed Director of the Kaiser-Wilhelm Institute in Berlin, succeeding Vogt. At the outbreak of World War II he was mobilized to join the Luftwaffe until 1941 when he returned to Berlin. He was arrested by American police and then was invited to join the U.S. Aeromedical Center. In 1949 he and Hallervorden were given laboratories in the Physiology Institute in Vienna and here he mapped out the tubero-hypophyseal pathways. He was a very humane and thoughtful person, who smuggled food to prisoners of war whilst he was in Holland.

HALLOPEAU DISEASE

1. Lichen sclerosis et atrophica. A chronic condition of the skin with white sclerotic areas and atrophic macules which may range from half to a few centimetres in diameter and which may coalesce to form atrophic plaques with irregular edges. Most commonly occurs in middle-aged to elderly women and may occur in the neck, axilla, trunk or limbs and sometimes in the perineal area. In the latter it may cause pruritus.

2. Pyodermatitis Vegetans. Lesions may involve the axilla, groin, genitalia, scalp and the lips and oral mucosa. It is believed to result from staphylococcal superinfection.

Henri Hallopeau (1842–1919) French dermatologist and physician. He was born in Paris and was an outstanding scholar at school, who won the history prize, beating Anatole Leroy-Beaulieu, who was later to become a very successful French writer. He commenced Medical School when he was 24 and initially was interested in neurological problems and pathology and became Professeur Agrégé in 1878 with two theses, one on neurological problems and the other on the use of mercury. His first hospital was Tenon, later Saint-Antoine and in 1884 he moved to St. Louis.

In the same year his book on Pathology was published and became the leading text on pathology in France and was translated into a number of other languages. On arriving at St. Louis Hospital he turned his attention to Dermatology and had a prolific output in papers written, perhaps owing something to his poor sleeping habits, since he would often wake in the middle of the night to work for one or two hours. He wrote 26 papers on mycosis fungoides alone and with his colleague, Emilé Leredde he wrote a book on Dermatology in 1900 which was widely acclaimed and included an attempt at classifying dermatological conditions according to their cause. When Fournier retired in 1902, Hallopeau vied with Gaucher for the vacant chair but lost by a single vote. An extremely pleasant person, he not only bore no grudge against Gaucher but attended Gaucher's inaugural lecture and supported his admission to the Academy of Medicine. He retired from St. Louis Hospital in 1907 but still maintained his interest in dermatology and attended the first session of the French Dermatological Society after the cessation of the First World War in 1919 and died a few days later.

HAM TEST

The definitive test for paroxysmal nocturnal hemoglobinuria (PNH). Lowering of pH results in complement lysis of red cells with the PNH defect.

Thomas Hales Ham (1905–1987) American physician born in Oklahoma City, brought up in Yonkers, New York and graduated from Cornell Medical School, M.D., in 1931. He did his medical residency at the New York Hospital and then went to the Thorndike Memorial Laboratory at Boston City Hospital where he worked with William Castle. He spent the next 16 years at Harvard and the Thorndike Laboratories, apart from his absence in the army during World War II. He moved to become Professor of Medicine at Western Reserve University, Cleveland in 1950. Always an innovator in medical education (he had introduced a clinical pathology course at Harvard emphasizing clinical cases and problem solving). He was a leading light in the Western Reserve Faculty which undertook the revolution in medical educational approach by breaking down department barriers to structure courses that were interdisciplinary and introduced students to patients from the very first day of their medical course. He was a founding father of the American Society of Hematology and pioneered the educational program which became a major drawcard for the Society's meetings. Undoubtedly one of the large reasons for his success was his personality with which he managed to imbue excitement and interest in both education and research into his colleagues and his many students. He was well known for his wit and sense of humor and "hamisms". Although mainly remembered internationally for his contributions to hemolytic anemias he co-authored the first paper with Castle on the role of extrinsic factor in the hemopoietic response in pernicious anemia.

HAMILTON SIGN

Hairs growing on the anti-tragus of the ear indicate normal androgenic function in males over 30.

J.B. Hamilton U.S. endocrinologist.

HAMMAN DISEASE

Spontaneous mediastinal emphysema.

HAMMAN SIGN

Crunching systolic sound heard over the sternal edge in mediastinal emphysema, often heard only after altering the patient's position.

HAMMAN-RICH SYNDROME

Idiopathic diffuse interstitial pulmonary fibrosis.

Louis V. Hamman (1877–1946) U.S. physician born in Baltimore, graduated M.D. Johns Hopkins in 1901 and interned at New York Hospital to return to Johns Hopkins in 1903 as Head of the new Phipps Tuberculosis Clinic. He was highly recommended for the job by Osler and with S. Wolman he studied the use of tuberculin in the diagnosis and treatment of tuberculosis. He introduced the glucose tolerance test for the diagnosis and management of diabetes and was one of the first to delineate clearly the symptomatology of coronary thrombosis. He identified and first described the condition of spontaneous mediastinal emphysema with its characteristic auscultatory findings (Hamman sign). He was an extremely kind and gentle person to whom patients and staff responded warmly. He was a superb teacher who excelled at the Clinicopathological Conference (CPC) held with Dr Rich and could always bring out the best in his students and interns. He died of a coronary thrombosis.

Arnold R. Rich (1893–1968) U.S. pathologist. He was born in Birmingham, Alabama, was schooled at a Military Academy in North Carolina and entered College at the University of Virginia. During his last year there he became interested in zoology where he investigated the proboscis of a flat worm which when separated from the body would ingest anything, but was selective when attached to the worm. He entered Johns Hopkins Medical School and there spent much of his time in the research laboratory, initially investigating blood coagulation with W.H. Howell. He had wanted to go into experimental surgery and Halstead suggested he spend a year in pathology with MacCallum. Thereafter he remained in the Pathology Department of Johns Hopkins, eventually becoming its Director and Professor of Pathology when MacCallum left. He made contributions to the classification of jaundice. A major portion of his research was devoted to pursuing the relationship between hypersensitivity and immunity and he demonstrated that peri-arteritis could result from hypersensitivity to drugs such as sulphonamides. He identified the Gaucher cell as a phagocyte and wrote substantial papers on experimental pancreatitis and cirrhosis. He contributed to morphological pathology, describing the characteristic lesion in the spleen in sickle cell anemia, the renal lesion peculiar to syphilis and interstitial fibrosis of the lung. Probably his most important role was as a teacher and the CPCs, first with W.S. Thayer, then with L. Hamman and finally A. McGhee Harvey were remembered by all students passing through Johns Hopkins. He was by American standards an eccentric, never arriving at work before 12. He was a fly fisherman, an engraver, composer and poet.

HAMMOND DISEASE

Congenital athetosis.

William A. Hammond (1828–1900) U.S. neurologist. A surgeon-general in the U.S. Army, he wrote a book on nervous disorders as well as describing athetosis. He was born in Maryland where his father

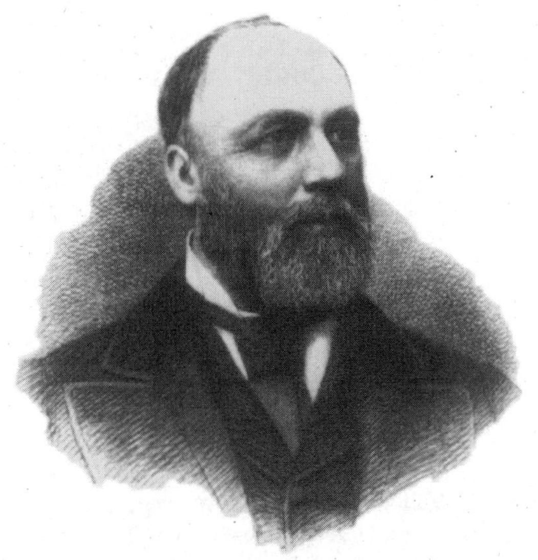

William A. Hammond (Courtesy of the Royal Society of Medicine, London, UK)

was a doctor. He entered the U.S. medical department as an assistant surgeon and fought the Sioux Indians, then became ill and convalesced in Europe where he studied military hospitals. He returned to the U.S. and a mutual interest in arrow ordeal poisons and snake venoms led to a friendship with Weir-Mitchell, and a joint publication in 1859 in the American Journal of Medicine. In 1860 he resigned from the army to be appointed to the Chair of

Anatomy and Physiology but re-entered the army when the American Civil War broke out. Lincoln appointed him Surgeon-General in 1862 and he founded the Army Medical Museum. With co-authors he wrote "The Medical and Surgical History of the War of the Rebellion" which was highly praised by Virchow. Unfortunately there was constant friction between him and the Secretary of War, Stanton, and Hammond was court-martialled and found guilty on a trumped up charge, which was quashed 14 years later by Act of Congress. On leaving the army he arrived in New York penniless and set up practice in neurology. He became Professor at the University of the City of New York in 1874 and in 1876 at Bellevue Hospital College and was one of the seven founders of the American Neurological Association. He was a playwright, novelist and lecturer as well as writing a neurology textbook. He died of heart disease in Washington.

HAND-SCHÜLLER-CHRISTIAN DISEASE

Histiocytosis X, characterized by a triad of defects in membranous bone, exophthalmos and polyuria, often with hepatosplenomegaly and lymphadenopathy.

v. LETTERER-SIWE DISEASE

Alfred Hand (1868–1949) U.S. pediatrician. In 1893 he found yellow deposits in the skull of a patient with polyuria and thought it was tuberculosis.

Artur Schüller (1874–1957) Austrian radiologist, born in Brunn, Czechoslovakia. His father was a specialist in otolaryngology, and a friend of Politzer. He was outstanding at school, especially in the humanities and music, and he entered medicine in Vienna aged 17. He graduated with the highest honors, being awarded a prize by Franz Josef at a special audience, which had only been given twice during the Emperor's 60 year reign. Holzknecht invited him to join his X-ray department and rapidly he fulfilled the promise of his undergraduate days by his careful analysis of X-ray examinations of the skull, which set out fundamental principles still forming the basis of this examination. In 1910 he performed experiments on dogs which suggested the practicality of cordotomy for pain relief. He also suggested the trans-sphenoidal nasal approach for pituitary operations. In 1909, aged 35, he was appointed University Professor in Vienna, where his colleagues were his former teachers Billroth, Nothnagel, Finsterer, Politzer, Krafft-Ebing and Wagner Juaregg.

When World War I came Schüller did much medical work for the army, and wrote a paper describing a patient with Hand-Schüller Disease in 1915. Following the war, Vienna changed from a city of prosperity to one of poverty and in the inflation which followed he found great difficulty in making ends meet. In order to eke out a living, he undertook postgraduate classes in private on X-ray diagnosis of disorders of the skull, ear, nose and throat and made a collection of almost every disorder known of the skull, which unfortunately was lost when he left Vienna. He wrote over 300 papers, monographs and books, and in one described the disorder osteoporosis circumscripta cranii, which is an early stage of Paget Disease of the skull and may be detected before any symptomatology. With the rise of Hitler, he left Vienna hurriedly in 1938, leaving most of his possessions behind. His two sons were prevented at the last moment from leaving. After a short time in England he went to Australia where at the age of 65 he commenced to build up a career. He worked in the X-ray department of St. Vincent's Hospital, Melbourne, where Dr. John O'Sullivan, who had been a pupil of his in Vienna, was an associate. He was much sought after as an X-ray Consultant and received X-rays from all over the country for his opinion. During the latter years he was troubled by depression and developed Parkinson Disease. His two sons died in a concentration camp.

Henry A. Christian (1876–1951) U.S. physician, born in Virginia, and graduated from Randolph-Mason College in 1895. He received his M.D. at Johns Hopkins in 1900 and worked with F.B. Mallory at the Boston City Hospital. In 1908 he was appointed Jersey Professor of Theory and Practice and became the first Physician in Chief to the Peter Bent Brigham, retiring in 1939. He reported a typical example of the disorder in 1919. He was an outstanding teacher and clinician who wrote a number of texts and guided many young people into academic medicine.

HANOT CIRRHOSIS

Primary biliary cirrhosis.

Victor C. Hanot (1844–1896) French physician who described cirrhotic jaundice (1875) and biliary cirrhosis. Whilst with Charcot, he published his first paper on rupture of the aorta and although he published in many areas of medicine, devoted most of his research to the study of liver disease and wrote on all aspects in clinical and pathological terms ranging from hemochromatosis to hepatic malignancies. He greatly influenced Gilbert (*v. supra*).

HANSEMANN MACROPHAGES

Large mononuclear cell with abundant cytoplasm and large intra-cytoplasmic inclusions with calcium and iron laden bodies termed Michaelis-Gutmann bodies. These cells are characteristic of malakoplakia (soft slab), an unusual granulomatous condition predominantly affecting the urinary tract. He reported malakoplakia in 1903, two years after he had first recognized it.

D.P. von Hansemann (1858–1920) German pathologist who introduced the theory of anaplasia or the changes in a cell to make it morphologically and functionally different from its fellows and thereby cancerous. He was born in Eupen and studied medicine at Berlin, Kiel and Leipzig, graduating M.D. in 1886. He became assistant to Virchow (*v. infra*) at the University of Berlin and became titular Professor of Anatomy and Pathology in 1897. He was an army pathologist in World War 1. He opposed the indiscriminate use of tuberculin in the treatment of tuberculosis.

HANSEN BACILLUS

Mycobacterium leprae.

HANSEN DISEASE

Leprosy.

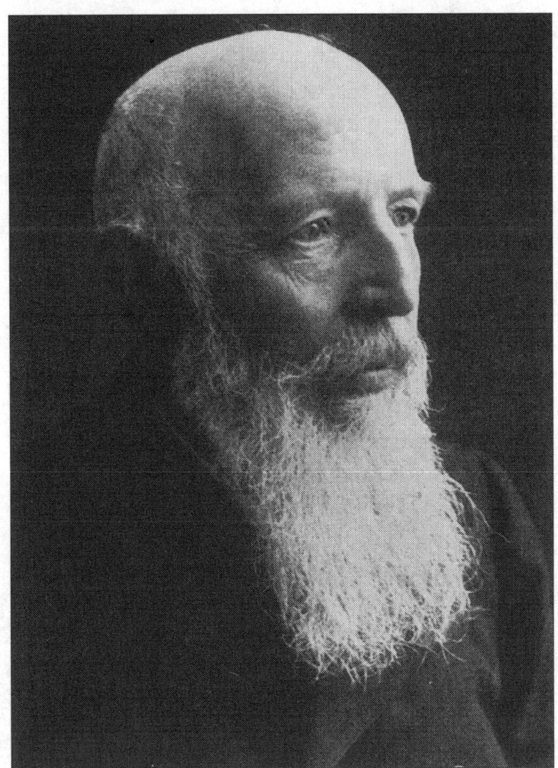

Armauer Hansen (Courtesy of Dr H. Stomorken and the Hansen Family, Norway)

Armauer Hansen (1841–1912) Norwegian bacteriologist from Bergen in Norway, he graduated from the University of Christiana (Oslo) in 1866. He noted the relationship between the lepra bacillus and leprosy (1871–4) but his work was initially not recognized, and Neisser (*v. infra*), who came to Bergen to examine his specimens, took samples back to Breslau where he succeeded in staining the bacillus and for a time Neisser was given priority.

HARADA SYNDROME

Uveo-meningoencephalitis – with predominant choroiditis, sometimes complicated by exudative detachment of the retina. There is an increase in cerebrospinal fluid (CSF) protein and white cells. It is perhaps related to Vogt-Koyanagi Syndrome (*v. infra*).

E. Harada Contemporary Japanese ophthalmologist.

HARLEY DISEASE

1. Paroxysmal hemoglobinuria.
2. Dressler syndrome (*v. supra*).

George Harley (1829–1896) Scottish physician. He was born in Haddington, in East Lothian, and entered Edinburgh Medical School when he was 17 years old. Whilst he was still a student at the maternity hospital, one of the expectant mothers died of a heart attack, and he successfully performed a Cesarean section without assistance or previous experience. He delivered a living child. Harley graduated that year and became a resident at the Royal Infirmary. He then went to Paris where he studied in the laboratories of Robin, Verdeil and Wurtz. There he observed that iron was a normal constituent of urine and that there was a pigment in urine which he called urohematin (presumably urobilinogen) which was derived from the breakdown products of the red cell. He next worked in the College de France with Magendie who retired a few months later and was replaced by Claude Bernard. Influenced by the latter's publications on the role of the liver in the production of diabetes, Harley commenced research with J. Bowman on the effects of infusing the portal circulation with substances such as alcohol, ammonia, and chloroform and established diabetes in animals. During this time he placed himself on a diet of asparagus laced with pepper and vinegar for three days and was said to have rendered himself diabetic for 14 days! He next spent two years in Germany at Würzburg where he worked with Professor Scherer, a recognized authority on urine pigments who had initially questioned his findings. After Harley had worked with him he agreed that his findings had been correct and that iron was a normal constituent in both blood and urine. Whilst there Harley worked with Kolliken in histology and with Virchow.

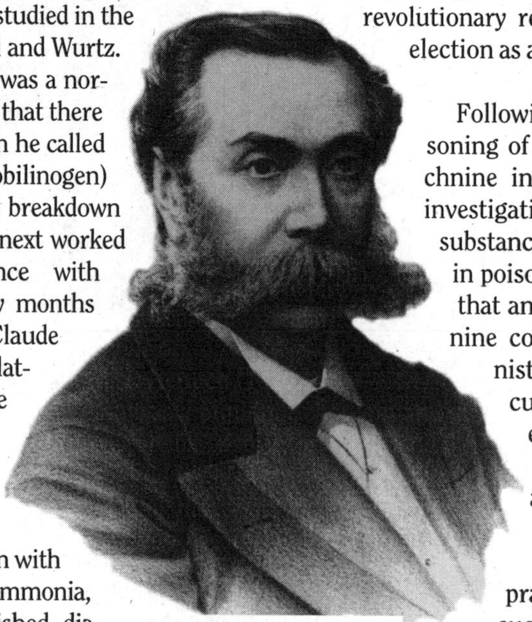

During this period he visited Würzburg, Giessen, Berlin, Vienna and Heidelberg where he worked in Bunsen's laboratory, acquiring the techniques of gas analysis. Whilst in Germany he published two important papers, one on urohematin and the other on urine analysis in a patient with the nephrotic syndrome. After leaving Germany he went to Italy, but stayed only a few days at the University of Padua where he was disappointed at the standard of the Faculty and returned to England in 1855 to become Curator of the anatomical museum at the University College and Lecturer on Practical Physiology and Histology. Soon after he published a paper which proved Magnus's theory that respired oxygen formed a chemical combination with blood constituents (namely hemoglobin). This was at the time revolutionary research and resulted in his election as a Fellow of the Royal Society.

George Harley (Courtesy of the Royal Society of Medicine, London, UK)

Following the famous Palmer poisoning of his friend Cooke with strychnine in 1856, Harley commenced investigations on the toxicology of this substance and developed an interest in poisons. He was the first to show that animals poisoned with strychnine could be saved by the administration of the arrow poison curare. He undertook some early research on the anatomy and physiology of the adrenals.

In 1856 he commenced practice, but initially had little success and in 12 months had seen only two patients. However, in December that year at a meeting of the Pathological Society, he suggested that an hepatic intestinal calculus was located there by ulcerating directly from the gall bladder into the duodenum. This theory greatly attracted the then President, Dr. Watson, who from then on used Harley as a consultant, not only in patients with liver disease, but also those with kidney trouble. Next he investigated the effects of the pancreas and showed that it had ingredients which could digest both starch and protein and therefore fulfilled the functions of the saliva and gastric secretion. In 1859 he was appointed Professor of Medical Jurisprudence at the University College. At that time he postulated that the reason why the stomach is not itself digested is because of a protective layer of alkaline mucus which is rapidly replaced.

His interest in arrow poison continued, and he also wrote concerning the effects of the ordeal poison, Calabar beans (physostigmine) and of long continued minute doses of arsenic. He had a flair for the original and was a great raconteur as demonstrated by his presentation contrasting the effects of the arrow poisons from Borneo, Antiar ("cardiac glycoside") and Guinea (curare) – "one poison produced a dead heart and a living body, and the other a dead body with a living heart". Through his interest in arrow poisons, he became interested in anthropology and wrote on the origin of the races in North and South America, postulating that they came from parts of Asia, especially Borneo and South America.

Like many of his day, he was interested in the unusual, and sometimes extraordinary manifestations of hysteria. In 1863 he published the story of a 33 year old woman who made an extraordinarily loud noise from her vagina by expelling gas, and demonstrated by gas analysis that this was simply air which had been previously sucked in by voluntary contractions of her abdominal muscles! He reported another instance "an extraordinary case of spasmodic cough in a girl aged 14 years". The number of times the girl coughed was counted at intervals by students especially allocated for the job as 70/minute. On reckoning, if this girl coughed only 12 out of 24 hours, she then coughed 40 000 times daily. It is recorded that with anti-spasmodic treatment she made a complete recovery!

In 1865 he published notes on two patients with intermittent hematuria and for the first time made the point that in some forms of malaria blood constituents were eliminated in the urine giving it a red or sometimes tea-like appearance without there being any red cells present on microscopic examination.

He wrote important textbooks of the day on histology and liver disease. One evening whilst working with his microscope he suffered a left retinal hemorrhage and this was followed by what is described as acute retinitis with glaucoma and an extirpation of the affected eye was recommended because the right eye had become involved (ophthalmitis sympathetica). He declined this, however, and kept himself in a totally dark room for nine months, during which time he did not even see his own hands! When he emerged from the room he made the following observations. Initially he was unable to judge even the shortest distances, and he found that he had lost the ability to distinguish colors. He reasoned that this explained why infants initially knock things over when they try to take hold of them. For the first month all mauves, blues, greens and yellows appeared to be white, whilst the grays, browns and reds all looked black. During his time in total darkness he made arrangements to dictate and in 1872 a book entitled "The Urine and its Derangements" was published and reprinted in America and translated into French and Italian.

Apart from his medical contributions he wrote a number of short stories and even tried to change the English language in a book entitled "The Simplification of English Spelling" where he advocated the omission of any redundant or duplicated consonant in a language except those in personal names. He read a paper on "Primitive writings in sticks and bones" where he attempted to trace the origin of writing among the native tribes of Australia and other primitives. He invented a number of time-saving devices in the laboratory including a simple attachment to convert a microscope from monocular to binocular. He also introduced the use of the sound in demonstrating the presence of calculi both in the gall bladder and in the ureter.

His magnum opus was his book "Diseases of the Liver" with the motto on the title page "True science is the key to wise practice". The book provided many illustrations whereby the current knowledge in physiological chemistry could be applied to patients' problems at the bedside. He constantly attempted to marry structure and function with the then known chemistry.

Harley was a strong protagonist of cremation and after a peculiar neurological problem towards the end of his life which resulted in difficulties in walking, he died suddenly. He was cremated at his own wish and buried at Woking cemetry.

HARRISON SULCUS OR GROOVE

Groove in the thorax extending laterally from the xiphisternum to the axillae, due to rickets.

Edwin Harrison (1766–1838) English physician, born in Lancashire, and studied medicine in Edinburgh. He described his sign in 1798. He became an F.R.S. and wrote a book on spinal disease in 1827 and made observations on spinal nerves in 1831.

HARTMANN POUCH

Dilatation of the neck of the gall bladder.

Henri Hartmann (1860–1952) French surgeon born in Paris. He wrote on large bowel surgery and established "Hartmann critical point" where the lowest sigmoid artery meets the superior rectal branch. He became Professor of Pathology, Paris Faculty of Medicine in 1909.

HARTMANN SOLUTION

Lactated Ringer solution for intravenous administration.

Alexis F. Hartmann (1898–1964) U.S. pediatrician in St. Louis.

HARTNUP DISEASE

Autosomal recessive disease with aminoaciduria, pellagra, skin rash and cerebellar features.

Hartnup was the surname of the first family described and investigated by Charles Dent at the Middlesex Hospital, London.

HASHIMOTO DISEASE, THYROIDITIS

Struma lymphomatosa – a goitre, often associated with mild hypothyroidism and thought to be autoimmune.

Hakaru Hashimoto (1881–1934) Japanese surgeon. He was born in the village of Midau, Nishi-tsuge in the Mie Prefecture, Japan. He and his family were medical practitioners and he entered the new medical school at Kyushu University in 1903. He was one of the first graduates of the University in 1907 and then worked in the surgical department with Professor Hauari Miyake from 1908–1912 and wrote his M.D. thesis on "Struma lymphomatosa". Since his account was published in a German surgical journal, his compatriots were unaware of his discovery. After obtaining his M.D. he went to Europe, spending 3 years in Berlin, Göttingen and London, and paid particular attention to renal tuberculosis. When World War I broke out he returned to Japan, and because his father died, went straight into the family practice and rapidly became a prosperous surgeon with a very highly regarded reputation especially for major abdominal surgery. He published two further papers, one on erysipelas and the other on penetrating wounds of the chest. He was a very fervent Buddhist and was fond of traditional Japanese theatre. He died of typhoid.

HASSALL CORPUSCLES

Characteristic lymphoid structures in the thymus.

Arthur H. Hassall (1817–1894). Born in Teddington, Middlesex, at the age of 29 he wrote the first English textbook on microscopic anatomy and also was well recognized as a Botanist. He became a physician at the Royal Free Hospital in London and practiced later on in the Isle of Wight where he died.

HAVERHILL FEVER

Erythema arthriticum epidemicum. An acute infection due to *Streptobacillus moniliformis* with fever, rash and polyarthritis.

Haverhill was the township in Massachusetts where the first outbreak occurred in 1926, attributed to contaminated milk. It is usually acquired by rat bite.

HAVERSIAN CANALS

Longitudinal canals in compact bone inter-connecting with one another.

Clopton Havers (1650–1702) English anatomist and physician. He went to Catherine Hall, Cambridge, graduated M.D. from Utrecht, Holland in 1685 and L.R.C.P. in 1687. He practiced as a physician in London and became F.R.S. in 1686. He studied bone growth and repair as well as its structure.

HAWTHORNE EFFECT*

This refers to a study undertaken to improve productivity by the Western Electric Company at its Hawthorne plant. Working conditions were changed in a number of ways, e.g., by shortening working hours or introducing rest periods. It soon became obvious that whatever experimental changes were made the girls would work more effectively. The greater interest shown to them caused them to be more motivated. This improvement in productivity has been compared to educational experiments where innovations make teachers more interested and students respond to their greater interest. The better results achieved may only be transitory.

* Roethlisberger, F.J. and Dickson, W.J. (1939) "Management and the Worker", Harvard University Press, Boston.

HAYEM-WIDAL SYNDROME

Acquired hemolytic anemia.

Georges Hayem (1841–1933) French physician and hematologist. Born in Paris. Professor of Therapeutics (1879–93) and clinical medicine (1897–1911) in Paris. He was one of the founders of hematology and wrote on digestion, the stomach and cholera, and described goats' milk anemia in 1889 as well as doing pioneer work with platelets introducing the first accurate platelet counts. He was said to have saved 30% of his patients in the cholera epidemic by giving them an isotonic saline solution to combat the dehydration and was later nicknamed Dr. Cholera. His textbook on hematology in 1900 was widely read.

G.F.I. Widal French physician

v. WIDAL TEST

HAYGARTH NODES

Fusiform joint swellings in rheumatoid arthritis. The middle and proximal joints are the most commonly affected.

John Haygarth (1740–1827) English physician, from Bath, who was one of the earliest epidemiologists, and documented the diseases occurring in Chester. He used smallpox as a means of immunization. He studied at St. John's College, Cambridge, and graduated M.B. in 1766. After studying in London and Edinburgh he was appointed physician at the Chester Infirmary where he investigated infectious diseases and the usefulness of isolation. In 1798 he moved to Bath and there published his works on rheumatism and rheumatic fever.

HEAD AREAS OR ZONES

Skin segments exhibiting hypersensitivity due to referred sensation from the viscera, e.g. shoulder tip pain with gall bladder disease.

Sir Henry Head (1861–1940) English neurologist. Head was a Quaker who gained a scholarship to Trinity College, Cambridge, where he graduated B.A. and then spent 2 years at the German University in Prague (where he introduced soccer) and at the University of Halle. His first paper was on nerve action potentials. He worked with Hering in Halle and in 1889 wrote on vagal respiratory effects. He then studied at the University College Hospital, London, and graduated in 1892. He examined pain referral from deep structures, which led him to a study of herpes zoster, and from this he went on to study dermatomes. In 1898 he was elected assistant physician to the London Hospital and continued in hospital and private practice until his retirement in 1925. His investigations were confined to the sensory system and he made many observations on himself after sectioning of the superficial ramus of his radial nerve. Among his contributions was the postulate of proteopathic and epicritic sensory systems to explain different susceptibilities of sensation – the first explanation of the nature of sensory dissociation.

He joined the lively debate on aphasia, opposing the Broca and Wernicke schools which supported localization of areas, but he introduced confusing terminology so that it was said if there was not chaos before Head there certainly was after.

Head was well known for a weakness for possessing omniscience on all subjects, particularly his own specialty. One day William Bullock, a bacteriologist, asked him over lunch at his hospital whether he had read Hagenheimer's new book on locomotor ataxia. Head replied he had only had time to glance at it. Bullock commented "Well, you have done better than the rest of us. There is no such book" ...! Head, however, was rarely put out by any eventuality and was a superb bedside teacher. One day in his ward with a large class of students he was examining a lady who whilst he was leaning down examining her heart, threw her arms around his neck and kissed him. Without a moment's hesitation he turned to the students and said, "Typical, gentlemen, typical".

He was editor of "Brain" from 1910–1925 and was knighted in 1927. He wrote a book of verses. In the latter years of his life he developed Parkinson Disease, which he coped with well, aided by Riddoch (*v. infra*).

HEAF GUN

Method of subcutaneous inoculation by atomizing the fluid to be injected with such force that it penetrates the skin. It is extremely useful for mass inoculation or surveys with Mantoux tests.

Frederick R.G. Heaf (1895–) British physician. Born in Desborough. He went to Medical School at Cambridge University and St. Thomas's Hospital, worked in various positions in Public Health becoming a Professor at the University of Wales in 1949. He had a lifelong interest in tuberculosis.

HEBERDEN ARTHRITIS

Degenerative disease of the terminal joints of the fingers with bony prominence dorsally (HEBERDEN NODES), and sometimes flexion deformities – often associated with osteoarthritis of weight-bearing joints.

HEBERDEN DISEASE

1. Arthritis (*v. supra*).
2. Angina pectoris.

HEBERDEN NODES

These consist of bony enlargements, usually twin tubercles, at the dorsal base of the terminal phalanges. When they first appear they may be tender but later they are non-tender and the overlying skin is normal.

HEBERDEN-ROSENBACH NODES (*v. supra*)

William Heberden Sn. (1710–1801) English physician, who was born in London in 1710 and in 1724 went to St. John's College in Cambridge where six years later he was elected a Fellow. He studied medicine in Cambridge and London and obtained his Doctor of Physic and then practiced in London at the University, giving an annual course in therapeutics. In 1746 he became a Fellow of the Royal College of Physicians and two years later was elected to the Royal Society. In 1766 he suggested the establishment of Medical Transactions to the College of Physicians, in which observations on cures and disease could be recorded. He was a very religious man and a leading Latin and Hebrew scholar. He gave classic accounts of angina and chicken pox and also described night blindness. He noted that tuberculosis often improved during pregnancy but not post-partum. Dr. Samuel Johnson referred to him as "Dr. Heberden ultimus

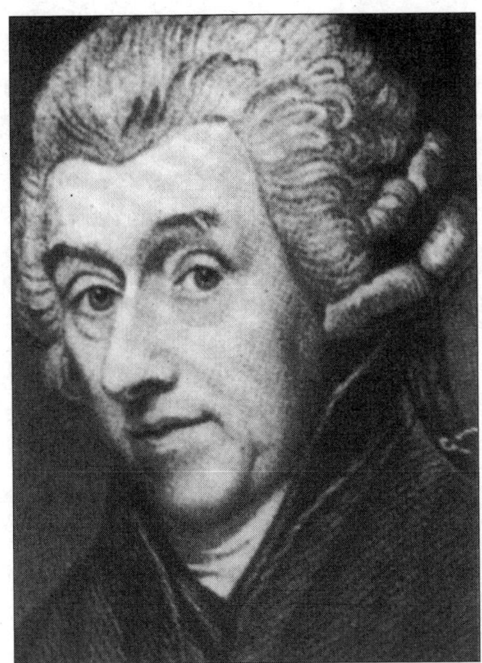

William Heberden Sn. (Reproduced from *"The Royal College of Physicians of London Portraits"* by G. Wolstenholme & D. Piper [Published by J & A Churchill Ltd. London 1964])

Romanorum – the last of our learned physicians". His son, W. Heberden, translated his commentaries on the history and cure of diseases from the original Latin into English and both versions were published one year after his death. W. Heberden Jr. (1769–1854) followed his father and wrote an Epitome of Paediatrics.

Ottomar Rosenbach (1851–1907) German physician.

v. ROSENBACH LAW and SIGN

HEBRA PRURIGO (Prurigo nodularis)

Chronic, recurrent, intensely pruritic papules and nodules on the trunk and limbs. No known cause, and very difficult to treat.

Ferdinand von Hebra (1818–1880) Viennese dermatologist who was born in Brunn (Brno). He graduated M.D. at Vienna in 1841 and worked in Vienna with Skoda. Initially he was allocated to the "rash-room", the most lowly regarded position with Skoda, which was crammed with severe skin disease and which most trainees regarded as a necessary evil to progress up the medical ladder. Hebra was immediately interested in trying to understand and improve the treatment of these conditions. He was greatly influenced by Rokitansky whose classification techniques he applied to the skin disorders and the resultant classification remained in place for almost a century. He emphasized the local factors in skin disease and was at constant odds with the constitutionalists who believed skin disease was all secondary to a general metabolic upset. He did not share the latter's therapeutic nihilism and applied active therapy successfully to many types of skin disorders. He was one of the doyens of dermatology and his book "Textbook of Skin Diseases" was translated into English, French, Italian and Russian, and for years to come would be the bible of dermatology. He first described dermatitis herpetiformis and wrote a classical account of tinea cruris.

HECKATHORN DISEASE

A rare form of factor VIII deficiency characterized by variable VIII-C levels but constantly abnormal prothrombin consumption test, inherited as a sex linked recessive and named after the first person in whom the disorder was recognized by Jessica Lewis and Oscar Ratnoff.

HEERFORDT DISEASE OR SYNDROME

Uveoparotid fever, characterised by uveitis, parotid enlargement, fever and often a 7th nerve palsy. There may be associated hyperalgesia, papilledema, meningism and pleocytosis in the cerebrospinal fluid due to sarcoidosis. Also called WALDENSTRÖM UVEOPAROTITIS.

Christian F. Heerfordt (1871–1953) Danish ophthalmologist.

HEFKE-TURNER SIGN

In inflammatory disease of the hip of children, X-ray shows a bending of the obturator line into the pelvis. Obturator sign.

H.W. Hefke (1897–) U.S. radiologist.

U.C. Turner U.S. surgeon.

HEGGLIN ANOMALY

v. MAY-HEGGLIN ANOMALY

HEIDENHAIN CELLS

Enterochromaffin cells of the gastric mucosa.

v. KULTSCHITZKY CELLS

Rudolph P.H. Heidenhain (1834–1897) German physiologist, Professor of Physiology at Breslau (now Wroclaw, Poland). Pavlov worked with him on pancreatic and gastric secretion. The Heidenhain pouch was similar to the Pavlov pouch but with the vagal nerves severed. Carl Weigert was influenced by him when he studied medicine in Breslau. He developed a technique for staining kidney cells by injecting indigo carmine into the blood, proposed a secretion theory for renal function and worked with du Bois Reymond in a study of mechanics and heat production of muscle contraction and did some work with Burger on hypnotism. He studied the effects of mechanical irritation in stimulating nerves, and the secretory nerves of glands. He enunciated the concept that the older the cell is, the smaller will be its nucleus and this led Arneth (*v. supra*) to develop his technique for polymorph lobe counts.

HEIDENHAIN SYNDROME

Presenile dementia associated with blindness, ataxia, dysarthria, athetotic movements and rigidity of all four limbs. Neuronal lesions with proliferation of astrocytes are seen in the cerebral cortex and to a lesser degree in the basal ganglion.

cf. JAKOB-CREUTZFELDT DISEASE

Adolf Heidenhain (1893–) German neurologist.

HEIM-KREYSIG SIGN

Systolic intercostal retraction due to adherent pericarditis.

cf. BROADBENT SIGN

Ernst L. Heim (1747–1834) German physician who worked in Berlin.

Friedrich L. Kreysig (1770–1839) German physician who worked in Dresden.

HEIMLICH MANEUVER

A sudden application of pressure subdiaphragmatically to the chest causing expulsion of air and dislodgement of a foreign body in the airways.

Henry J. Heimlich U.S. surgeon at Xavier University, Cincinnati, Ohio.

HEINE-MEDIN DISEASE

Infantile paralysis.

Jacob von Heine (1800–1879) German orthopedist who worked in Stuttgart. He wrote a monograph on congenital and acquired dislocation and first described acute poliomyelitis as well as spastic paraplegia in 1840.

Karl O. Medin (1847–1927) Swedish physician born in Axberg. He became Professor of Pediatrics in Stockholm and first described the epidemic nature of the disorder. He described the first epidemic of poliomyelitis in 1890.

HEINER SYNDROME

Chronic pulmonary disease, diarrhea, iron deficiency anemia and failure to thrive in early infancy with serum antibodies to cow's milk.

Douglas C. Heiner (1925–) U.S. pediatrician, born at Salt Like City in 1925, graduated M.D. McGill in 1950 and trained in pediatrics at the University of Pennsylvania Hospital, Philadelphia, and Boston Children's Medical Centre. He became Professor of Pediatrics at the University of California, Los Angeles, and has research interests in allergy, pulmonary hemosiderosis and celiac disease.

HEINZ BODIES

Deep purple small irregular bodies in red cells stained with crystal violet which represent denatured hemoglobin, seen characteristically in glucose-6-phosphate dehydrogenase deficiency following administration of oxidant drugs, e.g. primaquin, with unstable hemoglobins and post splenectomy, especially in patients with thalassemia.

Also called HEINZ-EHRLICH BODIES.

Robert Heinz (1865–1924) German physician and pharmacologist from Breslau (Wroclaw) who reported these in 1890 in the blood of guinea pigs treated with acetylphenylhydrazine. He was director of the Institute of Pharmacology at Erlangen. He worked on metallic colloids.

Paul Ehrlich (*v. supra*).

HEISTER VALVE

Spiral valve in the cystic duct.

Lorenz Heister (1683–1758) German anatomist and surgeon born in Frankfurt/Main who introduced the use of spinal braces and made the first postmortem section of appendicitis, introduced the term tracheotomy and wrote an illustrated textbook on surgery and is held by some to be the father of scientific surgery in Germany. He was educated at the University of Giessen (Germany), Amsterdam and Leiden in Holland and was taught by Ruysch and Boerhaave. He was Professor of Anatomy and Surgery in Altdorf, Switzerland (1710–19) and then 1719 at the University of Helinstedt (Germany).

HENDERSON-HASSELBALCH EQUATION

$$\text{Blood pH} = 6.1\ (\text{pK}) + \log_{10}\frac{(\text{Plasma bicarbonate conc.})}{(\text{Plasma carbonic acid conc.})}$$
$$= 7.4$$

Lawrence J. Henderson (1879–1942) U.S. biochemist at Harvard who developed nomograms to calculate pH values of blood. He graduated M.D. from Harvard in 1902 and then spent 2 years at the University of Strasburg until 1904 when he was appointed lecturer in biological chemistry at Harvard becoming Professor in 1919. He emphasized the relation of physical properties of matter to the existence of life. He commenced a course in 1911 on the history of science emphasizing the nature of scientific method and thinking. He also initiated a course in the medical curriculum aimed at improving and understanding human relationships.

Karl Hasselbalch (1874–1962) Danish biochemist and physician, who with Bohr and Krogh showed that the affinity of blood for oxygen varied with the pressure of carbon dioxide, in his pioneering work on blood pH.

HENLE, LOOP OF

Medullary portion of the nephron between the proximal and distal tubules of the collecting system of the kidney.

Friedrich G.J. Henle (1809–1885) German anatomist who was the greatest histologist of his time. Born of Jewish parents at Furth near Nuremberg, he was a prosector to J. Müller in Berlin and Professor of Anatomy at Zurich (1840), Heidelberg (1844) and Göttingen (1852–1885). He recognized that the cell was a physiological as well as a structural unit. He described and defined epithelial tissue as the lining tissue of body tubes and cavities, and also described columnar and ciliated forms. He described the muscle coat in small arteries and the tubules in the kidney and wrote the first accurate description of the cornea and the development of the larynx. He first connected cataracts and exanthemata with inflammation and demonstrated the importance of urinary casts in renal disease. He supported Müller's concept that fever was a symptom. He established a medical journal and wrote several books on anatomy and pathology. He was a superb lecturer, a poet and a fine musician, playing the violin, viola and violincello. He maintained it was a physician's duty to prevent and cure disease, that disease is a deviation from normal physiological processes and death the cessation of metabolism. He had a wide circle of friends, including Felix Mendelssohn and Humboldt.

HENNEBERG DISEASE

Metachromatic leukodystrophy. A demyelinating disease whose clinical features depend on age of onset. In the child, difficulty in walking with hypotonia and weakness and loss of reflexes may lead on to nystagmus and cerebellar signs, dementia and tonic seizures and eventually paralysis. In the adult, the patient may present with psychiatric features and presenile dementia.

HENNEBERG REFLEX

v. LAEHR-HENNEBERG HARD PALATE REFLEX

Richard Henneberg (1868–1962) German neurologist who worked in Berlin.

HENOCH-SCHÖNLEIN PURPURA

Purpuric eruption without thrombocytopenia, associated with glomerulonephritis, abdominal colic and intussusception, urticaria, and arthralgia.

Eduard H. Henoch (1820–1910) A German pediatrician who was a pupil of Schönlein and practiced in Berlin, wrote extensively on childhood illnesses and translated C. West's work into German. He retired in 1894 and his Chair was taken by O. Heubner (*v. infra*) who became the first named Professor of Pediatrics at a German University. He described the above in 1868 and in 1887 wrote the first description of purpura fulminans.

Johannes L. Schönlein (1793–1864) German physician. He was born in Bamberg, the son of a papermaker. He studied at the University of Landshift where Von Walther taught that the only way for medicine to progress was by the use of physics, chemistry and the natural sciences. From Landshift he went to Würzburg, graduating in 1816. He became Privatdozent in 1817 and Professor in 1824.

He was the founder of the Natural History School for the study and classification of medicine using similar methods to botany and zoology. He moved from Würzburg to Zurich in 1833 where he was the first Professor of Medicine and finally to Berlin in 1839. In his clinic at the Charité he was the first to lecture on medicine in German rather than Latin and introduced into Germany modern clinical examination, percussion, auscultation, examination of the blood and urine, chemical analysis and the use of the microscope. He wrote relatively little (his doctor's thesis and two papers of 1 and 3 pages respectively), but introduced the terms hemophilia and tuberculosis and described peliosis rheumatica (Schönlein Disease). He also discovered that a fungus caused favus (Achorion-Schönleini).

During his later years he affected the habits of a recluse and often avoided his patients or treated them with a degree of aloofness which was then fashionable. However, he was held in very high esteem by people such as Virchow and he had an immense influence on German medicine. At one time he threatened to resign because of some slight, but was persuaded to stay by the award of the Red Eagle Order with star and diamonds.

He conducted his teaching clinics in much the way patient presentations are made today with the history, physical findings, chemistry and microscopic findings being presented – he would check these findings and then develop the discussion with a diagnosis and discuss the etiology and therapy. If the patient died there would be a discussion of the pathological findings and any errors in diagnosis. He had a goitre for a number of years and retired because of poor health in 1859.

He was not one of the most sensitive of men, and when an elderly clinician tried to excuse his ignorance by pointing at his gray hair, Schönlein said "Donkeys are also gray". Virchow's succinct summation of his teaching was "little system, many facts".

HENRY LAW

The amount of gas in solution is proportional to the pressure of the gas.

William Henry (1774–1836) English chemist who was born in Manchester. He studied medicine in Edinburgh and practiced in Manchester. Elected F.R.S. in 1809.

HERING CANAL

Passage from the bile canaliculi to the smallest branch of the bile duct.

HERING-BREUER REFLEX

Impulses controlling respiration conducted by the vagus.

Karl E.K. Hering (1834–1918) German physiologist who was born in Altgersdorf and went to medical school at the University of Leipzig, graduating in 1858. As a medical student he greatly admired J. Müller. In 1860 he was appointed assistant to E. Wagner in the Polyclinic of Leipzig and during that time commenced his study on the physiology of vision. In 1865 he was appointed to C. Ludwig's former position in the Academy for Military Medicine in Vienna and there continued to develop his theories on vision but he also studied the histology of liver. Working with J. Breuer he developed the concept of an autonomic reflex control mechanism for respiration as well as describing the central control mechanisms for blood pressure which if abolished cause the "Hering waves".

In 1870 he was appointed to Purkinje's Chair in Prague and possibly was unpopular with the locals since he emphasized the importance of German science and German culture there and in 1882 was a very important factor in the foundation of the German University in Prague and as a consequence did not accept an invitation to move to Strasburg. When Ludwig died in 1895 he followed him to head the Physiological Institute in Leipzig and at the time was regarded as the authority in the physiology of vision. He was a good teacher but, like many in those days, welcomed controversy and public debate and for example when he was quite young (29) he attacked G. Meissner, then Professor at Göttingen, on careless mistakes in his studies on vision. In turn he himself was criticized by Helmholtz for some of his new approaches and ideas. He attracted many people to work with him including Henry Head from England and the famous German ophthalmologist C. von Hess and a well known physiologist W. Biedermann. His son, H.E. Hering (1866–1948), was also a well known German physiologist who in 1903 described auricular fibrillation (pulsus irregularis perpetuus) and discovered the carotid sinuses and their role in blood pressure in 1924.

Josef Breuer (1842–1925) Austrian psychiatrist and physiologist born in Vienna who, with Freud, introduced questioning under hypnosis. Jointly with Hering he studied the automatic regulation of breathing and showed that this was a function of expansion and contraction of the lungs which provided a normal stimulus for the vagi. He studied vestibular function and was trained in physiology in Vienna by E. Brucke. He practiced clinically and was the physician to many of the members of the medical faculty.

HERMANSKY-PUDLAK SYNDROME

Tyrosinase +ve occulocutaneous albinism, with accumulation of a ceroid bile pigment in macrophages and a bleeding tendency due to a platelet storage pool defect resulting in a prolonged bleeding time. Ultrastructural studies of the platelets show the absence of dense granules. It is an autosomal recessive condition.

F. Hermansky Czech physician.

P. Pudlak Czech physician.

HERS DISEASE

Glycogen storage disease (Type Vl of Cori) due to lack of phosphorylase resulting in hepatomegaly and hypoglycemia.

Henri-Gery Hers Belgian biochemist who is at present Emeritus Professor of Biochemistry of the University of Louvain. He worked in close collaboration with a Belgian Nobel laureate, Christiane de Duve, the discoverer of lysosomes. He specialized in lysosomal deficiency states and in particular in the various forms of glycogen storage disease.

HERXHEIMER REACTION

v. also JARISCH-HERXHEIMER REACTION

Acute exacerbation of syphilitic lesions within 6–10 hours of the initiation of treatment. The intensity of the reaction reflects the intensity of inflammation present, and the duration is usually short (2–4 hours).

Karl Herxheimer (1861–1944) German dermatologist. Born in Wiesbaden he trained with Neisser (*v. infra*) at Breslau and in 1885 joined his brother in practice in Frankfurt. He conducted his clinics at the Municipal Hospital, Sachsenhausen where his dramatic style and choice of controversial topics soon made him famous together with a series of publications on a variety of dermatological topics. He described chronic atrophic acrodermatitis. He observed his reaction in patients he had treated with mercury. He was Jewish and the Nazis transported him to the concentration camp at Theresienstadt where he died of dysentery and starvation.

HERYING SIGN

An infra-orbital shadow seen when the mouth is closed around a flashlight with empyema of the maxillary sinus.

Théodor Herying (1847–1925) Polish otolaryngologist.

HESS TEST

A test for capillary fragility using the sphygmomanometer cuff to raise venous pressure in the forearm and inspecting the skin for petechial eruptions after deflation.

Alfred F. Hess (1875–1933) U.S. physician. He graduated M.D. from the College of Physicians and Surgeons, Columbia University, New York, in 1901 and trained at Mt. Sinai Hospital and studied for a year in Europe returning to New York to practise in 1905. He spent his mornings at the Rockefeller Institute and his afternoons at the Babies Hospital or at Bellevue. He wrote on rickets and scurvy and showed that the missing factor in the latter was abundant in citrus fruits and tomatoes. He discovered that certain oils and foods became antirachitic on exposure to UV light and introduced treatment of rickets by use of sunlight and showed that rubella was caused by a virus. He wrote a book on both scurvy and rickets which contains interesting historical accounts of these disorders.

HESSELBACH TRIANGLE

Inguinal triangle.

Franz C. Hesselbach (1759–1816) German anatomist and surgeon born in Hammelburg. Professor of Anatomy and Surgery at Würzburg. He described the femoral hernia in 1798 and distinguished direct and indirect inguinal hernias in 1810.

HEUBNER-HERTER DISEASE

Infantile celiac disease

v. GEE DISEASE

Johan O. Heubner (1843–1926) German pediatrician who was born in Muhltroff, Vogtland and is said to have retained his Saxon accent and temperament throughout his life. He was a pupil of Wunderlich and became Professor of Pediatrics in Berlin in 1913. In 1898, with M. Rubner, he made the initial investigation on food requirements for normal and ill-nourished children which formed the foundation of later investigations in this area. He warned against too prolonged sterilization of milk and whilst in Leipzig recognized Behring's discovery of diphtheria antitoxin and was one of the first to use it in treatment. He isolated meningococci from the cerebrospinal fluid in 1896.

Christian A. Herter (1865–1910) U.S. physician. Born in Glenville, Connecticut. He graduated from medicine at the College of Physicians and Surgeons (Columbia University) in 1885. He worked with Welch in Baltimore, and Forrel in Zurich. He returned to the United States and initially practiced medicine primarily as a neurologist, writing a book in 1892 "The Diagnosis of Diseases of the Nervous System". He soon became interested in biochemical approaches, however, and in 1893 had the upper floor of his house remodelled so that he could carry out laboratory work.

He was especially interested in clinical problems connected with pathological conditions and one of his close associates was H.D. Dakin (*v. supra*). He investigated the role of bacteria in the gastrointestinal tract and developed techniques for measuring their products such as indol. He was commissioned by President Theodore Roosevelt to examine the possible effects of sodium benzoate in its use in food preservatives and from the investigations concluded that it was perfectly safe. From 1897 to 1902 he was Professor of Pathological Chemistry at the University of Bellevue Hospital Medical College. In 1903 he was appointed to the Chair of Pharmacology and Therapeutics at the College of Physicians and Surgeons and remained in that position until he died. He founded the *Journal of Biological Chemistry* (1905) which was the first journal of this nature in the English language and he was one of the founding trustees of the Rockefeller Institute as well as a founder of the American Society of Biological Chemists (1908).

He was interested in painting and the visual arts and in his final years was troubled with ill health so that he ceased practice, resigning as visiting physician to the New York City Hospital in 1904 after 10 years of service. He founded two lectureships, one at the University and Bellevue Hospital Medical College and the other at Johns Hopkins Medical School, which served to bring scientists from Europe to give lectures. In his address at the opening of the medical school at the College of Physicians and Surgeons at Columbia University in 1909 he said "I like to think of medicine in our day as an ever broadening and deepening river, fed by the limpid streams of pure science. The river at its borders has its eddies and currents, expressive of certain doubts and errors that fringe all progress; but it makes continuous advances on the way to the ocean of its destiny".

Despite his ill health he continued to work in his laboratory, but finally died of pneumonia.

HEYD SYNDROME

Hepatorenal syndrome.

Charles G. Heyd (1884–1970) U.S. surgeon.

v. AUSTIN FLINT.

HILL SIGN

Femoral artery pressure 20 mmHg > brachial pressure is seen in severe aortic regurgitation.

Sir Leonard E. Hill (1866–1952) English physician and physiologist. He was Professor of Physiology at the London Hospital and was knighted in 1930. He wrote a book on the physiology and pathology of the cerebral circulation in 1896 and on Caisson sickness in 1912. Together with Barnard he modified Riva-Rocci's original sphygmomanometer by using a pressure gauge instead of a mercury manometer. He won the Nobel Prize in 1923 with Myerhof for their discoveries of heat production and muscle metabolism.

HILTON LAW

The nerve trunk supplying a joint also supplies the overlying skin and the muscles that move the joint.

John Hilton (1804–1878) English surgeon and anatomist, born in Castle Hedingham in Essex, he commenced at Guy's Hospital in 1824 and gained his M.R.C.S. in 1827 and was appointed demonstrator in anatomy. In 1844 he was appointed assistant surgeon and ultimately resigned from the hospital in 1870. A very skilful observer and shrewd clinically, he could interest students in the most mundane topics and always managed to find some point overlooked by others so that he was highly regarded as a consultant. He was no scientist and opposed and ridiculed Darwin's ideas and although his rounds and lectures were always crowded, he was not liked by many students, whom he often hurt by sarcasm and jokes at their expense. His book "Rest and Pain" is still a classic.

HINES AND BROWN TEST

Cold pressor test. Immersion of one extremity in ice water for 1–3 minutes will normally increase the systolic and diastolic blood pressure by 15 mmHg. Failure to respond is due to a central or efferent sympathetic lesion.

Edgar A. Hines (1906–1978) U.S. physician at the Mayo Clinic. He was born in Seneca, South Carolina, and graduated M.D. in 1928 from the Medical College of the State of South Carolina. He entered the Mayo Graduate School of Medicine in 1931, and was appointed a consultant at the Mayo Clinic in medicine in 1935. He became Professor in the Mayo Graduate School of Medicine in 1950, retiring in 1962. He had a life-long interest in peripheral vascular disease and hypertension and introduced the use of the drug, thiocyanate, in the treatment of migraine and hypertension headaches.

George E. Brown (1885–1935) U.S. physician. Born in Grand Rapids, Michigan, he graduated M.D. from the University of Michigan in 1909. He practiced in Montana introducing the first fluoroscope there. During World War I he served in France with the Rockefeller Foundation and joined the Mayo Clinic in 1921 where he developed a special interest in peripheral vascular disease and the role of the sympathetic nervous system. He became an international authority and influenced many in this area (v. Allen).

HIPPEL-LINDAU DISEASE

Retinal angioma (von Hippel Disease) associated with cerebellar angioma (Lindau Disease) and sometimes angioma in other viscera.

Eugen von Hippel (1867–1939) German ophthalmologist. Born in Königsberg where his father was a Professor of Ophthalmology. At Heidelberg he studied medicine with Erb, pathology with Arnold and ophthalmology with von Leber (*v. infra*). He moved to Halle in 1909 and Göttingen in 1914 as Professor of Ophthalmology, retiring through ill health in 1934.

Arvid Lindau (1892–1958) Swedish pathologist. He studied with Aschoff in Freiburg and became Professor of Pathology in Lund University in 1933.

HIPPOCRATIC FACIES

Sunken facies seen in dehydration and shock.

HIPPOCRATIC FINGERS

Clubbed fingers.

HIPPOCRATIC OATH

Expression of ideals and philosophies by which a physician should practice medicine.

HIPPOCRATIC SUCCUSSION OR SPLASH

Splashing or gurgling sound heard when the patient's abdomen is shaken due to fluid in the stomach in pyloric obstruction; sometimes also applied to fluid in the pleural cavity.

Hippocrates (460–370 BC) Greek physician, often regarded as the founder of medicine, who initiated its ethical ideals and scientific basis. He is thought to have been born on Cos in the 18th Olympiad of an Ascelepiad family. He was first instructed in medicine by his father, then studied in Athens, Thrace, Thessaly and Macedonia. His influence was enormous – he established the ethical standards of the profession, separated medicine from philosophy and religion and sifted and synthesized current knowledge into a systematic science. He instituted careful observation and examination, and therefore description of disease which became the first scientific bedside medicine which was later taken up by Sydenham, Charcot and Osler. His case histories and descriptions of many disease processes are often not bettered by today's authors.

HIRSCHBERG REFLEX OR SIGN

Adduction reflex of the foot. Tickling the base of the plantar surface of the big toe may cause adduction of the foot in pyramidal lesions.

Leonard K. Hirschberg (1877–) U.S. neurologist who practiced in Baltimore.

HIRSCHSPRUNG DISEASE

Dilation of the colon due to lack of ganglion cells, causing obstruction at the rectum with resultant constipation and growth retardation.

Harald Hirschsprung (1830–1916) Danish pediatrician, he was born in Copenhagen and graduated in medicine there in 1855. He gained an official university teaching post in 1861 and in 1870 was appointed Head Physician at the Queen Louise Children's Hospital in Copenhagen. He became Professor of Pediatrics in 1877 until he retired in 1904. He published in many areas of pediatrics including intussusception, rickets, rheumatic nodules and the disease to which his name is attached, which he reported in 1887. Although other patients had been reported earlier, his was by far the most convincing account in which he described two children under the age of 12 months with clear descriptions of the clinical aspects and autopsy findings.

HIS-TAWARA BUNDLE

Atrioventricular bundle which conducts impulses to the heart from the sino-auricular node.

v. KENT, BUNDLE OF

HIS-TAWARA NODE

Atrioventricular node.

Wilhelm His Jr. (1863–1934) German physician, son of the embryologist, W. His of Basel who later became Professor of Anatomy at Leipzig (1872) and invented the microtome.

His Jr. was director of the first medical clinic in Berlin. As a medical student in Strasburg he investigated pyridine metabolism and discovered the bundle in 1893, when an assistant at the medical clinic in Leipzig. One year later he severed the bundle and demonstrated dissociation of auricular and ventricular beats. During the war he reported Trench Fever (1916) in Volhynia, Russia. Later he studied gout and arthritis. He was a sophisticated conversationalist, as well as a musician and painter.

Sunao Tawara (1873–1952) Japanese pathologist.

HOCHSINGER SIGN

In hypocalcemia compression of the inner aspect of the biceps causes the fist to close.

v. TROUSSEAU SIGN

Karl Hochsinger (1860–) Austrian pediatrician.

HODGKIN DISEASE

The most frequent form of lymphoma seen in western society.

Thomas Hodgkin (1798–1866) English physician, born in Tottenham. He was a staunch Quaker who graduated from Edinburgh in 1823 and became a member of the Royal College of Physicians in 1825, Curator of the Pathology Museum at Guy's Hospital and a demonstrator in pathology. He visited Paris as a medical student and studied with Laennec and

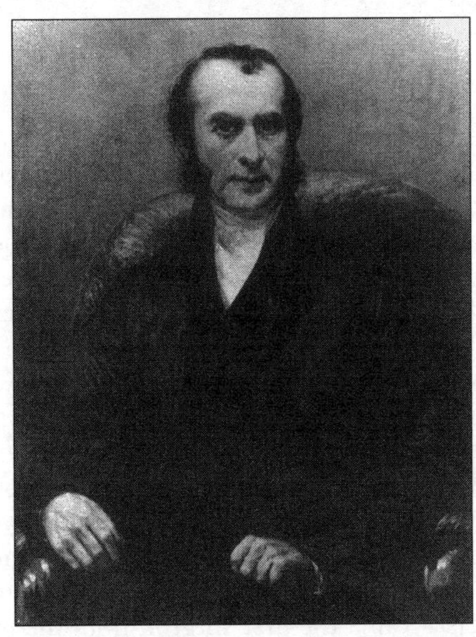

Thomas Hodgkin (Courtesy of the Gordon Museum, Guy's Hospital Medical School, London, UK)

took a stethoscope back to England and introduced it to Guy's Hospital. He was a lecturer in pathology for 10 years but resigned after being unsuccessful in his application for the post of assistant physician, Babington (*v. supra*) being preferred to him. This caused much debate at the time since Hodgkin had played a major role in establishing Guy's as an independent school of the highest quality and was affectionately regarded by his old students. He may never have made a success of practice; after sitting up all night with a very wealthy patient he was given a blank cheque and offended the patient by filling in 10 pounds, adding that he didn't look as if he could afford more. The patient never consulted with him again. It was said that it was so difficult to get him to take fees that many of his friends would not ask him to consult. He practiced in London at St. Thomas's for a while but became interested in philanthropy and whilst travelling the world with his friend Sir Moses Montefiore, he died with dysentery in Jaffa and was buried there. Apart from his description of the enlargement of the spleen and lymph nodes, he also wrote an original account of aortic regurgitation in 1829.

HODGSON DISEASE

Uniform aneurysmal dilatation of the aorta.

Joseph Hodgson (1788–1869) English surgeon born in Penrith, Cumberland. He was initially apprenticed to George Freer, a surgeon at Birmingham General Hospital and later trained at St. Bartholomew's Hospital, London. There in 1811 he gained the Jacksonian Prize and later expanded his essay to publish a book on "Wounds and Diseases of the Arteries and Veins" in 1815 which was one of the earliest works on vascular disease and techniques of ligation. He moved back to Birmingham in 1818 and became a surgeon to the Birmingham General Hospital in 1821. Amongst his patients was Sir Robert Peel, the Prime Minister and many years later in 1850 he attended him when he fell from his horse on Constitution Hill – a fall which was to be fatal. He became the first surgeon from the provinces to be elected president of the Royal College of Surgeons. Although a conservative in every sense of the word he was well liked, but was consistently opposed to all reforms, including the formation of a school of medicine in Birmingham.

HOEHNE SIGN

If uterine contractions cease during delivery the uterus may have ruptured.

O. Hoehne (1871–1932) German gynecologist. Born in Treuenbrietzen he studied medicine in Kiel, Rostock and graduated in Berlin in 1895. He was appointed Professor of Gynaecology in Greifswald in 1918. He died with multiple pulmonary emboli.

HOFFA DISEASE

Solitary traumatic lipoma of the knee. The infrapatellar fat pad is inflamed and causes tenderness and swelling on both sides of the patellar ligament.

Albert Hoffa (1859–1907) German orthopedic surgeon, born in Richmond, South Africa. He introduced operative techniques for treating congenital hip dislocation. He worked in Würzburg where he was Professor and then moved to Berlin. He founded the first journal of orthopedic surgery and published a book on the subject in 1891.

HOFFMAN ATROPHY

v. WERDNIG-HOFFMAN DISEASE

Infantile spinal muscular atrophy (also called Hoffman-Werdnig Disease).

HOFFMAN FINGER REFLEX OR SIGN

Finger reflex elicited by flicking the ring finger; flexion of the forefinger and thumb occur with any cause of hyper-reflexia including upper motor neurone lesions.

HOFFMAN SYNDROME

Muscle hypertrophy in association with weakness, slowness of movement and painful spasm seen in myxedematous adults.

Johann Hoffman (1857–1919) German neurologist. He was a student of Wilhelm Erb (*v. supra*) and succeeded him as Professor of Neurology at Heidelberg. He demonstrated his reflex in lectures after 1904 but it was first described in the literature by his student, Hans Curschmann (*v. supra*) in 1911. Curschmann had been Hoffman's assistant from 1901–1904.

G. Werdnig (*v. infra*).

HOLLY ANEMIA

Hypoplastic anemia of pregnancy which resolves when the pregnancy is completed.

F. Holly U.S. obstetrician.

HOLMES PHENOMENON OR SIGN

Rebound sign seen in cerebellar disease. The patient is asked to flex his arm with a clenched fist against the examiner's resistance by gripping the patient's wrist and placing his other arm between the patient's forearm and body. The examiner suddenly releases the wrist and in cerebellar disease the patient will not be able to stop flexion and will hit the examiner's intervening arm.

HOLMES-ADIE SYNDROME

v. ADIE SYNDROME

Sir Gordon M. Holmes (1876–1965) English neurologist. He was born in Dublin and graduated from Trinity College in medicine in 1898. He was a resident at the Richmond Asylum and undertook 2½ years postgraduate study in neurology in Germany. Initially he was in Berlin, but he said "it was all spoon feeding" and he went to Frankfurt-am-Main where he worked in the Senckenberg Institute with Edinger and also Weigert. Edinger (*v. supra*) suggested that he investigate the experimental model of Goltz, which was a dog who had had his brain extirpated, saying "I can't make anything of it"! It is possible that this experimental animal may have aroused his initial interest in the cerebellum. He said, "I might have become a German" for there was an effort to create a post for him in Frankfurt, but Ehrlich had just commenced his work on Salvarsan and it was decided that the money over the next two years go to that work. He therefore returned to London and became a resident medical officer at the National Hospital for Nervous Diseases in Queen's Square and remained attached to that hospital for the rest of his working life. In 1908 he commenced collaborating with Henry Head; this led to the first accurate account of the functions of the optic thalamus and its relation to the cerebral cortex. The two men complemented one another because Head was imaginative and enthusiastic as well as speculative, whereas Holmes insisted upon attention to detail and would never bend facts to fit a hypothesis. At times this led to clashes between the two, but they continued a close collaboration until the outbreak of the First World War when Holmes was appointed a consultant neurologist to the British Expeditionary Forces and was twice mentioned in despatches. During this time his observations on gunshot wounds re-awakened his interest in cerebellar disease; this culminated in his classical analysis of the symptoms of cerebellar lesions which were published in his Croonian Lectures to the Royal College of Physicians in 1922, where he added more cases of gunshot wounds to his First World War experience as well as patients with cerebellar tumors. He investigated amyotonia congenita with Collier and described the first removal of a suprarenal tumor (by P. Sargent) reversing virilism in the patient. He was editor of the Journal "Brain" for many years and was well known for aiding young neurologists by going over their manuscripts and ruthlessly abbreviating and improving the English.

He disliked medical politics and when forced to be on committees was said to vary between someone who was overwhelmingly bored to being forceful and bullying! He introduced to England the painstaking physical examination of a neurologist and even outstripped Gowers (*v. supra*) in his systematic collection of clinical data and its correlation with anatomy and pathology.

Outside of medicine he was interested in ecclesiastical Gothic architecture and the geology of Ireland and also the garden. Guests to his country cottage would be commandeered into performing such tasks as tree felling and trench digging. He was a keen golfer until shortly before his death. He was a martinet and together with his rather brusque manner these characteristics may have accounted for his late recognition in the honors list. He was knighted in 1951.

HOLMGREN TEST

Test for color blindness using colored wool.

Alarik F. Holmgren (1831–1897) Swedish physiologist who investigated color blindness with reference to railway and maritime conditions following a serious railway accident in Sweden in 1875 which he believed was due to color blindness. He was the first to demonstrate retinal action currents in 1865. He was Professor of Physiology at Uppsala University.

HOLT-ORAM SYNDROME

Autosomal dominant. Secundum atrial septal defect with bony abnormalities of the upper extremity resulting in short forearms and loss of opposition of the thumb or a thumb which looks finger-like.

Mary Holt Cardiologist, King's College Hospital, London.

Samuel Oram Cardiologist, King's College Hospital, London.

HOLTER MONITOR

This is a continuous and ambulatory technique for obtaining an uninterrupted record of the ECG for a period of 24 hours allowing later analysis. It is extremely valuable for monitoring for rhythm disturbances as well as detecting unsuspected episodes of ischemia during activity or sleep.

Norman J. Holter An electrical engineer from Montana, U.S.A.

HOMANS SIGN

Passive dorsiflexion of the foot may give pain in the calf when there is a deep venous thrombosis. Vigorous dorsiflexion of the foot is used by surgeons to expel clot from the veins and so this test may have its dangers.

John Homans (1877–1954) U.S. surgeon. He worked with Cushing at Johns Hopkins on experimental hypophysectomy and then became interested in peripheral vascular disease and wrote his monograph on it in 1939. He wrote a very successful "Textbook of Surgery" based on the Harvard surgical course which went through four editions. He was Professor of Surgery at Harvard at the Peter Bent Brigham Hospital. He died of a myocardial infarction.

HOOVER SIGN

1. A maneuver to distinguish organic hemiplegia from malingering or hysteria. When hands are placed under the patient's heels and he is asked to press on them with both his feet, pressure will be less on the paralyzed side. A hand is then placed on top of the non-paralyzed leg and the patient is asked to raise his leg. In organic hemiplegia there will be increase in pressure felt from the heel, in contradistinction to hysteria.
2. A hand is placed under the heel of the sound leg and the patient is asked to try to raise the paralyzed leg. The pressure on the hand of the heel of the sound leg is much greater in organic hemiplegia than in hysteria.

Charles F. Hoover (1865–1927) U.S. physician, born in Cleveland, Ohio, graduated from Harvard 1892 and worked in Vienna with Neusser and in Strasburg with F. Kraus. He came back to live in Cleveland and in 1907 was appointed Professor of Medicine at Western Reserve where he specialized in pulmonary and hepatic disease, investigating the action of the diaphragm in respiration.

HOPE MURMUR

Apical systolic bruit of mitral incompetence.

James Hope (1801–1841) English physician, born in Stockport, Cheshire. Hope spent 5 years studying medicine in Edinburgh, then a year at St. Bartholomew's Hospital, and then worked with Chromel in Paris, who was impressed with his sketches of

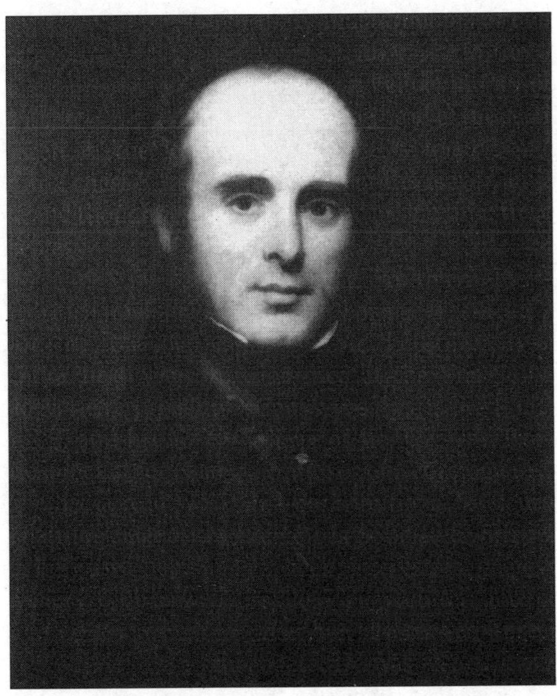

James Hope (Reproduced from *"The Royal College of Physicians of London Portraits"* by G. Wolstenholme & D. Piper [Published by J & A Churchill Ltd. London 1964]).

pathology specimens. He gained his licentiate of the Royal College of Physicians and enrolled at St. George's Hospital where he made many observations and set standards in auscultation and wrote "Diseases of the Heart and Great Vessels" in 1831, in which he gives concise descriptions of cardiac asthma, valvular disease and cardiac neurosis. He published an excellent pathology atlas which he illustrated with his own drawings. He became a physician at St. George's and died of tuberculosis.

HOPMANN POLYP

Nasal polyps.

Carl M. Hopmann (1844–1925) German otolaryngologist.

HOPPE-GOLDFLAM DISEASE

Myasthenia gravis.

Herman H. Hoppe (1867–1919) U.S. neurologist. He was born in Cincinnati of German American parentage, entered Xavier College, and then Ohio Medical College in 1886, graduating M.D. in 1889. After his internship he went to Strasburg where he studied pathology with von Recklinghausen and neurology with Oppenheim in Berlin. He returned to Cincinnati Medical School in 1892 and began working in neuro-psychiatry and became lecturer in nervous diseases at Ohio Medical College. When the University of Cincinnati Medical School was founded in 1900 he became Head of the Neurological Department; he visited Europe on a number of occasions and wrote papers on many neurological topics.

Samuel V. Goldflam (*v. supra*).

HORNER SYNDROME

Unilateral narrowing of the palpebral fissure, meosis, enophthalmos and reduction of sweating due to a lesion of the cervical sympathetic nerve.

Johann F. Horner (1831–1886) Swiss ophthalmologist who was born in Zurich. He commenced medicine in 1849 and was greatly influenced by the physiologist Carl Ludwig. He graduated in 1854 and then visited Munich and Vienna, becoming interested in ophthalmology. He worked with von Graefe (*v. supra*) and a close friendship resulted. He studied in Paris with Desmarres and returned to Zurich. In 1862 he was appointed Professor of Ophthalmology there. He established (1876) that a man with a red-green color blindness transmitted this anomaly to his male grandchildren through his daughter who was not color blind, similar to hemophilia, i.e. sex linked transmission.

HORSLEY SIGN

Axillary temperature is higher on the paralyzed side in middle meningeal hemorrhage.

Victor A.H. Horsley (1857–1916) English neurosurgeon. He graduated from the University of London in 1873 and initially performed a number of physiological studies including production of myxedema in monkeys by thyroidectomy. He studied cerebral function with Schafer at University College and Beevor at the Brown Institute. He was appointed surgeon to the National Hospital, Queen's Square, when he was 29, and introduced operative techniques for laminectomy and craniotomy and performed the first successful removal of a spinal tumor diagnosed by Gower. He successfully performed the first division of the sensory root of the Vth nerve in an endeavor to relieve trigeminal neuralgia. He was very active publicly in condemning the use of tobacco and alcohol and was very outspoken and dogmatic. He advocated muzzling of dogs to control rabies. Supposedly he was short with the nursing staff but strongly supported women's suffrage. He suggested experiments with saline and blood coagulation to L.C. Wooldridge which led to the introduction of normal saline solution. Horsley joined the medical corps in the Ist World War and after serving in Egypt and Gallipoli died in Mesopotamia of heat stroke.

HORTEGA CELL

Microglial cell

Pio del Rio Hortega (1882–1945) Spanish neuroanatomist. He was born in a Castilian village, Portillo, near Valladolid, and lived in a family castle, until his mother died, when the family moved to Valladolid, where he went to university and graduated in medicine. His graduation thesis was on tumors of nerve tissue, showing his early interest in neurology and after two years in general practice he went to Madrid to work with Cajal, who handed him on to Achucarro who had just returned to Cajal's laboratory from the United States. He improved the latter's staining techniques, was the first to describe centrosomes of ganglion cells, and identified two previously unrecognized cell types in the nervous system which Cajal had not been able to stain although he knew they were present and called them "the third element". One of these cell-types (microglia), Hortega showed to be wandering cells analogous to those of the monocyte reticulo-endothelial system, and believed them to be derived from blood elements in the early development of the brain. The other cell-type he identified was the oligodendroglia. Initially he withheld publication of some of this work because it ran contrary to Cajal's beliefs, but finally was persuaded to do so. Shortly after he found a note on his laboratory door from Cajal requesting that he leave. In 1926 he was appointed Director of the Junta Para Amplicion de Estudios and later Director of the Cancer Institute in Madrid where he stayed until the Civil War, when his Institute was demolished. He moved for a brief time with the Republican forces to Valencia, then to Paris where he worked in the laboratory of the neurosurgeon Clovis Vincent at the Pitié. After spending 18 months there he was invited by Cairns to work in his laboratory in Oxford. Here he is said to have tried very hard to be "English". He said, "I love you all, Oh God, not your draughts and your everlasting mutton". Melting point of mutton fat, he claimed, was too high for the intestinal cells to work and the rook's nest in the elms reminded him of senile plaques. His English was appalling but understandable "my section good, your section not good". He was invited back to Spain by Franco but stuck with his political principles and in 1940 went to Buenos Aires. Before leaving England he had discovered that he had a carcinoma of the penis which he alone knew since he had himself examined the biopsy specimens. He spent five years in Buenos Aires before he developed severe back pain, and dictated a biography he was preparing on Cajal when he could no longer hold a pen.

He was a very sensitive, excitable man, who delighted in the fine arts; he used to visit the Prado and make sketches and even painted oils of some of the paintings there. A lifelong friend was his constant companion, Nicholas Gomez y del Moral, who remained with him right till the end of his life, nursing him in his final illness. Following students' requests, he wrote an article for their publication and in it said "Histology is an odd-tasting dish, repulsive as a medicament to students, who must be examined in it, and little liked by physicians who consider their schooling finished. Taken in large quantities under compulsion it is not absorbed, but if tasted in little sips it finally becomes a delight to the palate, and even a cause for addiction." Other important works of his were the histological descriptions of the pineal gland and a book on cerebral tumors.

HORTON HEADACHE OR SYNDROME

Histamine cephalalgia.

Bayard T. Horton (1895–) U.S. physician at the Mayo Clinic. He described temporal arteritis in 1932 unaware of an earlier report by M. Schmidt. He was associated with the first report of a pulmonary arteriovenous aneurysm causing secondary polycythemia.

HOTTENTOT APRON

Overgrowth of labia minora seen in Hottentot tribe in South Africa.

HOTTENTOT BUSTLE

Excessive fat in the buttocks (*v. supra*).

HOUSSAY PHENOMENON

Amelioration of diabetes mellitus following ablation of the pituitary.

HOUSSAY SYNDROME

Improvement of the diabetic state in patients following pathological disease of the pituitary, causing hypopituitarism, usually due to a vascular or infiltrative cause (tuberculosis or sarcoidosis).

Bernardo A. Houssay (1889–1971) Argentinian physiologist who was born in Buenos Aires and graduated from the University there. He became Professor of Veterinary Physiology at Buenos Aires from 1910–1919, and was then appointed Professor of Medical Physiology and became Director of the Institute of Biology and Experimental Medicine. He received the Nobel Prize in Medicine in 1947, sharing it with Cori for his work on the influence of the anterior pituitary on diabetes. He showed that if one transplanted an ischemic kidney to a dog previously nephrectomized, hypertension followed, and that such kidneys contain an excess of renin, and thereby established a chemical cause for hypertension.

HOUSTON VALVES

Three transverse folds in the rectum.

John Houston (1802–1845) Irish surgeon. He graduated in medicine at Edinburgh University in 1826 and was appointed as a surgeon to the City of Dublin Hospital (Baggot Street) at the time of its opening in 1832. He introduced the microscope to Dublin medicine, publishing a paper on studies he had undertaken on cancer in 1844, in which he addressed the diagnostic possibilities of this approach. While he was attending his clinic at the hospital he had a stroke and died.

HOWELL-JOLLY BODY

Globular nuclear fragments in erythrocytes in peripheral blood of patients who have been splenectomized or with a megaloblastic anemia or atrophy of the spleen.

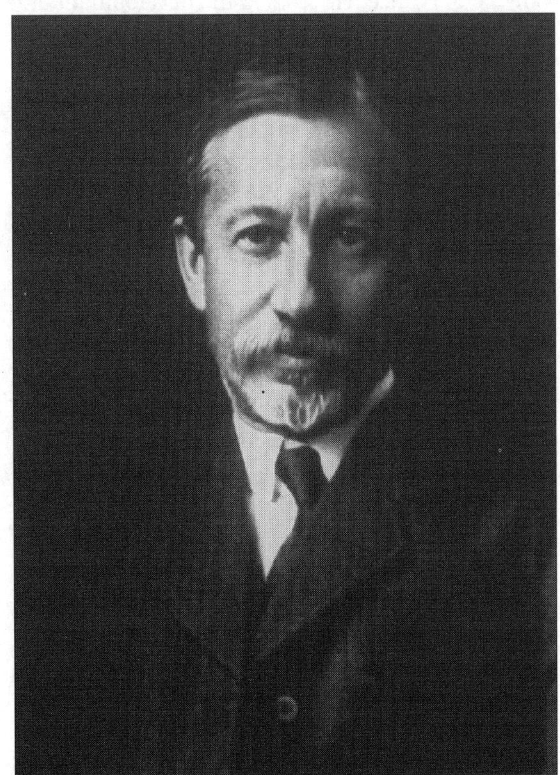

William H. Howell (Courtesy of the Royal Society of Medicine, London, UK)

William H. Howell (1860–1945) U.S. physiologist. He was born in Baltimore, majored in biology to gain his Ph.D. at Johns Hopkins University in 1884. In 1893 he was appointed Professor of Physiology at Johns Hopkins. He discovered and isolated heparin and carried out many important investigations on blood coagulation and the circulation. He wrote a textbook of physiology which was a standard text during his lifetime and was a major influence on many of the students at Hopkins.

Justin M. Jolly (1870–1953) French histologist. He interned with Dieulafoy.but right from the beginning was anxious to pursue a career in the laboratory. He entered the College of France where he studied with Ranvier and Malassez and from them he learnt histological techniques and the relationship of histology to physiology. He was the first of the hematologists in France to devote his studies to living tissue and to attempt to relate the morphology with the physiology and pathology. From 1925 to 1940, when he retired, he was a professor at the College of France. He studied the development and differentiation of the red and white cells and also of the lymphatic system, and in 1913 and 1917 presented the first films displaying mitosis in living cells, using microscopic moving pictures. Working with some members of the Curie Institute, Regaud and his pupil Lacassagne, he studied the effects of radiation on leukocytes and showed that a reduction in oxygen resulted in a strong inhibition of radio-sensitivity.

In 1923 he published his book "Technical Treatise of Haematology" which became a classical book in France and was used by innumerable students there. He was one of the founders of the Revue d'hematologie.

HOWSHIP LACUNAS

Osteoblast accumulation on surface of bone causing depressions and resorption.

HOWSHIP-ROMBERG SIGN OR SYNDROME

Pain or paraesthesia on the inner aspect of the thigh down to and often most severe at the knee due to obturator nerve compression.

John Howship (1781–1841) British surgeon. He worked at St. George's Hospital, London and developed osteomyelitis of the tibia and described the lacunae in the sequestrum of his own bone.

Moritz H. Romberg (1795–1873) German neurologist (*v. infra*).

HUCHARD DISEASE

Essential hypertension.

HUCHARD SIGN

In hypertensives the drop in heart rate on changing from standing to lying position is much less than in normals.

Henri Huchard (1844–1910) French physician of Auxon – a leading clinician of his day. He made contributions to therapeutics, disorders of the circulation, and especially arteriosclerosis. He first used the eponym STOKES-ADAMS disease.

HUGHES REFLEX

Downward movement of the penis when the prepuce or glans is pulled upward.

Charles H. Hughes (1839–1916) U.S. neurologist. He was born in St. Louis, Missouri, and went to medical school there, graduating from St. Louis Medical College in 1859. In 1867 he was appointed superintendent in an insane asylum in Fulton, Missouri, and for many years he was Professor of Psychiatry and Neurology at the Marion-Sims Medical College in St. Louis, which was largely founded by his efforts. He founded the Journal of Neurology and Psychiatry called "The alienist and neurologist" and was a pioneer of these subjects in the mid-west of the U.S.A.

HUGHES-STOVIN SYNDROME

Pulmonary artery aneurysms associated with pulmonary emboli, and peripheral venous thrombosis – most patients between 14–37 years old and male.

John P. Hughes British physician in Ipswich who was a medical registrar at the London Hospital when he reported this syndrome with his co-author.

Peter G.I. Stovin British pathologist who trained with Dorothy Russell (*v. infra*) and it was from working with her and his involvement with the cases to which his name is eponymously attached that he developed a lasting interest in cardio-thoracic pathology which he first pursued at the London Hospital and later at Papworth Hospital, Cambridge.

HUGHLINGS JACKSON EPILEPSY, FIT OR SYNDROME

v. JACKSONIAN CONVULSION, EPILEPSY, SEIZURE

HUGUIER DISEASE

Leiomyoma.

Pierre C. Huguier (1804–1874) French surgeon and gynecologist. Born in Sezanne and graduated M.D. in Paris in 1834. He invented one of the first uterine sounds and described the appearance of lymphogranuloma venereum involving the perineum. He was a surgeon at the Beaujon Hospital and Professor of Anatomy, School of Fine Arts, Paris.

HUNNER ULCER

Chronic vesical ulcer usually located at vertex of the bladder.

Guy L.R. Hunner (1868–1957) U.S. surgeon, and gynecologist. The obsessive compulsivenesss necessary for a successful life in medicine was displayed early, when as a young boy in Wisconsin he had a paper run, and would always place each paper out of the reach of snow or rain. When he grew older he used to accompany the local general practitioner, helping with anesthetics and doing odd jobs whenever he was able. Whilst at college he went on a camping trip to Yellowstone Park and met there some German doctors. He told them of his ambition and they in turn directed him to the recently founded Johns Hopkins Medical School and told him about a brilliant young gynecologist and obstetrician, Howard A. Kelly, who had come down from Philadelphia to head that department. Hunner sent for the application forms from Yellowstone Park and entered the first class of that medical school

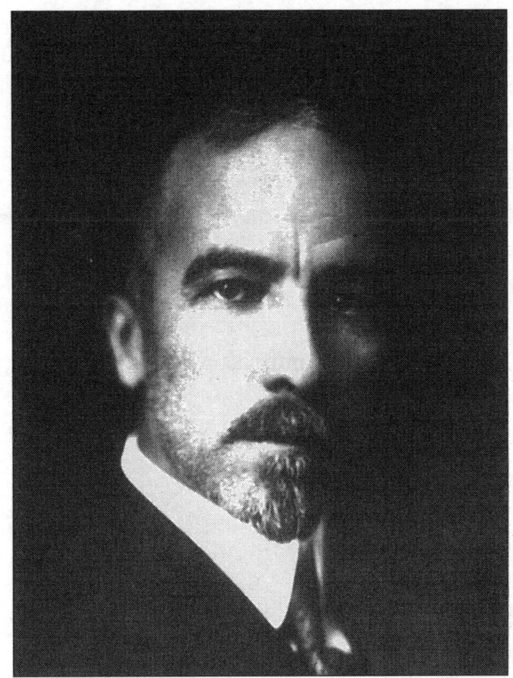

Guy L.R. Hunner (Courtesy of the Royal Society of Medicine, London, UK)

He later worked with Kelly, who had developed a technique for examining the bladder and ureters of women by inflating their bladder with air and using a cystoscope of his own invention. This became a very important part of the gynecological service and Hunner became particularly interested in it, and for some years was in charge of this section of the department.

He left in 1902 to go into private practice in Baltimore. Although he could not play an instrument himself, he was a keen lover of music and was a one man audience for a local chamber music group every Saturday night.

He was an extremely kindly person who frequently paid the hospital and nursing bills of needy patients out of his own pocket and sometimes invited patients to recuperate in his own home before they returned to their own surroundings. His house was not only a convalescent home for patients, but sick stray dogs were also nursed back to health there!

HUNT ATROPHY

Wasting of the small muscles of the hands without sensory loss.

HUNT NEURALGIA

Geniculate neuralgia

v. RAMSAY HUNT SYNDROME

HUNT TREMOR

Striocerebellar tremor.

James Ramsay Hunt (1874–1937) U.S. neurologist who graduated from University of Pennsylvania in 1893. He was appointed Professor of Neurology at Columbia University College of Physicians and Surgeons in 1931. He described the geniculate ganglion syndrome in 1907 and progressive cerebellar dysynergy in 1917. In 1914 he published a paper pointing out that 25% of people with fresh cerebral softening have carotid artery lesions, pointing the way to the recognition of cerebrovascular disease due to extracerebral vascular involvement.

HUNTER CANAL

Adductor canal.

HUNTERIAN CHANCRE

Syphilitic chancre.

John Hunter (1728–1793) Scottish surgeon, considered by many the greatest surgeon-anatomist of all time. "But why think? why not try the experiment?" He was born at Long Calderwood in Lanarkshire, Scotland. He was a very poor student at school and had little formal education prior to joining his brother William, who ran private courses in dissection of anatomy in the Great Windmill Hospital, London, and who had attracted considerable attention by that time. He joined his brother when he was aged 21 and spent the following years in the dissecting room, but was said to be some embarrassment to his brother because of his inability to express himself and his lack of formal education. He joined St. Bartholomew's Hospital in 1754 and was taught there by Percival Pott and by Cheselden at Chelsea Hospital. In 1755 he went to Oxford University, but could not stand the requirements in classic languages there and wrote of this time "Jessie Foot accuses me of not understanding the dead languages and I could teach him that on the dead body which he never knew in any language dead or living". He joined the Army in 1760 and went on the expedition to Belle Isle in 1761 and gained a great deal of experience in gun shot wounds.

His famous experiments on himself on venereal disease were said to have resulted in a delay of his marriage since the "cure" took three years. He conducted these experiments in 1767 using a lancet to make a puncture on his glans and prepuce, having dipped the lancet in a lesion from a prostitute. Unfortunately for Hunter, the patient from whom he obtained the specimen had both syphilis and gonorrhea and led him and others to believe that they were one and the same disease.

He married in 1771 and as his fame grew his surgical practice became immense. He established a unique collection of pathological specimens which resulted in the nucleus of the Hunterian museum of the Royal College of Surgeons, London.

Edward Jenner was initially his student and became a close friend who first noted that he was suffering from angina. Hunter's attacks were frequently precipitated by emotional upsets and he predicted correctly that one of these would cause his death. Following a meeting of the Board at St. George's Hospital at which he was angered by some of the discussion, he said nothing, left the room and turned to one of the physicians of the hospital, groaned and dropped dead.

HUNTER GLOSSITIS

Painful glossitis caused by B_{12} or folic acid deficiency with atrophy of the papillae and burning and pain particularly after condiments or citrus fruit.

William Hunter (1861–1937) Scottish physician. He was born in Ballantrae on the Ayrshire coast and studied medicine at Edinburgh University, where he had a brilliant undergraduate career, graduating in 1883. He served as a house physician at the Royal Infirmary, Edinburgh, and studied overseas at Leipzig, Vienna and Strasburg. From 1887–1890 he worked whole time on laboratory research at Cambridge, devoting himself to pernicious anemia. He was the first person to note that the alimentary and the nervous system were often affected in this disorder and he laid particular stress on the red, tender tongue which, together with oral sepsis, he regarded as being an essential in the disease. He also regarded the hemolytic element as being most important and made numerous observations on the excessive pigmentation and iron deposition in the liver.

In 1895 he joined Charing Cross Hospital and the London Fever Hospital and remained there for his active life. In the 1st World War he served in Serbia in 1915 and was responsible for organizing the control of a serious epidemic of typhus. He recognized that the essential problem was the eradication of lice, and with his team developed techniques known as the "Serbian Barrel" and the "de-lousing train" which were highly successful and were used in other theaters of war. After a demonstration of his train and pressure steam disinfectant to a group of Army experts, one of the younger medical officers asked "Will it kill a weevil, sir?" "A weevil" said Hunter, completely nonplussed, but ready to bluff it out – "a weevil – has anyone got a weevil?" No one obliged, and the crisis passed. Hunter turned to a colleague and whispered, "Most amazing! What is a weevil, anyway?"

Although his work on pernicious anemia was largely astray, he even questioned Ehrlich's observation that megaloblastosis was related to the anemia, he was a sound clinician and a good teacher of medical students, who wrote an interesting book entitled "On the History of Charing Cross Hospital". He was also one of the early proponents of the mouth as the site of focal sepsis and so probably was responsible for more teeth being extracted than any other person in medical and dental history!

HUNTER SYNDROME

Similar to Hurler syndrome but mental deterioration is less rapid, and there is no gibbus or corneal clouding. X-linked recessive (1:40 000) mucopolysaccharidosis due to iduronate sulphatase deficiency. Abnormal granules are found in the lymphocytes and occasionally neutrophils and chondroitin sulphate B and heparitin sulphate are excreted in the urine.

Charles H. Hunter (1872–1955) Canadian physician who was Professor of Medicine at the University of Manitoba who described the condition in 1917.

HUNTINGTON CHOREA

Autosomal dominant – usually has onset in middle age with uncontrollable tics, progressive chorea and mental deterioration.

George S. Huntington (1851–1916) U.S. physician, born in East Hampton, Long Island N.Y., son and grandson of physicians. After training with his father, he went to the College of Physicians and Surgeons in Columbia University, graduating in 1871. He returned to general practice in East Hampton and wrote his paper on hereditary chorea there, having first been aware of the condition when he made rounds with his father.

HURLER SYNDROME

Gargoylism – autosomal recessive mucopolysaccharidosis with hunchback, mental retardation, clouding of the cornea and deafness, hepatosplenomegaly, and enlarged tongue, due to x-L-iduronidase deficiency. Heparitin sulphate and chondroitin sulphate B are excreted in the urine and anomalous granules are found in the lymphocytes and sometimes in the neutrophils. Its incidence is 1:10 000 and the child usually dies before puberty.

cf. HUNTER SYNDROME

Gertrud Hurler German pediatrician who described the condition in 1919.

HURTHLE CELL ADENOMA

Thyroid adenoma composed of Hurthle cells (large epithelial cells with acidophilic cytoplasm).

K.W. Hurthle (1860–1945) German histologist.

HUTCHINSON TRIAD

8th nerve deafness; notched teeth and interstitial keratitis seen in congenital syphilis.

HUTCHINSON-BOECK DISEASE

v. BESNIER-BOECK DISEASE

HUTCHINSON-BOECK FRECKLE

Melanotic freckle.

HUTCHINSON-BOECK PUPIL

Fixed dilated pupil due to 3rd nerve lesion.

HUTCHINSON-BOECK TEETH

Notched incisor teeth in congenital syphilis.

HUTCHINSON-GILFORD DISEASE OR SYNDROME

Progeria – early senescence in children with large skull, bird-like features, atrophy of skin, loss of subcutaneous fat, high serum lipid levels and early atherosclerotic changes in the vessels.

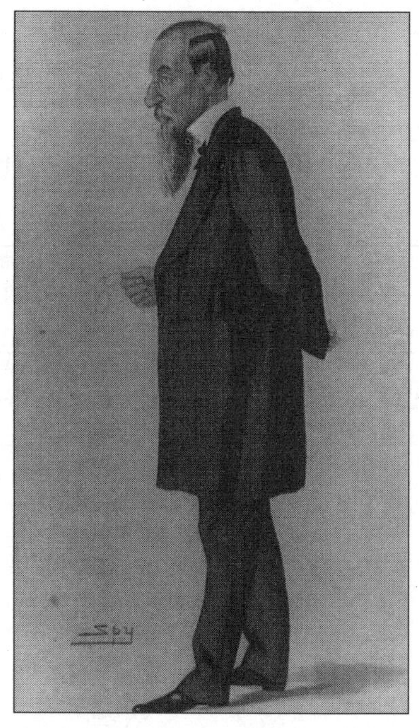

Sir Jonathan Hutchinson
(From a sketch in Vanity Fair by Spy)

Sir Jonathan Hutchinson (1828–1913) English surgeon, born in Selby, Yorkshire. He studied first in the York School of Medicine and Surgery, then at St. Bartholomew's Hospital. He was surgeon to the London Hospital (1859–83), and Professor of Surgery at Royal College of Surgeons (1879–83). He worked at the Blackfriars Hospital for skin diseases and was elected to the staff in 1867. He trained many dermatologists and was a member of the Dermatological Society of London. In 1851 he studied ophthalmology at Moorfields in London.

He wrote the 10 volume "Archives of Surgery" (1885–99) entirely by himself. He was elected F.R.S. in 1882 and knighted in 1908 for distinguished service to medicine. He was a Quaker, and knew Hodgkin. Syphilis was one of his major interests and it is said that he saw more than 1 million patients with this disorder in his life time. He recognized that Raynaud Disease had numerous causes including scleroderma, occupational, etc. and also described varicella gangerola

L.P.M. Boeck (*v. supra*).

Hastings Gilford (1861–1941) English surgeon. He studied medicine at Guy's Hospital and graduated in 1887 when he went into general practice in Reading and was rapidly recognized for his skills as an obstetrician and pediatrician, which resulted in him going into consultant practice and he gained his F.R.C.S in 1889. He was an enthusiastic contributor to scientific meetings and to journals and published his classical paper on progeria in The Lancet in 1914, and maintained an interest throughout his life in endocrinology and introduced the term progeria. He was one of the early environmentalists, contending that cancer was not caused by an outside agency acting on the cells, but by a disorder of the cells stimulated by civilized man's unnatural ways of living. He displayed a continuous interest in the ageing process and its relationship to cancer, which formed the basis of Hunterian lectures he gave in 1913, and under the pen name John Cope set out his views for the edification of the lay public. Although somewhat unconventional for his time, he was very highly esteemed by his local colleagues and was well liked by young and old.

HUTCHINSON TUMOR

Adrenal neuroblastoma with prominent skull metastasis, exophthalmos, periorbital discoloration.

Sir Robert G. Hutchinson (1871–1943) British radiologist. His father was a minister of religion, but there were numerous doctors in his family, including his grandfather. He graduated from Glasgow University in 1925 and trained in radiology at the Western Infirmary and the Holt Radium Institute, Manchester. He was radiologist at the Royal Alexandra Infirmary, Paisley, when he died following injuries in a motor car accident. He made a number of contributions to the radiology literature including the use of radium in the treatment of carcinoma of the bladder and in the management of carcinoma of the breast.

HYDE DISEASE

Prurigo nodularis.

James N. Hyde (1840–1910) U.S. dermatologist. He served as a surgeon in the U.S. navy during the Civil War and for 3 years after its cessation. He was Professor of Skin, Venereal and Genito-Urinary Diseases at the Rush Medical College in Chicago for 31 years and made numerous contributions to the literature of dermatology, including a textbook which went through eight editions.

I

IMERSLUND-GRÄSBECK SYNDROME

Autosomal recessive megaloblastic anemia in children associated with malabsorption of vitamin B_{12}, proteinuria and aminoaciduria. Urinary tract abnormalities are frequent, e.g. double ureters.

Olga Imerslund Norwegian pediatrician, Pediatric Department, Rikshospitalet, Oslo.

Ralph Gräsbeck (1930–) Finnish pediatrician, Helsinki.

IMRIE SIGN

Facial flushing in the first 48 hours of acute pancreatitis, usually lasting for 24 hours. The patient is afebrile but may have other features, e.g. upper abdominal pain and vomiting.

C.W. Imrie Surgeon, Royal Infirmary, Glasgow.

IRU KANDJI SYNDROME

This refers to a syndrome resulting from a jelly fish sting. The patient experiences general symptoms with shock, muscle pains which may often be agonising in the back, abdominal wall and chest, vomiting, headache and sweating. The site of the muscle pains has no relationship to the area of the sting and recovery is usual in 24–48 hours. There may be little evidence on inspection, of the original wound.

Iru Kandji An Aboriginal tribe which formerly inhabited coastal regions of Queensland from Mowbray River in the north to Trinity Inlet, near Cairns in the south.

ISAACS GRANULES

Solitary refractile granules seen in normal unstained erythrocytes and in supravitally stained wet preparation.

R. Isaacs (1891–) U.S. physician who, together with C. Sturgis, first showed that stomach extract contained a factor active in the treatment of pernicious anemia.

ISAACS SYNDROME

This is a rare manifestation of peripheral polyneuropathy resulting from continuous repetitive discharges in motor fibres with a generalized neuromyotonia or muscle rigidity. It is another form of the stiff man syndrome.

Hyam Isaacs (1927–) South African neurophysiologist. He was born in Johannesburg and graduated from the University of Witwatersrand in 1950. He undertook his post-graduate training in the United Kingdom, working with Sir Charles Simons and Professor Ritchie Russel, and in 1957 described for the first time noradrenaline secretion by neuroblastomas. In 1960 he worked for a year with Dr. Brian McArdle (*v. infra*) at Guy's Hospital. He returned to South Africa in 1961, developing the first clinical electromyographic laboratory there and describing his syndrome in the same year. He continues to be very productive in the areas of muscle pathophysiology and has published extensively on malignant hyperthermia and various forms of muscular dystrophy. He is currently head of the Neuromuscular Research Laboratory in the Department of Physiology at the University of Witwatersrand.

ISAMBERT DISEASE

Tuberculous ulceration of the larynx and pharynx.

Emile Isambert (1827–1876) French physician.

ISHIHARA TEST

Test for color blindness.

Shinobu Ishihara (1879–1959) Japanese ophthalmologist who graduated from Tokyo University and studied in Germany from 1912–1914. He developed his tests in 1917 and became Professor at Tokyo University in 1922.

IVEMARK SYNDROME

Absence of the spleen and abnormal cardiac development, e.g. situs inversus, cor biloculare.

Björn I. Ivemark (1925–) Swedish pathologist.

IVY METHOD OR TEST

Test for skin bleeding time using multiple sites of skin puncture on the forearm combined with compression to elevate venous pressure to 40 mmHg.

Andrew C. Ivy (1893–) American physiologist, born in Farmington, Missouri, gained his Ph.D. University of Chicago and graduated M.D. from Rush Medical College in 1922. He was Professor of Physiology at Northwestern University Medical School from 1925–1946. He made contributions to the study of gastric secretion (proving there was a humoral mechanism) and uterine function and was one of the founders of the journal Gastroenterology. He was head of a team to investigate war crimes of German physicians and scientists and his report clearly established their involvement in many degrading and immoral experiments.

Later in life he became associated with a controversial cancer treatment (Krebiozen).

J

JACCOUD ARTHRITIS

Progressive periarticular fibrosis with subsequent pain and loss of mobility and deformity without erosions following recurrent rheumatic fever. Today it is more commonly seen with lupus erythematosus.

JACCOUD DISSOCIATED FEVER

Febrile meningitis with a slow pulse rate seen in patients with tuberculous meningitis.

JACCOUD SIGN

Prominence of the aorta in the suprasternal notch, seen in aortic dilation.

Sigismond Jaccoud (1830–1913) French physician who was born in Geneva and studied medicine in Paris graduating in 1859. He practiced in Paris and became Professor of Internal Pathology in 1876.

JACKSON SYNDROME

Paralysis of 10th, 11th and 12th cranial nerves unilaterally due to a nuclear or radicular lesion.

JACKSONIAN CONVULSION, EPILEPSY, SEIZURE

Focal seizure involving spasmodic contraction of peripheral muscles and spreading centripetally, initially confined to one limb but sometimes proceeding to a generalized fit with loss of consciousness.

John Hughlings Jackson (1835–1911) English neurologist. Jackson was born at Providence Green, York, the son of a farmer. He studied medicine in York and at St. Bartholomew's Hospital, London. In 1856 he qualified and worked with Thomas Laycock at the York Dispensary. The latter was especially interested in the brain, the conscious state, the spoken word and print. Sir Jonathan Hutchinson encouraged Jackson to continue with medicine rather than philosophy and he was appointed to Moorfields Eye Hospital where he became familiar with the ophthalmoscope, which he popularized in English neurology. In 1862 he joined the staff of the National Hospital in Queen Square, founded in 1860 with Brown Séquard as Physician-in-Chief. His interest in seizures may have stemmed from his experiences with his wife and a cousin who had Jacksonian epilepsy and died at an early age. He enunciated a number of fundamental principles concerning the brain functions, motor and sensory, involuntary and voluntary movement and seizures and the gradation of movement. He made numerous contributions to the understanding of aphasia and was one of the founding editors of "Brain" in 1878.

He was somewhat of an eccentric. He had a taste for thrillers which were bound in yellow. He would buy a book, rip it in half and put one half in his pocket and leave the store. One day he bought one from a stall on a pier at Brighton and sat down on a bench with a nervous elderly lady. He unwrapped the book, tore off one yellow cover and threw it into the sea, and then tore off the other. The lady began to appear alarmed. He then tore the book in two, stuffing the last half in one of his pockets. The lady started to get up. Jackson turned to her and said "Don't be alarmed, Madam. They are lunatics who don't do this." The old lady fled down the pier.

After his wife died he became a recluse and suffered from vertigo and migraine. He died in 1911 of pneumonia.

JACOD SYNDROME OR TRIAD

Optic atrophy, total ophthalmoplegia and trigeminal neuralgia due to a space-occupying lesion in the petrosphenoid space, usually secondary to a tumor in the nasopharynx.

cf. GODTFREDSEN SYNDROME

Maurice Jacod (1880–) French neurologist who described this triad in 1921.

JAFFÉ-LICHTENSTEIN DISEASE OR SYNDROME

Monostotic form of fibrous dysplasia.

Henry L. Jaffé (1896–1979) U.S. pathologist. Born in New York, he graduated from the University School of Medicine there in 1920 and trained in pathology at the Montefiore Hospital. He largely devoted his life to the study of bone pathology. He was fond of music and a keen gardener.

Louis Lichtenstein (1906–1977) He was born in New York and graduated M.D. from Yale in 1929. He trained in pathology at the Mt. Sinai Hospital in New York and initially worked as an Instructor in Pathology at Louisiana State University before returning to New York to the Hospital for Joint Diseases with Jaffé. He later moved to California but retired to Palm Springs, Florida, where he died.

JAKOB-CREUTZFELDT DISEASE

Progressive encephalopathy, frequently familial, characterized by the gradual onset of pyramidal signs with later development of extrapyramidal signs and muscular atrophy. It commences in middle or late life and is commonly associated with mental deterioration and psychosis; thought to be due to a slow virus.

Alfons M. Jakob (1884–1931) Born in Bavaria, Ashaffenburg-am-Main, the son of a shopkeeper. He looked after the shop as a boy and is said to have increased its profitability by raising the prices of the goods. He trained in Munich and Strasburg, graduating in 1909 to do clinical work with Kraeplin and laboratory work with Nissl and Alzheimer. He then went to Hamburg-Friedrichsberg to work with Josef Kaes. After serving in the German Army in World War I, he returned to Hamburg and on Kaes' death he took his post of Prosector in 1930. Under Jakob's guidance the department grew rapidly. He had a large private practice and worked with the Hamburg neurologist Max Nonne. He made notable contributions to knowledge on concussion and secondary nerve degeneration and rapidly became a doyen of neuropathology. His work was praised by Cajal. He made numerous studies of the pathology of neurosyphilis and wrote an important monograph on extrapyramidal disease. He first recognized Alpers Disease, (*v. supra*) and accounts of this were published by three of his students, Souza (Madrid), Freedom (Baltimore), and Alpers in Philadelphia. His laboratory attracted postgraduates from Japan, Russia and Portugal and Italy as well as the U.S.A. He made a lecture tour of the U.S.A. and South America where he wrote a paper on the neuropathology of yellow fever. His productivity was remarkable for one in private practice, particularly as he suffered from chronic osteomyelitis during the last 7 years of life. This eventually caused a retroperitoneal abscess and paralytic ileus from which he died following operation.

Hans G. Creutzfeldt (1885–1964) First described the above disorder in a young woman whom he investigated whilst he was working in Spielmeyer's unit in Munich, as "a peculiar nodule forming disease of the nervous system". A few months later Jakob published three more cases which he called "spastic pseudosclerosis".

JANEWAY LESION

Skin lesion seen in bacterial endocarditis, with a profuse reddish eruption on the palms of the hands and soles of the feet which may be slightly nodular. They may be tender and purple in color and fade to brown in a few days.

Edward G. Janeway (1841–1911) U.S. physician. He was born in New Brunswick, New Jersey, and followed Austin Flint as Professor of Medicine at Bellevue Hospital Medical College. He was the first person in the U.S.A. to practice consultant medicine in a full time capacity within an institution. He was an outstanding clinician and became Health Commissioner in New York (1875–81) and established the first infectious disease hospital in Manhattan. His son, T.C. Janeway, was Professor of Medicine at Johns Hopkins (1914–1917).

JANSEN SYNDROME

Congenital metaphyseal dysostosis – a very rare dysplasia causing dwarfism, mental retardation, short lower extremities, widely spaced exophthalmic eyes and funnel chest. Patients usually do not survive childhood.

Murk Jansen (1867–1935) Dutch orthopedic surgeon. He graduated in 1900 from the University of Leyden. He founded an orthopedic hospital there and this was largely financed by him.

JARISCH-HERXHEIMER REACTION

v. HERXHEIMER REACTION

Adolph Jarisch (1850–1902) Austrian dermatologist. He was born in Vienna, entered the Faculty of Medicine in 1868 and whilst still a student in 1871 published his work on inorganic components of blood. He graduated in 1873 and in 1876 became F. Hebra's assistant and remained in that position until Hebra died (1880). He remained in Vienna until 1888 when he was nominated Associate Professor of Dermatology in Innsbruck and in 1892 he moved to Graz where in 1901 he was promoted to a full Professorship. Perhaps his most influential publication was his "Textbook of Skin Diseases" which was said to be the best written in the German language, in which he accorded priority and recognition to other people's work in an extensive bibliography. He published on many areas of skin disease and syphilis. He died of typhoid fever after a brief illness of a few days.

JELLINEK SIGN

Increased pigmentation of the lids and area around the eyes in hyperthyroidism.

Stefan Jellinek (1871–1968) Austrian physician with a special interest in electropathology.

JENDRASSIK MANEUVER

Reinforcement to facilitate testing of tendon reflexes. The patient is asked to hook their fingers together in a "monkey grip" and then to pull strongly in abduction.

Ernst Jendrassik (1858–1921) Hungarian physician.

JENNERIAN VACCINATION

Vaccination of cowpox to prevent smallpox.

Sir Edward Jenner (1749–1823) English physician, born in Berkeley, the son of the Vicar of Berkeley. Although initially interested in classics, he decided he wanted to do medicine and was apprenticed at the age of 13 to Mr. Ludlow, a surgeon at Lodbury near Bristol, and stayed with him for 6 years. He is said to have discussed smallpox with a young dairy maid who told him, "I cannot take it for I have had cowpox".

At 21 he went to London where he studied with John Hunter. They subsequently corresponded regularly until Hunter's sudden death. One of Hunter's letters to him on September 25th, 1778, clearly shows the closeness of their friendship:

"Dear Jenner,

I know I was at a loss to account for your silence and I was sorry for the cause. I can easily conceive how you must feel for you have two passions to cope with, viz. that of being disappointed in love, and that of being defeated; but both will wear out, perhaps the first the soonest. I know I was glad when I heard you was married to a woman of fortune; but "let her go, never mind her". I shall employ you with hedgehogs, for I do know how far I might trust mine. I want you to get a hedgehog in the beginning of winter and weigh him; put him in your garden and let him have some leaves, hay or straw to cover himself with, which he will do; then weigh him in the Spring and see what he has lost. Secondly I want you to kill one at the beginning of Winter to see how fat he is, and another in Spring to see what he has lost of his fat. Thirdly, when the weather is very cold, and about the month of January, I could wish you would observe their heat … so much at present for hedgehogs. I beg pardon – examine the stomach and intestines.

Ever yours, J. Hunter."

Jenner returned to Berkeley to become a busy country practitioner but carried on animal experiments and made observations on the cuckoo which he reported to the Royal Society of London (to which he was elected as a Fellow). He made observations of angina pectoris but did not publish these because he felt it might have worried John Hunter, then a sufferer.

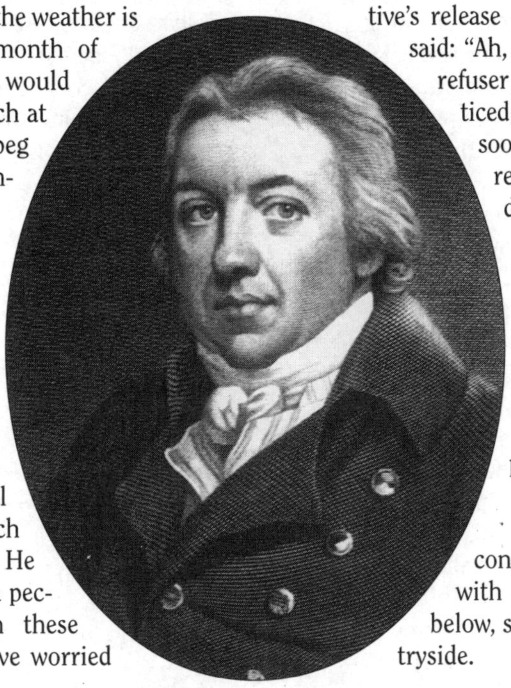

Sir Edward Jenner (Courtesy of the Royal Society of Medicine, London, UK)

In 1796 cowpox appeared on a farm in his practice and he took pus from the sore of a dairy maid and vaccinated James Phipps, a healthy boy of eight. The boy developed a small pustular sore – six weeks later Jenner inoculated the boy with variolus lymph and smallpox did not ensue. He successfully performed the experiment on three more patients and submitted a paper to the Royal Society who advised him not to present the paper "lest it should injure his established credit". However, Jenner went ahead and published the work in London in 1798, "Inquiry into the causes and effects of the Variolae Vaccinae" which recounted 23 cases. This discovery aroused much controversy.

It was, however, enthusiastically supported by most famous people of the day – Thomas Jefferson, who had several family members vaccinated – Napoleon, who ordered all his soldiers to be vaccinated, and the Empress of Russia, who urged vaccination for all her subjects. Jenner became world famous. In 1802 the English Parliament voted him 10 000 pounds, in 1807 an additional 20 000 pounds, and in 1808 formed the National Vaccine Establishment under his direction. During the Napoleonic Wars he wrote to Napoleon to request a relative's release (Captain Milman). Napoleon said: "Ah, c'est Jenner, je ne peut rien refuser à Jenner". In 1802 he practiced for a while in London, but soon he tired of it again and returned to Berkeley where he died of a stroke and was buried in the parish church. He was apparently a prototype of the English country gentleman of his day, but gentle and kind, and built a cottage for his first vaccination patient, James Phipps, and personally planted the rose garden.

Apart from his scientific contributions, he also dabbled with poetry, a sample of which is below, showing his love of the countryside.

Signs of Rain

The hollow winds begin to blow,
The clouds look black, the glass is low,
The soot falls down, the spaniels sleep,
And spiders from their cobwebs creep.
Last night the sun went pale to bed,
The moon in haloes hid her head,
The boding shepherd heaves a sigh,
For, see! a rainbow spans the sky;
The walls are damp, the ditches smell,
Closed is the pink-eyed pimpernel;
Hard how the chairs and tables crack!
Old Betty's joints are on the rack;
Her corns with shooting pains torment her
And to her bed untimely send her.

Loud quack the ducks, the peacocks cry,
The distant hills are looking nigh;
How restless are the snorting swine!
The busy flies disturb the kine;
Low o'er the grass the swallow wings;
The cricket, too, how sharp he sings!
Puss on the hearth with velvet paws;

Sits wiping o'er her whiskered jaws;
Through the clear stream the fishes rise,
And nimbly catch the incautious flies;
The glow-worms, numerous and bright,
Illumed the dewy dell last night;
At dusk the squalid toad was seen
Hopping and crawling o'er the green;

The whirling dust the wind obeys,
And in the rapid eddy plays;
The frog has changed his yellow vest,
And in a russet coat is dressed;
Though June, the air is cold and still,
The merry blackbird's voice is shrill;
My dog, so altered in his taste,
Quits muttonbones on grass to feast;
And see yon rooks, how odd their flight!
They imitate the gliding kite,
And seem precipitate to fall,
As if they felt the piercing ball.

Twill surely rain – I see with sorrow
Our jaunt must be put off tomorrow.

Sir Edward Jenner, M.D.

JENSEN RETINOPATHY OR DISEASE

Juxtapapillary choroiditis.

Edmund Z. Jensen (1861–1950) Danish ophthalmologist.

JERVELL AND LANGE-NIELSEN SYNDROME

Autosomal recessive, sensory deafness and mutism with prolonged QT interval, recurrent syncope and sudden death.

Anton J. Jervell (1901–) Norwegian physician.

Friedrik Lange-Nielsen Norwegian physician.

JEUNE SYNDROME

Skeletal dysplasia characterized by a long narrow thorax, present at birth and sometimes improving with age. Polydactyly with variable shortening of the extremities, hands and feet is present at birth and persists. The ribs are short and horizontally oriented with irregular costochondral junctions and an abnormal sternum giving a bell-shaped chest. Progressive renal disease occurs and occasionally involvement of other organs, e.g. liver, heart, retina, teeth, nails and pancreas.

Mathis Jeune (1910–) French pediatrician from Lyons.

JOB SYNDROME

Recurrent staphylococcal abscesses.

Book of Job Old Testament.

JOD-BASEDOW PHENOMENON

Hyperthyroidism induced by exogenous iodine.

Jod German for iodine

K.A. von Basedow

v. BASEDOW DISEASE.

JOFFROY REFLEX

Pressure on the buttocks causes twitching in the gluteal muscles in spastic paralysis.

JOFFROY SIGN

Failure to wrinkle the forehead when the patient is asked to bend the head and look up; seen in thyrotoxicosis.

A. Joffroy (1844–1908) French neuropsychiatrist who made contributions to the understanding of syringomyelia. Together with Charcot he recognized that the anterior horn cells were damaged in poliomyelitis.

JORDANS ANOMALY

Vacuoles in neutrophils and monocytes and sometimes eosinophils and basophils which stain for fat with Sudan III. These have been reported in some families with progressive muscular dystrophy of the Erb type (*v. supra*).

Godefridus H.W. Jordans (1902–1979) Dutch physician who initially trained with Van den Bergh (*v. infra*) in Utrecht and then became physician at St. Joseph Hospital in Eindhoven in 1932 where he introduced and directed Radiology as well as being the head of the clinical laboratory. He was the director of the hospital from 1932 until 1953 as well as having a very busy practice. When he started, the hospital had 131 beds and by 1953 this had risen to 330. The number had reached 600 when he retired in 1970. His medical colleagues as a token of their appreciation published his medical papers in book form in 1991.

JOSEPH DISEASE OR JOSEPH-MACHADO DISEASE

Slowly progressive cerebellar ataxia commencing in the second decade with other features suggestive of oliveopontine atrophy, e.g. extrapyramidal rigidity and opthalmoplegia and sometimes peripheral neuropathy.

Described in the JOSEPH and MACHADO families of Portuguese descent in the Azores Islands.

JOSEPH SYNDROME

Hereditary defect in renal tubular reabsorption resulting in proteinuria, accompanied by increased excretion of glycine and hydroxyproline with the onset of epilepsy early in life.

R. Joseph French pediatrician.

JÜNGLING DISEASE

Osteitis cystica multiplex caused by sarcoidosis.

Otto Jüngling (1884–1944) German surgeon.

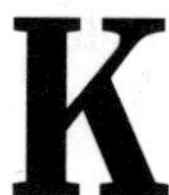

KAHLER DISEASE

Multiple myeloma.

Otto Kahler (1849–1893) Austrian physician, Professor of Medicine at the German University in Prague. He described syringomyelia. Together with Arnold Pick (*v. infra*) he elucidated the anatomical course of the posterior nerve roots which enter the posterior columns so that fibres at higher levels displace those from lower levels medially – "Kahler-Pick" law. Kahler preached the gospel of Charcot's approach to clinical medicine and neurology to Middle Europe. He then moved to Vienna, taking Friedrich Kraus with him as assistant. After a year in Vienna Kahler developed cancer of the tongue. Kraus took over his lectures and established himself as a brilliant teacher, laying the foundation for his appointment to Berlin.

KALISCHER DISEASE

v. STURGE-WEBER DISEASE

Otto Kalischer (1842–1910) German physician.

KALA-AZAR

An infectious febrile disorder which has protean manifestations. It may cause skin lesions and hepatosplenomegaly. It has a wide distribution throughout the world but is particularly prevalent in India, China, East Africa, the southern parts of the former USSR, and South America. The infectious agent is the protozoan *Leishmania* (*v. infra*) *donovani* (*v. supra*).

Kala is Hindi for black and azar is Assamese for fever.

KALLMANN SYNDROME

Familial hypogonadism with or without anosmia. Inherited as a sex-linked recessive or as an autosomal transmission with expression only in the male. Often characterized by microphallus or cryptorchidism.

Franz J. Kallmann (1897–1965) U.S. psychiatrist. He graduated from Breslau and was a resident at the All Saints Hospital and later trained in Berlin in psychiatry where he became interested in genetics. He moved to New York in 1936 and became Professor of Psychiatry at Columbia University.

KANAVEL SIGN

A tenderness in the centre of the hypothenar eminence may reflect ulnar bursitis.

Allen B. Kanavel (1874–1938) U.S. surgeon. He was born in Sedgewick, Kansas, the son of a Methodist minister and attended Northwestern University Medical School, from where he graduated in 1899. He spent six months in Vienna doing postgraduate work and then interned at Cook County Hospital, Chicago. He was associated with both Cook County Hospital and the Department of Surgery at Northwestern University Medical School until the time of his death. He was Professor of Surgery at Northwestern University Medical School from 1919–1938, and he was associate editor of "Surgery, Gynaecology and Obstetrics" from 1905–1935 and editor from 1935–1938.

He served with the American Army in the 1st World War at the Surgeon-General's Office in Washington but he went to France in September 1918 as assistant to the Chief Consultant in Surgery of the American Expeditionary Forces. Early in his career he became interested in the treatment of hand infections and his formula for investigation in medicine was constant pursuit of intelligently directed thought. He used to keep a soap box in his apartment where he would put notes and observations he made on infections of the hand. He gathered this information for some 10 years, directing his attention both to the anatomy of the hand and to patients with hand problems. In 1912 he published a monograph on this subject which has been regarded as a milestone in hand surgery. He was particularly helpful to young people whom he felt had a future in surgery, and although his last few years were dogged by bad health, with frequent attacks of glaucoma making reading difficult, he continued to exert influence in the surgical world through his editorship of the Journal of Surgery, Gynaecology and Obstetrics.

He was an excellent speaker and a fine raconteur who loved all games, particularly golf or bridge, enjoyed hiking, fishing and had an interest in geology and astronomy. He died as a result of an accident near Mojave in California.

KANTOR STRING SIGN

Narrowing of the lumen resulting in a thin line of barium ending at the ileo-cecal junction, seen in Crohn regional ileitis, in ileal tuberculosis, endometriosis, actinomycosis or enterogenous cysts.

John L. Kantor American radiologist who published his sign in 1934.

KAPOSI DISEASE

1. Xeroderma pigmentosum.
2. Kaposi sarcoma. Hemorrhagic sarcoma often seen on the lower limb and involving the liver and now recognized to occur more commonly in immunosuppressed patients with Acquired Immune Deficiency Syndrome (AIDS).
3. Eczema vaccinatum. A vesicular eruption due to herpes simplex or vaccinia occurring more commonly in people with atopy or icthyosis.

Moritz Kaposi (1837–1902) Viennese dermatologist who was born in Kaposvár in Hungary and his family name was Kohn. His family was unable to

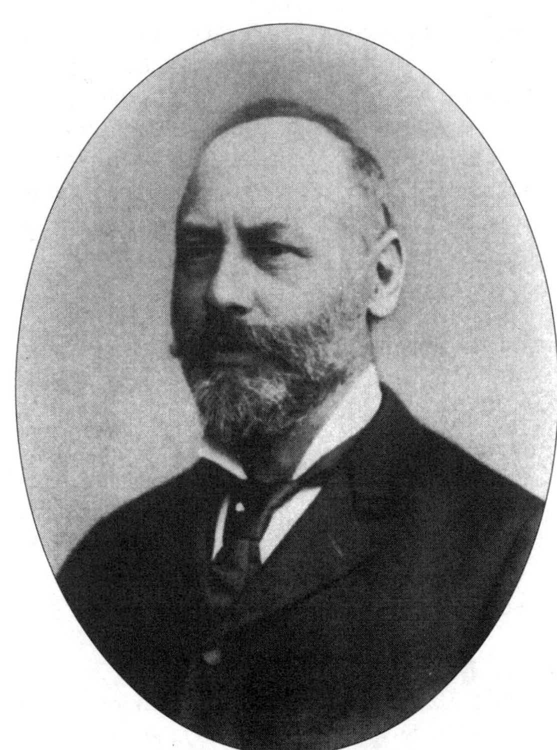

Moritz Kaposi (Courtesy of the Royal Society of Medicine, London, UK)

support him and he had to work his way through medical school, graduating M.D. in 1861 in Vienna. He changed his name from Kohn to Kaposi which was a derivation of his birth place and may have related to his becoming a Catholic. He became Von Hebra's (*v. supra*) assistant and later his son-in-law. He completed Von Hebra's "Textbook of Dermatology" and wrote another. He was clearly the outstanding dermatologist of his day and dominated the dermatology meetings he attended in Vienna. He conducted lecture clinics following Hebra's format but he was more didactic and was not so universally accepted. It was said that he appeared conceited and one observer commented that he never responded to a question with "I don't know" as the answer. One English visitor said of his presentations, "He does not forget mustard in his sandwiches, and true to his nationality – for he is Hungarian by birth – makes them extra pungent now and then".

He established dermatitis herpetiformis (first described by Von Hebra) as an entity and also lymphodermia perniciosa and lichen ruber moniliformis. With Hebra, Brett and Bateman he wrote some of the early descriptions of lupus erythematosus of the skin and he noted the systemic involvement in 1872. In 1875 he described the rash as "butterfly". He described rhinoscleroma and rhinophyma and in his book related skin disease to the body as a whole.

KARTAGENER SYNDROME OR TRIAD

Transposition of the viscera and malformation of the sinuses producing sinusitis and bronchiectasis. Bronchial biopsy shows abnormal cilia characterized by loss of the dynein arms in the cilia which are immotile, resulting in recurrent infection and bronchiectasis. Males may be infertile because of immotile sperms.

Manes Kartagener (1897–1975) He was born in Galizien, Czechoslovakia, the son of a rabbi. He migrated to Switzerland in 1916 and worked in Zurich and Basel becoming an assistant of Professor Löffler in Zurich and became his protégé. His main areas of interest were respiratory medicine and cardiology and he reported his syndrome in 1935. He used this as evidence to support his own belief that bronchiectasis had a congenital origin.

KASABACH-MERRITT SYNDROME

Giant capillary hemangioma with thrombocytopenia and purpura believed to be secondary to disseminated intravascular coagulation within the vascular abnormality.

Haig H. Kasabach (1898–1943) U.S. radiologist. He was born in Sivas, Turkey, the son of a highly placed government official in the Armenian community there. His family was deported during World War I and Haig was beaten by the Turks and left for dead. He recovered and made his way back to Sivas where he was taken in by his former teachers at the American missionary school and here he recovered from pneumonia. When the Turks learnt of his presence he left for Amasia where the widow of his eldest brother, who had been killed by the Turks, lived. He became a music teacher in a government school in Amasia after World War I and helped his sister to establish an Armenian school. In 1920 he migrated to the United States and worked his way through medical school at Ann Arbor in the University of Michigan, graduating M.D. in 1926. He joined the Radiology Department there and moved to the Presbyterian Hospital, New York in 1929. He became an Assistant Professor of Radiology at Columbia University but in 1942 developed hypertension and possibly because of this an acoustic neuroma was not diagnosed as early as it might have been and he died in the Neurological Institute, New York.

Katharine K. Merritt (1886–) U.S. pediatrician.

KASHIN-BECK (BEK) DISEASE OR UROV DISEASE

Generalized osteoarthrosis in children and adolescents limited to certain geographical areas in Asia – the alternative name is Urov disease, because it was first recognized among settlers near the Urov River. It is thought to be due to ingestion of wheat infested with a fungus *(Fusarium sporotrichiella).*

Nikolai I. Kashin (1825–1872) Russian physician.

E.V. Beck (Bek) Russian physician.

KAST SYNDROME

Chrondroma associated with multiple cavernous hemangiomas – sometimes the patients show pigmentation. It may be a variant of Maffucci Syndrome (*v. infra*).

Alfred Kast (1856–1903) German physician. He was born in Illenau in Baden and studied medicine in Heidelberg, Freiburg and Leipzig, graduating in 1879, and was an assistant to Erb in Heidelberg, then worked with Cohnheim in pathology in Leipzig. He returned to Freiburg as clinical assistant to Baumler. In 1888 he became director of the new Eppendorf Hospital in Hamburg and in 1892 was appointed Professor of Medicine in Breslau

(Wroclaw). He introduced phenacetin and the sulphonal group of drugs (1888) which were widely used as hypnotics before they were replaced by barbiturates. Together with Rumpel he published a beautifully illustrated atlas of pathology and published widely on neurology and pharmacology.

KATZ-WACHTEL SIGN

High voltage complex in mid-precordial ECG leads seen in ventricular septal defect (V.S.D.).

L.N. Katz (1897–) U.S. physician. Born in Pinsk, Poland, migrated to the U.S.A. and was naturalized in 1904. He graduated M.D. from the Western Reserve University in 1921 and interned at the Cleveland City hospital. He was appointed director of the cardiovascular institute, Michael Reese Hospital, Chicago in 1930 and attending physician in 1947. He has numerous publications on electrocardiography and arrhythmias.

H. Wachtel U.S. physician.

KAUFFMANN SYNDROME

Autosomal recessive disorder, characterized by post axial polydactyly, congenital heart defects and hydrometrocolpos. (cf. ELLIS-VAN CREVELD SYNDROME.) It is found in the Lancaster County Amish. Only one patient has all three manifestations and polydactyly is the only marker observed so far in males.

Robert L. Kauffmann U.S. geneticist.

KAWASAKI SYNDROME

Febrile mucocutaneous lymph node syndrome – febrile illness of unknown etiology occurring mainly in children under 5 years consisting of fever, erythema, edema and desquamation of hands and feet, oropharyngeal inflammation, injected conjunctiva, lymphadenopathy and high incidence of coronary artery aneurysm subsequently (15–30%).

T. Kawasaki Japanese pediatrician.

KAYSER-FLEISCHER RING

Ring of brown pigment seen in the outer border of the iris due to copper deposition in hepato-lenticular degeneration or Wilson disease (*v. infra*). It may require slit lamp examination to be seen.

Bernard Kayser (1869–1954) German ophthalmologist. He was born in the Hanseatic town of Bremen, graduated in 1893 in Berlin and became an assistant doctor in Tübingen. He then joined the North German Lloyd Shipping Company as a ship's doctor and went to work in Brazil as a general practitioner for 2½ years. He returned to work in general practice in Brandenburg and Bremen when he became interested in ophthalmology. In 1903 he specialized in ophthalmology and moved to Stuttgart where he remained for the rest of his life. He was for many years the editor of the essay section of the Klin. Mbl. Augenhk. and published some of his original work in that journal, including megalokornea. He was one of the pioneers in treatment of eye diseases in Stuttgart and although shy and a very reserved man, became the best known ophthalmologist in that part of Germany.

Bruno Fleischer (1874–1965) German ophthalmologist. He was born in Stuttgart and studied medicine in Tübingen, Geneva and Berlin. He worked in Tübingen from 1898 and described the corneal ring in 1903. He became a Professor in 1909. He recognized that this sign was associated with a cirrhosis and a neuro-psychiatric disorder but his work was overshadowed by that of Kinnier Wilson which was published in the same year, 1912. He moved to Erlangen in 1920, remaining there until his death. He was described as being one of the best examples of the old school of professor, being always proper and independent but with pointed and strong opinions. He was punctiliously exact but a stimulating colleague who was loved by his students even though he was somewhat of a hawk in examinations!

KEARNS-SAYRE SYNDROME

Progressive external ophthalmoplegia often with cardiac defects and pigmentary degeneration of the retina and proximal muscle weakness. Muscle biopsy discloses abnormal mitochondria and these have been shown to be due to mitochondrial DNA deletions.

Thomas P. Kearns (1922–) He was born in Louisville, Kentucky, and graduated M.D. from the University of Minnesota in 1952. He was a resident at the Mayo Clinic where he stayed throughout his professional life. He was appointed Professor of Ophthalmology at the Mayo Medical School in 1973, retiring in 1987.

George P. Sayre (1911–) U.S. pathologist. He was born in Glen Ridge, New Jersey, and graduated M.D. from McGill University, Montreal in 1938. He entered the Mayo Graduate School in 1939 as a resident in pathology and remained in the Pathology Department thereafter, apart from four years with the U.S. Army Medical Corps, where he served in New Guinea and the Philippines. He has a particular interest in neuropathology and the pathology of cerebrovascular disease. He became an Associate Professor of Pathology in 1958 and retired in 1975.

KEHR SIGN

Splenic rupture may cause pain and hyperasthesia over the left shoulder.

Hans Kehr (1862–1916) German surgeon. He was born in Weltershausen and studied medicine in Freiburg, Jena, Halle and Berlin. He was assistant to Meusel in Gotha for two years and set up private practice in Halberstadt as a surgeon in 1888. In 1895 he was made professor and in 1905 he was appointed Privy Councillor. In 1910 he went to Berlin to concentrate purely on bile duct surgery and his interest in music and the arts. He wrote a book on gallstone surgery and died of septicemia following an injury to his finger during surgery. He selected a verse of Wagner for his tombstone.

KEHRER REFLEX

v. KISCH REFLEX

Auriculopalpebral reflex.

Ferdinand A. Kehrer (1883–) German neurologist who worked in Münster.

KEITH NODE

or

KEITH-FLACK NODE

Sino-atrial node.

Sir Arthur Keith (1866–1955) He was born at Quarry Farm, near Aberdeen. He was not outstanding as a schoolboy scholar but on entering medical school soon showed his abilities and while studying medicine at Marischal College, in Aberdeen, he twice topped the anatomy classes, and for prizes was given Darwin's "The Origin of the Species" and the following year, 1886, Tyler's "Anthropology". These two books greatly influenced his career. He graduated in 1888 as M.B. from the University of Aberdeen. He spent a period in general practice and then went to Thailand as the medical officer for a gold mine and as a plant collector assistant in the Botanical Survey of the Malay Peninsula. During his 3 years in Thailand, he collected 500 plants which were later used in Ridley's Flora, but his real interest was in monkeys and apes. He spent a time studying with His at Leipzig. He returned to England and published his book "An Introduction to the Study of Anthropoid Apes" in 1896 and was appointed demonstrator of anatomy at the London Hospital. At this time he studied the functional anatomy of respiration, morphology of the pelvic floor, the acquisition of the upright posture and the structure and development of the heart. His interest in the heart led him to meet and become a life-long friend of the internationally famous cardiologist James McKenzie, and from then on he examined many of the hearts which McKenzie sent him, asking for anatomical reasons for their clinical problems. During the course of these investigations he noted that where the superior vena cava entered the right auricle (the sulcus terminalus) there was a localized area of tissue in which nerve fibres terminated. Martin Flack had been working with him on the anatomy of the mole's heart, and together they published the discovery of the sino-atrial node in 1907. At this time he wrote his textbook "Human Embryology and Morphology" which became a standard text of the day and went through many editions.

In 1908 he was appointed Curator of the Museum of the Royal College of Surgeons in London. There he continued his work on congenital disabilities of the heart and its embryological development and he wrote extensively on the endocrinology of racial characteristics and on anthropological topics. Under his direction the Hunterian Museum was greatly expanded and his own interests brought there much human anthropological material from all over the world. He became a leading authority on human remains and developed a number of methodological techniques for their measurement and identification. He published his first book on anthropology "Ancient Types of Man" in 1911, but his monograph in 1915 entitled "The Antiquity of Man" established for him a worldwide reputation, as one of the greatest anthropologists of his day.

In 1933 ill health forced his resignation from his position at the College of Surgeons but in view of his services he was appointed Master of the Buckston Brown Research Farm at Downe near Darwin's old house "Down House". There he continued to be very active and was a guiding light to a number of younger experimental surgeons working at the farm. In 1935 he re-evaluated his 1914 interpretation of the Piltdown "fossil" the nature of which had always puzzled him and on which he had spent considerable time and thought. He never fully accepted the Piltdown "mosaic of neanthropic and simian features". When this find was exposed as a fraud, it is easy to imagine the mental turmoil that he must have gone through, but he said that the major tragedy to him was "loss of faith in the testimony of our fellow workers".

An extraordinarily active and creative man, he made more than 500 publications, was much sought after by the popular press and engaged in several public debates largely revolving around his Darwinian beliefs and agnosticism.

He was tall and thin, with aquiline features, a prominent forehead and engaging and searching eyes and spoke softly with a somewhat piping voice and distinct Scottish burr. Although he presented a diffident exterior, he was well aware of his abilities and strengths and had the flair which made him an excellent teacher who was persuasive rather than didactic and who maintained personal contact with his students. His most distinguished pupil was Frederick Wood Jones, for whom he had the highest regard. McKenzie said of him "whenever Keith looks at anything, he sees something no-one else has noticed; and when he sees it he begins to wonder why".

Martin Flack (1882–1931) English physiologist, he was born in the village of Borden, Kent. His family was poor and he had to support his education by bursaries and scholarships which he attained throughout his undergraduate career. He commenced studying medicine at Oxford University and then did his clinical work at the London Hospital where his potential was recognized by Sir Leonard Hill and Sir Arthur Keith with whom he collaborated in the work on the sino-auricular node already discussed. He worked with Sir Leonard Hill on physiology of respiration and following his graduation in 1909 he attained a Fellowship which enabled him to work with Kronecker in Berne and also with Professor Fredericque in Lieges. He returned to work with Hill on physiology of the heart and respiration. In 1915 he was appointed Head of the Department of Medical Research, which the Air Ministry had recently established. Here he made a number of notable contributions including the supply of oxygen to pilots who were flying at high altitudes, and in setting up a pro forma for a series of tests to establish the physical fitness of flyers. This approach was adopted by many air forces in different parts of the world. Apart from first discovering the anatomy of the auricular node, he first proved the function of the node by showing that local cooling caused dramatic lowering of the heart rate. As a child, Flack had rheumatic fever which left valvular lesions and he developed subacute bacterial endocarditis and after a protracted illness, died.

KELL SYSTEM BLOOD GROUP

Occurs in 10% of Caucasian population and may be associated with hemolytic reaction, particularly after multiple transfusions. It is named after the first patient in whom this antigen was recognized, Mrs. Kell.

KELLER OPERATION

Arthroplasty of the first metatarsophalangeal joint to correct hallux valgus or hallux rigidus.

William L. Keller (1874–1959) U.S. surgeon, who also introduced pleurectomy.

KELLY-PATERSON SYNDROME

v. PATERSON-KELLY SYNDROME

v. PLUMMER-VINSON SYNDROME

KEMPNER RICE DIET

Low sodium diet originally used in treatment of hypertension.

Walter Kempner (1903–) U.S. physician. He was born in Berlin with a father and mother who had both been assistants to Robert Koch and Koch was the godfather of his brother, who became the American Deputy Chief Counsel during the Nuremberg war trials. He graduated from Heidelberg University in 1926 and worked in Berlin at the Kaiser Wilhelm Institute in Warburg's laboratory until 1934. He also held a post from 1928 to 1933 as assistant physician in the University of Berlin School of Medicine in Professor Gustav von Bergmann's department. In 1934, he was recruited to the Department of Medicine, Duke University as its first full-time appointment to develop teaching and medical research. In 1939, he introduced his rice diet initially in the treatment of chronic glomerulonephritis with uremia. This new therapeutic approach was important for a number of reasons, but perhaps the most important was that it showed that the hitherto fatal condition of malignant hypertension could have its effects dramatically reversed by this approach. Furthermore, using his diet he established the principles of low protein diet for renal failure and showed that its low cholesterol content could lower blood cholesterol levels and that it was also of benefit in diabetic control. He was finally appointed Professor of Medicine at Duke in 1952 and became Emeritus in 1972. The principles he established with his dietary approach are now largely accepted in modern medical therapy.

KENDALL COMPOUND A–F

Various forms of adrenocortical steroid hormones, e.g. B is corticosterone, F is cortisol.

Edward C. Kendall (1886–1972) U.S. scientist who was born in South Norwalk, Connecticut. He graduated Ph.D. from Columbia University in 1910 and studied thyroid disorders at the University of Cincinnati gaining his D.Sc. there. In 1914 he was appointed to the Mayo Clinic as head of Biochemistry and became a Professor in the Mayo Graduate School of Medicine in 1921. He isolated thyroxine and crystallized glutathione. His investigation of the adrenocortical hormones resulted in the demonstration of partial synthesis of "cortisone". For this work he, his Mayo associate Philip Hench and the Swiss chemist Tadeus Reichstein, were awarded the Nobel Prize in Physiology and Medicine in 1950. One of his earlier graduate students was Albert Szent-Györgi. After retiring from Rochester in 1951 he was appointed as visiting professor at the James Forrestal Research Institute of Princeton University where he remained until he died.

KENT, BUNDLE OF

Narrow band of muscle conductive tissue connecting the auricle and ventricle – more commonly called the Bundle of His, but first described by Kent in 1892.

v. HIS-TAWARA BUNDLE

Albert F. Kent (1863–1958) English physiologist who graduated in natural science from Magdalen College, Oxford in 1886 then worked in physiology departments in Manchester, Oxford and St. Thomas's Hospital, London, where he helped establish the radiology department. In 1899 he was appointed the first Professor of Physiology at University College, Bristol, and he was one of the most vigorous proponents to establish a university there which eventuated in 1909. He resigned from his Chair there in 1918 and devoted the remainder of his working life to studying industrial hygiene. He continued his interest in cardiac histology to the end, establishing a laboratory in his home and leaving behind thousands of sections.

KERLEY B LINES *or*

KERLEY LINES

Horizontal lines usually best seen in the lower zones of the lungs peripherally in a chest X-ray. A sign of congestive cardiac failure and thought to be due to fluid in the interlobular septa.

Sir Peter Kerley (1900–1978) British radiologist who was born in Dundalk, Southern Ireland. He graduated in 1923 and spent the next year in Vienna, the then centre of radiology. He returned to Cambridge and gained his D.M.R.E. and his M.D., University of Ireland, in 1939. The joint author of an authoritative text on radiology, he had a ready wit, enjoyed life outdoors and had a flair for diagnosing the unusual. A great raconteur he was a popular clubman at White's and the Travellers' Club as well as a fine golfer.

KERNIG SIGN

Flexion of the thigh at the hip and extension of the leg causes pain and spasm of the hamstrings in meningeal irritation due to meningitis, encephalitis or subarachnoid hemorrhage.

Vladimir M. Kernig (1840–1917) Russian physician in St. Petersburg (Leningrad).

KERNOHAN SYNDROME *or*

KERNOHAN-WOLTMAN SYNDROME

v. WOLTMAN-KERNOHAN SYNDROME

False localizing sign due to pressure from a cerebral lesion, e.g. a tumor causing herniation of the temporal lobe through the tentorial incisura with the contralateral cerebral peduncle being squeezed by the tentorium resulting in homolateral hemiparesis. (Also called CRUZ PHENOMENON)

James W. Kernohan (1897–1981) Born in Moyasset, County Antrim, Northern Ireland. Graduated from Queen's University, Belfast in 1920 and gained a B.Sc. and a Diploma of Public Health the following year. He migrated to the United States in 1922 to become a Fellow in Pathology at the Mayo Clinic. He became head of the section of Anatomical Pathology from 1943 to 1955 and was elected President of the staff of the Mayo Clinic in 1952. He was a fine golfer and at one time the champion of his club.

Henry W. Woltman (1889–1964) U.S. neurologist. He was born at Westfield, Wisconsin and graduated M.D. from the University of Minnesota in 1913. He interned at the University of Minnesota hospitals and served as a First Lieutenant in the Medical Corps of the U.S. Army from 1917–1919 and became Professor of Neurology in 1931. He made a number of contributions to neurology, in particular the changes associated with pernicious anemia. He had a keen interest in geology and became a highly skilled gem cutter and polisher and collected a number of local semi-precious stones, particularly agate. He was also a fine wood worker. He died of a cardiac arrest due to calcific aortic stenosis.

KETRON-GOODMAN VARIANT

v. WORINGER-KOLOPP DISEASE

This is a disseminated form of Pagetoid reticulosis (Woringer-Kolopp disease), a rare skin disorder which resembles mycosis fungoides.

Lloyd W. Ketron U.S. dermatologist who worked at Johns Hopkins Medical School.

M.H. Goodman U.S. dermatologist.

KIDD SYSTEM BLOOD GROUP

Named after the family surname in whom it was first identified.

KIENBÖCK ATROPHY

Acute atrophy of bone seen distally in inflammatory diseases.

KIENBÖCK DISEASE

Osteochondrosis of the lunate bone.

Robert Kienböck (1871–1953) Austrian radiologist who introduced the use of dosage in administering X-ray therapy. He graduated from the University of Vienna in 1895 and after spending a year in London and Paris became an assistant to von Schrotter and commenced using X-rays in 1897. He developed their use diagnostically and therapeutically, which eventually led to an independent department of radiology being established in 1904. In 1910 he fell off his horse and fractured his skull and he changed into a quiet and withdrawn man and concentrated mainly on diagnostic use of X-rays, publishing an 8 volume work on the diagnosis of disorders of bones and joints. However, he suffered another attack of severe depression which lasted for many years.

In 1933 he resigned from being President of the German Roentgen Society since he received a letter from the secretary of that Society informing him that the current German political situtation demanded all officers and lecturers of the congress to be of the Aryan race exclusively. His brother, Otto, was a leading member of the Austrian Christian Socialist Party and President of the Austrian National Bank. Their mother was of Jewish descent. As a result of this episode members of the Austrian Roentgen Society unanimously decided that they would not attend the Bremen congress. Members of the Hungarian Roentgen Society also withdrew from the congress.

KIESSELBACH AREA OR TRIANGLE

Thin area of nasal septum which may be the site of epistaxis or perforation.

Wilhelm Kiesselbach (1839–1902) German otolaryngologist who worked in Erlangen.

KIKUCHI NECROTIZING LYMPHADENITIS

This lymphadenopathy was first described in Japan but has now been recognized throughout the world. It characteristically affects the cervical lymph nodes of young women and must be distinguished from malignant lymphoma since its course is usually self-limited, although some have developed lupus erythematosus. The patient often presents with fever and the nodes are sometimes tender.

M. Kikuchi Japanese pathologist.

KIMMELSTIEL-WILSON KIDNEY

Nodular diabetic glomerulosclerosis.

KIMMELSTIEL-WILSON SYNDROME

Nephrotic syndrome in diabetes.

Paul Kimmelstiel (1900–1970) U.S. pathologist born in Germany and migrated to the U.S. to work in Boston.

Clifford Wilson (1906–) English physician. He studied medicine at Oxford and the London Hospital graduating in 1933 and becoming a Professor of Medicine at London University.

KINNIER WILSON SIGN

v. WILSON SIGN

KIRSCHNER TRACTION

Skeletal traction using Kirschner wires.

KIRSCHNER WIRE

Wire inserted through holes drilled in bone to exert traction.

Martin Kirschner (1879–1942) German surgeon, Professor of Surgery, University of Heidelberg, a pupil of Trendelenburg he performed the first successful pulmonary artery embolectomy (v. Trendelenburg).

KISCH REFLEX (KEHRER REFLEX)

Auriculopalpebral reflex. Reflex closing of the eye in response to a loud noise.

Bruno Kisch (1890–) German physiologist.

KJELDAHL METHOD

Method of measuring total nitrogen in organic compounds.

Johan G.C. Kjeldahl (1849–1900) Danish chemist who described his technique in 1883.

KLATSKIN TUMOR

Sclerosing bile duct carcinoma, classically occurs at the bifurcation of the hepatic ducts and presents as extrahepatic obstruction. The tumor is often small, localized and slowly growing, metastasing late.

Gerald Klatskin U.S. gastroenterologist, Yale University.

KLEBS DISEASE

Glomerulonephritis.

KLEBSIELLA PNEUMONIAE

Capsulated Gram negative bacteria which infects the respiratory tract, also called Friedlander bacillus.

KLEBS-LOEFFLER BACILLUS

Corynebacterium diphtheriae.

Theodor A.E. Klebs (1834–1913) German bacteriologist. He was born in Königsberg, East Prussia, and studied first at Königsberg with Rathke and Helmholtz and then at Würzburg where he was influenced by Kolliken and Virchow. He followed Virchow to Berlin and graduated there with a thesis on tuberculosis and became one of Virchow's early assistants in Berlin. He held numerous Chairs of Pathology (Berne, 1866; Würzburg, 1871; Prague, 1873; Zurich, 1882 and finally at the Rush Medical College, Chicago, 1896).

He returned to Europe in 1900, working successively in Hannover, Berlin, Lausanne, and Berne. He was one of the great pioneer proponents of the bacterial theory of infection. He was not an easy man, being readily ruffled and upset, and although he made many initial discoveries, often failed to follow them up. He introduced paraffin embedding for tissue sectioning in 1869. Apart from being the first to identify a number of infectious bacteria, he wrote two text books of pathology and a classical monograph on gunshot wounds following his experiences in the Franco-Prussian War and showed that traumatic septicemia was bacterial in origin. He recognized hemorrhagic pancreatitis as a cause of sudden death and was one of the first experimental pathologists to produce cardiac valve disease experimentally. He invented a technique for obtaining a pure culture of bacteria, employing a subsampling technique (Darwinising or cloning technique). He invented a filter impervious to bacteria and was the first to employ solid culture media.

Together with Gerlach, Klebs made numerous observations on tuberculosis and was the first to produce bovine infections by feeding with milk. With Naunyn and Schmiedeberg he founded the Archiv. für experimentalle Pathologie und Pharmakologie in 1872.

He is said by one of his students to have stated, "I was the first to see and partially describe many pathogenic bacteria but I had no success with those methods which yielded conclusive evidence."

Friedrich A.J. Loeffler (Löffler) (1852–1915) German bacteriologist, born in Frankfurt-am-Oder, he was a surgeon in the Prussian army for a number of years before becoming Professor of Hygiene at Greifswald in 1888. He discovered the bacteria causing swine erysipelas and glanders and proved that foot and mouth disease was due to a filterable virus. He established the causal relationship of

Corynebacterium diphtheria with diphtheria in 1884 although Klebs had first isolated the organism.

He was a pupil of a number of very distinguished teachers including Reichert, du Bois-Reymond, Virchow, A.W. Hoffman, Traube, Frerichs, von Bardeleben, von Langenbeck and Robert Koch. Of the latter he had the fondest memories and said, "The memory of those days, when he still worked in this room, Koch in the centre and we about him; when almost daily new wonders in bacteriology arose before our astounded vision and we, following the brilliant example of our Chief, worked from morn till eve and scarcely had regard to our bodily needs – the memory of that time will remain unforgettable to us. Then it was that we learnt what it means to observe and work accurately and with energy to pursue the problems laid before us."

In 1891 he discovered *Bacillus typhimurium* which caused an epidemic among mice in the Institute of Greifswald, and afterwards was used to combat mice plagues which threatened to destroy harvests in Thessaly (1892) and elsewhere. He was the first to demonstrate that when animals have recovered from a bacterial disease (mouse septicemia) they are immune to a second infection from the same organism in a similar fashion to that known for non-bacterial diseases such as measles and smallpox. He made many advances in techniques of microbiology, both from the point of view of staining of bacteria and in the development of media to cultivate the bacteria.

KLEIN-WAARDENBURG SYNDROME

Patchy areas of pigment loss in the skin together with a broad-based nose, a white forelock, and heterochromia of the iris, meeting of the eyebrows in the midline of the forehead. There may be a nerve deafness and the inheritance is autosomal dominant with variable expressivity.

David Klein (1908–) Swiss ophthalmologist and geneticist. He was born in Falkau, then in the Austro-Hungarian empire. He studied medicine at Freiburg and the University of Basel, where he graduated in 1934. He then worked at the Rheinhau Psychiatric Clinic in Zurich and became an assistant to Professor A. Franceschetti at the ophthalmological clinic in Geneva, where he became a full professor in 1970. He wrote many articles on genetics and also was the co-author of three books. There has been some argument as to whether Klein's and Waardenburg syndrome (*v. infra*) are one and the same since in the initial description by Klein the patient had a limb malformation.

Petrus J. Waardenburg (*v. infra*)

KLEINE-LEVIN SYNDROME

Periodic attacks of sleep and hunger with amnesia for periods of the attacks, related to narcolepsy.

Willi Kleine German psychiatrist.

Max Levin (1901–) U.S. neurologist.

KLINE TEST

Serum test for syphilis.

Benjamin S. Kline (1886–1968) U.S. pathologist.

KLINEFELTER SYNDROME

(Also called KLINEFELTER-REIFENSTEIN-ALBRIGHT SYNDROME)

Feminization with reduced testicle size and gynecomastica with one Y but more than one X chromosome.

Harry F. Klinefelter (1912–) U.S. physician who was born in Baltimore and graduated from Johns Hopkins Medical School in 1937. He worked at Harvard University in 1941–42 with Fuller Albright and then returned in 1943 to Johns Hopkins Medical School where in 1965 he became the Associate Professor of Medicine. He had a life-long interest in investigation of areas of rheumatology, endocrinology and alcoholism.

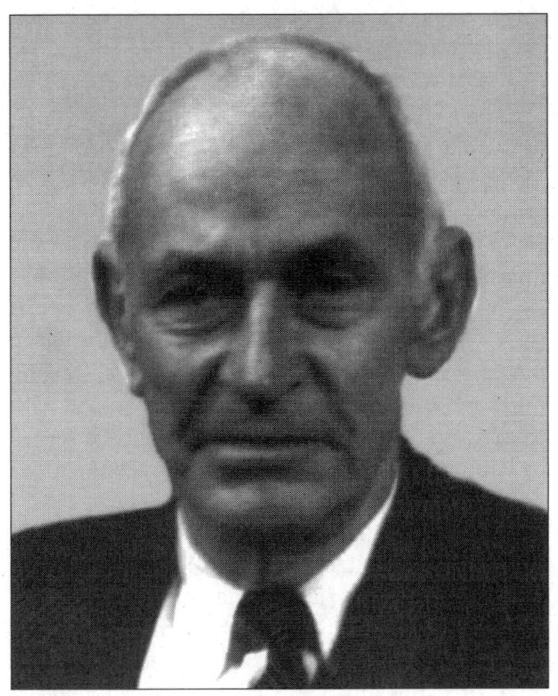

Harry F. Klinefelter
(Courtesy of Dr Klinefelter)

He considered the syndrome named after him to be another of Albright's (*v. supra*) discoveries and describes the way it came about as follows – whilst a travelling Fellow at Harvard from Johns Hopkins he initially worked with Howard Means, on a study of oxygen consumption of the adrenal cortex using a Warburg apparatus. "After many unsuccessful attempts at this and after breaking several valuable pieces of apparatus, I asked Dr. Means if I might work with Dr. Fuller Albright in clinical endocrinology; Dr. Means readily acceded to my request. The next week, at Dr. Albright's famous Saturday morning clinic, the first patient I saw was a 19 year old black man with gynecomastica and small testes. Dr. Albright had no clear ideas about this disorder and suggested that I work on it. During the remaining six months of my fellowship we found eight other patients with the condition and worked hard to try to fit together the different pieces of the puzzle." He concludes, "This is really another of Dr. Albright's diseases: he unselfishly allowed my name to come first on the list of authors."

Edward C. Reifenstein (*v. infra*).

Fuller Albright (*v. supra*).

KLIPPEL-FEIL SYNDROME OR DEFORMITY

Congenital fusion of the bodies of two or more cervical vertebrae producing a short neck and sometimes results in neurological deficits due to platybasia.

KLIPPEL-TRÉNAUNAY-WEBER SYNDROME

Cutaneous hemangioma of a limb which may extend to the trunk. As the child grows the involved limb may hypertrophy and various veins may appear. There is often mild mental retardation.

KLIPPEL-WEIL SIGN

Passive extension of a flexion contracture of the fingers results in involuntary flexion of the fingers and abduction of the thumb in pyramidal tract disease.

Maurice Klippel (1858–1942) French neurologist and psychiatrist who was born in Mulhouse. He studied in Paris and graduated in 1889. J. Lhermitte (*v. infra*) trained with him and wrote his obituary. He was appointed head of the medical department at the Hôpital Tenon in Paris in 1902, retiring in 1924. He was a prolific writer and submitted one article in the year of his death.

André Feil (1884–) French neurologist.

Paul Trénaunay (1875–) French neurologist.

Frederick P. Weber (1863–1962) British physician (*v. infra*).

Mathieu P. Weil (1884–) French physician.

KLUMPKE PARALYSIS

Lower brachial plexus paralysis.

Augusta Dejerine-Klumpke (1859–1927) French neurologist. She came from a well-to-do San Francisco family and became the wife of Dejerine. She was profoundly influenced by Vulpian in Paris, who warned her of the difficulties for a woman studying medicine. She became the first woman to receive the title "Interne des Hôpitaux" (1887) in face of great opposition. After her husband died she continued on his practice and their joint work (v. Dejerine).

KNOOP THEORY

The theory that fat is catabolised by B oxidation.

Franz Knoop (1875–) German physiologist who worked in Freiburg. As well as studying the metabolism of fat he showed that the ability of the liver to produce amino acids from ingested protein was limited.

KOCH LAW OR POSTULATE

Four criteria are required to establish that an organism causes a disease.

1. The organism must be demonstrated to be present in patients with the disease.
2. The organism must be cultured.
3. The pure culture must cause the disease in susceptible animals.
4. It must be recovered from (3) and re-grown in pure culture.

KOCH PHENOMENON

Delayed hypersensitivity response.

KOCH-WEEKS BACILLUS

Haemophilus aegypticus causes Koch-Weeks conjunctivitis.

Robert Koch (1843–1910) German bacteriologist. Born in Clausthal, Hannover, he went to school in his local town and took his medical degree at Göttingen (1866) where J. Henle influenced him greatly, in particular his theory of contagion. He fought in the Franco-Prussian War and afterwards became a district physician at Wollstein where he undertook studies with his microscope, first making observations on anthrax. He presented this to a group gathered together by Professor of Botany, F. Cohn, and including Weigert, Auerbach, Traube and Cohnheim, who were greatly impressed. Cohn had Koch's paper published, showing that anthrax was the cause of the disease and could be cultured in pure form outside the animal for several generations and then subsequently infect an animal with the disease. These findings were violently disputed by Paul Bart, but were confirmed by Pasteur.

In 1877 Koch published his fixation, staining and the photographic techniques for identification and comparison of bacteria, and then his great paper on bacterial infections in trauma. He published techniques for obtaining pure cultures and in 1882 he discovered the tubercle bacillus by special culture and staining techniques and in this paper enunciated Koch's postulates. In 1883 Koch, as the Head of the German Cholera Commission, went to India and Egypt, and discovered the cholera vibrio – and found the organism of Egyptian ophthalmia – infectious conjunctivitis, the Koch-Weeks bacillus. In 1885 he became Professor of Hygiene and Bacteriology at the University of Berlin, where amongst his students were Welch, Pfeiffer, Loeffler, and Kitasato.

Koch made a number of journeys to Africa to investigate tropical diseases with much success. He initially felt tuberculin would be a cure for tuberculosis and this was his one error, but somewhat mollified by the fact that it became an important means of diagnosis and screening populations for the disease.

Koch received the Nobel Prize in 1905 in Medicine and Physiology and was elected to the Prussian Academy of Science, but attracted wide criticism when he fell in love with a young actress and divorced his wife to marry her. Rumors were even circulated that he had sold his patent on tuberculin to Behringwerke and allowed it to be tried in patients before it had been properly proved in order to have sufficient money to support his second wife. A tablet which had been placed on the walls of his home by his fellow citizens of Clausthal was torn down. He died of heart disease and his body was cremated at his request and the ashes deposited in his Institute. Prior to his investigations only anthrax and relapsing fever had been established with reasonable certainty as being bacterial in origin.

John E. Weeks (1853–1949) U.S. ophthalmologist. Born in Painesville, Ohio he graduated M.D. in 1881 from the University of Michigan. He interned in New York and trained with Herman Knapp at the Ophthalmic and Aural Institute until 1884 when he spent a year in Berlin. He returned to New York where he isolated the bacillus causing epidemic conjunctivitis in 1886. He was an excellent surgeon and wrote 2 text books on the eye, one of which was a standard text for many years. He retired to Portland, Oregon where he rapidly became prominent in the University of Oregon Medical School donating the funds for a library building. He was a keen fisherman and golfer.

KOCHER INCISION

Oblique abdominal incision paralleling the thoracic cage on the right side of the abdomen for cholecystectomy.

KOCHER MANEUVER

Technique for reduction of a dislocated shoulder.

KOCHER SYNDROME

Splenomegaly with or without lymphocytosis and lymphadenopathy in thyrotoxicosis.

KOCHER-DEBRÉ-SEMALAIGNE SYNDROME

Hypothyroidism in children may be associated with muscular enlargement to give the appearance of an infant Hercules.

Theodor Kocher (1841–1917) Swiss surgeon whose name is given to the Kocher Institute in Berne. He was born in Berne and graduated in medicine from the University there. He was a student of Langenback and Billroth. From 1866–72 he was assistant to Professor Lucke at Berne, where Lucke operated on 10 patients with goitre and 9 died. He succeeded Lucke as Professor of Surgery in Berne in 1872 and in 1874 published his first 13 goitre operations with only 2 deaths. He did much experimental work on the thyroid gland and was the first to excise the thyroid for goitre in 1878. He performed this operation over 2000 times and had only a 4½% mortality, truly remarkable when the era in which he was undertaking the operation is considered. He described myxedema following thyroidectomy, "Cachexia strumipriva" which occurred in 30 out of 100 thyroidectomies. He undertook much experimental work on animals and was interested in the physiology of the brain and the spinal cord. He evolved a hydrodynamic theory for the effect of gunshot wounds and attempted in 1912 to accelerate hemostasis in internal hemorrhage by injecting a sterile coagulating fluid which had been derived by Fonio from platelets. Above all he was extremely painstaking and careful and at all times a calm and imperturbable operator. He was a complete master of dissection and maintained total asepsis at all times. He wrote an important textbook on operative surgery and made contributions to almost all areas including such things as hernias, shoulder dislocation and abdominal operations for resection and anastomosis of bowel loops and for the fashioning of colostomies.

His methods were somewhat similar to those of Lister and Halstead in that he relied on absolute precision and care rather than speed and show, and this was vindicated by his low mortality figures.

Probably three men, Lister, Halstead and Kocher, did more to improve operative mortality than any other surgeons of their time and ended the days when surgeons were regarded as good only if they were quick, rapid and spectacular. He won the Nobel Prize for his work on the thyroid gland in 1909 and the Kocher Institute in Berne was established as a permanent memorial to him. He retired as Professor of Surgery in 1911.

Robert Debré French pediatrician (*v. supra*).

Georges Semalaigne French pediatrician who worked with R. Debré.

KOEBNER RESPONSE

The occurrence of psoriasis following trauma of the skin e.g. a scratch. Later widened to include lichen planus, warts and vitiligo.

Heinrich Koebner (1838–1904) German dermatologist who trained with von Hebra in Vienna and Hardy in Paris. He established a research orientated skin clinic in Breslau (Wroclaw). With a flair for the dramatic he always attracted an interested audience and is reported to have demonstrated various skin infections resulting from self inoculation from afflicted patients' skin to his forearms and chest. During his lecture demonstration he exposed the various parts of his anatomy to convince his audience. He rapidly assembled a large clinic and was particularly interested in tuberculosis, syphilis and leprosy. He was succeeded by Oscar Simon with whom Neisser trained and who in turn succeeded him when Simon died with carcinoma of the stomach in 1882.

KÖHLER DISEASE

Aseptic necrosis of the navicular bone.

Alban Köhler (1874–1947) German radiologist. He was born in Pesta, Germany, and worked in Wiesbaden. He described his condition in 1908 and wrote a book on radiology (1910) and one on the history of military medicine. He also introduced technical modifications to improve X-ray visualization of the heart.

KOHLMEIER-DEGOS SYNDROME

v. DEGOS SYNDROME

W. Kohlmeier German dermatologist.

KOMMERELL DIVERTICULUM

Swelling of the descending aorta at the origin of an aberrant right subclavian artery which passes posteriorly to the esophagus.

B. Kommerell German radiologist.

KÖNIG DISEASE

Osteochondritis dissecans.

Franz König.(1832–1910) German surgeon, who described the disease in 1905. He was born in Rotenburg on Fulda in Hesse.

He graduated in 1855 from the University of Marburg and after a short term in the medical clinic there he went to Berlin to work with Professor Langenbeck and the ophthalmologist Graefe, and in 1858 he became assistant to Roser, the Professor of Surgery at Marburg. In 1860 he went to Hanau as medical officer for health and surgeon to the hospital. Whilst there he published a number of clinical case reports as well as new operative approaches to problems in the lung and rectum. He became best known, however, for his work on joint resection and was appointed Professor of Surgery at the University of Rostock where he remained until 1875. He was then appointed Professor of Surgery at Göttingen until 1895 when he succeeded Professor Bardeleben at the University of Berlin. He retired in 1904, initially to Jena, but returned to Berlin where he continued to take a prominent part in medical societies and meetings. He was the author of a successful textbook on surgery which was published in many languages and described the disease to which his name is attached in 1905. He was a poor, perhaps boring speaker because he developed each problem in minute detail, but he was outstanding in clinical practice, always putting the patient first and treating clinic and private patients equally. He demanded the same high standards of his colleagues and assistants, and in particular insisted that any operation, no matter how minor, be justified, berating those who did not do so. By some he was called the conscience of German surgery, by others he was heartily disliked for his almost tyrannical demarcations of what he considered ill-practice.

KOPLIK SPOTS

Red spots surrounding the opening of the parotid duct which precede the skin eruption of measles.

Henry Koplik (1858–1927) U.S. pediatrician from New York and Mt. Sinai Hospital, reported the spots in 1898 and published a book on pediatrics in 1902. He was born in New York, graduating M.D. from Columbia University, N.Y. in 1881 and then studied in Berlin, Vienna and Prague. He established the first sterilized milk depot for infants in the U.S. and was one of the founders of the American Pediatric Society. He died of a coronary thrombosis.

KORO

An acute anxiety reaction in males, mainly seen in Chinese migrants to Malaya. The patient has a sudden panic reaction and fears that his penis is shrinking into his abdomen, and to prevent this has his penis grasped, either by him or a friend. He has a fear of impending death. Koro has very rarely been reported in Caucasian whites. Koro is probably Indonesian in origin and means shrinking tortoise.

KOROTKOFF (KOROTKOV) SOUNDS

Sounds heard through the stethoscope on eliciting blood pressure, using a Riva-Rocci sphygmomanometer.

Nicolai S. Korotkoff (1874–1920) Russian surgeon who introduced the auscultatory technique in blood pressure measurement in 1905. This observation followed his use of the stethoscope to ensure that no blood was flowing below pressure exerted by a cuff or ligature even though no pulses were present. He was introduced to the use of the stethoscope in vascular disease by his teacher, the surgeon Nicolai I. Pirogoff, who used it to distinguish aneurysms from solid tumors. He had served as a surgeon in the Russian-Japanese war in 1904 and returned to study at the Surgical Clinic of the Military Academy of Medicine in St. Petersburg. Here he studied the problem of post-traumatic vascular aneurysm and gained his M.D. on the subject in 1910.

KORSAKOFF PSYCHOSIS

A mental state classically seen in alcoholics with recent memory loss and confabulation.

Sergei S. Korsakoff (1853–1900) Russian neuropsychiatrist. The first great Russian psychiatrist, the son of the manager of a glass factory, he studied at the University of Moscow, graduating in 1875. From 1876–9 he was with Kozlevnikov's clinic for nervous disease, and his M.D. thesis "Alcoholic Paralysis" was awarded in 1887. In 1892 he was appointed Superintendent of a new University Psychiatric Clinic and Professor Extraordinarius, and at this time studied with Meynert in Vienna. Apart from his studies on alcoholic psychosis he introduced the concept of paranoia and wrote an excellent textbook on psychiatry.

He was a leader in more humane patient management with his use of "no restraint" principles. This was not popular with hospital personnel. "The less restraint for the patient, the more restraint for the doctor", and as a result the doctor must "give more attention and devotion to the patient". He was a great humanitarian and addressed students, "First of all, I wish that all students recognize the absolute necessity of education, that they deeply love science and knowledge, and that they despise ignorance ... For the great privilege of being educated, students must be ready to sacrifice, even to pay with their lives if necessary, for the good of the country and for the ideals of mankind."

KOSTMANN DISEASE OR SYNDROME

Congenital agranulocytosis. The patient has a predilection to develop acute leukemia. Chromosome studies in the non-leukemic phase have shown abnormalities. It appears to be autosomal recessive.

Rolf Kostmann (1909–) Swedish pediatrician, Clinical Director of Division of Pediatrics, Norrkoping, Sweden. He undertook this investigation whilst he was Director of the Division of Pediatrics of the Army Hospital in Boden. The initial children came from a district in Norrbotten, the northern-most province of Sweden.

KOZHEVNIKOV EPILEPSY

Chronic focal epilepsy (epilepsia partialis continua) associated with chronic focal inflammatory pathology in the brain. In Russia it is thought to be related to tick borne viruses isolated from cerebral tissue removed at surgery.

Alexei I. Kozhevnikov (1836–1902) Russian neurologist and psychiatrist, born in Ryazan and graduated M.D. from Moscow University in 1860 and studied neurology in Russia, then in Europe, especially in Germany but also in England, and with Charcot in France, where he reported the pathology of amyotrophic lateral sclerosis. When he returned home he became the first academic neuropathologist and psychiatrist in Russia, was appointed Professor of Nervous and Mental Disease in Moscow and rapidly introduced more humane approaches to the treatment of the insane and promoted this throughout Russia and wrote a popular textbook. His most famous pupil and assistant was Korsakoff. He died of cancer.

KRABBE DISEASE

1. Globoid leukodystrophy.
2. Sturge-Weber Syndrome (*v. infra*).

Knud H. Krabbe (1885–1965) Danish neurologist based in Copenhagen, Chief Physician, Neurology Department, Kommune Hospital from 1933. He was interested in comparative anatomy and studied the morphogenesis of the brain of submammalian species and described "familial infantile diffuse sclerosis" in 1934. He championed the theory that many cerebral hemorrhages were secondary to vascular malformation. In later life he developed Parkinson disease.

KRAEPELIN-MOREL DISEASE

Schizophrenia.

Emil Kraepelin (1856–1926) German psychiatrist. He was born in Strelitz, Micklenburg, studied medicine at Leipzig and Würzburg and decided to become a psychiatrist when still a student. He graduated in 1878 and was an assistant to von Gudden (who in 1886 was killed by the mad King Ludwig while trying to prevent him from suicide) in Munich and to Flechsig in Leipzig. He became Professor of Psychiatry at Dorpat and moved to Heidelberg in 1890 and then to Munich as Professor and Director of the Psychiatric Institute. His major contributions were in the classification of psychiatric illness. He was often opposed by Wernicke (*v. infra*).

Nissl worked with him in Heidelberg and Alzheimer joined him there in 1902 and then moved with him to Munich. Initially Kraepelin was reluctant to undertake histological studies in psychoses, but the studies of Vogt and Brodmann on cortical structure and function convinced him to commence in 1905. In 1911 he attached the eponym Alzheimer Disease to pre-senile dementia. Other students of his included A. Jakob, H. Spatz and R. Barany.

He was a fierce campaigner against alcohol and investigated the psychiatric effects of alcohol. He was a pioneer of experimental psychiatry and founded a museum setting out the inhumane treatment of the insane.

Bénédict A. Morel (1809–1873) French psychiatrist.

KRAUSE CORPUSCLE

Nerve ending receptor.

Wilhelm J.F. Krause (1833–1910) German anatomist who worked in Göttingen and Berlin.

KREBS CYCLE

Tricarboxylic acid cycle.

KREBS-HENSELEIT CYCLE

Ornithine citrulline arginine urea cycle.

Hans A. Krebs (1900–) English biochemist, formerly Professor of Biochemistry, University of Oxford and Nobel Prize winner. He was born in Hildesheim, Germany, and studied medicine at Göttingen, Freiburg, Munich and Berlin, graduating from Hamburg in 1925. In 1926 as an assistant at Warburg's department in the Kaiser Wilhelm Institute of Biology in Berlin, he began work on the determination of amino acids. He returned to hospital work in 1930 at Professor Thannhauser's clinic in Freiburg and in 1932 became privatdozent and established the ornithine-arginine cycle in urea metabolism in the liver. A few months later his appointment was terminated due to the Nazis and he migrated to England, where he was invited to work at Cambridge with Sir F. Gowland Hopkins. In 1935 he became lecturer in biochemistry at the University of Sheffield where he elucidated the tricarboxylic acid cycle. He worked in the field of nutritional requirements (vitamins A and C) during the war and in 1945 was appointed Professor of Biochemistry at Sheffield. In 1947 he was elected F.R.S. He won the Nobel Prize in 1953 and was appointed to Oxford in 1954.

K. Henseleit (1907–) German physician.

KREZSIG SIGN

v. HEIM-KREZSIG SIGN

KRUKENBERG TUMOR

Bilateral ovarian carcinoma, commonly used to denote ovarian secondaries from a gastric carcinoma.

Friedrich E. Krukenberg (1871–1946) German pathologist who was born in Halle, Germany. He studied medicine at Halle and Marburg and for a while was an assistant to the physiologist Axenfeld. His father was a judge and his brother was a well known orthopedic surgeon.

KUFS DISEASE

Late onset juvenile amaurotic familial idiocy.

Hugo Kufs (1871–1955) German neurologist. He was born near Leipzig and graduated in medicine from the University there. He spent a short time in the City Hospital in Chemnitz and then entered the state service of the Saxon Mental Institutes, Sonnenstein, Hockweitzschen and Hubertusburg. He initiated there work in histopathology of the nervous system and wrote an excellent paper on tuberose sclerosis in 1913 which resulted in his appointment as Prosector in the Leipzig-Dösen Institution in 1919, where he was given a newly established laboratory. He became a Professor in 1925 and worked there until he retired in 1936. He continued in the Clinic for Nervous Diseases in Leipzig and in 1943 his home was destroyed during its bombardment. Following the Second World War he had to spend 2½ years in Naumburg but in 1946 returned to work in Leipzig, where he remained active until 1954. His investigations covered most aspects of neuropathology and he made a number of contributions, particularly in the areas of Niemann-Picks disease (*v. infra*), Alzheimer's disease (*v. supra*) and Hippel-Lindau disease (*v. supra*).

KUGELBERG-WELANDER SYNDROME

Juvenile spinal muscular atrophy or chronic proximal muscular atrophy commencing in the lower limbs. It is usually autosomal recessive, but some families with autosomal dominant inheritance have been described. Some families also have Werdnig-Hoffman disease (*v. infra*) and so the conditions may be related.

Eric Kugelberg (1913–1983) Swedish neurologist. He was born in Stockholm and studied medicine at the Karolinska Institute. He was appointed the first Professor of Neurophysiology there in 1948 and in 1954 became Chairman of Neurology.

Lisa Welander (1909–) Swedish neurologist.

KULTSCHITZKY (KULCHITSKY) CARCINOMA

Carcinoid tumor.

KULTSCHITZKY CELLS

Argentaffin cells between the crypts of Lieberkühn (*v. infra*) in the intestinal mucosa.

KULTSCHITZKY K CELL

Neural crest cells from which small cell (oat cell) carcinoma of the lung is believed to be derived.

Nicolai Kultschitzky (1856–1925) Russian histologist. He was born at Kronstadt and studied medicine at the University of Kharkov in 1879. He was appointed Professor of Histology at the University of Kharkov in 1893 and resigned in 1910 because he felt a younger person should be given an opportunity. In 1912 he was appointed to the Ministry of Irrigation and in 1912 a representative of the Ministry of Education in Kasan. In 1914 he was appointed to the same position in St. Petersburg where he became known to the Czar who in 1915 appointed him as a Senator and in 1916 made him Minister of Education which post he held at the time of the 1917 revolution. He was imprisoned at that time, but, unlike his fellow ministers, he was allowed to return to his home at Kharkov and there commenced to earn his living by manufacturing soap. In the days when he first commenced studying histology, one had to use soap for embedding tissues and the first technique to be learnt was how to make soap. He walked his family all the way from Kharkov to Sebastopol and escaped in 1918. He finally migrated to London where he arrived without any money in 1921 and was appointed to the Anatomy Department of University College as a lecturer in histology and there he commenced his studies on nerve endings in muscle. He greatly influenced the brilliant young Australian investigator, John I. Hunter, and dedicated his last paper on nerve endings in lizard muscles to the memory of his young friend who died so early in life. He was one of the pioneers of neuropathology and wrote an important textbook on histology and microscopical techniques, as well as inventing modifications of staining techniques which were widely used in their day. A very modest and painstaking investigator, he used to say "Young men can afford to make mistakes, they have time to correct them, but that is not possible for me".

KÜMMELL DISEASE

Compression fracture of the vertebra giving traumatic spondylitis.

Hermann Kümmell (1857–1937) Born in Corbach he graduated in medicine in 1875 and worked as a surgeon from 1883 at the Hamburg-Eppendorf Hospital. He wrote on all areas of surgery and was an early advocate of appendicectomy for acute appendicitis. With E. Schiffle he used X-rays to successfully treat skin lupus. When Hamburg University was established he was made its first Professor of Surgery.

KÜNTSCHNER NAIL

Stainless steel rod used for intramedullary fixation of fractures of the femur and tibia.

Gerhard Küntschner (1902–1972) German surgeon. He studied at Würzburg, Hamburg and graduated from Jena in 1926. Initially he trained in radiology but changed to surgery and became Professor at Kiel in 1942. In World War II he was on the Eastern front and the use of his nail resulted in an earlier return to active service in some but complications through infection in many. After the war he became Medical Director of the Hafer hospital in Hamburg and on retiring spent some time in Spain.

KUPFFER CELLS

Macrophages in the hepatic sinusoids.

Karl W. von Kupffer (1829–1902) German anatomist, born in Lister (Kurland) he went to medical school in Dorpat, graduating there in 1854 and joined the Anatomy Department working with Bidder. In 1865 he moved to Kiel, becoming Professor of Anatomy there in 1867. In 1876 he moved to Königsberg and in 1880 he replaced Bischoff in Munich where he stayed until he retired through ill health in 1899. One of the great anatomists of his day, his work covered fields of histology, zoology, anthropology and ontogeny. Outwardly he was an elegant, dignified and stiff person but in his private circle of friends he displayed a keen sense of humor.

KURU

This is a progressive cerebellar disorder with truncal ataxia which pursues a rapid course with death within 12 months. Towards the end of the disorder there may be extra-pyramidal features and pseudobulbar and bulbar signs as well as frontal lobe dysfunction and sometimes dementia. Death usually results from intercurrent infection or direct pathological involvement of the medulla. This disorder was found in the Fore people in the Okapa district of the Eastern Highlands of Papua New Guinea. It was the first human encephalopathy to be shown to be transmissible and secondary to a slow virus. This work was the basis for the award of the Nobel Prize to Gadjusek. It was a direct result of cannibalism and following the cessation of this practice in 1956, there was a progressivc decrease in the disorder's incidence.

Kuru is a native word meaning "laughing death".

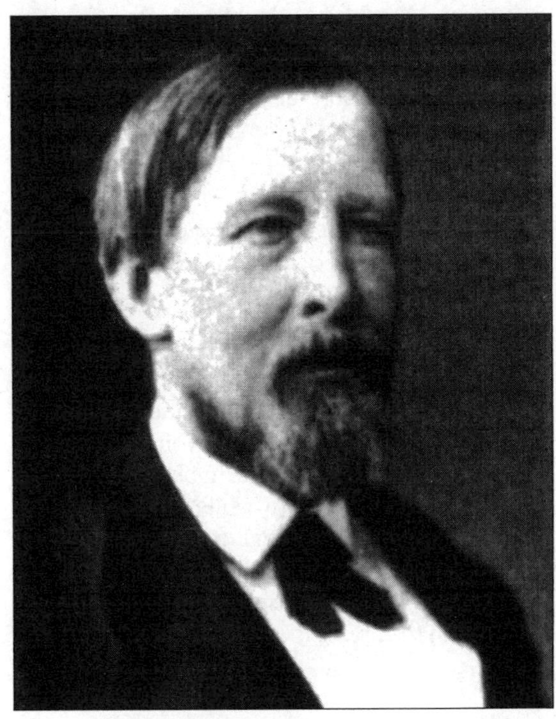

Adolf Kussmaul (Courtesy Bibliothèque Nationale et Universitaire, Strasbourg)

KUSKOKWIN DISEASE

Stiffness and ankylosis of joints in the Yupik Eskimos.

Kuskokwin Town in south-west Alaska.

KUSSMAUL DISEASE

Polyarteritis nodosa.

(Also called KUSSMAUL-MAIER DISEASE)

KUSSMAUL RESPIRATION

Rapid deep respiration seen in diabetic keto-acidosis.

KUSSMAUL SIGN

Paradoxical rise in the jugular venous pressure on inspiration in constrictive pericarditis or chronic obstructive airways disease.

Adolf Kussmaul (1822–1902) German physician who was born near Graben, Karlsruhe, and studied at Heidelberg. After graduating he served 2 years as an Army surgeon, was a general practitioner for some years and then undertook a doctorate at Würzburg. Virchow was lecturing there and this was the reason Kussmaul chose to study at Würzburg where he gained his doctorate in 1855. He was the first to describe periarteritis nodosa and progressive bulbar paralysis and to diagnose mesenteric embolism and to attempt esophagoscopy and gastroscopy. He wrote a book on aphasia which was a landmark in its time. He introduced pleural tapping and gastric lavage. He was always precise and very alert and often complained that none of his colleagues could write good German. He was successively Professor of Medicine at Heidelberg (1857), Erlangen (1859), Freiberg (1859) and Strasburg (1876) and wrote an autobiography.

Rudolf Maier (1824–1888) German physician.

KVEIM ANTIGEN

Lymph node extract from patients with sarcoidosis.

KVEIM TEST

Intradermal injection of Kveim antigen which results in formation of a granuloma in patients with sarcoidosis.

Morten A. Kveim (1892–) Norwegian pathologist.

KWASHIORKOR

Protein malnutrition. The child is often 1½–2 years and is apathetic, with skin lesions which may resemble pellagra with a reddish hue in blacks. Their hair is fine and may be red to white. Kwashiorkor is Ghanian and has been said to mean "displaced child" or "the disease the child gets when the next baby is born" or "the disease suffered by a child displaced from the breast" or "the red or brown boy".

KYRLE DISEASE

Disease of hair follicles due to keratin plugs. Hyperkeratosis follicularis.

Joseph Kyrle (1880–1926) Austrian dermatologist, born in Schärding, Austria, the son of a chemist. He graduated from medical school in Graz in 1904 and entered the Pathology Institute in Vienna under the direction of Professor Weichelbaum in 1905. Two years later he became assistant in Finger's clinic. In 1917 he was offered the Chair of Dermatology in Basel, but he did not accept it and in 1918 he became Associate Professor of Dermatology and Syphilis in Vienna. He again was invited to go to Basel in 1922, but once more refused the offer. He was a very fine lecturer and was particularly kindly and helpful to young colleagues. His ambition to become Professor of Dermatology in Vienna was never realized when he died of a hypernephroma.

L

LAEHR-HENNEBERG HARD PALATE REFLEX

Tickling of the hard palate results in contraction of the orbicularis oris and lowering of the upper lip in pseudo bulbar palsy.

H.H. Laehr (1820–1905) Editor of Allgemeine Zeitschrift für Psychiatrie. He wrote a detailed history of psychiatry and compiled a list of asylums in German countries of his time.

R. Henneberg German neurologist, worked with Bielschowsky in Berlin.

LAENNEC CIRRHOSIS

Micronodular cirrhosis most commonly associated with heavy alcoholic intake.

René T.H. Laennec (1781–1826) French physician. He was inventor of the stethoscope and modern auscultatory techniques. Born in Quimper, Brittany, the son of a lawyer, who was also a poet of little note, Laennec went to live with his uncle after his mother died when he was six. His uncle was a physician in Nantes and at the age of fourteen Laennec commenced an apprenticeship in medicine with him. He served in the Civil War as a regimental sergeant and as a surgeon. In 1801 he went to Paris and studied under Corvisart, Napoleon's favourite physician, who revived percussion. Laennec graduated in 1804 and became an assistant, with his friend Bayle, to Dupuytren (*v. supra*). He trained as an anatomical pathologist, and published a number of papers including one with Bayle on tuberculosis. He was the first to describe the sub-deltoid bursa and studied the fibrous capsule of the liver and he gave a clear clinical and anatomical description of peritonitis.

He was a physician at Beaujon (1806) and in 1814 at the Salpêtrière, then a military hospital, and Chief of Services at the Hôpital Necker (1816). In 1816 he invented and named the stethoscope (Greek for examining the chest). He got the idea from some children playing near the Louvre who applied their ears to two ends of long pieces of wood to listen to the transmission of sounds of pin scratches etc. The following day he rolled up a piece of paper, tying it with some string, and applied it to a patient's heart. He next made an instrument out of a wooden cylinder 30 cm long (he was an expert carpenter). He wrote two books which were masterpieces of description of diseases of the chest and heart, although the section on the heart in both books was not nearly as significant as that of the chest because so little of the physiology of the heart was understood at the time (Laennec attributed the 2nd sound to auricular function after the closure of the pulmonary and aortic valves).

His studies on tuberculosis were monumental. He first recognized the unity of this condition which had previously been thought to be a number of different diseases. He wrote the first descriptions of bronchiectasis and cirrhosis, and classified pulmonary conditions. He introduced many terms still used today; for example, pectoriloquy, rales and aegophony, and described bronchial and vesicular breathing. In short, he perfected the art of physical examination of the chest. Ill health (tuberculosis) caused him to retire to Kerlouarnec in Brittany. After two years he returned to Paris where he became Professor at the College de France and Head of the Medical Clinic at the Charité, but he became ill again, and again retired to Brittany, where he died. He was a quiet and modest man who was a superb clinician and whose teachings remain a corner-stone of modern medical training and practice.

LAFORA DISEASE

Progressive familial myoclonic epilepsy. An autosomal recessive disorder characterized by fits, mental deterioration and dementia starting in the second decade. Autopsy reveals Lafora bodies most frequently in the dentate nucleus and the basal ganglia. The bodies are fibrillar deposits of polyglucosan in the endoplasmic reticulum.

G. Rodriquez Lafora (1887–) Spanish physician, who was a pupil of Cajal.

LAMBERT-EATON SYNDROME

Myasthenic syndrome commonly associated with an underlying malignancy, in particular carcinoma of the lung, characterized by proximal weakness, often paresthesiae, and sensory neuropathy, and absent tendon reflexes which can be made to appear after contracting the muscles against pressure.

Edward H. Lambert (1915–) U.S. neurophysiologist at the Mayo Clinic. He graduated M.D. from the University of Illinois in 1939 and Ph.D. in physiology in 1944. Most of his career has been spent at the Mayo Clinic where he founded the Electromyography Laboratory in 1947 and became Professor of Physiology at the Mayo Graduate School, University of Minnesota, in 1958. He moved to the University of Minnesota in 1985, where he is Professor of Physiology. During the 2nd World War he collaborated in the development of the G suit to prevent blackouts in fliers. In 1956 Eaton approached him to measure the reflexes in myxedema and this led to his interest in the neuromuscular system. Whilst investigating a series of patients with myasthenia he noted a group of patients who were distinctive on electromyography in that stimulation at frequencies higher than 10 Hz or voluntary exercise for a brief period markedly facilitated their response so that the evoked action potential became normal in amplitude unlike that seen in classical myasthenia. Over the years he has made a number of contributions to electromyography and introduced the resistant wire strain gauge manometer to measure intra-arterial pressure which, combined with cardiac catheterization, was an important step towards the development of open heart surgery.

Lee M. Eaton (1905–1958) U.S. neurologist, Mayo Clinic. Born in Owineco, Illinois, graduated M.D. University of Chicago in 1932 and went to the Mayo Clinic in 1933 as a fellow, becoming Professor there in 1950. His major research was in neuromuscular disease, especially myasthenia gravis and polymyositis.

LAMBLIA

Giardia (*v. supra*).

LAMBLIASIS

Giardiasis.

Wilhelm D. Lambl (1824–1895) Bohemian physician. He was born in Kharkou but practiced in Prague. He described warty-like lesion on the mitral and aortic valves possibly due to microthrombi or mucoid degeneration. These were termed "Lambl excrescences".

LANCEFIELD GROUPS

A classification of *Streptococcus*.

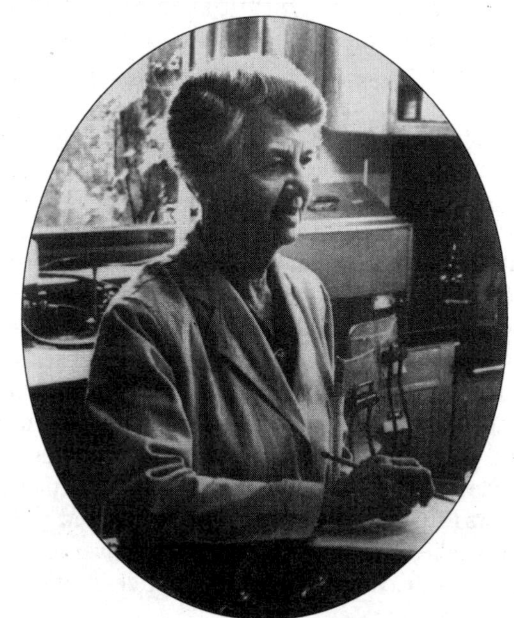

Rebecca C. Lancefield
(Courtesy of E. Scholze, New York)

Rebecca C. Lancefield (1895–1981) U.S. bacteriologist who was born at Fort Wadsworth, New York, and gained her Ph.D. in immunology and bacteriology at Columbia University in 1925. She worked as a technical assistant at the Rockefeller Institute from 1918–19, was an instructor in bacteriology at the University of Oregon until 1922 and then returned to the Rockefeller Institute where she became a Professor of Microbiology in 1958–65. She worked for most of her life on various aspects of the *Streptococcus*.

LANCEREAUX DIABETES

Diabetes mellitus and extreme emaciation.

LANCEREAUX LAW

Marantic thrombosis occurs at sites of maximal stasis.

Étienne Lancereaux (1829–1910) French physician, born in Brécy-Brières in the Ardennes of poor means, he was admitted as an intern in 1857 and hospital physician in 1869, and Agrégé in 1872. He made a number of original observations based on autopsy studies related to symptoms and clinical observations he made during the patient's life. He was a student of Claude Bernard and published important works on cerebral thrombosis and embolism and on meningeal hemorrhage, but his most important contribution was the linking of diseases of the pancreas with diabetes. He explained important clinical features of the onset of diabetes such as weight loss, intense thirst and craving for food, and its rapid course as being associated with inadequacy or destruction of the pancreas, a view proven by von Hering and Minkowski. He wrote extensively on toxins and diseases of liver, and gout. He attributed cirrhosis to a specific toxin, believed that it occurred only in wine drinkers and suggested it was potassium bisulphate rather than alcohol. He published a number of books and monographs, including an atlas of pathology, a book on syphilis and a series of clinical lectures. He died after a short illness with pneumonia.

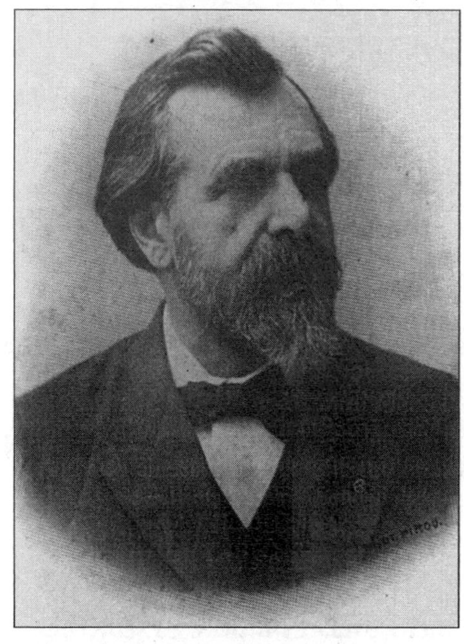

Étienne Lancereaux (Courtesy of the Royal Society of Medicine, London, UK)

LANCISI SIGN

'V' wave in the jugular venous pulse with tricuspid incompetence.

Giovanni M. Lancisi (1654–1720) Italian physician to a number of Popes including Clement XI who gave him the works of Eustachius (*v. supra*) made in copper plates in 1522 and forgotten in the Vatican library, which he edited and published in 1714. He was a notable epidemiologist and described epidemics of influenza and of malaria in 1690–5 and 1715, and was the first to suggest that malaria was transmitted by the mosquito and proposed the drainage of marshy regions to control it. He first described vegetations on cardiac valves and cardiac syphilis, wrote on cardiac disease and aneurysms, and set out a classification of cardiac disease.

LANDAU REFLEX OR RESPONSE

When a baby is held in the air, face facing the floor, with the examiner's hands around the chest, his head and back normally extend slightly. In hypertonia, this is exaggerated, and in hypotonia the baby drops itself around the examiner's hands.

A. Landau German pediatrician who described the test in 1923.

LANDIS-GIBBON TEST

If one heats the opposite hand or foot vasodilatation will occur in the other limb if there is vasospasm but not if there is obliterative vascular disease.

Eugene M. Landis (1901–) U.S. physiologist who introduced the direct measurement of capillary pressure.

John H. Gibbon (1903–) U.S. surgeon, inventor of the heart-lung machine in 1939 and first to use it in open heart surgery in 1954 in Philadelphia.

LANDOLT RING

Incomplete circle used to test visual acuity.

Edmund Landolt (1846–1926) French ophthalmologist who wrote an important text on the subject. Born in Aarau, son of a Swiss minister, his graduating thesis was on the anatomy of the retina and he became Horner's first assistant. At the outbreak of the Franco-Prussian War he joined the Swiss Ambulance and accompanied the ill-fated army of Bourbaki and caught typhoid fever while looking after the French soldiers interned in Switzerland. After the war, at Horner's insistence, he embarked on several years study in Italy, France, England, the United States and Germany. He was an expert linguist and worked with Sichel, Helmholtz, Knapp and Graefe. The two he admired most were Horner (*v. supra*) and Snellen of Utrecht.

He came to Paris in 1874 and established himself as a brilliant ophthalmic surgeon and superb teacher, attracting French students as well as trainees from Germany, England and the U.S.A. and teaching them in their native tongue. He invented or perfected many instruments and developed many operative techniques for cataracts, strabismus, as well as contributing to the basic physiology of visual acuity, refraction and accommodation. He was co-author with L. de Wecker of a 4 volume textbook of ophthalmology (1880–9)

He was one of the founders of the Archives d'ophthalmologie and contributed more than 400 papers to the literature. He died in cardio-renal failure with edema and pulmonary effusions.

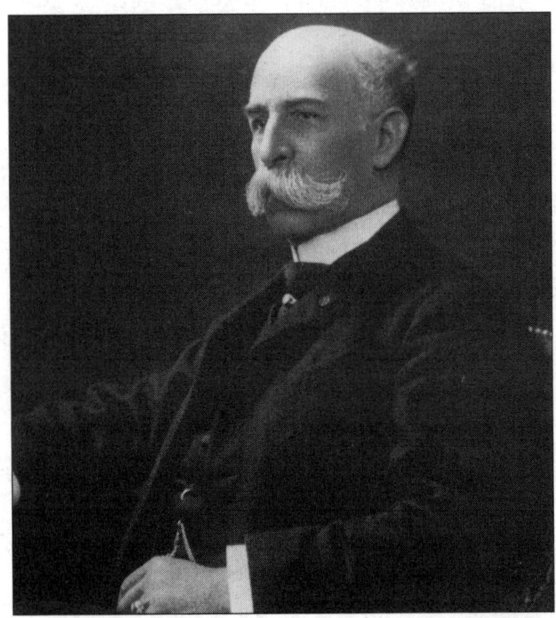

Edmund Landolt (Courtesy of the Royal Society of Medicine, London, UK)

LANDOUZY DISEASE

Leptospirosis.

Purpura.

LANDOUZY-DEJERINE DYSTROPHY

v. DEJERINE-LANDOUZY DYSTROPHY

Louis T.J. Landouzy

v. DEJERINE-LANDOUZY DYSTROPHY.

J.J. Dejerine (*v. supra*)

LANDRY-GUILLAIN-BARRÉ SYNDROME

v. GUILLAIN-BARRÉ SYNDROME

Jean B.O. Landry de Thézillat (1826–1865) French physician. He was born in Limoges and had an uncle who was a psychiatrist and neurologist. When 24 he was Externe des Hôpitaux in Paris. He volunteered to help in a cholera epidemic in L'Oise and a medal was made for him by the grateful population. In 1852 he interned with Sandras and Gubler at l'Hôtel Dieu and Hôpital Beaujon and whilst an intern he proposed that both active and passive muscle movements required afferent impulses. He wrote a description of posterior column ataxia independently of, but 4 years later than, Romberg. He described ascending paralysis in 1859 (Kussmaul also reported two patients in that year), and included in his description three manifestations: (1) ascending paralysis without sensory signs or symptoms; (2) ascending paralysis with concomitant anesthesia and analgesia; and (3) a progressive generalized disorder with paralysis and sensory signs. His name became attached to the ascending form only. This was his last contribution. In 1857 he married Claire Giustigniani, a lady of great beauty and social standing, but little money. When his father died he also had to look after the other members of his family. He therefore moved to a spa at Auteuil and there he made an excellent living. He was a generous and modest man, who was a distinguished musician and accomplished singer. He was also an expert dancer and a favorite of the salons, and his portrait was painted by E. Corbet in 1864. He was a fine horseman, hunter and alpinist and was interested in geology and crystals. He went to give aid to a cholera epidemic in the Paris suburbs in 1865, contracted the disease and died shortly after with Charcot in attendance.

LANDSTEINER CLASSIFICATION

Major blood groups system A, B, O and AB.

Karl Landsteiner (1868–1943) U.S. pathologist and founder of serology. He introduced blood grouping techniques by hemagglutination. Born in Vienna, he graduated in 1891 and then studied chemistry with Emil Fischer, returning to Vienna to become an assistant in an Institute of Pathology in 1898. In 1900 he discovered isoagglutinins in human blood and demonstrated specific blood groups the following year, which established safe techniques for blood transfusions. He introduced dark field illumination to identify spirochetes in 1906. In 1909 with Popper he demonstrated transmission of poliomyelitis to monkeys by intraspinal injection. After World War I he went to the Hague and then in 1922 to the Rockefeller Institute. He developed techniques for coupling simple compounds to proteins and demonstrated antibody specificity to chemical structure of the antigen. In 1927 he discovered the M and N systems and in 1940 with A.S. Wiener the Rh (Rhesus) factor. He developed techniques in animals using simple chemical compounds to study contact dermatitis, and drug allergies. He won the Nobel Prize in 1930. In his laboratory he was authoritarian and energetic but outside he was diffident and shy. When he spoke to an audience he was stimulating and brief. He was a fine pianist. He died of a coronary thrombosis at work in his laboratory at the Rockefeller Institute.

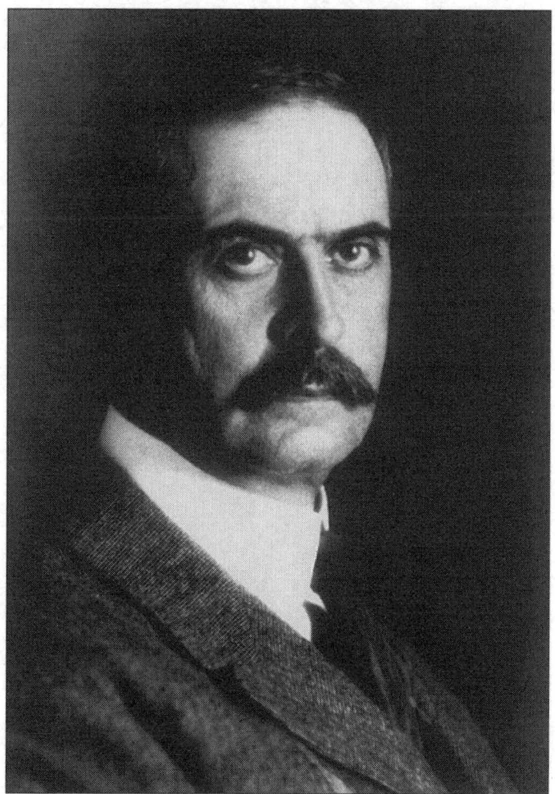

Karl Landsteiner (Courtesy of the Royal Society of Medicine, London, UK)

LANGENDORF PREPARATIONS

Isolated heart perfused with oxygenated Ringer or equivalent solution.

Oskar Langendorf (1853–1909) German physiologist. Originally from Breslau (Wroclaw), he was an assistant with Wittich and then Herman at Königsberg and in 1890 succeeded H. Aubertat at the University of Rostock. He studied the location and function of the respiratory center as well as the function of ganglia in nerve transmission and digestion, but won world wide recognition for his studies on the isolated heart.

LANGER LINES

Cleavage lines of the skin.

Carl von Langer (1819–1887) Austrian anatomist. He was born in Vienna, but went to school in Pilsen and Prague and studied medicine at Prague, where he was influenced particularly by Hyrtl. He moved from Prague university to Vienna and following his graduation there became assistant to the Professor of Anatomy at the time, Berres. When the latter died in 1844, Hyrtl was appointed to his Chair, and Langer became his assistant. He studied the development of the mammary gland and comparative anatomy. In 1853 he moved to the University of Pest to become Professor of Zoology and there studied the vascular system of some invertebrates. In 1856 he was appointed to the Imperial Josephsakademie in Vienna as Professor of Human Anatomy and stayed there until 1869 when the Academy was dissolved. Here he published on the structure and function of joints and wrote a textbook on systematic and topographical anatomy. His investigations on cleavage lines commenced when he observed that if he punched circular holes in the skin of cadavers they became elliptical. He was then appointed to a second chair of Anatomy in Vienna where he taught with Hyrtl. From 1871–74 he was Dean of the Medical Faculty and in 1875 was appointed Rector (Vice-Chancellor). When Rokitansky died he was appointed referee of the Minister of Education.

LANGERHANS ADENOMA

Insulinoma.

LANGERHANS CELLS

These cells of the epidermis are concerned with immune response and are involved in contact dermatitis and process antigen and move into the lymphatics. The dendritic aurophilic Langerhans cell sometimes contains structures called Langerhans granules which are tubulo-vesicular structures with characteristic periodicity on electron microscopy. The function of the granules is unknown.

LANGERHANS, ISLET OF

Cells in pancreas producing insulin.

Paul Langerhans (1847–1888) German pathologist and biologist. In 1868 using the technique taught to him by Cohnheim, he stained a sample of human skin with gold chloride and described the dendritic cells in the skin which now bear his name and

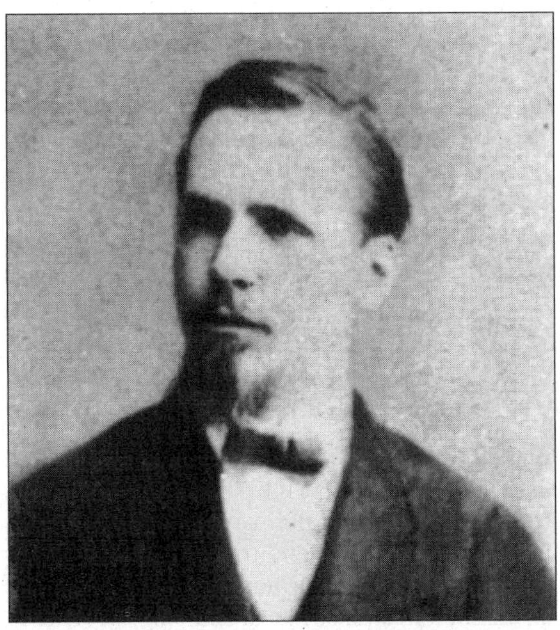

Paul Langerhans (Courtesy of the Royal Society of Medicine, London, UK)

which from their morphology he believed to be nerve cells. It was during his studies for his doctorate at the Berlin Pathological Institute that he made his second important contribution (1869), the description of the islet cells of the pancreas.

He travelled to the Middle East and served as a physician during the Franco-Prussian War and in 1871 was made Prosector in Pathology in Freiburg and later became a full professor. He published a number of papers in Virchow's archives but moved to Madeira because of pulmonary tuberculosis. During his stay in Madeira he became interested in the marine fauna off the Portuguese coast and made important observations on the classification of invertebrates. He proposed the name Virchowia for one of the four new genera of worms which he described to honor his former teacher and friend, and he gave a lecture to the Royal Academy in Berlin on these topics in 1887. He had initially studied at Jena where he fell under the spell of Ernst Haeckel, one of the great zoologists of his day. Thus Langerhans' name will always be linked with both medicine and zoology.

He died following an infection and renal disease, and was buried in Madeira in the cemetery of the English church.

LANGHANS GIANT CELL

Multinucleated foreign body giant cell.

Theodor Langhans (1839–1915) German pathologist and anatomist born in Usingen. He studied medicine at Göttingen, Berlin and Würzburg and worked in Switzerland. He described the cytotrophoblastic layer in the chorionic villi. In 1867 he described the giant cells in tuberculosis.

LARON DWARFISM

These dwarfs lack the receptor for growth hormone on their cell membranes. As a result their phenotype is similar to pituitary dwarfs but they have normal levels of growth hormone. Inherited as an autosomal recessive.

Zevi Laron (1927–) Israeli pediatrician and endocrinologist. He was born in Cernauti, Romania. After the Second World War he commenced medical studies at Timiswara in Romania but transferred to the Hadassah Hebrew University in Jerusalem graduating M.D. in 1954. He studied pediatrics at the University of Pittsburgh and later Harvard before returning to Israel where he became the Director of an Institute of Paediatric and Adolescent Endocrinology in 1958 and described his syndrome in 1960. He became Professor of Paediatrics at Tel Aviv University in 1971.

LARREY SIGN

Pain in the sacroiliac region when the patient sits down suddenly on a hard seat. Sign of sacroileitis.

Dominique J. Larrey (1766–1842) French surgeon. Larrey was born in Bordeaux and trained initially with his uncle, Alexis Larrey of Toulouse. He next studied in Paris with Louis and Desault, the latter teaching him the principles of wound debridement. He then joined the Navy for a brief period, visiting Newfoundland as a surgeon of a man-of-war, returning to Paris to enter the College de Chirurgie. In 1792 he joined the army of the Rhine, took part in all of Napoleon's campaigns, and was at the latter's side at Waterloo at the end of which he was captured and sentenced to death. Fortunately a Prussian surgeon recognized him, having attended a lecture of his 6 years previously, and he was later released at Blucher's instigation since he had saved the life of Blucher's son in Austria.

He invented the flying ambulances for attending and collecting wounded on the battlefields, and became Professor at the École de Médecine Militaire at Val-de-Grâce. He introduced the concept of taking the hospital to the wounded and giving first aid on the battlefield – three times wounded, he performed 200 amputations in 24 hours at Borodino. He was the first to describe trench foot, to observe that Egyptian ophthalmia (trachoma) was contagious, and to amputate at the hip. He considered trephining essential in depressed fractures of the skull and advocated removal of foreign bodies near wounds of the skull or those that were quite distant if they could be located by a probe or gum elastic catheter. He observed that injury to the brain caused contralateral paralysis, loss of memory and aphasia, and that paresis due to a cerebellar lesion was homolateral and sometimes associated with respiratory failure (syncope). He noted Jacksonian epilepsy which in one case was cured by operation and in another due to an abscess over a carious tooth which could be precipitated by pressure.

He was admired by all for his humanity and humor and Napoleon left 100 000 francs in his will to Larrey, describing him as "C'est l'homme le plus vertueux que j'ai connu".

LARSEN SYNDROME

Short stature with "double jointedness" and congenital dislocation of elbows, hips and knees, with a flat facies, depressed nasal bridge and shortened fingers. A mild form is inherited as an autosomal dominant and a more severe one as a recessive.

Loren Larsen (1914–) U.S. orthopedic surgeon who was born in Idaho and studied medicine in Chicago graduating from the Rush Medical College in 1941. He trained in orthopedics in San Francisco where he became Surgeon-in-Chief at the Shriners' Hospital for Crippled Children in 1968 until his retirement in 1980.

LARSEN-JOHANSSON DISEASE

(Also called SINDING-LARSEN DISEASE)

Osteochondrosis involving apex of patella.

Christian M.F. Sinding-Larsen (1866–1930) Norwegian surgeon.

Sven Johansson (1880–) Swedish surgeon.

LASÈGUE SIGN

Straight leg raising sign which is elicited with the patient supine, the leg is kept straight at the knee and flexed at the hip, passively. When the foot is slowly lifted only a few centimeters there is pain at the level of the sciatic notch. The leg is lowered, and the hip again passively flexed, but with flexion of the knee at the same time. The thigh can be flexed without any pain at all. A positive result suggests a neural lesion.

Ernest C. Lasègue (1816–1883) French physician. Born in Paris and shared rooms with Claude Bernard in the Latin Quarter where they were often short of money to pay the rent, since they had spent it on buying experimental animals to study. He initially wanted to study philosophy but hearing a lecture by Trousseau at the Hôpital Necker changed to medicine and became Trousseau's favorite pupil and close associate. He obtained his M.D. in 1847 and was sent by the French government to investigate a cholera epidemic in South Russia. He was physician at the Salpêtrière, Pitié and Necker hospitals and was Trousseau's Chef de Clinique from 1852–54.

He was interested in psychosomatic disease and studied hysteria, malingering, dipsomania, paranoia (Lasègue disease), catalepsy, exhibitionism and described folie à deux. He made one of the earliest descriptions of cerebro-vascular accidents and emphasized that once one had occurred the patient was predisposed to recurrence.

He had a celebrated exchange with Virchow, saying of Virchow's Cellular Pathologie (1858) that disease of the cells was only a fragment of pathology. Virchow replied that the only critics he worried about were competent ones and that thus far he had not heard from them. Lasègue's retort was that innovators like Virchow were like knights who feel they are fastest in the saddle because they have sharp spurs. He enjoyed classical music, and is said to have thought of his sign while trying to answer a question posed by the Inspector-General Dujardin-Baumetz on how to discover a malingerer who was simulating sciatica and noted that his son-in-law was tuning a violin, and compared the sciatic nerve with a violin string, but on the stretch. He was an extremely witty man who took great pains in understanding his patients and their history. He died of diabetes.

LASSA FEVER

Pyrexia, myalgia, purpura, pneumonia, with cardiac and renal involvement with 10% incidence of VIIIth nerve damage, due to viral infection which is carried by rodents.

Lassa, Africa.

LASSAR PASTE

Starch, zinc oxide and acetylsalicylic acid paste.

Oskar Lassar (1849–1907) German dermatologist in Berlin who advocated public baths for people who were poor in large cities. Born in Hamburg, he studied at Heidelberg, Göttingen, Strasburg and Berlin, and received his M.D. in Würzburg in 1872. He worked for some years in physiology and pathology before becoming one of Germany's best known dermatologists. He died in a motor car accident.

LAURENCE-MOON (BIEDL-BARDET) SYNDROME

Retinitis pigmentosa, obesity, hypogonadotrophism, hypogonadism, polydactyly and mental deficiency, probably recessive inheritance.

John Z. Laurence (1830–1874) English ophthalmologist. He graduated from University College, London in 1854 and studied surgery. He went to Utrecht to learn refraction technique and widely promoted the use of the ophthalmoscope in England. He was the founder of the Royal Eye Hospital and founder and editor of Ophthalmic Review, the first English journal devoted to ophthalmology.

Arthur Biedl (1869–1933) Born in Hungary, he studied medicine in Vienna graduating in 1892. He trained in experimental pathology in Vienna and was one of the pioneers in endocrine investigation. In 1913 he was appointed Professor of Experimental Pathology at the University of Prague.

Robert C. Moon (1844–1914) English ophthalmologist who was born in Brighton, England and as a youth helped his father who was blind, to develop a print (Moon type) to help people with diminished vision to read. After graduation Robert joined John Laurence and wrote a book on ophthalmology with him as well as reporting this syndrome. In 1879 he migrated to the U.S.A. and practiced in Philadelphia where he instigated the Moon Press for the blind.

Georges Bardet (1885–) French physician.

LAVERAN BODIES

Malarial parasites in red cells.

Charles L.A.A. Laveran (1845–1922) French physician, born in Paris, son of an army surgeon, who graduated from Strasburg in 1867. He served in the Franco-Prussian War and while an army surgeon in Algeria in 1880 discovered the malarial parasites and described them in red cells, although his initial discovery was met with much scepticism. He demonstrated the parasites to a number of Italian scientists 2 years later. In 1891 he was appointed Professor of Military Hygiene at Val-de-Grace where his father had been Director, but by 1895 he was moved to a purely administrative position in Lille and Nantes because his independence had offended some of the politicians. He resigned the service in 1895 and joined the Pasteur Institute initially on a volunteer basis. He won the Nobel Prize in 1907. He wrote on military medicine, hygiene and trypanosomes and other parasites.

LEBER DISEASE OR OPTIC ATROPHY

Sex linked recessive optic atrophy usually of acute onset in young males with loss of central vision.

Theodor von Leber (1840–1917) German ophthalmologist. He was born in Karlsruhe and graduated in medicine in 1862 and then worked as Knapp's assistant in Heidelberg. After studying physiology in Vienna he went to work for Von Graeffe in Berlin and was appointed Professor of Ophthalmology in Göttingen in 1871. He studied diabetic disorders in the eye and defects of circulation and discovered the excretion of intra-ocular fluid by the ciliary body. He was Professor of Ophthalmology at the University of Heidelberg.

LEDDERHOSE DISEASE

Dupuytren contracture involving the plantar aponeurosis. May be associated with classical Dupuytren contracture or with Peyronie syndrome.

Georg Ledderhose (1855–1925) German surgeon who in 1876 discovered glycosamin whilst working on cartilage with F. Hoppe-Seyler in Strasburg.

LEDERER ACUTE ANEMIA

Acute hemolytic anemia with rapid onset and recovery in children.

Max Lederer (1855–1952) U.S. pathologist.

LEE AND WHITE METHOD

Whole blood clotting time method.

Roger I. Lee U.S physician, Massachusetts General Hospital.

Paul D. White

v. BLAND-WHITE-GARLAND SYNDROME

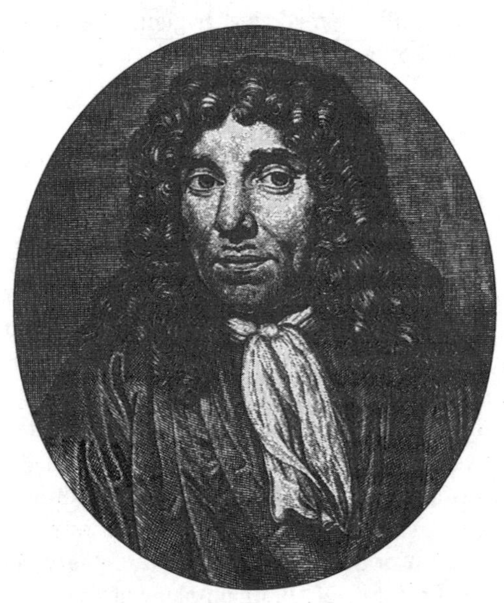

Anthony van Leeuwenhoek (Courtesy of the Royal Society of Medicine, London, UK)

LEEUWENHOEK DISEASE

Respiratory myoclonus – this results in shortness of breath and epigastric pulsations. Hiccups (singultus) are not heard. Antony van Leeuwenhoek complained of these symptoms in 1723 – cardiac palpitations were diagnosed but he doubted the diagnosis as his arterial pulse was slower and more regular than his epigastric pulsations which he felt were diaphragmatic in origin.

Anthony van Leeuwenhoek (1632–1723) A draper who devoted his spare time to the study of biology and microscopy. He made his own microscopes, grinding the lenses himself and was elected F.R.S. in 1680. He sent 26 microscopes to London as a present to the Royal Society and sent 375 scientific papers to the same body. He was the first to describe spermatozoa, red blood corpuscles, to see protozoa and he described giardia lamblia in his own stools. He reported the striped nature of voluntary muscle, the sarcolemma and the structure of the lens. He was sent specimens from the East India Company and was visited by Peter the Great on his European tour in 1689. He introduced histological staining in 1719 using saffron to examine muscle fibres.

LEGAL DISEASE

Paroxysmal pain and tenderness in the scalp in the region of the auriculo-temporal nerve associated with pharyngitis and otitis.

Emmo Legal (1859–1922) German physician who devised a test for acetonuria (1882).

LEGG-CALVÉ-PERTHES DISEASE

or

LEGG-CALVÉ-PERTHES-WALDENSTRÖM DISEASE OR SYNDROME

or

LEGG-PERTHES DISEASE

Osteochondritis deformans juvenilis – epiphyseal involvement, e.g. hip or tibial tubercle in young children 5–10 years.

Arthur T. Legg (1874–1939) U.S. orthopedic surgeon. He graduated from Harvard Medical School, Boston, in 1900 and when he was a junior assistant surgeon at Children's Hospital in Boston he described the disorder named after him in an article entitled "An obscure affliction of the hip joint" which was published in 1910. He became an instructor in orthopedic surgery at Harvard from 1917–1931 when he was promoted to assistant Professor of Orthopaedic Surgery. He died of a heart attack at the Harvard Club.

Jacques Calvé (1895–1954) French orthopedic surgeon who described the condition in 1910 whilst working at the Marine Hospital at Berck (*v. supra*).

Georg C. Perthes (1869–1927) German surgeon, Professor of Surgery, Tübingen, who independently described the condition in 1913 and stressed the non-tuberculous nature of the condition (*v. infra*).

Johann H. Waldenström (*v. infra*)

LEGIONNAIRES DISEASE

Epidemic of severe and often fatal pneumonia which occurred following a convention of legionnaires (retired servicemen) in Philadelphia in 1976, due to a Gram negative bacillus.

LEIGH SYNDROME OR DISEASE

Subacute necrotizing encephalomyelopathy. This occurs in infancy or early childhood and results in spasticity, psychomotor repression, seizures and brainstem dysfunction and death. Two biochemical defects not coexistent have been described, one cytochrome oxidase deficiency, the other pyruvate dehydrogenase complex deficiency. Some families show autosomal recessive inheritance pedigrees, others X-linked recessive.

Denis Leigh (1915–   ) English neuropathologist.

LEINER DISEASE

Erythroderma desquamation (generalized seborrheic dermatitis) in infants with severe diarrhea, recurrent local and systemic infection and marked wasting and central nervous system deficiency.

Karl Leiner (1871–1930) An Austrian pediatrician who was educated in Prague and graduated in Vienna in 1898. He immediately commenced his interest in pediatrics and was the assistant for many years with Knopfelmacher. In 1920 he was appointed the director of the Maultner-Markhof Children's Hospital in Vienna. He was the first to use an intracutaneous technique for the vaccination of smallpox and was the first to recognize its relationship to post-vaccinial encephalitis. He investigated poliomyelitis and other viruses and bacteria at the Weichselbaum Institute. He combined the skills of a consultant physician with that of a laboratory worker and scientific investigator. One of his clinical observations was the association of annular erythema in patients with rheumatic fever and endocarditis. He was an entertaining teacher who was equally at home with German and English and described the condition named after him in the British Journal of Children's Diseases in 1908.

LEISHMAN STAIN

Romanovsky type stain for peripheral blood films and bone marrow preparations.

LEISHMANIA BRASILIENSIS

Species of leishmaniasis found in South America.

LEISHMANIA DONOVANI

Protozoa causing leishmaniasis.

LEISHMAN-DONOVAN BODIES

Inclusions of protozoa seen in macrophages in a variety of organs but especially liver and spleen in the disorder Kala azar or leishmaniasis.

Sir William B. Leishman (1865–1926) Scottish pathologist, born in Glasgow, son of the Professor of Obstetrics, graduated in 1886 in Glasgow and joined the Army, serving in India 1890–1897 and seeing active service with the Waziristan expedition. When he returned to England he joined Professor Almroth Wright in the Laboratory and Army Medical School at Netley and played a major role with him in developing an effective anti-typhoid vaccine which was to save many lives in the 1914–18 war. It was at this time that he modified the Romanovsky (*v. infra*) stain to develop his staining technique which is still used in many laboratories and which enabled him to identify the bodies bearing his name in an autopsy examination of a soldier who had contracted the infection at Dum Dum, near Calcutta, and was invalided home to Netley where he died. He succeeded Wright as Professor of Pathology of the Army Medical School in London. He was knighted in 1909, elected F.R.S. in 1910, honorary physician to the King in 1912. He developed a technique for measuring phagocytosis and described the development cycle of the *Spirochaeta duttoni* in the African tick. He was an unassuming man, a fine teacher and an accomplished musician and artist.

Charles Donovan (1863–1951) British physician, student at Trinity College, Dublin, and graduated M.D. in 1899 and in 1901 joined the Indian Medical Service and served on the Northwest Frontier and in the Tirch Expeditionary Force, seeing action at Dargai and in the Baru Valley. He was appointed as Professor of Physiology at the Madras Medical College and became an inspiring teacher there. He retired in 1920. Outspoken and direct, though affectionately regarded by his colleagues and students, he was clearly something of a showman, being the kind of lecturer to enter his class in a black academic gown, accompanied by his assistants. He was a keen butterfly collector and an enthusiastic laboratory worker. A major in the Indian Army Medical Corps, he found the Leishman-Donovan Bodies in a specimen obtained by splenic puncture whilst the patient was still living, in 1903 in Madras. He also independently discovered the cause of granuloma inguinale (Donovanosis).

LENNERT LYMPHOMA

Malignant lymphoma with a major component of epithelioid histiocytes, which is now called lymphoepithelioid cell lymphoma, a special type of low grade T cell lymphoma. It has to be differentiated from other malignant lymphomas which may have a high content of epithelioid cells (e.g. Hodgkin lymphoma, angio-immunoblastic lymphoma, lymphoplasmacytic lymphoma) and some inflammatory lymph node lesions (e.g. Whipple disease). It is usually seen in the elderly, sometimes with involvement of the tonsils, but mostly with generalized lymphadenopathy and splenomegaly.

Karl Lennert (1921–) German histopathologist, born in Furth, Bavaria. He studied medicine in Erlangen (1939–1945) and was attracted to hematology by N. Henning. He joined the department of pathology and studied blood cell morphology comparing smears, imprints and sections stained by hematological techniques, e.g. Giemsa. Later he applied these techniques to lymph nodes and he discovered that he could distinguish epithelioid cells from normal histiocytes by the formers' oxyphilia. This led to the description of Lennert lymphoma in 1952. He became head of pathology in Kiel in 1963 and as a result of his work on lymph nodes he developed with Stein and Kaiserling a classification of lymphomas in 1974 which became known as the Kiel classification. He is a pianist who often acts as an accompanist.

LENNOX SYNDROME

or

LENNOX-GASTAUT SYNDROME

Myoclonic and akinetic seizures in young children often associated with a petit mal type pattern in the electroencephalogram. Usually commences before the age of 6 with sudden drop attacks, tonic fits and head nods ("cornflake fits") and often has a poor prognosis with progressive mental deterioration.

William G. Lennox (1884–1960) U.S. neurologist. He became Associate Professor of Neurology at Harvard University and wrote a definitive two-volume textbook "Epilepsy and Related Disorders".

Henri Gastaut (1915–) French neurobiologist born in Monaco and graduated M.D. University of Marseilles in 1945. His major interests have been the study of electroencephalography and brain function and epilepsy. He was appointed Professor of Anatomical Pathology in 1952 and Director of the Regional Centre for Epileptic Children in 1960.

LENOBLE AND AUBINEAU SYNDROME

Heredofamilial syndrome of congenital nystagmus, with muscle fasciculations spontaneously elicited by cold, tremors of the head and limbs, vasomotor abnormalities and increased reflexes.

E. Lenoble French physician.

Ernest Aubineau (1871–) French physician.

LEPRECHAUNISM

This is a rare congenital condition in which there has usually been intra-uterine growth retardation and at birth there is marked deficiency of subcutaneous fat, phallic enlargement and pachydermia, acanthosis nigricans and hypertrichosis as well as prominent rugae around the mouth and anus. There is a failure to thrive and the patients often have severe recurrent hypoglycemia. The child often does not survive infancy.

Leprechaun A figure in Irish mythology which equates to a fairy but is usually thought of as a dwarf-like individual with elderly and rather distorted visage.

LÉRI DISEASE

Thickening of fingers and toes limiting movement, mongoloid facies and short stature called pleonosteosis.

LÉRI SIGN

Absence of normal elbow flexion following passive flexion of fingers and forcible wrist flexion in spastic hemiplegia.

LÉRI TYPE OF OSTEOPETROSIS

Melorheostosis – candle bone disease – a very rare bone disorder.

André Léri (1875–1930) French physician who worked in Paris. A neurologist, he studied vision and was President of the French Ophthalmological Society.

LERICHE SYNDROME 1

Impotence due to atheromatous involvement or occlusion of the aortic bifurcation often associated with claudication in the buttocks and reduction or absence of the femoral pulses.

LERICHE SYNDROME 2

(Also called SUDECK-LERICHE SYNDROME)
v. SUDECK ATROPHY

René Leriche (1879–1955) French surgeon, son of a Roanne lawyer, initially at Lyons (1920) and in 1924 Professor of Surgery, Strasburg. In 1927 he was elected honorary Fellow of the Royal College of Surgeons in England. He was especially interested in vascular surgery, introduced periarterial sympathectomy; arteriectomy for arterial thrombosis, and wrote on bone disorders, fractures and pain. In 1938 he moved to Paris to become Professeur au College de France, held previously by Laennec, Magendie, Claude Bernard, Brown-Séquard, d'Arsonval and Charles Nicholle and to whose memory he dedicated his book "La Chirurgie de la Doleur".

His home had a fine collection of objets d'art from his patients, one of whom was Matisse. He emphasized the importance of linking physiology and surgery and regarding the patient as a whole rather than concentrating on operative techniques. He himself was a first rate technical surgeon with a great flair for teaching and innovation and this attracted to him people like Wertheim and De Bakey. He was a bon vivant who loved the cuisine and wine of his country. Described as having a Napoleonic figure (he was small, round and lively, and often wore a spotted bow tie), he would arrive to start his clinic before 8, driving at high speed, often on the wrong side of the road, turning round to talk with passengers. He was a superb speaker who never required notes.

LERMANS-MEANS SCRATCH

Rub heard at the left sternal edge in thyrotoxicosis, possibly due to increased blood flow.

J. Lermans (1902–) U.S. physician.

James H. Means (1885–1967) U.S. physician who had a life-long interest in metabolism and wrote on many topics including the effect of drugs on body heat. He was Professor of Medicine at Harvard University and worked at the Massachusetts General Hospital. He was an authority on thyroid disease and together with Robley Evans, a physicist at the Massachusetts Institute of Technology (MIT), introduced radio-labelled iodine as a test for thyroid function. He graduated as an M.D. from Harvard in 1911 and was influenced by Walter Cannon (*v. supra*) and Lawrence Henderson (*v. supra*) but was induced to pursue a career in academic medicine when an intern by David Edsall, then the Professor of Medicine. Means founded the famous Mallin krodt research ward, Ward 4, at the Massachusetts General Hospital, where many famous clinical investigators worked and were trained.

LERMOYEZ SYNDROME

Periods of diminished hearing followed by vertigo after which hearing returns.

Marcel Lermoyez (1858–1929) French otolaryngologist, born in Cambria, the son of a roadway and bridge engineer. He was orphaned when 16. He was tutored by Leblane, a distinguished member of the Institute of Archaeology. He was a brilliant schoolboy and interested in art and music (he wrote an opera), and on graduation he interned with Gouguenheim at the Lareboisière – then the only ear, nose and throat service. He wrote a book "Physiology of the Voice of the Song and the Health of the Singer" in 1885 and followed this with more physiological studies of speech. In 1892 he founded the journal "Annale des Maladies des Oreilles et du Larynx". In 1893 he spent some time with Politzer in Vienna and returned and wrote a book "Otolaryngo-rhinology – the Teaching and Practice of the Faculty of Medicine of Vienna" which contained much of his own experience as well, and which helped found the French School of Otolaryngology. In 1898 he was appointed to St. Antoine and he created an otolaryngology service there. He wrote on most aspects of his speciality. One interesting article was devoted to the bactericidal properties of nasal mucus. He was good surgically and contributed here as well as to the theoretical aspects of his subject. He was extremely productive in all fields until the death of his son, who had followed his father into ear, nose and throat surgery in 1923. After this he withdrew completely and remained depressed until his death. He was probably the most influential force in founding otolaryngology as a speciality in France.

LESCH-NYHAN SYNDROME

Sex-linked recessive deficiency of hypoxanthine-guanine phosphoribosyl transferase. Mental deficiency associated with a striking propensity to self mutilation and hyperuricemia.

Michael Lesch (1939–) U.S. physician, born in New York and graduated M.D. from Johns Hopkins in 1964. Professor of Medicine and Chief of Cardiology, Northwestern University, Chicago, U.S.A.

William L. Nyhan (1926–) U.S. pediatrician at University of California School of Medicine, San Diego.

LESER-TRÉLAT SIGN

Sudden onset of seborrheic dermatosis (senile warts) with malignant tumors. Tumors of the gastrointestinal tract have been the most commonly reported.

Edmund Leser (1828–1916) German surgeon.

Ulysse Trélat (1828–1890) French surgeon.

LETTERER-SIWE DISEASE

Disorder of infancy and early childhood characterized by skin infiltrates, splenomegaly and bone tumors and erosions seen on X-ray. A disorder of histiocytes possibly related to eosinophilic granuloma.

Erich Letterer (1895–) German pathologist who worked in Tübingen.

Sturre A. Siwe (1897–1966) Professor of Paediatrics at Lund, Sweden.

LE VEEN SHUNT

Procedure for relieving ascites by implanting a valved conduit subcutaneously connecting the peritoneal cavity to the great veins.

Harry H. Le Veen (1914–) U.S. gastroenterologist, Veterans Administration Hospital, Brooklyn, N.Y.

LÉVI-LORAIN DWARFISM

(Also called LÉVI SYNDROME and LORAIN-LÉVI SYNDROME)

Pituitary dwarf.

Leopold Lévi (1868–1933) French endocrinologist. Born in the Saint-Antoine district of Paris of modest means, he became a student at L'Hôpital Saint-Antoine and was influenced by Hanot. He then trained in surgery with Marchand at the Hotel Dieu and histopathology especially neurological at Salpêtrière and bacteriology with Roux at the Pasteur Institute. Hanot's clinic held the greatest interest for him, and Levi held Hanot in the highest esteem.

Initially he published on many topics, writing a chapter on therapeutic approaches to liver disease for a book edited by Debove and Achard and on cerebral and pulmonary edema, but he soon returned to studying the endocrine glands and in 1908 wrote a book on the pathophysiology of the thyroid and pituitary, with a preface by Achard. He worked tirelessly on the inter-relationship of the endocrine glands. He worked in the Rothschild Clinic from 1906–1914, and then after the war with Achard at Beaujon and then Cochin and finally at the Institut Prophylactique.

He was a fine clinical investigator and an inspiring teacher – a little deaf, with a faint lisp, but his enthusiastic presentation and friendliness overcame these difficulties.

He had a special interest in ophthalmology especially the effects of the endocrines on the eye. Following a trip to the U.S. he established a medical service for the Paris Transport Agency. He died suddenly 24 hours after developing intestinal obstruction.

Paul J. Lorain (1827–1875) French physician who in a letter prefacing a thesis by F. de la Cour (1871) described idiopathic lack of growth in a child. He was born in Paris but was educated in Lyons. He joined the Faculty of Medicine in Paris in 1860 and won a gold medal for his work in the cholera epidemic in 1866. He was appointed Professor of the History of Medicine in Paris in 1873.

LEVIN TUBE

One of the original tubes used to sample gastric and duodenal contents, usually passed intranasally.

Abraham L. Levin (1880–1940) U.S. physician. He was born in Poland and served in the Russian Army before migrating to the United States and gaining his M.D. at Tulane Medical College in 1907. He became a Captain in the U.S. Medical Corps in the U.S. army in the 1st World War and served as a gastroenterologist at the hospital in Camp Beauregard. He became an Associate Professor in Gastroenterology at Tulane and in 1931 was appointed Clinical Professor at Louisiana State University Medical Center. In 1921 he introduced his duodenal tube and was the author of many articles on gastroenterology.

LEVINE GRADATION OF CARDIAC MURMURS

Six grades – Grade 1 where the murmur is barely audible, Grade 6 so loud it can be heard without the stethoscope.

LEVINE SIGN

In myocardial infarction the patient will often describe the pain by the illustration of clenching his fist.

Samuel A. Levine (1891–1966) U.S. cardiologist. He was born in Lomza, Poland, coming to the U.S.A. with his parents in 1894 and naturalized in 1896. He graduated M.D. from Harvard in 1914. He wrote a well known text book "Clinical Heart Disease". He was Professor of Medicine, Harvard Medical School and physician at the Peter Bent Brigham Hospital, Boston. He was a fine clinician. This applies to so many of the names in this book but this story in a letter to the New Engl. Journal* illustrates an aspect which makes up a shrewd clinician, and the use of experience and thoughtfulness in treating the patient and not the disease. "In the early Spring of 1944, a 50-year-old man was admitted to the Peter Bent Brigham Hospital because of a second myocardial infarction. His course was uneventful. After about two weeks of bed rest, his physician, Dr. Samuel A. Levine, told the intern to let the patient out of bed, begin ambulation and discharge him during the following week. The astonished intern asked Dr. Levine why he was departing from the then usual practice of keeping such a patient hospitalized for six weeks. Dr. Levine pointed out that the patient's professional career – a seasonal one – would be jeopardized if he were not able to begin work very soon. He added that his knowledge of what caused heart attacks and what factors promoted or inhibited recovery was at best uncertain. 'If patients smoke, I tell them to stop. If they don't smoke, I suggest they start. I try to change some factor in their lives, but I'm certainly not sure that six weeks of rest is as important for this artist's future life as letting him get back to his work. Even though that work is physically vigorous'." The patient was Arthur Fiedler, who died in 1979 at the age of 85.

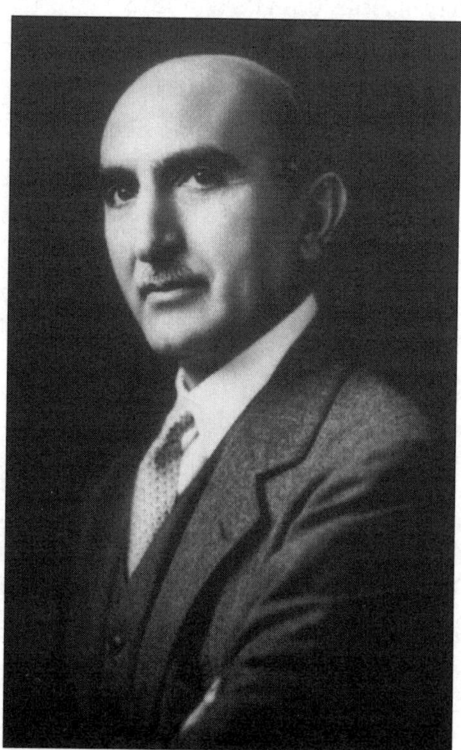

Samuel A. Levine (Courtesy of the Royal Society of Medicine, London, UK)

* J.H. Scheinberg, New Engl. J. Med. 301:668, 1979.

LÉVY-ROUSSY SYNDROME

v. ROUSSY-LÉVY DISEASE

Hereditary spinocerebellar degeneration with lower limb muscular atrophy with loss of deep reflexes and sometimes upgoing toes on examination of the plantar reflex. Cerebellar signs are often mild with truncal ataxia being the most prominent.

Gabrielle Lévy (1886–1934) French neurologist. She worked for a number of years at the Salpêtrière, where she was particularly influenced by Pierre Marie and Charles Foix. She had a particular passion for neuropathology and was helped in the studies by being fluent in a number of languages other than French. She went to work at the Paul-Brousse Hospital at Ville-Juif, under the direction of Lhermitte (*v. infra*). She made a number of important contributions particularly on the late manifestations of sleeping sickness, which formed her inaugural thesis in 1922 and from which she undoubtedly developed her interests in muscle movement and extrapyramidal disorders. She wrote on the role of radiological investigations in neurological problems and worked with Lhermitte on nystagmus. She died suddenly whilst correcting her proofs on her article on hereditary ataxia to which her name is attached.

Gustave Roussy (1874–1948) French pathologist who held many distinguished positions including Professor of Pathology at the Faculté de Médecine de Paris (1926), Director of Institut du Cancer (1930) and Rector of Université de Paris (1937). In 1940 during the German occupation he was dismissed from his posts without reason but reinstated on liberation. He interned with Pierre Marie and Jules Dejerine and from then on studied neurology. He described the thalamic syndrome with Dejerine and showed the syndrome could follow thrombosis of the thalamic branch of the posterior cerebral artery. He undertook pioneer work on the reflex areas of defecation and urination and during the 1st World War wrote an important book with Lhermitte (*v. infra*) on spinal cord injuries. He investigated the hypothalamic and pituitary pathways. He contributed to improvement of social conditions and was an influential teacher.

LEWIS DISEASE

Diminished glycogen storage in the liver due to decreased glycogen synthetase or UDPG-glycogen transglucosidase.

George M. Lewis British pediatrician. He trained in pediatrics at Leeds in England and was influenced by Professor Lathe, Professor of Biochemistry at Leeds University. He was in charge of investigating a pair of identical twins, one of whom was spastic and mentally retarded, and both of whom had fasting hypoglycemia. His investigations suggested a glycogen storage problem and a liver biopsy showed the absence of the enzyme glycogen synthetase. The clinical importance of the finding was the early realization that hypoglycemia in the neonate could occur undiagnosed and the shortage of liver glycogen stores could lead to early brain damage. He is currently Consultant Pediatrician at St. Mary's Hospital in Portsmouth.

LEWIS SYSTEM BLOOD GROUP

Occurs in 22% of population – termed Le^a. Le^a people are non-secretors. It was first recognized in Mrs Lewis.

LEYDEN CRYSTAL

v. CHARCOT-LEYDEN CRYSTALS

LEYDEN-MÖBIUS DYSTROPHY

Muscular dystrophy involving pelvic girdle and thighs with wasting in the legs, onset in childhood and progresses with occasional facial involvement.

Ernst V. von Leyden (1832–1910) German physician born in Danzig (Gdansk) and was a pupil of Schönlein, and Traube. He wrote on tabes and poliomyelitis and established sanatoria for the treatment of tuberculosis. He succeeded Frerichs to the Chair of Medicine in Berlin in 1885 at the Charité. He was asked to treat the Czar Alexander in Prussia in 1899, and he founded the Schrift für klinische Medizin with Frerichs in 1879. He was especially interested in neurology and his lectures greatly influenced L. Edinger. H. Nothnagel was his assistant when he was at Königsberg.

Paul J. Möbius (1853–1907) (*v. infra*).

LEYDIG CELL

Interstitial cell of testis in which androgens are produced.

Franz von Leydig (1821–1908) German histologist, who investigated these cells in 1850 and wrote on cell membrane. Initially of Tübingen, later at Bonn he wrote on neural tissue and his work influenced the great Norwegian zoologist and polar explorer F. Nansen who some believe shared with W. His and A. Forel priority in establishing the anatomical entity of the nerve cell.

LHERMITTE SIGN

Flexion of neck gives electric shock-like sensations in the extremities in disseminated sclerosis (Barber Chair Phenomenon).

LHERMITTE SYNDROME

Anterior internuclear ophthalmoplegia. Nystagmus and paralysis of abduction on looking laterally, characteristically seen in disseminated sclerosis.

Jacques J. Lhermitte (1877–1959) French neurologist and neuro-psychiatrist. Wrote on myoclonus, spinal injuries and Huntington chorea, and internuclear paralysis. Born at Mon-Saint-Père Aisne, the son of an artist. He went to Paris after early education at St. Etienne and graduated in medicine in 1907 and specialized immediately in neurology. He made a special study of spinal injuries during the 1st World War and became interested in neuropsychiatry and published on visual hallucinations of the self. He became Clinical Director at the Salpêtrière. He was one of the great clinical neurologists of his day, with great enthusiasm which infected his younger contemporaries. He was deeply religious and explored the common territory between theology and medicine, and this led to interesting studies on demoniacal possession and stigmatization. He died peacefully in his sleep.

LIBMAN-SACKS ENDOCARDITIS OR DISEASE

Non-infective verrucous endocarditis, classically seen in lupus erythematosus but the lesions are rarely sufficient to cause signs.

Emanuel Libman (1872–1946) U.S. physician, born in New York and physician at Mt. Sinai Hospital, graduated M.D. 1894 from the College of Physicians and Surgeons, Columbia University. Interned at Mt. Sinai and then went overseas to work in Escherich's laboratory and thereafter pursued clinical bacteriology. He returned to Mt. Sinai to his initial appointment as associate pathologist and combined his great talents of clinical observation with his pathology skills and made many basic contributions to sub-acute endocarditis, blood culture and blood stream infections. His pupils included Leo Buerger, A.E. Cohn, A.A. Epstein and others. He became Clinical Professor of Medicine at Columbia University.

Benjamin Sacks (1873–1939) U.S. physician, a pupil of Libman, also wrote on Hindu medicine.

LIDDLE SYNDROME

Familial renal disorder characterized by hypertension, hypokalemic alkalosis and deficient aldosterone secretion, responding to triamterene but not spironolactone or dexamethasone.

Grant W. Liddle (1921–1989) U.S. endocrinologist. Born in American Fork, Utah, a small agricultural community on the road south from Salt Lake City, where the descendants of Mormon pioneers "make the desert bloom like a rose". They held that "the glory of God is intelligence" and gave Liddle a seriousness of purpose which remained with him for life. After majoring in Sociology at the University of Utah, he graduated M.D. from the University of California Medical School in 1948. Initially interested in psychiatry, he changed to that of endocrinology after observing the remarkable response of a female patient with diabetic ketoacidosis following rehydration and insulin overnight. He spent his endocrine fellowship years with Lesley Bennett at the University of California (San Francisco) (UCSF), and with Fred Bartter (*v. supra*) at N.I.H. He was recruited to Vanderbilt Medical School to develop a Division of Endocrinology in 1956 and his meticulous rounds, conducted six days a week, were legendary. Over the next 12 years he unravelled the pathophysiology of Cushing's disease, developed the dexamethasone and metyrapone tests of pituitary-adrenal function and was the first to recognize and describe the secretion of hormones by non-endocrine tumors ("ectopic" ACTH secretion). His major contributions were intellectual and conceptual, perhaps reflecting his pre-medical training and his capacity of intense concentration. The story goes that when his contingent of 20, on evening endocrine rounds, was prevented from crossing the road to the Veterans' Hospital by extremely heavy rain, Liddle strode forward, held a hand aloft, and the rain ceased. His fellows regarded this as more than coincidence! He was Professor and Chairman of Medicine at Vanderbilt and Co-director of the Division of Endocrinology when a car accident in 1983 left him hemiplegic and aphasic.

LIEBERKÜHN GLANDS

Intestinal glands.

Johann N. Lieberkühn (1711–1756) German anatomist who was born in Berlin. He studied medicine in Halle, Jena, Leiden, Paris and London. He practiced in Berlin. He described them in 1745 but they were originally discovered by Malpighi in 1688. He invented a reflector microscope in 1738. He was elected F.R.S. in 1741 following his demonstration of his technique for injecting anatomical specimens in London.

LIGNAC-DE TONI-FANCONI SYNDROME

(Also called LIGNAC-FANCONI SYNDROME)

v. FANCONI SYNDROME

Georges O.E. Lignac (1891–1954) Dutch pediatrician.

LILLIPUTIAN HALLUCINATION

Hallucination where objects and people seem diminutive.

Lilliput, the land of little people, described in Gulliver's Travels, by J. Swift.

LINDAU DISEASE

v. HIPPEL-LINDAU DISEASE

LINDSAY NAILS

Brown pigmentation of nails in chronic renal failure. Sometimes called half and half nails, around 50% of nail is white but the distal portion is brown.

P.G. Lindsay U.S. physician.

LIPSCHÜTZ BODY

Eosinophilic nuclear inclusion seen in cells infected by virus, e.g. herpes simplex or zoster, cytomegalovirus, etc.

Benjamin Lipschütz (1878–1931) Austrian dermatologist. He described a non-venereal ulcer of the vulva which was rapidly spreading and thought due to Bacillus crassi sometimes called Lipschutz ulcer. He was born in Brody and studied medicine in Vienna but learnt his bacteriology at the Pasteur Institute in Paris in 1907. He applied this knowledge to his study of skin disorders.

LISCH NODULES

Lisch nodules are transparent yellow or brown prominences on the iris surface. They are found in more than 90% of all school-age patients with peripheral neurofibromatosis (von Recklinghausen disease (*v. infra*)).

Karl Lisch (1907–) Austrian ophthalmologist who was born in Kirchbichl, a village in the North Tyrol, the son of a general practitioner who had an interest in ophthalmology. He went to the nearest high school in Kufstein, and in 1925 commenced his medical studies at the University of Innsbruck. He graduated M.D. in 1931. He undertook his residency in ophthalmology at the First University Eye Clinic in Vienna, which was directed by J. Meller. After a year as an unpaid trainee in the University of Vienna Pharmacological and Neurological Institute, he continued in ophthalmology at the University Eye Clinic in Innsbruck and went to Munich in 1935 where he was initially an assistant to the University Eye Clinic and later became senior physician. He published his paper describing the nodules in 1937. He worked at the University Eye Clinic in Munich throughout World War II and in 1947 became Chief Physician of the Eye Department of the hospital of Wörgl, a small town only a mile from his birth place, and remained in that position until his retirement in 1980. He attracted patients from all over Austria, Germany and Italy and in his homeland of the North Tyrol, he was called the "Ophthalmological Pope".

Lisch continues to work in private practice. He has published in almost every area of ophthalmology and has described another condition called Lisch Syndrome, which combines a pellucid iris with nystagmus. He has two sons, one of whom is a professor of ophthalmology in Germany. While ophthalmology remains his main interest, he enjoys swimming, bicycling and skiing in his Tyrolean mountains.

LISSAUER FASCICULUS OR TRACT

Tract from the dorsal root which runs in the spinal cord – fasciculus propius.

LISSAUER PARALYSIS

General paralysis of the insane, rapid in onset with fits and monoplegia.

Heinrich Lissauer (1861–1891) German neurologist who worked in Breslau (Wroclaw).

LISTERIA MONOCYTOGENES

Gram positive bacillus causing meningitis, lymphadenopathy and pyrexia. It may present as a cerebritis and is more usually seen in immunosuppressed patients.

Joseph Lister (Baron Lord Lister) (1827–1912) English surgeon who introduced antiseptic principles into surgery. He was born in Upton, Essex, the son of a wealthy Quaker who was a wine merchant with a keen interest in optics and invented an achromatic lens which advanced the science and probably influenced Lister's early interest in microscopy. Lister entered University College, London, in 1844, to study medicine. At that time it was known as the Godless University because both Oxford and Cambridge required students to take an oath and subscribe to the 39 Articles of the Church of England. It was only in 1858 that dissenters from the Church of England were granted degrees at Oxford or Cambridge.

Lister graduated B.A. 1847 and M.B. 1852. He impressed Wharton Jones and Sharpy, and under their encouragement he published articles on muscle histology and the dilator and sphincter muscles of the iris. He then joined Professor Syme in Edinburgh in 1854 and in 1855 was appointed lecturer in surgery at the College of Physicians and assistant surgeon to the Royal Infirmary. He wrote weekly summaries of Syme's lectures for The Lancet, and in 1856 married Syme's eldest daughter, and in so doing had to resign from the Society of Friends to join the Church of England. His work continued and he wrote on vessel injury, coagulation and inflammation, and in 1860 was appointed Regius Professor of Surgery at the University of Glasgow and was elected F.R.S. Here he noted the high surgical mortality related to sepsis and that simple fractures healed rapidly whereas compound fractures were often infected and resulted in gangrene and death.

He revived the Hippocratic principle of healing by first intention and observed this only occurred in the absence of infection. The Professor of Chemistry, T. Anderson, told him of the work of Louis Pasteur. In 1865 he commenced treatment of wounds with carbolic acid with a resultant reduction of wound infection, which he reported in The Lancet in 1867, "On a new method of treating compound fractures". His discovery was widely publicized and was strongly opposed by the senior surgeons of the U.K. but was supported by Thiersch of Leipzig and Volkmann of Halle, and Billroth in Vienna.

In 1867 he returned to Edinburgh as Professor of Surgery where he continued his work on antiseptic techniques and examined ligatures and found soaking them in carbolic acid prevented infection and resultant breakdown of wounds. He made a trip to Germany in 1875 and his views were fully accepted there.

In 1877 Lister returned to London to King's College Hospital but unlike Edinburgh where his lectures were filled with students, he found his classes became smaller and smaller, because the students found that if they put forward Lister's views they failed their exams and soon only a small number attended, usually ones who had already passed.

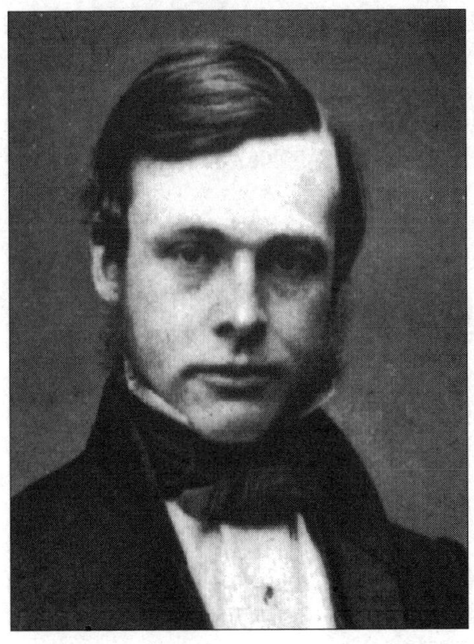

Joseph Lister, aged 28 (Reproduced from *"Lord Lister"* by Sir Rickman John Godlee [Published by McMillan & Co. St Martin's St., London, 1917])

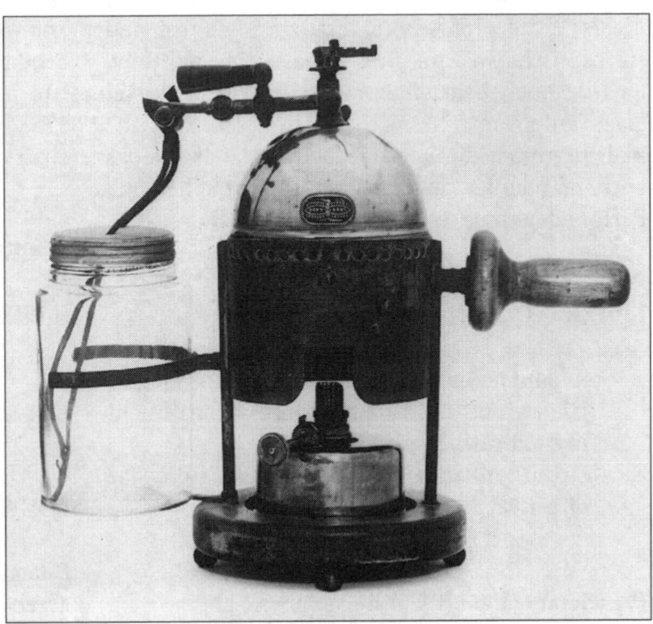

The Lister spray
(Courtesy of the Gordon Museum, Guy's Hospital, London)

His introduction into surgery of the concepts of absolute cleanliness and antisepsis which laid the foundations for the advancement of modern surgery was eventually recognized at home. In 1883 he was created a Baronet; in 1885 he received the Prussian Pour le Merite; President of the Royal Society in 1897, he became Lord Lister in 1903 and became one of the first 12 to receive Edward VII's new Order of Merit.

As a surgeon he was not a brilliant technician but concentrated meticulously on details and principles to reduce morbidity and mortality with surgical procedures. He was a rather retiring and quiet man, who did not show outwardly resentment of much of the controversy which resulted from attacks on his methods by his surgical colleagues. His funeral service was held in Westminster Abbey. Only two other medical men have their graves there, Thomas Willis and John Hunter.

LITTLE AREA

Region on nasal septum where blood vessels con verge and is a frequent source of troublesome nose bleeding which may require cauterization.

James L. Little (1836–1885) Born in New York he became Professor of Surgery at the University of Vermont.

LITTLE DISEASE

Spastic paraplegia.

William J. Little (1810–1894) Physician at the London Hospital. He had had infantile paralysis with resultant talipes equinovarus. This was corrected by an operation by Louis Stromeyer of Hanover, Germany and he named his third son Louis Stromeyer Little. The latter became a prominent surgeon who pioneered the use of intravenous saline for cholera.

LITTRÉ GLANDS

Urethral glands.

Alexis Littré (1658–1726) French anatomist and surgeon who was the first to advocate colostomy for intestinal obstruction and to describe a Meckel diverticulum in a hernial sac. His treatise on the male urethra in 1719 referred to the glands. He was born in Lourdes and studied at Montpellier and Paris and became Professor of Anatomy there.

LIVIERATO SIGN

1. Abdomino-cardiac sign. A blow to the epigastric area of the abdomen causes enlargement of right cardiac area of dullness.
2. Ortho-cardiac sign. Enlargement of right side of cardiac border when the patient stands up compared to lying supine.

P. Livierato (1860–1936) Italian physician.

LOBELIA

Plant *Lobelia inflata* which contains the alkaloid lobeline which is used as an expectorant and as a respiratory stimulus in the newborn. The alkaloid like nicotine acts on the chemoreceptors.

Matthaeus Lobelius or **L'Obel** (1538–1616) Flemish botanist, born in Lille and studied medicine at Louvain and Montpellier, graduating in 1568. He became physician to William of Orange and migrated to England and became physician and botanist to James the First.

LOBSTEIN DISEASE

Osteogenesis imperfecta.

Jean G.C.F.M. Lobstein (1777–1835) Alsatian pathologist, Professor of Pathology at Strasburg, who described the condition in 1833 and wrote a book on pathology. He discovered the accessory ganglion of the great splanchnic nerve above the diaphragm. He wrote a two volume book in 1833 on pathology, commencing with the ancient Egyptians and concluding with Corvisart. He coined the word arteriosclerosis in a section on arterial disease in the 2nd volume and in this same volume described the condition to which his name is attached, but which had been previously described by O.J. Ekman in 1788. His appointment in 1819 established the first chair of anatomical pathology in the world.

LOCKE-RINGER SOLUTION

v. RINGER SOLUTION

F.S. Locke (1871–1949) English physiologist.

LOEWI SIGN

Dilatation of the pupil following a weak solution of adrenaline described in patients with thyrotoxicosis and pancreatitis.

Otto Loewi (1893–1961) U.S. pharmacologist, born in Frankfurt-am-Main, the son of a wealthy wine merchant. He studied medicine at Strasburg where he found most of the lectures boring but in the last year he was excited by Naunyn, and work in the laboratory of Schmiedeberg, a pioneer in pharmacology. He spent some time with Hofmeister to improve his biochemistry and then went to a tuberculosis clinic of Van Noorden in Frankfurt but seeing the numbers of young people dying he decided that laboratory work attracted him and joined the Department of Pharmacology under H.H. Meyer whom he followed to Vienna. In 1909 he became Professor of Pharmacology in Graz.

He showed that animals could grow adequately on a diet of enzyme digest and therefore they could synthesize protein from smaller molecules. With Frölich in Vienna he showed that small doses of cocaine potentiated the response of sympathetic end-organs to adrenaline and nerve stimulation. He stressed the role of cations and Ca^{++} in muscle contraction, and first demonstrated that neural impulses could be transmitted by a chemical substance and for this won the Nobel Prize with Sir Henry Dale.

In 1938, being Jewish, he was imprisoned by the Nazis, but was released after two months and he migrated to the United States where he was appointed Research Professor at New York University. He was a lively teacher who "never ceased to wonder". He was elected Foreign Member of the Royal Society of London in 1954.

LÖFFLER DISEASE

or

LÖFFLER SYNDROME

Transient pulmonary infiltrates associated with eosinophilia, often due to the passage of *Ascarides* larvae through the lungs, but can be caused by other parasites and allergens including drugs.

LÖFFLER ENDOCARDITIS

Restrictive cardiomyopathy with prominent eosinophil infiltration and myocardial damage and fibrosis. Probably identical to tropical endomyocardial fibrosis. It is associated with the hypereosinophilic syndrome which occurs predominantly in Caucasian males with persistent eosinophilia and can involve other organs, lungs, brain and liver.

Wilhelm Löffler (1887–1972) Swiss physician, born in Basel. Trained in Geneva, Basel and Vienna – studied the formation of urea and succeeded Nageli as Professor of Medicine at the University of Zurich in 1921. A well-rounded clinical investigator equally at home in the laboratory or ward, he introduced the mass X-ray surveys in Switzerland and was one of the first to use insulin. He first described diffuse mural endocarditis – endocarditis parietalis fibroplastica with eosinophilia, giving congestive cardiac failure. A renowned teacher of the scientific method in clinical medicine.

LÖFGREN SYNDROME

Erythema nodosum, hilar lymphadenopathy and acute iritis seen in sarcoidosis.

Sven Löfgren (1910–1978) Swedish chest physician who was born in Stockholm and studied medicine there. He joined the staff at St. Goran's Hospital and was influenced by Westergren and especially Schaumann who were his senior colleagues. He succeeded Westergren as head of the pulmonary clinic but it was Schaumann to whom he owed most. This was reflected by his office on the walls of which were hung a number of Schaumann's paintings and he used Schaumann's old roll-top desk. His work greatly improved the clinical understanding of sarcoid and he was a worthy successor of the man whose name in Sweden (Schaumann) was eponymous for sarcoidosis.

LONDE ATROPHY

v. FAZIO-LONDE DISEASE

LOOSER ZONES

Pseudofractures seen in osteomalacia usually best seen in the angle of the scapula.

LOOSER-MILKMAN SYNDROME

v. MILKMAN SYNDROME

Emil Looser (1877–1936) Swiss surgeon who practised in Zurich.

LORAIN-LEVI SYNDROME

v. LEVI-LORAIN DWARFISM

LOUIS, ANGLE OF

v. LUDWIG

Angle of sternum at the level of the 2nd intercostal space.

Antoine Louis (1723–1792) French surgeon at the Hôpital de la Charité, Paris, who was co-inventor of the guillotine (*v. supra*) and a pioneer of medical statistics.

LOUIS-BAR SYNDROME

Ataxia telangiectasia. This is characterized by progressive cerebellar ataxia, cutaneous and sometimes ocular telangiectasia and recurrent respiratory infections and there is a 10–15% incidence of malignancies (lymphomas, leukemias and gastrointestinal cancer). Thymus derived lymphocyte function is abnormal and IgA and IgE levels are often greatly reduced and chromosome abnormalities have been reported with many involving chromosome 14.

Denise Louis-Bar Belgian neuro-pathologist.

LOWE SYNDROME

Oculocerebrorenal syndrome. X-linked recessive – growth and mental retardation, bilateral cataracts, metabolic acidosis, proteinuria and amino-aciduria, rickets and hypotonia.

Charles V. Lowe (1921–) U.S. pediatrician. Born in Pelham, New York, and graduated from Yale University M.D. in 1945. He did his residency at the Children's Hospital in Boston and became Associate Professor of Pediatrics at the New York State University in Buffalo in 1951–55, becoming a Research Professor in 1955–65. Currently he is a specialist assisting Child Health Affairs Office of the Assistant Secretary of Health which appointment he took up in 1974.

LOWN-GANONG-LEVINE SYNDROME

Paroxysmal supra-ventricular tachycardia with a short PR interval and normal QRS (compare WOLFF-PARKINSON-WHITE SYNDROME).

Bernard Lown (1921–) U.S. cardiologist, Peter Bent Brigham Hospital, Boston. He has pioneered the use of defibrillation as a treatment of ventricular fibrillation. He is a leading campaigner in opposition to the use of nuclear weapons and recently shared the Nobel Prize for Peace.

William F. Ganong U.S. physiologist, born in Northampton, Massachusetts. He graduated from Harvard in 1945. He became Professor of Physiology at the University of California School of Medicine, San Francisco in 1964. His main interests are in neuro-endocrine regulatory mechanisms especially related to the adrenal gland and aldosterone.

Samuel Levine (*v. supra*).

LUBARSCH-PICK SYNDROME

Scleroderma macroglossia and skeletal muscle involvement with amyloid and scleroderma.

Otto Lubarsch (1860–1933) German pathologist who, with F. Henke, wrote a 12 volume book on histopathology.

Ludwig Pick (1868–1944) German pathologist who wrote an account of Niemann-Pick disease (*v. infra*). He was Professor of Pathology at Rostock in 1894 and later director of the Anatomical Pathology Institute in Berlin. He introduced the term hypernephroma to describe Grawitz tumors.

LUCAS-CHAMPONNIÈRE DISEASE

Chronic pseudomembranous bronchitis.

Justin M.M. Lucas Championnière (1843–1913) French surgeon with an interest in anthropology. He was born in Saint-Leonard and graduated M.D. Paris 1872 and won his Agrégé in 1874. He demonstrated that prehistoric flints could produce trephine holes in a skull in 30–50 minutes. He was an ardent supporter of Lister and worked with him in Edinburgh before graduating and introduced antiseptic surgery to France. He was a pupil of Broca and did much for surgical techniques, especially involving bone. He published a classical monograph on treatment of hernias in 1887. He performed the first valvotomy to relieve aortic stenosis in 1913.

LUCIANI TRIAD

Weakness, hypotonia and ataxia due to cerebellar disease.

Luigi Luciani (1840–1919) Born in Ascoli Piceno, Italy, a nephew of G.A. Vecchi, the patriot. At 22 he commenced medical studies at the University of Bologna and graduated M.B. in 1868. He became Vella's assistant at the Physiological Institute and spent 1½ years in Leipzig with Ludwig whom he regarded as his greatest influence. He was Professor of Physiology at Siena then Florence and finally Rome. He made early contributions on the automatic activity of the heart and respiratory centre, but his monumental work was on cerebellar function in dogs and apes, in which he created cerebellar lesions and observed the resultant ataxia and discoordination. He wrote a textbook on physiology which was translated into English. He was elected Rector of the University of Rome from 1905 until he died from a chronic genito-urinary disease.

LUDER-SHELDON SYNDROME

Hereditary renal disorder with abnormal tubular function causing glycosuria and aminoaciduria and resultant dwarfism and rickets. Autosomal dominant.

Joseph Luder British pediatrician.

Sir Wilfred Sheldon (1901–) British pediatrician.

LUDWIG, ANGLE OF

v. LOUIS

Daniel Ludwig (1625–1680) German anatomist.

LUDWIG ANGINA

Cellulitis of the submandibular space usually due to an anaerobic bacteria.

Wilhelm F. von Ludwig (1790–1865) He was born near Stuttgart in the Duchy of Würtemberg and initially was an apprentice to a surgeon and later studied medicine at the University of Tübingen where he graduated in 1811. His then ruler, Frederick II, joined Napoleon against Prussia, Austria and Russia and Ludwig was an assistant surgeon in the army on the Russian front. After the Battle of Vilna he was imprisoned by the Russians for two years. In 1816 he returned to Tübingen to become Professor of Surgery and Midwifery and personal physician to King Frederick. In 1836 he published his first paper which was on Ludwig angina which occurred in Queen Catherine of Würtemberg. This was his only notable clinical observation. He suffered with cataracts and renal stones, and when he died left the majority of his fortune to found a hospital for the poor in Würtemberg which was opened in 1874.

LUFT SYNDROME

Progressive weight loss despite increased food intake, increased perspiration, muscular wasting and weakness, absent deep reflexes and increased metabolic rate with normal thyroid function due to mitochondrial abnormality which results in uncoupling of oxidative phosphorylation and morphological abnormality of the mitochondria.

Rolf Luft (1914–) Swedish endocrinologist. Born in Stockholm and graduated M.D. from the Karolinska Institute in 1940. He was appointed Professor of Endocrinology at the Karolinska Institute in 1949–61 and Professor of Internal Medicine in 1966. His major interest has been in diabetes and he has investigated many aspects of metabolism and pituitary and adrenal interactions.

LUGOL IODINE

Iodine solution.

Jean G.A. Lugol (1786–1851) French physician, his daughter married Paul Broca (*v. supra*). Born in Montauban, Tarn-en-Garonne, and graduated M.D. from Paris in 1812. Seven years later he gained appointment to the Hôpital St. Louis. He was much interested in tuberculosis and gave a paper to the Royal Academy of Sciences of Paris in 1829 in which he advocated the use of fresh air, exercise, cold bathing and drugs. He advocated the use of his

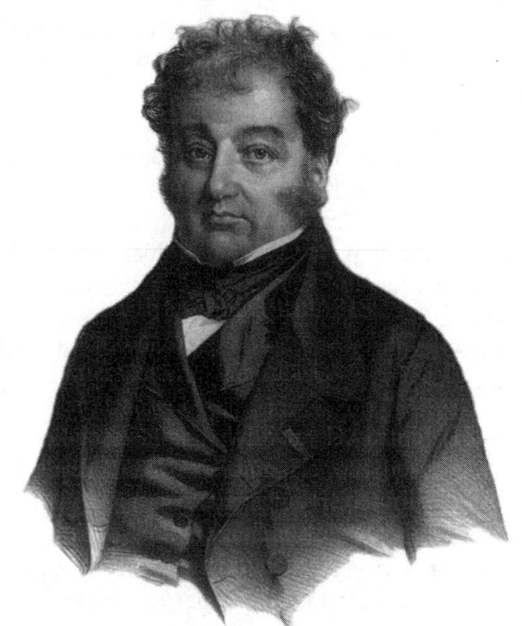

Jean G.A. Lugol (Courtesy of the Royal Society of Medicine, London, UK)

iodine solution, which consists of 5% iodine, 10% potassium iodine and distilled water, in tuberculosis. These works were published in 1831 and initially attracted much attention. The use of iodine was not found to be of value in tuberculosis, although his solution was later used in thyrotoxicosis by H.S. Plummer in 1924 (*v. infra*).

LUSCHKA FORAMEN

Foramen of 4th ventricle.

LUSCHKA, JOINTS OF

Articulation between lateral aspects of adjacent cervical vertebral bodies (C2–7).

Hubert von Luschka (1820–1875) German anatomist. He was born in Konstanz and studied medicine at Freiberg and Heidelberg graduating in 1844. He became Professor of Anatomy at Tübingen in 1849 and remained there until his death. He described the foramen in 1859. He investigated the anatomy of the larynx and the physiology of voice production, and first described polyposis of the colon.

LUTEMBACHER SYNDROME

Mitral stenosis combined with atrial septal defect.

René Lutembacher (1884–1936) French cardiologist who was greatly influenced by Vasquez (*v. infra*). Born in Jouy-en-Josas, graduated in Paris in 1912 and described his syndrome in 1916. He wrote numerous articles on cardiology with a particular emphasis on the distinction of functional from organic heart disease. He was Physician, Centre du Cardiologie de Seine-et-Dise (France).

LUTHERAN BLOOD GROUP

Antibodies developed in a patient who has been multiple-transfused which were directed against the red cells of a donor called Lutheran.

LUTZ-SPLENDORE-ALMEIDA DISEASE

South American blastomycosis.

Adolfo Lutz (1855–1940) Brazilian physician.

Alphonso Splendore Italian physician.

Floriano P. de Almeida Brazilian physician.

LUYS BODY LESION

Hemiballismus due to lesions involving the subthalamic nucleus.

Jules B. Luys (1828–1897) French neurologist. Born in Paris. His thesis in 1857 was on the microscopic pathology of tuberculosis. In 1862 he was Médecin des Hôpitaux and Chef de Service at the Salpêtrière and the Charité, and succeeded Marie as Director of the Maison de Sante Esquirol at Tury-sur-Seine. He was also director of the lunatic asylum at Ivy.

When 37 he completed his first and most important book of the nervous system and in it he described two structures which are still named after him, the subthalamic nucleus and the median centre of the thalamus. He made important contributions on the function of the thalamus and recognized four centers, each mediating one of the senses, the anterior or olfactory centre, the middle or optic, the median or somesthetic centre and the posterior or acoustic center. He initiated a 3-dimensional approach to the structures of the brain and he was one of the first to use photographs to illustrate the anatomy.

He was primarily a clinician and studied insanity, hysteria and hypnotism. He was elected to membership of the Academy of Medicine in 1877 and awarded Légion d'Honneur the same year, being promoted to officer in 1895. He founded and edited L'Encéphale, a journal devoted to nervous diseases. As he grew older his scientific contributions fell away and his reputation was hurt by his investigations into hypnotism in which he allowed himself to be imposed upon and indeed duped by his subjects. His own honesty and integrity were not in question.

LYELL SYNDROME

Toxic epidermal necrolysis giving an appearance of scalding of the skin – sometimes secondary to staphylococcal infection.

Alan Lyell English dermatologist. He graduated from Cambridge and St. Thomas's Hospital in London and became the head of dermatology at the Glasgow Royal Infirmary.

LYME ARTHRITIS

Characterized by brief recurrent attacks of asymmetric oligo-articular pain, and swelling involving the large joints. There is sometimes migratory polyarthritis in large and small joints. Preceding the attack is an annular skin lesion: erythema chronicum migrans. Cardiac conduction anomalies may occur and there may be neurological involvement. It is infectious with the tick as a vector. The organism is a spirochaete *Borrelia burgdorferi*. First recognized because of patients from Lyme, Connecticut.

LYNCH SYNDROME I

Familial colonic cancer not associated with polyposis. Inheritance is autosomal dominant and there is a predominance of it being sited proximally with frequent synchronous or metachronous carcinomas of the colon.

LYNCH SYNDROME II

This syndrome is similar to Lynch I but the families also have a propensity to other primary cancers, particularly endometrial and ovarian in origin, but others reported include pancreas, urological tract, nasopharynx.

Henry T. Lynch (1928–) U.S. oncologist. He was born in Boston and after attaining his Masters degree in Clinical Psychology at the University of Denver commenced a Ph.D. in Psychology and Genetics but on gaining admission to Medical School did not complete his degree. He graduated M.D. from the University of Texas Medical School at Galveston and undertook residency training at the University of Nebraska College of Medicine intending to become a cardiologist. As a resident he was asked to see an alcoholic with delirium tremens who told him that the reason he drank was "because everyone in his family dies of cancer". He investigated and reported this family and changed his career orientation to oncology. He has now published extensively in this area as well as in medical genetics and has occupied the Chairmanship of the Department of Preventive Medicine at Creighton University School of Medicine in California since 1970.

LYON HYPOTHESIS

Only one of the two X-chromosomes is genetically active in female cells.

Mary Lyon English geneticist.

M

MADELUNG DEFORMITY

Dorsal dislocation of the head of the ulna resulting in a deformity at the wrist.

Otto W. Madelung (1846–1926) German surgeon. He was born in Gotha and studied medicine in Bonn, Berlin and Tübingen, and graduated in 1869. He was assistant at the mental hospital in Siegburg when the Franco-Prussian war broke out and he then worked in the military hospital in Diez. After the war he worked with W. Buschs in Bonn and at the Pathological Institute of Rindfleisch. He remained at the University of Bonn and eventually became Associate Professor in 1881. In 1882 he was appointed to the Chair of Surgery in Rostock and in 1894 succeeded Luckes in Strasburg. In 1920 he left Strasburg as the last of the German lecturers, the French having two years earlier forced him to retire from his position. He then moved to Göttingen where he remained until he died.

He wrote extensively on many areas of surgery and was especially interested in injuries and diseases of the pancreas, liver and bile ducts as well as Dupuytren contracture and the deformity he described.

MAFFUCCI SYNDROME

Enchondromatosis and cutaneous hemangiomas.

Angelo Maffucci (1847–1903) Italian pathologist of Genoa who became Professor of Pathological Anatomy in Pisa, undertook important early work in tuberculosis and isolated the bacteria causing avian tuberculosis *(B. gallinaceous)*.

MAGENDIE FORAMEN

Median foramen in the 4th ventricle.

MAGENDIE LAW

Sometimes called BELL-MAGENDIE LAW (v. Bell). Anterior spinal roots are motor and posterior are sensory.

François Magendie (1783–1855) French physiologist, "Medicine is a science in the making" (une science à faire). He described himself as a chiffonier (a ragpicker) and in fact he was a data collector who did not try to link what he found with hypotheses and sought to explain all his findings in terms of physics and chemistry.

Magendie was the son of a surgeon and was born in Bordeaux, but during the Revolution in 1791 the family moved to Paris. He entered medical training at 16, and worked at the Hôtel Dieu with Boyer and then with Fr. Xavier Bichat and G. Dupuytren. He remained a practicing physician all his life but turned increasingly to physiology and general pathology at the College de France while continuing to practice and teach at the Hôtel Dieu. His father was an ardent republican who followed Rousseau's belief that the first education ought to be purely negative and Magendie received no schooling until he was ten. His father later persuaded Citizen Boyer, who became Napoleon's personal surgeon, to take his son as a pupil and François soon became an excellent anatomist and gave courses on the subject. In 1801 Napoleon, then first Consul, passed a statute reforming medical education and stipulated that no-one could practice medicine without a diploma. Even Boyer and Dupuytren had to be examined and Magendie wrote his thesis on the soft palate.

He was the first modern experimental physiologist and he founded the first journal devoted entirely to physiology, *"Journal de Physiologie Expérimentale"*. He proved Bell law by severing the anterior and posterior roots of spinal nerves in a litter of puppies. Stimulation of the posterior roots caused pain. He investigated the mechanism of deglutition and vomiting and the function of the cerebellum. He recognized that fluids were absorbed by blood vessels as well as lymphatics, with Poiseuille he noted that the blood pressure rises on expiration, and he destroyed the concepts of points of election for venesection (it was previously widely held that the site of venesection was important in its efficacy in various maladies) by showing that the effects were the same whatever the site of removal.

He introduced the use of bromine and iodine by his examination of the pharmacological activities of these elements and also the alkaloids morphine, strychnine and emetine. He demonstrated anaphylaxis experimentally for the first time showing that rabbits died after a second injection of egg albumin.

He was a friendly and witty man who was a fine teacher and a staunch opponent. Most of his experiments involved vivisection and he was an obvious target of the anti-vivisectionists, especially as many of his experiments would seem to be cruel by modern criteria. Nonetheless his contributions were extremely important and he led the way for Claude Bernard to follow.

MAGNAN SIGN

Crawling sensation under the skin as seen in cocaine addiction.

Valentin J.J. Magnan (1835–1916) French psychiatrist. Surviving a bout of cholera, he became one of the leaders of the French school of organic psychiatry and amongst those influenced by him were the Russian Merzheivsky (with whom Bekhterev worked) and C. von Economo.

MAIN SYNDROME

Manipulation by the patient to cause argument over management.

T.F. Main U.S. psychiatrist.

MAJOCCHI DISEASE OR PURPURA

Usually annular in appearance and most common in lower limbs with hemorrhagic and pigmented areas secondary to a vasculitis which gives an atrophic and telangiectasic appearance.

Domenico Majocchi (1849–1929) Italian physician. Initially he trained in surgery at the University of Rome but soon became interested in the specialty of dermatology and syphilis. He was appointed Professor of Dermatology in Parma in 1880 and finally Bologna in 1891 until he retired in 1924.

MALGAIGNE BULGINGS OR SWELLING

Bilateral groin swelling when the abdominal musculature is weak.

Joseph F. Malgaigne (1806–1865) French anatomist and surgeon who worked in Paris.

MALLORY BODIES

Acidophilic hyaline bodies in the hepatocyte consistent with alcohol ingestion in cirrhosis. Also seen in prolonged cholestasis (e.g. primary biliary cirrhosis) but in this case usually situated more peripherally.

Frank B. Mallory (1862–1941) U.S. pathologist from Cleveland, Ohio, graduated from Harvard in 1890 and in 1891 was appointed assistant pathologist at the Boston City Hospital under W.T. Councilman (*v. supra*). In 1893 he worked with Chiari (*v. supra*) in Prague and then Ziegler in Freiburg, returning to the U.S.A. to the Boston City Hospital. He made many contributions to pathology techniques and studied the function and origin of the histiocyte. He confirmed by Koch postulate that the whooping cough bacillus first discovered by Bordet was indeed the causative organism. He made important contributions to tumor classification, especially meningiomas, and cirrhosis. He was foundation editor of the American Journal of Pathology in 1925, having been previously editor of its predecessor, the Journal of Medical Research, and was Professor of Pathology at the Harvard Medical School (1928– 1932). With J.H. Wright he wrote "Pathological Technique" which was pre-eminent in the English-speaking world and which was a major

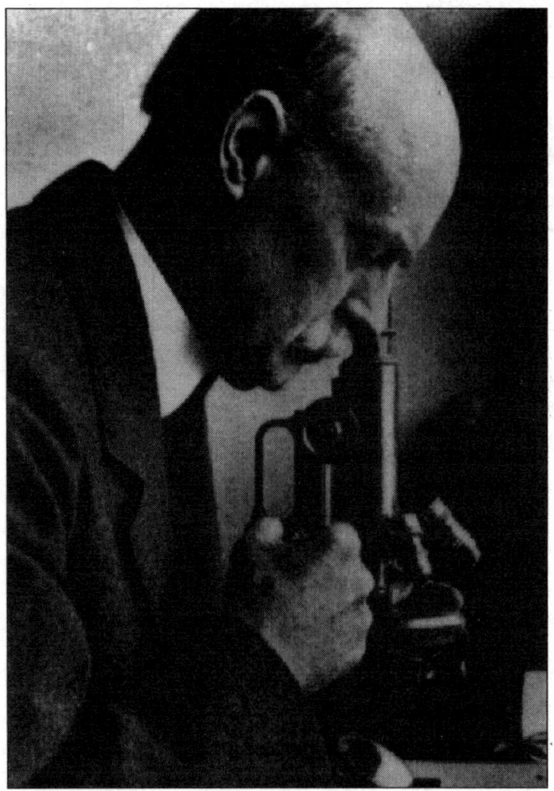

Frank B. Mallory (Reproduced from the *American Journal of Pathology,* Vol. IX, Suppl. 1933, p. 659)

force in improving staining techniques and stain standardization. He gave this advice to a colleague engaged in a scientific argument of some rancour, "I never found that arguing did much good. If my facts were not convincing I went to work to find others which were." One year after he retired a new pathology building at the Boston City Hospital was named after him. He was held in great affection by over 100 pathologists he had personally trained.

MALLORY-WEISS SYNDROME

Hematemesis due to a tear in the esophagus following forceful vomiting.

v. BOERHAAVE SYNDROME

George Kenneth Mallory (1900–) U.S. pathologist. Born in Boston the son of Frank B. Mallory (*v. supra*). He graduated M.D. Harvard in 1926 and trained in Pathology at the Boston City Hospital becoming pathologist in chief and Director of the Mallory Institute in 1951 and Professor of Pathology, Boston University.

Soma Weiss (1899–1942) U.S. physician. The son of a widely respected architect and engineer who worked for the Hungarian Government he was born in Bestereze, Hungary. During the First World War he went to the Royal Hungarian University in Budapest and worked as demonstrator and research fellow in physiology and biochemistry but migrated to the United States in 1920. He attended medical school at Cornell University Medical College, New York, and graduated M.D. in 1923. One of his early mentors, teacher and later friend was Eugene Du Bois. He interned for two years at the Bellevue Hospital and also worked on the action of digitalis and so had good clinical and pharmacological grounding and training. He joined the Thorndike Memorial Laboratory at the Boston City Hospital in 1925 where he was influenced by its first director, Francis W. Peabody, and later by George Minot (*v. supra*) who recommended him to be in charge of the two Harvard medical services at the Boston City Hospital. In 1939 he left this post to become Professor of Medicine at the Peter Bent Brigham Hospital where he remained until his death from a subarachnoid hemorrhage due to a berry aneurysm three years later. He combined his shrewd clinical skills, perhaps exemplified by his aphorism "a diagnosis is easy as long as you think of it", with basic scientific knowledge which he applied to diagnosis of his patients and to research into the mechanisms of ill health. He was a superb teacher at the bedside with special emphasis on therapeutic approaches to a patient's problems.

MALPIGHIAN CORPUSCLE

Lymph nodules in the spleen.

Marcello Malpighi (1628–1694) Professor of Anatomy at Bologna, Pisa and Messina and physician to Pope Innocent XII. He was the founder of histology, and of descriptive embryology, in describing the development of the chick embryo. He established the presence of capillaries and described the Malpighian layer of the skin. He accurately described the anatomy of the lung, and made many of the initial observations on the structure of the liver, kidney and spleen. He was a very fair and sympathetic person who was very kind to patients but suffered from a family feud with a neighbouring clan and constant verbal attacks by a Pisan colleague, Borelli. His description of the anatomy of the silkworm was an important contribution to biology.

MALTA FEVER

v. BRUCELLOSIS

Island of Malta.

MALTHUSIANISM

The concept that the world's population will outgrow the food supply.

Thomas R. Malthus (1766–1834) Guildford, England. He was perhaps the first true statistician whose theories and conclusions might lend weight to the saying "lies, damned lies and statistics". He was a clergyman who became a Fellow of Jesus College, Cambridge but resigned in 1804 because he married.

MANSONELLA

A Filarial worm transmitted by mosquitoes.

MANSONIA

The mosquito which is the vector of *Wucheria malayi*, and *Wucheria bancrofti*.

Sir Patrick Manson (1844–1922) Scottish physician and pioneer in tropical medicine. Born in Cromlet Hill, Aberdeenshire, Scotland. He graduated M.D. at Aberdeen in 1866. The same year he went to the Far East to Formosa for 5 years and then spent four years in Amoy, China. He returned to England in 1875 and gained attention with an article on filaria.

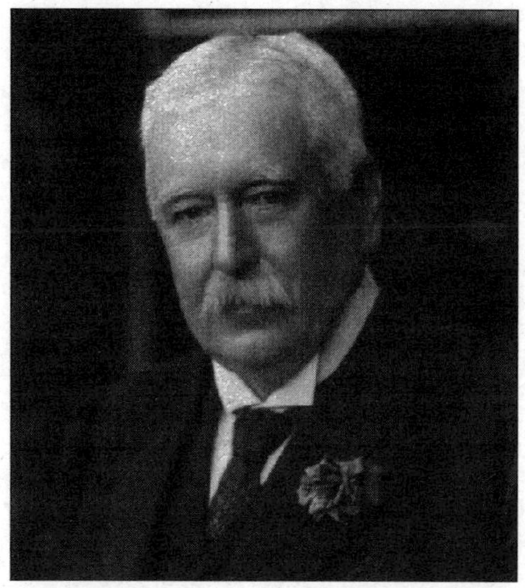

Sir Patrick Manson (Courtesy of the Royal Society of Medicine, London, UK)

He returned to China and discovered the life cycle of *Filaria bancrofti* in the mosquito. He discovered eggs of a previously unrecognized lung fluke in a patient with hemoptysis. He had an expensive Persian rug in his office, and the patient inadvertently coughed and expectorated on his precious rug. Manson was appalled until he noted the parasite whilst inspecting the rug for damage, and he immediately took a specimen onto a slide and demonstrated the fluke!

In 1883 he moved to Hong Kong, established an enormous medical practice and accumulated a considerable personal fortune. He retired in 1889 to an estate in Scotland but that year lost most of his fortunes through depreciation of Chinese currency, so went to London and recommenced practice and lectured on tropical medicine. He carried out experiments at home with mice, rats, birds and mosquitoes and became convinced that they transmitted malaria just as they did filaria but could not prove it. He passed the idea on to a young doctor from India, Ross, who proved the theory and won the Nobel Prize. Manson confirmed the transmission by receiving some mosquitoes from Italy which had fed on a patient with malaria and allowing them to bite his son, who two weeks later got malaria. Manson was the major force behind the founding of the London School of Tropical Medicine.

MANTOUX TEST

Intradermal injection of tuberculin results in a delayed hyper-sensitivity reaction in a person previously exposed to tuberculosis or immunised with Bacillus Calmette-Guerin (v. B.C.G. VACCINE).

Charles Mantoux (1877–1947) French physician. He graduated from the University of Paris, a student of Broca, Sire and Hutinel. For reasons of health he settled in Cannes, but continued to work in Paris during the long vacation periods given to people in sanatoriums. In 1908 he presented his first work on intradermal reactions to the Academy of Science and published an article on this in 1910. He showed that his intradermal reaction test was more sensitive than the older Pirquet subcutaneous tests using tuberculin and over the years the intradermal test completely replaced the subcutaneous approach of Pirquet. He developed a test for screening cattle for tuberculosis and applied this to pigs and horses. This was of great practical benefit with regards to public health, and he developed the test in the guinea pig for experimental studies of the rate of development of the allergic reaction. He undertook radiological studies of the disorder with Maingot and wrote extensively on pleural effusion, and on the fever of tuberculosis. He was one of the earliest clinicians to employ artificial pneumothorax and study its effects on lung cavities. All of this work was done away from major universities and institutions.

MARBURG DISEASE

African Hemorrhagic Fever or Green Monkey disease. Acute febrile illness with a high mortality and associated rash, coma, pancreatitis, hepatitis and hemorrhagic manifestations. Marburg is where the first outbreak occurred following the introduction of green monkeys (*Cercopithecus aethiops*) from Uganda.

Marburg, Germany

MARCHESANI SYNDROME

Short stature, brachydactylia, spherophakia (spherical lens with increased saggital and decreased equatorial diameter) and resultant myopia and glaucoma.

Oswald Marchesani (1900–1952) German ophthalmologist. He was born in Schwaz in the Tyrol. He went to medical school in Innsbruck and Freiburg, graduating from Innsbruck in 1923. He became an assistant at the Eye Hospital at the University of Innsbruck. Four years later he went to Munich to work with Professor K. Wessely. He became a Professor of Ophthalmology in 1936 in Münster, Germany. In 1945 he moved to the Chair in Hamburg. Initially he studied sympathetic ophthalmia and worked on uveitis. He was an enthusiastic skier and mountaineer.

MARCHIAFAVA-BIGNAMI SYNDROME

Degeneration of corpus callosum in alcoholics resulting in convulsions and focal motor abnormalities, usually seen in middle aged or elderly alcoholics, and attributed to drinking "rough" red wine.

MARCHIAFAVA-MICHELI SYNDROME

Paroxysmal nocturnal hemoglobinuria. An intravascular hemolytic anemia which is usually more severe during the night, resulting in the patient passing dark urine in the morning (v. HAM TEST).

Ettore Marchiafava (1847–1935) Born in Rome, he was a pathologist, physician and neurologist. He graduated in 1872 and for some years was assistant to T. Crudelli in pathology. In 1883 he was appointed as Professor of Pathology at the Royal University of Rome, and in 1917 Professor of Medicine until his retirement in 1921. He did much work on malaria and established the life cycle of *Plasmodium falciparum* as well as differentiating the three types of malarial parasites: tertian, quartan and aestino-autumnal, with Celli. He published an editorial on the effects of alcohol on the brain and gave the first description of syphilitic cerebral arteritis. Personal physician to three Popes and the House of Savoy, he won the Manson Medal for his research in tropical medicine. He was a highly successful medical practitioner and a very modest and cultured man.

Amico Bignami (1862–1929) Italian pathologist. Born in Bologna, he graduated in Rome in 1882 where he became Assistant Professor of Pathology in 1906. Apart from his work on brain pathology, he investigated acromegaly and leukemia, but subsequently devoted himself to malaria. In 1898 he produced malaria in man by infecting himself, allowing an infected mosquito to bite him. He is remarkable that of all the people in this field he is one of the few who took no part in the many disputes for precedence which many of his colleagues in malarial research indulged in!

He published a detailed study of Horace's references to wine.

Ferdinando Micheli (1872–1936) Italian physician. A student of C. Bozzolo of Turin, he rapidly gained international recognition for his work on congenital hemolytic anemias and his advocation of splenectomy. He worked at Siena and Florence and was appointed Professor of Medicine in Turin in 1921.

MARCUS GUNN DOTS

Small punctate reflections from the retina, particularly from the macula region in healthy people.

MARCUS GUNN PHENOMENON

Unilateral congenital ptosis – chewing or lateral movement of the jaw causes elevation of the eyelid.

Robert Marcus Gunn (1850–1909) Scottish ophthalmologist. He was born in Culgower in Sutherlandshire, Scotland. He graduated from medical school at Edinburgh University in 1873, where he was a contemporary of Robert Louis Stevenson, whom he knew. The teachers there who most influenced him were Syme and Lister and he was attracted into ophthalmology by Walker and Argyll Robertson (*v. supra*).

After graduation he visited Moorfields Eye Hospital and worked in comparative anatomy with Professor Shafer at University College, London. He then obtained a job at the Perth District Asylum and undertook a survey of their fundi occuli employing direct ophthalmoscopy which he had taught himself. He found that there was no difference in the changes he observed in the mentally defective compared with a similar sample of normal people. In 1874 he left for Vienna and spent 6 months there working with a number of people, but being particularly impressed with Jaeger, whom he considered superior to Arlt or Stellwag (*v. infra*) as a teacher. He then returned to Moorfields Eye Hospital and as a resident medical officer produced a number of reforms which resulted in superior case records and better results in cataract operations which were probably due to his introduction of the sterile principles, having indelibly imprinted on his mind the remark of Syme concerning Lister's patients in Edinburgh – "we are told of pus, we fear pus, we expect pus – but we see no pus".

In 1879 he went to Australia to collect specimens of the eyes of marsupials and his work on comparative anatomy of the eye attracted Sir William Bowman (*v. supra*). He examined the zoological material collected in the Challenger expedition. He was appointed Assistant Surgeon to the Moorfields Eye Hospital in 1883 and when he died he was senior surgeon of that hospital. An excellent surgeon, he was even more highly regarded for his abilities in examining the eye with the ophthalmoscope and introduced the use of a magnifying glass to examine the cornea and iris which became the loupe, now standardly used. He made one of the best and earliest descriptions of vessel changes in the retina and was one of the first to observe the poor prognosis of soft exudates in the retina, commenting – "in my experience it is most exceptional to see an old case of albuminuric retinitis; this latter affection seems to occur at a late stage of the general disease, so that death supervenes before the retinal changes have existed very long". He introduced systematized teaching of eye disorders, and it was this exercise which drew his attention to the prognostic significance of the above sign since he found it unusual for him to be able to show the same patient 12 months after he had observed soft exudates. He was keen on outdoor life, collected fossils, concentrating mainly on plants and fishes of the Jurassic period in the red sandstone systems from Scotland to Dorsetshire and a large number of his specimens were taken in by the British Museum. One of his students and admirers was E. Nettleship (*v. infra*).

MARDEN-WALKER SYNDROME

Kyphoscoliosis, arachnodactyly, micrognathia, with immobile facies and joint contractures. There is also cerebellar hypoplasia, blepharophiamosis and cataracts.

Phillip M. Marden (1937–) U.S. pediatrician.

William A. Walker (1937–) U.S. pediatrician.

MAREY LAW

Increased pressure in the aortic arch or the carotid sinus results in bradycardia and vice versa.

Etienne J. Marey (1830–1904) French physiologist. He improved recording techniques to study muscle contraction and used the movie camera to study human movement. He examined the pulse and invented a sphygmograph to record it graphically. He worked with A. Chauveau on heart physiology.

MARFAN SYNDROME

A disorder of collagen and elastic tissue. The patient has a characteristically long and narrow face with a high arched palate, an arm span greater than height, double jointedness, often subluxation of the lens, aortic regurgitation and a propensity to dissection of the aorta.

Antoine B.J. Marfan (1858–1942) French pediatrician, born in Castelnaudary, the son of a provincial medical practitioner who was of modest means and who initially opposed his son studying medicine. He finally acquiesced and Marfan entered the medical school at Toulouse and after two years went to Paris in 1879 and was an extern of the hospitals in 1880, working the following year with Lasègue (*v. supra*) and became an intern in 1882. He undertook military service and graduated with a silver medal in 1886. He was made Agrégé to the Faculty in 1892 and until 1901 deputized for Grancher during the winter terms. He was made Head of the Diphtheria Service at the Hospital for Sick Children and in 1910 was named Professor of Therapeutics and then appointed Foundation Professor of Hygiene at the Clinic of Infantile Diseases in Paris in 1914. In 1920 his Chair was moved to the Hospice des Enfants-Assistés.

His doctoral thesis entitled "Troubles and gastric lesions in pulmonary tuberculosis" commenced a life long interest on the subject from which was developed the so-called Marfan Law which stated that pulmonary tuberculosis was rare following the healing of local tuberculous lesions due to the development of immunity. He derived this from a series of observations which led him to say that "One rarely records pulmonary tuberculosis in people who during their childhood had been attacked by the disease and in whom the lesions had healed before the age of 15 years. This healing having taken place before any other site of tuberculosis had been recognized clinically." It was these observations that inspired Calmette to develop his B.C.G. vaccine (*v. supra*). He was one of the first to recognize the importance of skin reactions and when Pirquet developed his technique for skin testing for tuberculosis he immediately employed this in his clinical studies which became classics. He became interested in pediatrics when he deputized for Grancher at the Hospital for Sick Children and wrote many important papers on diphtheria and also on nutritional aspects including an important book "Infant Feeding and Nutrition" which was published in 1889 and he later published other books on pediatrics. He studied the detrimental effects of feeding infants goat's milk and studied rickets extensively. He was undoubtedly the pioneer of clinical pediatrics in France and an outstanding international figure of the day.

He was particularly grateful to his teachers, Lasègue and Michel Peter. He stated: "In medicine it is always necessary to start with the observation of the sick and to always return to this as this is the paramount means of verification. Observe methodically and vigorously without neglecting any exploratory procedure using all that can be provided by physical examination, chemical studies, bacteriological findings and experiment, one must compare the facts observed during life and the lesions revealed by autopsy."

Apart from his life in medicine he was an extremely cultivated man with interests in art and literature and greatly enjoyed concerts and his visits to Italy where he had a particular interest in Venetian painting. After he retired he wrote a biography of his friend Emile Broca and of his father as well as a study of Lauraguais. Amongst his friends were Lermoyez, Florand, Broca and Lepage.

From the time he replaced Grancher at the Clinic of Sick Children he organized a clinic for child nutrition, discussing the problems with the young mothers, incorporating rules of milk feeding which were passed on through his many pupils to other clinics. He created a post of a social worker in 1914 thanks to the help of Madame Nageotte and Getting, and the first appointment was Mlle. Oelcker. He took a very active part in promoting the welfare of children. He was a member since its foundation of the governing body of the Society for the Preservation of Infants against Tuberculosis, which he had called Grancher and which at the time of his death had approximately 6000 pupils every year from all parts of France. In his will he left a considerable fortune to this institution.

MARIE ATAXIA

Hereditary ataxia, with onset in early adult life and with features of cerebellar pyramidal tract and posterior column involvement (another source says no posterior column involvement), and sometimes an associated optic atrophy and 3rd nerve palsy but no skeletal deformities.

cf. FRIEDRICH ATAXIA, and

cf. LEVY-ROUSSY SYNDROME

MARIE-BAMBERGER DISEASE

Hypertrophic pulmonary osteoarthropathy.

MARIE-FOIX RETRACTION SIGN

Squeezing of the toes or forcing the foot downward causing dorsiflexion of the ankle and flexion of the knee and hip in upper motor neurone paralysis.

MARIE-STRÜMPELL ARTHRITIS, DISEASE

Rheumatoid arthritis, principally affecting the spine.

MARIE-STRÜMPELL ENCEPHALITIS

Acute infantile hemiplegia.

MARIE-TOOTH DISEASE

v. CHARCOT-MARIE-TOOTH DISEASE

Pierre Marie (1853–1940) First a student of law but changed to medicine and became an intern at the age of 25. His M.D. thesis was on thyrotoxic tremor. He worked with Charcot and made many classical descriptions of new clinical disorders which established him as a world famed neurologist. He wrote one of the early descriptions of acromegaly. He moved to the Hôpital de Bicêtre in 1897 and published extensively on aphasia, opposing the views of Broca and Wernicke concerning the localization of speech. He dissected one of Broca's specimens which he had left untouched and showed the lesion to involve far more than Broca's area. His pupils included C. Foix and G. Roussy. When 65 years old he succeeded Charcot's lineage of Raymond, Brissaud and Dejerine at the Salpêtrière in 1918. He retired in 1925.

Eugen Bamberger (*v. supra*).

Charles Foix (*v. supra*).

Ernst A.G.G. von Strümpell (1853–1925) Born in Neu Autz Kurland (Courland), a Baltic province of

Russia, and lived initially in Dorpat (Estonia) where his father was Professor of Philosophy and became a fine violinist. He spent a term in philosophy in Prague and then changed to medicine, first at Dorpat at the German University and then Leipzig where his father had moved to a Chair. There his teachers were Wunderlich, Thiersch, Crede and Carl Ludwig (who invented the kymograph drum). He graduated in 1875 and was appointed an assistant at Wunderlich's clinic. In 1877–78 in Vienna he met Johannes Brahms and he was impressed by Meynert and Benedikt. In 1878 he became Privatdozent and met Wagner, Cohnheim, Weigert and Erb. His first lectures were on infectious disease and only one student attended, who left when the lecturer entered the classroom. When Erb moved to Heidelberg in 1883 Strümpell moved also and became Director of the Medical Clinic with Möbius as his assistant. He was appointed Professor of Medicine at Erlangen (1886–1903) then Breslau (Wroclaw) (1903–1909), went to Vienna in 1909, then gained his final appointment at Leipzig, replacing G.H. Curselmann in 1910 and remaining there until his death.

He wrote a very famous textbook of medicine based on his own experience, which was the definitive text of internal medicine in Germany at the time. He described a number of disease entities including hereditary spinal spastic paralysis, Strümpell-Lorain Disease. He was an optimistic and kind person devoted to his patients and a liberal in life whilst respecting tradition. His flair for music gave him personal contact with many of the period's outstanding artists.

Howard H. Tooth (*v. supra*, Charcot).

MARIN AMAT SYNDROME

Automatic closure of one eye when patients with lower motor neurone 7th nerve palsy open their mouth.

Also termed REVERSE MARCUS GUNN.

Manuel Marin Amat Spanish physician.

MARINESCO HAND OR SIGN

Cold blue edematous hand seen in neurological lesions such as syringomyelia, giving trophic changes.

MARINESCO-SJÖGREN-GARLAND SYNDROME

Congenital cerebellar ataxia with hypertension, cataract, mental retardation and some skeletal deformities.

Georges Marinesco (1865–1938) Romanian physician. Born in Bucharest and after finishing medical school he went to the Salpêtrière to work with Charcot and there was associated with Pierre Marie, Babinski and Raymond. Later he worked with Weigert at Frankfurt and then du Bois-Reymond at Berlin. After 9 years abroad mainly in Paris, he returned home to the Pantelimon Hospital. In 1897 a Chair of Clinical Neurology was established for him at the University of Bucharest. He contributed to many areas of neurology, in particular to the juvenile form of amaurotic family idiocy, and hereditary conditions such as Friedrich ataxia and published over 250 papers and several books. He founded the Romanian school of neurology and was a fine teacher who introduced the modern approaches he had learnt in Paris to his country.

Karl G.T. Sjögren (*v. infra*).

Hugh Garland English neurologist.

MARIOTTE BLIND SPOT

Optical blind spot.

Edmé Mariotte (1620–1684) French physicist; he showed that the red light reflex is due to the reflection of light from the retina and demonstrated the blind spot in 1684.

MARJOLIN ULCER

Malignant ulcer superimposed on a previous scar or benign ulcer.

Jean N. Marjolin (1812–1895) French surgeon at Hôpital Sainte-Eugénie, Paris.

MAROTEAUX-LAMY SYNDROME

Gargoylism similar to Hurler syndrome but without any mental retardation and characterized by excessive urinary excretion of chondroitin sulphate B in the urine. It is also called mucopolysaccharidosis VI and is inherited as an autosomal recessive.

Pierre Maroteaux (1926–) French pediatrician. He was born in Versailles and graduated in Paris in 1952. A pupil of Lamy, he succeeded him to become Professor of Medical Genetics in Paris. A pioneer in medical genetics he was a protégé of Debré, at the Hôpital des Enfants Malades in Paris and worked with Weil on hereditary hemolytic anemias. He was appointed Professor of Medical Genetics in 1950.

Maurice E.J. Lamy (1895–1975) French pediatrician.

MARTINOTTI CELLS

Cells in the cerebral cortex.

Giovanni Martinotti (1857–1928) Italian pathologist. He graduated in medicine at Turin in 1880 where he was influenced by Bizzozero to study pathology. He was appointed Professor in Modena (1890), Siena (1891) and finally Bologna in 1893.

MARTORELL SYNDROME

Aortic arch syndrome.

v. TAKAYASU DISEASE

MARTORELL ULCER

Hypertensive ischemic leg ulcer.

Fernando Martorell Otzet (20th century) Spanish vascular surgeon who described ischemic leg ulcers with arterial disease secondary to hypertension. He founded an angiology department in Barcelona and has been a prolific writer publishing 15 books and founded the journal "Angiologia".

MASSON BODY

Macrophages and fibrin in pulmonary alveoli in organising pneumonia.

Pierre Masson (1880–1958) Canadian pathologist who also introduced a staining procedure for connective tissue (Masson Stain). He graduated in 1909 from the University of Paris and spent 5 years in the Pasteur Institute and after the 1st World War became the youngest Professor to occupy the Chair of Pathology in Strasburg, which had become French. He migrated to Canada in 1927 to the Chair of Pathology of the University of Montreal. He wrote a book on tumors and made many original advances in histo-pathological techniques.

MASTER TEST

Exercise test for screening of coronary disease by taking ECG before and after exercise.

Arthur M. Master (1895–1973) U.S. physician, born in New York City and graduated M.D. Cornell in 1921. He trained at Mt. Sinai Hospital, N.Y. and then worked with Sir Thomas Lewis in London before returning to become head of cardiology at Mt. Sinai. He served with the U.S. Navy in World War II in the Solomon Islands.

MASUGI NEPHROTOXIC NEPHRITIS

Animal model of glomerulonephritis.

Matazo Masugi (1896–1947). Born in Otsu, Shiga Prefecture, Japan, graduated Tokyo University Faculty of Medicine in 1921, associate professor Department of Pathology, Chiba Medical School, 1924, studied under Professor Ludwig Aschoff of Freiburg University in 1925, then Professor Rössle,

Department of Pathology, Basel University in 1926. Returned to Japan in 1927, Professor of Department of Pathology, Chiba Medical School, and started work on experimental nephritis. Injected kidney homogenates into peritoneal cavities of rabbits, then rabbit serum into rats produced nephritis. Later sensitized ducks with rabbit kidney homogenates, injected duck serum into rabbits and after 4–11 days observed onset of Masugi nephritis.

MAURER DOTS

Red dots due to *Plasmodium falciparum* malaria seen in red cells stained with Leishman stain.

Georg Maurer (1909–) German physician who worked in Sumatra in the Dutch East Indies (Indonesia).

MAURIAC SYNDROME

Growth retardation, obesity and hepatomegaly in juvenile diabetes mellitus.

Pierre Mauriac (1832–1905) French physician born in Saint-Aquilia. He worked on circulatory diseases and syphilis and its treatment and was on the staff of the Hôpital Midi from 1868–1897. He died in Pontours.

MAY-GRUNWALD STAIN

Romanovsky stain for peripheral blood film and bone marrow preparations.

MAY-HEGGLIN ANOMALY

Autosomal dominant. Döhle bodies are present in the granulocytic series and there is marked variation in platelet size and sometimes thrombocytopenia. Usually the anomaly is asymptomatic. May first described the white cell changes in 1809 and Hegglin recognized the associated platelet anomaly in 1945.

Richard May (1863–1936) German pathologist who worked in Munich.

Ludwig Grünwald (1863–) German otolaryngologist who was the first to use a surgical approach to infections of the ethnoid and sphenoid bones and to nasal sinusitis.

Robert Hegglin (1907–) Swiss pediatrician in Zurich.

MAYER REFLEX

With the patient's hand supinated and relaxed, firmly flex the metacarpophalangeal joint of the ring finger. Normally the thumb will appose and adduct. The response is absent in pyramidal tract disease.

Karl Mayer (1862–1931) Austrian neurologist.

MAZZONI CORPUSCLE

Golgi corpuscle.

Vittori Mazzoni (1880–1940) Italian physiologist.

MECKEL DIVERTICULUM

This is the persistence of the intra-abdominal part of the vitello-intestinal duct, which normally completely disappears. Vestigial remnants of the structure can take on a number of forms but the one best known is that of an out-pouching or diverticulum from the intestine which is said to be found two feet from the ileo-cecal valve in 2% of people and to be 2 inches long. It may contain cells similar to that found in the stomach or pancreas and cause complications such as perforation, hemorrhage from peptic ulceration, intussusception or intestinal obstruction.

MECKEL SYNDROME

v. GRUBER SYNDROME

Johann F. Meckel (the younger) (1781–1833) He came from a distinguished medical family. His grandfather, J.F. Meckel (1714–1774), was Professor of Anatomy, Botany and Obstetrics in Berlin and first described the spheno-palatine ganglion (Meckel ganglion) and the dural space which contains the Gasserian ganglion (Meckel cave). His father, P.F. Meckel (1756–1803), was Professor of Anatomy and Surgery at Halle, where he was born. He studied medicine there and at Göttingen, Würzburg and Vienna, and graduated M.D. at Halle in 1802. He then studied in Holland, France, Italy, Germany and England, returning home in 1806, succeeding his father in the Chair of Anatomy and Surgery in 1808. He discovered the first branchial cartilage, sometimes called Meckel cartilage. He wrote important books on human anatomy and pathology, and atlases of human abnormalities.

MEDJUGORJE MACULOPATHY

Central visual loss following gazing at the sun, e.g. during an eclipse – solar retinopathy.

Medjugorje A village in Yugoslavia where six teenagers reported seeing the Virgin Mary and received messages of peace daily by looking at a hilltop behind which the sun was setting.

MEES LINES

Transverse white lines in the nails distal to the cuticle in arsenical poisoning. It is also seen after thallium ingestion, cancer chemotherapy, febrile illnesses, Hodgkin disease and other systemic disorders, e.g. severe cardiac disease.

R.A. Mees Dutch physician who reported this sign associated with arsenical poisoning in 1919.

MEIBOMIAN CYST

Chalazion. Retention cyst or infection of the conjunctival gland.

Heinrich Meibom (1638–1700) German physician who was born in Lübeck. In 1666 he described the conjunctival glands. He taught archeology, geometry and philosophy as well as medicine. He was Professor of Medicine, History and Poetry at Helmstadt.

MEIGE DISEASE

v. MILROY DISEASE (sometimes called NONNE-MILROY-MEIGE DISEASE)

Henri Meige (1866–1940) French physician who described familial edema in 1899. A student of Charcot, he helped edit a publication with him which showed the facial appearance of many patients with nervous disorders. He investigated and published on diseases occurring in ancient Egypt and wrote on Charcot's artistic accomplishments.

MEIGS SYNDROME

Ovarian fibroma or neoplasm associated with ascites and hydrothorax. The pleura is normal and removal of the tumor usually results in resolution of the effusion.

Joseph V. Meigs (1892–1963) U.S. obstetrician and gynecologist. He was born in Lowell, Massachusetts and on leaving Princeton in 1915 went to Harvard and graduated M.D. in 1919. He became Professor of Gynaecology at Harvard and director of the gynaecology department at the Massachusetts General Hospital. He died of a coronary thrombosis.

MEISSNER CORPUSCLE

Sensory end organ.

MEISSNER PLEXUS

Submucosal nervous plexus of the intestine.

Georg Meissner (1829–1905) German anatomist and physiologist. He was born in Hannover and studied medicine in Göttingen. One of his teachers there was R. Wagner who created his interest in the natural sciences and with whom he went as a student on a zoological trip to Trieste. One of his friends as a student was the famous surgeon, Billroth (*v. supra*).

He was a pupil of J. Müller in Berlin and the latter influenced him greatly. In 1855 he was appointed Professor of Anatomy and Physiology in Basel and as his interests became more physiological, he returned to Göttingen to succeed his former teacher R. Wagner, in 1860.

At Göttingen he became a great friend and worked with the famous anatomist J. Henle (*v. supra*). In 1853 he discovered the tactile end organs in the skin and conceived that pressure changes triggered neural responses. This involved him with an argument concerning priority with his old teacher, Wagner, whom Meissner nonetheless continued to respect. In 1862 he described the mesenteric plexus. He described the breakdown of protein into smaller protein components in the stomach. Perhaps because of acrimonious diatribes against him by E. Brücke and W. Kühne, and more importantly the famous Berlin physiologist, du Bois-Reymond, he published nothing after 1872 until his death, although he had at this time achieved considerable fame for his development of a technique for preserving whole organs without the use of disinfectants. This involved the employment of aseptic surgery to remove the particular organ and the use of heat sterilization of the containers and enabled him to preserve these organs without putrification for years. This work was reported by a colleague Rosenbach, although he himself had presented his findings at a number of scientific meetings.

MELENEY SYNERGISTIC GANGRENE

This is a postoperative form of gangrene with a chronic enlarging ulcer due to infection with microaerophilic *Streptococcus* and *Staphylococcus aureus*.

MELENEY ULCER

Chronic skin ulcers due to mixed bacterial infection.

Frank L. Meleney (1889–1963) He graduated in 1916 from Columbia University College of Physicians and Surgeons in New York and served in the U.S. army corps in World War 1. He spent four years in Peking with the Rockefeller Foundation as a surgeon, returning to New York in 1925 to rejoin the Columbia University as an associate in surgery, becoming Professor of Clinical Surgery in 1950. He was particularly interested in research into bacteria and introduced the use of bacitracin following work with Miss Balbina Johnson. The first patient he treated with the antibiotic was a little girl called "Tracy" and hence the name for the new antibiotic. He wrote two books on surgical infections and retired to Miami in 1955 and died there of a coronary occlusion.

MELKERSSON-ROSENTHAL SYNDROME

Characterized by facial palsy in 30%, a scrotal tongue and facial lip swelling which looks like angioneurotic edema but when present for some time may be granulomatous on biopsy. There may be a familial incidence and migraine may be a feature.

Ernst Melkersson (1898–1932) Swedish physician.

Curt Rosenthal German neurologist and psychiatrist.

MELTZER SYNDROME

Vasculitis, arthritis and renal disturbances secondary to a circulating mixed cryoglobulin (IgM and IgG usually with Rheumatoid Factor activity). There may be an associated peripheral neuritis, and hepatitis may follow.

Martin Meltzer (1930–) U.S. physician, New York.

MENDELIAN DOMINANT

Autosomal dominant inheritance according to Mendel Laws.

Gregor Mendel (1822–1884) Austrian monk and botanist. The Abbot of Brün published his observations in an obscure journal in 1866. Born in Heizendorf, Moravia, he entered the Augustinian Order as a novice in 1843 at Alt-Brün. He studied at the University of Vienna for two years before returning to Brün to teach school children and during this time studied the hybridization of peas. He became Abbot in 1868 and had to cease his work. His work was rediscovered 35 years later when H. de Vries, C. Correus and E. Tschermak simultaneously confirmed his results. His work is the foundation stone of genetics as we know it today.

MENDELSON SYNDROME

Aspiration of gastric contents causing chemical pneumonia, which occurs whilst the patient is anesthetized due to abolition of the laryngeal reflexes.

Curtis L. Mendelson (1913–) U.S. obstetrician.

MENDENHALL SYNDROME

Short stature, somatic abnormalities and severe insulin resistant diabetes.

E.N. Mendenhall U.S. physician.

MÉNÉTRIER DISEASE

Giant gastric hypertrophy with hypoproteinemia and diarrhea and protein losing enteropathy. Also called giant hypertrophic gastritis. It was the first condition in which protein losing enteropathy was discovered – there is an 8% incidence of carcinoma and multiple endocrine adenomas have been found in some patients.

Pierre E. Ménétrier (1859–1935) French histopathologist. He described it in 1888 "polyadénomes en nappe". He wrote a highly regarded book on cancer which went to many editions and which dwelt on etiological aspects of cancer, especially carcinogenic forces such as X-rays and chemicals such as tar. He studied experimental cancers in mice and championed the idea of pre-cancerous states. He collected objets d'art and became Professor of Medical History in the Paris Faculty in 1920. He died in a car accident.

MENGO VIRUS

Encephalomyocarditis virus.

Mengo A district in Uganda, Africa.

MENIÈRE SYNDROME OR DISEASE

Attacks of nausea, vomiting and vertigo associated with progressive loss of hearing. Sometimes with tinnitus and nystagmus.

Prosper Menière (1799–1862) French ear, nose and throat specialist. He was born in Angers on the Loire, son of a tradesman, and went to Paris to study medicine in 1819. He graduated in 1826 and was assistant to Baron Dupuytren at the Hôtel Dieu during the civil disturbances of 1830, when more than 2000 injured rioters were treated in the Parisian hospitals. He was Assistant Professor in the Faculty of Medicine when he was asked by the government to determine whether the Duchess de Berry was pregnant. She was the wife of the murdered Duc de Berry, son of Charles X, and had considerable support for the accession of her own son to the throne. Menière determined that she was pregnant but it was found that this was the result of a secret marriage to an Italian, and popular support melted away. She was no longer a problem to the government of the day, who released her and Menière went with her to Naples. In 1835 he went to Aude and Haute-Garonne to control a cholera epidemic. In 1838 he was appointed Physician-in-Chief at the Institute for deaf mutes, a year after an unsuccessful application to become Professor of Medicine and Hygiene. He was a friend of Bakac and Victor Hugo, and wrote on medical references by Latin poets as well as devoting himself to the study of audiology. In 1838 he married Mademoiselle Becquerel, who was related to Anton Becquerel, who discovered radioactivity. Menière based his observations on recurrent labrynthine vertigo which he published in 1861 on the findings of M.J.P. Flourius who in 1820 in experiments on birds, had distinguished between the function of hearing and balance of the inner ear, and the function of the individual semi-circular canals. He died of pneumonia.

MENKES SYNDROME

1. Maple syrup urine disease.
2. Kinky hair disease.

John H. Menkes (1928–) U.S. pediatrician/ neurologist. He was born in Vienna but emigrated with his parents to the U.S.A. to escape the Nazis. He graduated M.D. from Johns Hopkins in 1954 and then interned at the Boston Children's Hospital. He has written a number of novels as well as a textbook of pediatric neurology and became Professor of Pediatric Neurology at U.C.L.A. in 1984.

MENZBACHER-PELIZAEUS DISEASE

v. PELIZAEUS-MENZBACHER DISEASE

MERKEL DISC, CORPUSCLE OR CELL

Sensory end organ.

MERKEL TUMOR

Tumor of Merkel cells. A malignant tumor of the skin with features similar to malignant carcinoid and small cell lung cancer.

Friedrich S. Merkel (1845–1919) German anatomist who wrote a 3 volume book on human anatomy. He experimented with osmium tetroxide staining and described these cells in the skin of the nose of a mole and later they were found in human skin. He followed Henle (*v. supra*) as Director of the Institute of Anatomy at Göttingen in 1885.

METCHNIKOFF THEORY

Phagocytosis leads to inflammation and immunity.

Ilia I. Metchnikoff (1845–1916) Born in Kharcov and graduated in zoology and the natural sciences from Kharcov University. He was Docent at Odessa and Lecturer in Zoology in St. Petersburg, returning as Professor of Zoology at Odessa in 1873. He resigned in protest at the repressive policies of the Russians and from then on held no further university appointments. He went to Messina in 1883, enjoying its wealth of marine life and observed that when he introduced a splinter into a transparent starfish larva, a number of cells surrounded it. This was the initial observation which set him on the path to discover phagocytosis. Virchow, visiting Messina, was greatly impressed by his work.

He next noted that when a transparent fresh water crustacean *Daphnia* was attacked by a fungus it produced cells which attacked the spores of the fungus and destroyed them. He then applied this to protection against bacterial infection and called these cells phagocytes – a term suggested to him in Vienna. In 1888 he returned to Odessa to head a bacteriological laboratory there, but in 1890 he returned to Paris to the Pasteur Institute, where he worked on embryology, comparative anatomy and anthropology. In 1895 he showed that bacteriolysis could take place in vitro as well as in vivo as Pfeiffer had originally shown and with Roux he inoculated higher apes with syphilis (1903). He wrote books on the comparative pathology of inflammation and immunity in infectious disease, and won the Nobel Prize in 1908. He was impressed by the apparent old age attained by peasants in the Balkans following a trip there and felt this was due to their diet of yoghurt which he advocated as a health food. Later investigations showed this to be fanciful and that perhaps they merely looked older than their real age!

MEYER LOOP

Optic radiation which curves around the inferior loop of the lateral ventricle beneath the temporal cortex and reaches the calcarine fssure.

Adolf Meyer (1866–1950) U.S. psychiatrist and neurologist. Born in Niederweiningen near Zurich, Switzerland, he graduated M.D. in Zurich. He worked in many centers in Europe and migrated to the U.S.A. in 1892. He held positions as pathologist and as a psychiatrist, becoming Professor of Psychiatry at Cornell in 1904 and went to Johns Hopkins as head of the newly founded Phipps Psychiatric Clinic, becoming Professor of Psychiatry in 1910. He retired in 1941.

MEYNET NODOSITIES

Nodules attached to tendon sheath and joint capsules in rheumatoid arthritis.

Paul C.H Meynet (1831–1892) French physician from Lyons.

MIBELLI DISEASE

Angiokeratoma Mibelli.

Vittorio Mibelli (1860–1910) Italian dermatologist who described angiokeratoma in 1891 and porokeratosis in 1893, but both were previously described, the former by Cottle in 1877, the latter by Neumann in 1875.

MICHAELIS CONSTANT

K_m – the substrate concentration in moles/l at which an enzyme reaction proceeds at half its maximal rate.

Leonor Michaelis (1875–1949) U.S. biochemist and physician, who studied at the University of Berlin and Freiburg, graduating from the latter, M.D. in 1897 and worked as Ehrlich's assistant in Berlin in 1898–1899. He became the director of laboratories of the Berlin Municipal Hospital from 1906–1922 when he went to Nagoya, Japan, as Professor of Biochemistry 1922–1926, from where he moved to Johns Hopkins for 3 years and then to the Rockefeller Institute 1929–1940. He developed the equation with Menten to explain the relationship of the concentration of reactants on enzyme catalyzed reactions. He discovered Janus Green and was the pioneer of the permanent wave since he found that keratin was soluble in thioglycolic acid. He died in New York City.

MICHAELIS-GUTMANN BODIES

Basophilic inclusions in histiocytes seen in malakoplakia, a chronic infection characteristically in the renal tract, e.g. bladder. These inclusions are calcium and iron laden lysosomes in large mononuclear cells called Hansemann Macrophages.

v. HANSEMANN MACROPHAGES

L. Michaelis German pathologist who published jointly on malakoplakia in 1902 with Gutmann.

C. Gutmann (1872–) German pathologist.

MICHEL FLECKS OR SPOTS

Loss of pigment in iris associated with chronic iritis.

J. von Michel (1843–1911) German ophthalmologist.

MICHELI SYNDROME

v. MARCHIAFAVA-MICHELI SYNDROME

MIKULICZ CELL

Large vacuolated phagocyte with small pyknotic nucleus seen in rhinoscleroma.

MIKULICZ DISEASE OR SYNDROME

Enlargement of salivary and lacrimal glands secondary to sarcoidosis, lymphoma or tuberculosis associated with dry mouth and dry eyes but no arthritis, cf. Sjögren Syndrome.

Johann von Mikulicz-Radecki (1850–1905) German surgeon. Professor of Surgery, Breslau (Wroclaw). Born in Czernowitz, Poland, he graduated in Vienna in 1878. He was Billroth's assistant until 1881, Professor of Surgery at Cracow in 1882, Professor of Surgery at Königsberg in 1887 and at Breslau in 1890. He used a gauze mask and was one of the first to use gloves* during surgery. He pioneered surgical approaches to the esophagus and was the first to use the electric esophagoscope invented by Leiter in 1880, and the first to suture a perforated gastric ulcer.

Sauerbruch was his protégé, who devised a pressure chamber which enabled Mikulicz and he to become the originators of modern thoracic surgery, since they could operate without causing collapse of the lungs.

Mikulicz made Breslau an international center for surgery. Perhaps because of his origins he was frequently consulted by people from Latvia or neighbouring areas. One time he corrected a phimosis (narrowing of the prepucial opening) of the son of a nobleman, who after the success of the operation had a banquet in his honor. By midnight only half the courses were served and Mikulicz felt satiated, but on the stroke of midnight 12 barbers with assistants entered, shaved their guests and refreshed them with hot and cold compresses and then withdrew for the banquet to continue.

He was a perfectionist and a sentimentalist who loved music and was an able pianist. When he realized he was dying of cancer he asked Sauerbruch to write his obituary, which he himself edited!

** Rubber gloves were subsequently introduced by Halstead to protect the hand of his head nurse who was sensitive to the antiseptics and with whom Halstead was enamoured and later married. They were designed by the tyre millionaire Goodyear who was a good friend of Halstead.*

MILIAN EAR SIGN

Ear involvement seen in facial erysipelas.

Gaston Milian (1871–1945) French dermatologist. Born at Vitry-le-Francois into a family of modest means he gained bursaries to support him studying medicine in Paris. Interne des Hôpitaux in 1895 he was greatly influenced by Fournier and in 1919 was appointed to Hôpital Saint-Louis where he devoted his life to the study of syphilis and other skin diseases. He developed progressive paralysis and died quadriplegic.

MILKMAN DISEASE OR SYNDROME

Osteomalacia due to decreased tubular reabsorption of phosphate often on an hereditary basis (autosomal recessive).

(Also called LOOSER-MILKMAN SYNDROME)

v. LOOSER ZONES

Louis A. Milkman (1895–1951) U.S. radiologist. Born in Scranton, Pennsylvania. Graduated from Temple University School of Medicine, Philadelphia in 1919. He served in the armed forces in the 1st World War and later specialized in radiology. He was on the Faculty of St. Thomas's College which is now the University of Scranton. He died following a myocardial infarction.

MILLARD-GUBLER SYNDROME

6th and 7th nerve palsy with contralateral hemiplegia due to a lesion in the pons.

cf. WEBER SYNDROME

Auguste L.J. Millard (1830–1915) French physician.

Adolphe M. Gubler (1821–1879) French physician who was Intern des Hôpitaux in 1845 and in 1849 wrote one of the first descriptions of syphilitic gumma of the liver and described the liver lesions in congenital syphilis. He obtained his Agrégé in 1853 for a thesis on the "Theories of the production of cirrhosis of the liver" and in 1856 published his first work on hemiplegia. The following year he drew attention to flushing of the cheeks in relation to pneumonia and popularized this sign which had been described earlier. He was one of the first to emphasize the importance of examining the patient's urine, both chemically and microscopically, and drew attention to the significance of the presence of hyaline and granular casts. Throughout his life he had an interest in botany and in 1868 was appointed Professor of Therapeutics in the Faculty of Medicine. A cheerful individual, he was above all a clinical investigator who endeavored to apply the most recent scientific advances to the treatment of his patients. He drew attention to forms of paralysis which followed infections and trained Landry at the Hôpital Beaujon.

MILLER-ABBOTT TUBE

Double lumen tube for passage into stomach and into small intestine for sampling gastrointestinal fluid or for therapeutic aspiration in intestinal obstruction.

Thomas Grier Miller (1886–) U.S. physician. He was born in Statesville, North Carolina, and graduated in medicine from the University of Pennsylvania in 1911. He interned at the University of Pennsylvania Hospital and then commenced clinical investigation in the Department of Medicine, but this was interrupted by the 1st World War where he served in the army as a captain. He returned to the University of Pennsylvania and in 1928 established the first gastrointestinal clinic and remained its head until his retirement. He published on many areas of medicine, but concentrated mainly on gastroenterology and in 1934 commenced a series of papers with W.O. Abbott and W.G. Carr on intubation and studies of the small intestine which became classics and were made possible by the invention of the double lumen tube. This arose when Abbott was unable to keep a tube with one distended balloon at a fixed point of the duodenum and Miller suggested that a second open tube be tied to the bag to see if this would make sampling easier.

William O. Abbott (1902–1943) U.S. physician. He graduated from the University of Pennsylvania School of Medicine, Philadelphia in 1928 and was a physician in the gastrointestinal section of the medical clinic at the hospital of the University of Pennsylvania. He joined the U.S. army as a major in the Medical Reserve Corps in May 1942, but was honorably discharged with physical disability in September of the same year and died of leukemia.This may have followed the X-ray exposure he would have received in screening the position of the tube in the volunteers and patients he investigated. He was a nephew of William Osler, the W.O. of his name. A witty man he once wrote in a patient's chart as an intern, "The patient is a 53 year old spinster who, during her youth, had symptoms from all her organs. As an adult she had her organs removed one by one. Now she is a mere shell with symptoms where her organs used to be." One of the trainees of Miller and Abbott was Franz Ingelfinger.

MILLER FISHER SYNDROME

Thought to be a variant of Guillain-Barré Syndrome with optic nerve and/or 3rd nerve involvement but usually characterized by:

1. Ophthalmoplegia
2. Ataxia
3. Areflexia

Miller Fisher (1910–) Canadian neurologist who worked at the Montreal General Hospital, and then at the Massachusetts General Hospital and has written extensively on cerebrovascular accidents.

MILROY DISEASE

Congenital or familial lymphedema of the legs due to inadequate lymph flow through an anatomically abnormal lymphatic system.

William F. Milroy (1855–1942) U.S. physician. He was born in New York City and graduated from Columbia University in 1882 and after his internship practiced in Omaha and described the disorder in 1892. He was appointed Professor of Clinical Medicine in 1891 and retired in 1933. The eponym Milroy Disease was given to it by Sir William Osler in his textbook. In 1857 H. Meige of France also described similar patients and in France the disorder is sometimes called Meige Disease (*v. supra*) or Nonne-Milroy-Meige in Germany (*v. infra*).

MINEMATA DISEASE

Mercurial poisoning resultant from eating contaminated shellfish and fish from Minemata Bay, Japan, secondary to industrial pollution.

cf. HAFF DISEASE

MINKOWSKI-CHAUFFARD HEMOLYTIC JAUNDICE

Hereditary spherocytosis.

Oskar Minkowski (1858–1931) Born in Kowno, Lithuania in 1885, he was a Privatdozent in Königsberg. In 1891 he moved to Strasburg as an Extraordinary Professor. In 1900 he went to Cologne to be the Director of the hospital and became Professor of the Academy of that city. He finally moved to Breslau where he succeeded Ernst Strümpell (*v. infra*) as Professor of Medicine. His major contribution was to the understanding of diabetes. He recognized the association of acidosis with diabetic coma and showed that pancreatectomized dogs developed diabetes and concluded that the pancreas must contain a substance necessary for carbohydrate metabolism. He was a sound teacher and a well liked clinician and the noted French neurosurgeon Clovis Vincent trained with him.

Anatole M.E. Chauffard (1855–1932) French physician whose father was a Professor of the Medical Faculty of Paris and whose grandfather was a well known practitioner in Aignon. He interned at Broussais and then worked at Cochin and finally Saint-Antoine hospital where he took up a clinical chair in 1911 after being named Professor in 1909. He was an exceptional clinician and teacher but was equally at home in general pathology. His major investigative work was in liver disease where he contributed descriptive pathology as well as introducing in France the use of emetine for the treatment of amebic abscesses and defining the anaphylactic nature of events following rupture of hydatid cysts. He described the important diagnostic features of hereditary spherocytosis, viz. dominantly inherited hemolytic anemia with spherocytes and increased red cell fragility.

MINOR DISEASE

Hemorrhage into the spinal cord. Sudden onset of back pain with paraparesis or paraplegia usually seen with vascular malformation (v. FOIX-ALAJOUANINE SYNDROME), blood dyscrasias and patients on anticoagulants.

MINOR SWEAT TEST

Test of autonomic system. The skin is painted with iodine solution and dusted with starch powder, and the subject then drinks hot fluid after taking aspirin.

MINOR TREMOR

Essential tremor.

Lazar S. Minor (1855–   ) Russian neurologist. A student of A. Kozhevnikov whose obituary he wrote.

MINOT-MURPHY DIET

Raw liver fed to patients with pernicious anemia resulting in remission.

George R. Minot (1885–1950) U.S. physician. Noted hematologist who made numerous contributions to hematology especially in the field of anemias and bleeding disorders. He won the Nobel Prize for the successful treatment of pernicious anemia.

Graduated from Harvard in 1912. Interned at Massachusetts General Hospital and then Johns Hopkins Hospital in 1913, returning to the Massachusetts General in 1915. In 1921 he developed diabetes and became progressively worse until the introduction of insulin in 1922 which restored him to work. He became Director of the Thorndike Memorial Laboratory of the Boston City Hospital in 1927 and Professor of Medicine, Harvard. He was an outstanding teacher and investigator who whilst seemingly relaxed and prepared to give lengthy time to discussion with young investigators, put in prodigious time to his work. Not only did he possess the desire to explain the previously inexplicable but he imparted this to the younger people who worked with him on whom he impressed his urge to alleviate suffering and disability and his intense enthusiasm for teaching. He stated "to solve problems, an active, creative imagination and scientific curiosity are necessary tools".

Among his protégés were Soma Weiss, William Castle, Chester Keefer, Hale Ham, Maxwell Finland

and Eugene Stead, all of whom have left their own mark on American medicine and medical education.

William P. Murphy (1892–) U.S. physician. Worked with Minot as a Harvard undergraduate in the investigation of dietary treatment of pernicious anemia, winning the Nobel Prize in 1934 together with Minot and Whipple. G.H. Whipple (*v. infra*) had observed that liver was the most efficient food to enable dogs rendered anemic by exsanguination to restore their hemoglobin most rapidly. Minot reasoned that in pernicious anemia, nutritional liver would be the best foodstuff to give them, and together with Murphy exhibited liver to his patients with pernicious anemia.

MITSUDA REACTION

Lepromin test.

Kenonke Mitsuda Japanese physician.

MIYAGAWANELLA

Unique species of micro-organisms better known as chlamydia. These are obligatory intracellular parasites and are bacteria-like. They cause psittacosis, lymphoma venereum, trachoma, non-gonococcal urethritis, cervicitis, salpingitis and inclusion conjunctivitis.

Yoneji Miyagawa (1885–1959) Japanese bacteriologist.

MÖBIUS DISEASE

Ophthalmoplegic migraine.

MÖBIUS SIGN

Weakness of convergence seen in thyrotoxicosis.

MÖBIUS SYNDROME

Congenital facial diplegia, congenital occulofacial paralysis, infantile nuclear aplasia. Congenital bilateral facial palsy associated with 3rd and 6th nerve palsies. Mental deficit and 8th nerve disorders are also frequent and sometimes there are accompanying myopathic features.

MÖBIUS-LEYDEN DYSTROPHY

v. LEYDEN-MÖBIUS DYSTROPHY

Paul J. Möbius (1853–1907) German neurologist who was assistant to E.A.G.G. von Strümpell in Heidelberg. Born in Leipzig, first studied philosophy and theology and then medicine, graduating in 1877. Worked with Strümpell in Leipzig and then in Heidelberg, becoming Privatdozent in 1883 but gave up teaching in 1893. He wrote several books on neurology and had broader interests, and made pathological studies on Rousseau, Nietzsche and Goethe. He was a brilliant clinician. A male chauvinist, he wrote on the weakmindedness of women. He developed the concept of endogenous and exogenous disease states.

MOLLARET MENINGITIS

Benign recurrent endothelial-leukocytic meningitis. Sudden attack of fever and meningeal signs with an increased CSF pressure and characterized by pleocytosis with endothelial cells, leukocytes and lymphocytes. Spontaneous cure results without residual signs and an attack usually lasts only 2–3 days.

Pierre Mollaret (1898–) French physician.

MÖLLER GLOSSITIS

Chronic superficial glossitis sometimes extending to cheeks and palate, seen usually in women.

MÖLLER-BARLOW DISEASE

v. BARLOW DISEASE

Julius O.L. Möller (1819–1887) German physician who first described acute rickets combined with scurvy in 1859.

Thomas Barlow (*v. supra*).

MONAKOW SYNDROME

Contralateral hemiplegia, hemianesthesia and hemianopia following thrombosis of the anterior choroidal artery.

Konstantin von Monakow (1853–1930) Russian neurologist. He investigated functional areas of the cerebral cortex and made fundamental contributions to the red nucleus. Born on a family estate, Brobietzova in Vologda, north of Moscow. His father was a nobleman who was a censor of the political press during the reign of Nicholas I and Alexander II, and in 1863 for political reasons sold his property and migrated to Dresden and later to Paris, and finally Zurich, where he became naturalized.

He was not a good scholar as a schoolboy, became at odds with his father and left home at 17, and against his father's wishes enrolled in medicine. While still an undergraduate he went to Hitzig, then the Director of the Burgholzli asylum near Zurich, who sent him on a survey of the administration of German asylums. During this he visited von Gudden in Munich, who showed him his newly invented microtome and the sections of a rabbit's brain, showing atrophy of the superior colliculus after its eye on the opposite side had been removed at birth.

In 1877 he returned to Munich and then studied at Würzburg but he was in financial straits and so took a job as a ship's doctor on a boat to Brazil and on his return was appointed physician to the Cantonal Asylum, St. Dorminsberg, near Ragaz. In 1879 he removed the occipital lobes of two newborn rabbits and a year later found that the lateral geniculate nuclei were completely degenerated while the rest of the thalamus was intact. He spent 3 months in Berlin in 1885 attending lectures by Westphal, Oppenheim, Virchow, du Bois-Reymond and Munk, and then returned to Zurich. He entered practice with a private research laboratory which was eventually incorporated into the University of Zurich. He made classical studies on the visual and auditory pathways and the functional relationship of the thalamus. He examined localization and integration of function in the cortex. He was something of an eccentric, very heavily built, with a high pitched voice, an avid reader, who in his younger days was a bon vivant but settled down and became very involved with philosophy and religion. He was not interested in medical politics and is said to have attended only one faculty meeting, marking the occasion by wearing a Russian blouse and boots. His life was sufficiently flamboyant for the poetess Maria Waser to write his biography in the form of a novel. He retired in 1928 and died of uremia secondary to prostatic enlargement and refusing treatment. He had requested in his will that his spinal cord be examined to explain long standing wasting of his thenar eminence. Unfortunately his spinal cord was lost!

MÖNCKEBERG ARTERIOSCLEROSIS OR SCLEROSIS

Seen in arteries with well developed muscular coat (e.g. the radial and temporal arteries) with medial degeneration and replacement by calcium giving readily felt thickening – medial sclerosis.

Johann G. Mönckeberg (1877–1925) German pathologist. He was born in Hamburg, his father being a Senator of the then free city. After graduation he worked as the assistant to E. Frankel at the Eppendorf Hospital and it was whilst he was under his guidance that he wrote his famous paper on atherosclerosis. In 1903 he was appointed first assistant to Weigert in Frankfurt and in 1904 moved to work with Boström in Giessen where he was promoted to Associate Professor in 1908. In 1912 he was appointed Professor of Pathology at Düsseldorf where he succeeded Lubarsch. In 1916 he was appointed Professor of Pathology at Strasburg where he succeeded Hans Chiari. When the French occupied Strasburg, he was expelled although at the time he was extremely ill with influenza and took some time recuperating in Freiburg before he succeeded Baumgarten to the Chair in Tübingen and in 1922 he moved once more to follow Ribbert in Bonn. He had another episode of influenza in 1923 and although he was asked to move to Hamburg to follow his old teacher Frankel, he was so sick that he refused. He developed chronic renal disease and died with uremia. His main contributions were the pathology of the vascular system including studies on the conducting system in the heart.

MONDOR DISEASE

Thrombophlebitis often affecting the thoraco-epigastric vein when it results in swelling over the breast (similar in appearance to lymphatic obstruction) which may be mistaken for cancer.

Henri Mondor (1885–1962) French surgeon. Born in the small village of Saint-Cernin where he was educated. He went to Paris in 1903 to study medicine and graduated in 1908. He worked with Henri Hartmann, Charles Waltham and J-L. Favre. In 1914 he volunteered and worked in the Army Medical Corps at the front throughout the war. He became agrégé in 1923 and in 1938 was appointed Professor of Pathological Surgery and in 1941 Professor of Surgery. He collected books and had a great interest in medical history.

MONGE DISEASE

Mountain sickness.

Carlos Monge (1884–1970) Peruvian physician. He was born in Lima, Peru, and graduated from San Marcos University San Fernando Medical School in 1911. He spent a year in England in 1912 studying at the School of Tropical Medicine and returned to Peru to gain his Ph.D. in 1913. Initially he worked on leishmaniasis, Carrion disease, leprosy and other tropical illnesses. He commenced his work on chronic mountain sickness in 1925, organizing the first medical expedition to the mining towns, La Oroya and Morococha, in the Peruvian Andes in 1927 and publishing his famous monograph in 1928 "La Enfermedad de los Andes". In 1931 he was appointed Professor of Medicine at San Fernando Medical School and he founded the National Institute of Andean Biology and became its Director in 1934. He remained Professor of Medicine until he retired in 1957. During his final years he suffered with Paget disease.

MONIZ SIGN

Forceful plantar flexion at the ankle may result in dorsiflexion of the toes in pyramidal tract lesions.

Antonio Egas Moniz (1874–1955) Portuguese neurologist. He studied medicine at the University of Coimbra, graduating in 1899. He studied neurology at Bordeaux and Paris and was appointed Professor of Neurology at Coimbra, then Professor of Neurology in Lisbon in 1911. He introduced cerebral arteriography and leukotomy. He was active in politics and served as a deputy in Lisbon from 1903–1917. He won the Nobel Prize in 1949 for his contribution to neurological physiology and neurosurgery.

His real name was Antonio Caetano de Abrea Freire and he was born on his family's farm in Avanca in northern Portugal. His godfather named him Egas Moniz after the hero of Portuguese resistance against the Moors. Moniz initially was heavily involved in politics and he was Minister of Foreign Affairs and Ambassador to Spain after the monarchy was overthrown. At the end of World War I he was Portugal's signatory to the Treaty of Versailles. Although he had written a book on the physiology and pathology of sex, and also after World War I a monograph on neurology in war, it was only when his party was defeated that he concentrated on neurology, and when 52 he conceived the idea of cerebral angiography. He was the author of several other works including an autobiography. He was an urbane man who loved good living and suffered from gout. At 65 he was shot in his office by one of his schizophrenic patients but he recovered to die peacefully on the farm on which he was born.

MONNARET PULSE

Bradycardia associated with jaundice.

Jules Monnaret (1810–1868) French physician.

MONRO FORAMEN

Foramen of Monro – interventricular foramen between lateral and third ventricles.

Alexander Monro (1733–1817) Scottish anatomist. Succeeded his father (primus) as Professor of Anatomy in Edinburgh in 1758. Like his father, he was a gifted teacher and made many studies of the lymphatics and nervous system. In 1808 his son (tertius) succeeded him as Professor of Anatomy at Edinburgh University. He, however, was less noted than his father or grandfather, and Charles Darwin is quoted as saying "made his lectures on human anatomy as dull as he was himself". The first Alexander Monro was a student of Boerhaave and appointed as Professor of Anatomy at Edinburgh in 1720, so there was an Alexander Monro as Professor of Anatomy there from 1720 until 1846!

MONTGOMERY GLANDS

Apocrine sweat glands in the areola of the nipple.

MONTGOMERY TUBERCLES

Swelling of Montgomery glands during pregnancy and lactation.

William F. Montgomery (1797–1859) Irish obstetrician who graduated M.B. from Trinity College, Dublin, in 1825. His major book "On the Signs of Pregnancy" was published in 1837 in London but he wrote on other aspects of obstetrics and a student text on therapeutics. Although recognized internationally he never became "Master" of the Rotunda Lying-in Hospital but he became the first Professor of Midwifery in Dublin. Rather vain of his appearance he usually wore a white tie with a diamond shirt stud.

MOON MOLARS

Cusps of first molars look like mulberries as a result of congenital syphilis.

Henry Moon (1845–1892) English dental surgeon at Guy's Hospital. He was appointed assistant dental surgeon in 1868 and in 1880 became the Lecturer in Dental Surgery and senior dentist but ill health forced his early retirement in 1887. Apart from his work on teeth abnormalities he stressed the importance of milk and white flour in providing calcium for adequate tooth development.

MOORE LIGHTNING STREAKS

Flashes of lightning seen on the temporal side of the eye due to intra-ocular causes.

MOORE SYNDROME

Abdominal epilepsy.

Matthew T. Moore (1901–) U.S. neurologist and neuro-psychiatrist, born in Philadelphia and graduated M.D. Temple University in 1927. Professor and neuropathologist, Graduate School of Medicine, University of Pennsylvania. His research interests included schizophrenic degenerative disorders of the brain and cerebrovascular disease.

MOOREN ULCER

Rodent ulcer of the cornea.

Albert Mooren (1828–1899) German ophthalmologist. He was born in Oedt on the lower Rhine and studied ophthalmology with A. von Graefe, graduating in medicine in 1854. He worked for a while in his home town, but he moved to Düsseldorf and became director of the Eye Hospital there in 1862 and remained in that position until he retired in 1883. After his retirement he continued in private practice in Düsseldorf. From 1863–1878 he was consulting ophthalmologist and surgeon at the "Institut Ophthalmologique" in Liege.

His major interests were in operative procedures in ophthalmology and he was the first to undertake operations on the lens in order to treat myopia. He contracted malaria whilst at the International Medical Congress in America and was seriously ill with it from 1887–1888.

MORAX-AXENFELD BACILLUS

Moraxella lacunata – the cause of Morax-Axenfeld conjunctivitis, chronic conjunctivitis.

Victor Morax (1866–1935) French ophthalmologist. A native of Switzerland, he studied medicine at Freiburg and Paris and became an ophthalmic surgeon at the Hopital Laboisière as well as working at the Pasteur Institute. He described the organism causing chronic conjunctivitis simultaneously with Axenfeld, and wrote a book with Henri Huchard "Traité des névroses".

Karl T.P. Axenfeld (1867–1930) German ophthalmologist who published a definitive article on metastatic ophthalmia in 1899 and worked in Freiburg.

MOREL-KRAEPELIN DISEASE

Schizophrenia.

v. KRAEPELIN-MOREL DISEASE

MORGAGNI FORAMEN

Areas between the diaphragm and sternum and costal margin which may be the site of diaphragmatic hernia.

MORGAGNI-ADAMS-STOKES SYNDROME

v. STOKES-ADAMS SYNDROME

Giovanni B. Morgagni (1682–1771) Italian anatomist and pathologist. He published "Seats and causes of disease investigated by the means of anatomy" in 1761, the same year as Auerbruggen's "New invention to detect hidden diseases of the chest by way of percussion". Morgagni was born in Forli. As a youth he wrote poetry, graduated aged 19 from medical school at Bologna and continued in anatomy. He was an excellent teacher and a prolific writer. He was a student of Valsalva, later Professor at Padua 1715–1771, and published his life work when he was 79. This was the first time correlation was made between the pathology found at postmortem and clinical findings. He was the first to describe cerebral gumma and diseases of heart valves, and recorded the first instance of heart block. He described the Stokes-Adams attacks in a patient who was a merchant of Padua "When visiting by way of consultation, I found with such a rarity of the pulse that within the 60th part of an hour the pulsations were only 22 – and this rareness which was perpetual ... was perceived to be even more considerable, as often as even two (epileptic) attacks were at hand – so that the physicians were never deceived from the increase of the rareness they foretold a paroxysm to be coming on." He described syphilitic aneurysms, acute yellow atrophy, that intracerebral infection could follow ear infection, and he proved Valsalva's contention that the cerebral lesion in stroke causing paralysis is on the opposite side of the brain. He described Fallot tetralogy, aortic coarctation and pneumonia with consolidation. He believed in contagion and would not dissect patients with tuberculosis or smallpox. Virchow considered that Morgagni introduced modern pathology "with him begins modern medicine". Morgagni was an active and practicing clinician, as well as a historian and philosopher.

MORO REFLEX OR RESPONSE

Seen in first 6 months of life – a loud noise or passive movement of the child's head results in abduction and extention of all extremities and fanning of all digits but flexion of thumb and first finger followed by flexion and adduction of the extremities. Absence under 6 months of age suggests diffuse central nervous system damage and asymmetric responses are seen with all forms of palsies – its presence after 6 months of age suggests cortical disturbance.

Ernst Moro (1874–1951) Austrian pediatrician, born in Lalbach. He studied skin responses and described the skin reactions to tuberculin. He first isolated *Lactobacillus acidophilus*.

MORQUIO SYNDROME

(Also called MORQUIO-BRAILSFORD DISEASE)

Mucopolysaccharidosis Type IV. Inherited as an autosomal recessive, it results in dwarfism, and bone deformities, with failure of development of the trunk and normal growth of the extremities. Mental impairment may occur but neurological problems usually result from secondary neural compression. Keratin sulphate is excreted in large amounts in the urine. Its incidence is 1:40 000.

v. HURLER SYNDROME

Luis Morquio (1867–1935) Uruguayan pediatrician, born in Montevideo and commenced studying medicine there in 1887, graduating from the faculty in 1892. He undertook his postgraduate work in Paris at Grancher's Clinic for Sick Children where he worked for Marfan (*v. supra*) and attended clinics of Charcot, Potain and Dieulafoy as well as Hayem and Lancereaux (*v. supra*). He returned to Uruguay in 1894 and commenced practice as a pediatrician as well as undertaking academic duties, becoming Professor in 1900. He was an outstanding pediatrician in Uruguay and had many honors conferred on him, including the Legion of Honour from France and in 1930 was appointed Director of the Institute of Clinical Paediatrics in Montevideo.

James F. Brailsford (1888–1961) British radiologist. He was born in Birmingham. He was working as an accountant/clerk when because of his interest in photography he applied for a job to do work in this area in the pathology and bacteriology department in Birmingham University. It was here that the then medical officer of health for Birmingham, Dr. (later Sir) John Robertson employed him to photograph specimens he had obtained from animals with tuberculosis. As Brailsford says, "photography was the means by which I secured the greatest friend of my life". He was appointed special investigator to the medical officer of health, and with Robertson studied the terrible conditions of the slums where tuberculosis had an incidence four times greater than in the better suburbs and helped Robertson in his campaign against the disease. W.A. Cadbury was the Chairman of Birmingham Public Health Committee and learning of his desire to do medicine, subsidized him so that he could take a medical course. The 1st World War, however, commenced, and Brailsford joined the R.A.M.C. as a radiographer and at the end of the war returned to his medical studies and graduated from the University of Birmingham in 1923. He was soon appointed as radiologist to the Queen's Hospital and St. Chad's Hospital, Birmingham, and rapidly established a fine reputation and in 1934 published his book "Radiology of Bones and Joints" which became a standard text and went through many editions.

He had a superb collection of plant and bird life photographs and was the first President of the British Association of Radiologists. His very strength of individualist activity and uncompromising approach also led him at times to misjudgements. He was bitterly opposed to the use of deep X-ray therapy for example. He publicly opposed mass radiology and the development of thoracic surgery, saying in one of his last articles that a radiograph that led to an operation was a bad radiograph. He was never slow to put his views to both speech and paper and as a result was embroiled in constant controversy.

MORTON METATARSALGIA

Pain between 3rd and 4th toes due to a neurofibroma of the digital branches of the medial and lateral plantar nerves.

Thomas G. Morton (1835–1903) U.S. surgeon, described this in 1876. He was one of the first to remove an inflamed appendix after a correct diagnosis with the patient surviving in 1877.

MORTON SYNDROME

Tenderness in the base of 2nd metatarsal bone, callosities beneath 2nd and 3rd metatarsals and hypertrophy of the 2nd metatarsal due to a short 1st metatarsal bone.

Dudley J. Morton (1884–1960) U.S. orthopedic surgeon.

MORVAN DISEASE

Syringomyelia with trophic changes in the extremities.

Augustin M. Morvan (1819–1917) French physician. He described it in 1883.

MOSCHOWITZ SYNDROME

Thrombotic thrombocytopenic purpura.

MOSCHOWITZ TEST OR SIGN

The leg is elevated and a tourniquet applied for 5 minutes. After the tourniquet is removed and the leg lowered to the horizontal a hyperemic blush occurs in 2–5 seconds. Delayed blushing is suggestive of arterial occlusive disease.

Eli Moschowitz (1879–1964) U.S. physician in New York who wrote a definitive article on pulmonary hypertension in 1927.

MOTT CELL

Grape cell. A histiocyte which has ingested material (? lipid), giving it an intracytoplasmic appearance like a bunch of grapes.

MOTT LAW OF ANTICIPATION

Hereditary disease may appear earlier in successive generations.

Sir Frederick W. Mott (1853–1926) British neuropathologist, born in Brighton, England, he graduated in 1881 from medical school at University College, London. In 1883 he became assistant Professor of Physiology in Liverpool but returned to London in 1884 and lectured in physiology and pathology and was appointed as a physician and finally pathologist in charge at the Maudsley Hospital, London (until 1923) when he moved to Birmingham as Lecturer in Morbid Psychology and was pathologist to the London county asylums.

He described the cell which he termed a morula cell in a monograph on sleeping sickness in 1906. He wrote a number of monographs, one being on war neurosis and shell shock, and undertook research on nerve pathways, especially those related to eye movements. He was particularly interested in higher center expression of disease and emphasized these effects in syphilis, myxedema and acute anemia states. Whilst at the Charing Cross Hospital, London he became friends with William Hunter (*v. supra*) but disagreed with him on the pathogenesis of pernicious anemia saying Hunter argued from one post-mortem whilst he Mott had performed 3! He was editor of Archives of Neurology and Psychiatry.

MOYNIHAN SYMPTOM COMPLEX

Hunger pain 3–4 hours after eating suggesting duodenal ulcer.

Berkeley G.A. Moynihan (Baron Lord Moynihan) (1865–1936) English surgeon, born in Malta and studied medicine in Leeds, London and Berlin. Professor of Surgery at Leeds. His outstanding contributions were to abdominal surgery and he popularized gastroenterostomy for peptic ulcer.

MUCHA-HABERMANN DISEASE

Pityriasis lichenoides et varioliformis acuta.

Viktor Mucha (1877–1919) Austrian dermatologist who worked with Landsteiner on dark field illumination to diagnose syphilis.

Rudolph Habermann (1884–1941) German dermatologist.

MUEHRCKE LINES

Two parallel white lines separated by normal nail seen in hypo-albuminemia.

Robert S. Muehrcke U.S. renal physician.

MÜLLER DUCT

or

MÜLLERIAN DUCT

Paramesonephric duct.

Johannes Peter Müller (1801–1858) German anatomist and physiologist. He was born in the town of Coblenz when it was occupied by French troops. His father was a shoemaker. He was initially going to study for the Catholic Church but changed to medicine. He graduated at Bonn in 1822 and spent 18 months in Berlin with Rudolphi, who taught him that the scientific approach of experiment and observation was the best approach to solving scientific problems rather than philosophical speculation. He returned to Bonn where he was at first Privatdozent (1824) then assistant Professor (1828) and finally Professor of Anatomy and Physiology (1830). In 1833, on the death of Rudolphi, he was appointed to Berlin and remained there until he died.

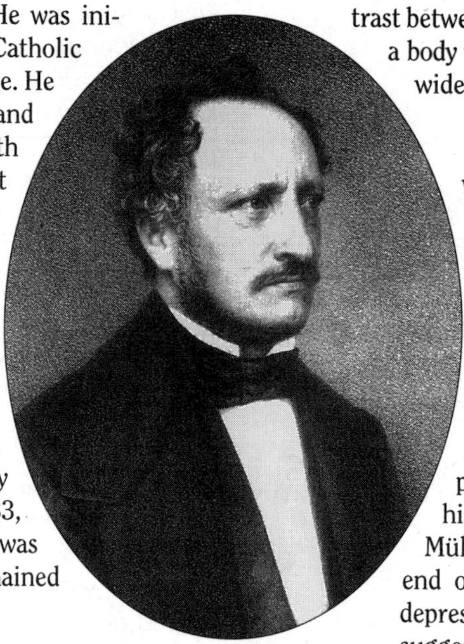

Johannes Peter Müller (Courtesy of the Royal Society of Medicine, London, UK)

Although he believed in the scientific process, he was a religious man who believed that all forms of nature had proceeded from the creative spirit of God and had not arisen through chance. When he was in Bonn in 1826 he published a work on ghosts. He made no major discoveries but his work was sound and above all he was an inspiring teacher who made contributions to all areas of the natural sciences. In 1834 he founded Müller's Archives and published a book on physiology which contained much of his and his students' work. He left an enormous number of students, many of whom made major contributions; some of these were Schwann, Henle, Du Bois-Reymond, Helmholtz and Virchow. Virchow had a particularly high regard for him and was much influenced by his approach and he wrote an interesting eulogy on Müller. He describes him as behaving like a preacher in a lecture and being very intolerant of any interruptions or disturbances, staring coldly at the offender until he left the lecture theatre. Virchow wrote of him, "What a contrast, when the usually cold and stern face suddenly changed into an expression of kind benevolence, and the eyes laughed more than the face, like warm sun rays piercing through clouds. In those moments, Müller was a captivating individual and one became conscious of the spiritual greatness of man. Physically one was also aware of the contrast between the great, wonderful head and a body whose only prominence was the wide shoulders."

Müller's main contributions were the introduction of the use of the microscope in the examination of tumors, studies on nerve transmission and color appreciation. He demonstrated the bristle cells of the internal ear and the whole of the fine anatomy of glandular and cartilaginous tissues as well as comparative work on fish. He made his embryological discovery of the Müllerian duct in 1825. Towards the end of his life he suffered bouts of depression and died suddenly, some suggest by his own hand. An enormous crowd attended his funeral; among his former students carrying his coffin was the famous biologist Ernst H. Haeckel and Alexander von Humboldt delivered the graveside eulogy.

MÜLLER MUSCLE

1. Orbital muscle.
2. Tensal muscle.
3. Innermost portion of the ciliary muscle.

Heinrich Müller (1820–1864) German anatomist who with R.A. Kolliken first measured action currents in cardiac muscle. He discovered visual purple.

MÜLLER SYNDROME

Hypercholesterolemia, xanthelasma, xanthomas and cardiac disease. Essential hypercholesterolemia inherited as an autosomal dominant.

C. Müller (1886–) Norwegian physician.

MUNCHAUSEN SYNDROME

Malingerer who employs vivid and imaginative symptoms to obtain medical care, hospitalization and/or drugs, and when discovered transfers his/her allegiance to another hospital or town.

Baron Hieronymus K.F.Freiherr von Munchausen (1720–1797) German traveller and soldier who told a number of preposterous stories to guests at his estate in Hesse about his heroic exploits. These were published by an impecunious family friend, R.E. Raspe, in England in a book "Baron Munchausen's Narrative of His Marvellous Travels and Campaigns in Russia". The name was given to this syndrome by Richard Asher.

MUNCHMEYER DISEASE

Progressive myositis ossificans.

Ernst Munchmeyer (1846–1880) German physician.

MURPHY SIGN

1. Sign of cholecystitis. After deep palpation under the mid point of the right subcostal margin the patient is asked to inspire with resultant pain.
2. Pinch tenderness over the costovertebral angle in perinephric abscess.

John B. Murphy (1857–1916) U.S. surgeon. Born in Appleton, Wisconsin, he became Professor of Surgery at Northwestern University, Chicago, from 1895–1916. A protégé of Christian Finger, after interning in Cook County Hospital and a brief period in practice he went to Vienna to work with Billroth in 1882, and afterwards visited Berlin and Heidelberg. He did much pioneering work on intestinal anastomosis including anastomosis of the gall bladder to the intestine. In 1896 he was the first person to successfully unite a femoral artery severed by a gunshot wound. He had previously undertaken much experimentation on end-to-end resections of arteries and veins. In his technique he invaginated the intima outside the adventitia of the vessel. This resulted in a narrowing of the lumen and of 13 cases only 4 were successful. He was a pioneer in the use of bone grafting and made contributions to the understanding and management of ankylosis as well as independently proposing artificial pneumothorax to manage unilateral lung disease in tuberculosis. A child he had been treating with tuberculosis died in a car accident and at autopsy he found that several tubercular cavities were healing on one side of the lung which was collapsed by the disease. He had a curiously harsh and strident voice but he nonetheless could fire the enthusiasm in his audience and was a fine clinical teacher as well as a painstaking operator.

A tall man with a parted red beard, with outspoken views, his flamboyant character and appearance made him good copy for the news media which upset the local conservatives and older surgeons. He was troubled throughout his life with recurrences of tuberculosis.

MURRAY VALLEY ENCEPHALITIS

Acute viral encephalitis seen in the Murray River valley area in Australia. Thought to be endemic in the water bird life and vector to be the mosquito. Also called Australia X Disease.

Murray Valley Area in Northwestern Victoria, through which flows the Murray River where the State of Victoria borders the State of New South Wales.

MUSSET SIGN

v. supra, DE MUSSET.

McARDLE SYNDROME OR DISEASE

Weakness and cramping in muscles after exercise due to a phosphorylase deficiency resulting in an accumulation of glycogen in muscle, also called glycogen storage disease type V.

Brian McArdle (1911–) He was born in London and studied medicine at Guy's Hospital, graduating in 1933. After working at a number of London hospitals including Guy's, he joined the Department of Medicine at Cambridge in 1936 and became interested in periodic paralysis. In 1939 he moved to Medical Research Council Unit at the National Hospital for Nervous Diseases, Queen Square, where he had intended to work on muscle disorders, but with the outbreak of the war he turned to investigation of motion sickness and its treatment and studied ability to work in very hot conditions as part of an applied physiology project for the armed forces.

After the war he returned to Guy's Hospital and remained there until his retirement. His major research interests were muscle metabolism and its disorders and demyelinating disease.

McBURNEY POINT

A point midway between the umbilicus and the anterior superior iliac spine – often the site of maximum tenderness in acute appendicitis.

McBURNEY SIGN

Maximum tenderness over McBurney point in acute appendicitis.

Charles McBurney (1845–1913) U.S. surgeon, born in Roxbury, Massachusetts. After graduating in arts from Harvard in 1866, he went to New York and obtained his M.D. from the College of Physicians and Surgeons in 1870. He spent 2 years in Europe and commenced practice in New York in 1873, gaining appointment as an assistant demonstrator in anatomy at the College of Physicians and Surgeons. He was elected assistant surgeon to the Bellevue Hospital in 1880, and in 1888 was appointed the Surgeon-in-Chief at the Roosevelt Hospital. He reported his sign in 1889 and rapidly made his hospital one of the centres of surgical excellence in the world of its day. He published numerous papers and was a keen hunter and fisherman. He died of a coronary thrombosis while on a hunting trip.

McCARTHY REFLEX

Tapping the outside edge of the supraorbital ridge results in closure of the eye unilaterally or bilaterally with lesions above the facial nucleus. No response is elicited with lesions at or below the 7th nucleus.

Daniel J. McCarthy (1874–1965) U.S. neurologist.

MACLEOD SYNDROME

v. SWYER-JAMES SYNDROME

W.M. Macleod British chest physician.

MacCORMAC REFLEX

Crossed adduction of the opposite thigh following elicitation of the knee jerk.

William MacCormac (1836–1901) Irish surgeon from Belfast who followed Lister's principles. He served in the Franco-Prussian and Turco-Serbian wars and pioneered surgery of intraperitoneal rupture of the bladder.

McNAGHTEN RULE

A person may claim insanity as a defense to a crime he has committed, if he can show that at the time he committed the crime he was suffering from a defect of reason and that the defect of reason was such that he either did not know the nature and quality of his act, or that what he was doing was wrong.

Daniel McNaghten A Scot born between 1810–16, the illegitimate son of a poor farmer's daughter and a Glaswegian woodturner with whom he became apprenticed, but was refused a partnership by his father who feared it might prejudice the chances of his legitimate offspring. Daniel then established his own business in Glasgow but after an illness in 1834 he began to have difficulty sleeping and in 1837 his behavior was so strange that he was asked to leave his rooming house and he slept at his shop. He developed increasing delusions of persecution and in 1841 tried to sell his business believing he was pursued by Jesuits and the Tories and even went to France to try to escape, but without success. He believed Sir Robert Peel, the then Prime Minister of Great Britain, had the power to stop this persecution, but would not. On January 20th, 1843, he shot Edward Drummond, Robert Peel's secretary, mistaking him for Peel. Drummond died five days later and McNaghten was tried for murder, but declared insane by the judge and permanently committed to an insane asylum.

N

NABOTHIAN CYST

Cystic distension of the mucous gland (NABOTHIAN GLAND) of the cervix uteri.

Martin Naboth (1675–1721) Born in Kalau, Saxony. He studied in Leipzig, graduating in medicine in 1703. He was initially in general practice but studied anatomy and became Professor of Chemistry in Leipzig in 1707, the year he described his cysts.

NAEGELI LEUKEMIA

Myelomonocytic leukemia – many cells in the peripheral blood are morphologically of the myeloid series.

Otto Naegeli (1871–1938) Swiss hematologist who was Professor of Medicine at Tübingen in Germany and then at Zurich University, retiring in 1937, to be followed by W. Löffler. He made many contributions to hematological diagnostic methods and leukemia, and reported the leukopenia in typhus as well as writing a textbook on blood disorders.

NAFFZIGER SYNDROME

Scalenus anterior syndrome. Numbness and tingling along ulnar border of the forearm which may be relieved by elevation. There may be associated wasting of the thenar eminence.

NAFFZIGER TEST

1. Pressure on the jugular vein results in increased cerebrospinal fluid pressure and may cause pain in the case of a herniated disc.
2. Pressure on the scalenus anticus muscle at the base of the neck causes tingling in the hand in the scalenus anticus syndrome.

Howard C. Naffziger (1884–1961) U.S. neurosurgeon, born in Nevada City, California, graduated from the University of California in 1909 and joined the faculty as an instructor in surgery in 1912 to become Professor of Neurological Surgery and Chairman of the department. During the 1st World War he was detailed on special duty in Washington DC but later served with the expeditionary force in France. During World War II he commanded U.S. Hospital No. 30 in the Far East and maintained his interest in that area, being Chairman of W.H.O. Mission (Medical) to the Philippines and Visiting Professor in Taiwan. He died of reticulum cell sarcoma.

NAGEOTTE-BABINSKI SYNDROME

v. BABINSKI-NAGEOTTE SYNDROME

NEFTEL DISEASE

Atremia – hysterical inability to walk but normal performance of all movements lying down.

William B. Neftel (1830–1906) U.S. physician. He was born in Russia and graduated in St. Petersburg in 1852 and joined the army serving as a surgeon at the Crimean War in the Imperial Guard. In 1865 he went to New York where he introduced electrotherapy. His wife was Princess Nadine of Georgia and grand-daughter of its King George XIII.

NEGRI BODIES

Acidophilic inclusion bodies in the cytoplasm of nerve cells, diagnostic of rabies.

Adelchi Negri (1867–1912) Italian microbiologist who was born in Perugia and attended medical school at Pavia where he graduated in 1900 to become assistant to Golgi (*v. supra*) at the Pathological Institute. In 1908 he was appointed Professor of Microbiology at the University of Pavia and held that position until he died in 1912.

From 1899–1902 he worked mainly on the structure of red blood corpuscles and the origin of blood platelets as well as the cytology of glandular structures in mammals and the changes which took place in blood elements during clotting. In 1903 he commenced his work on rabies and soon recognized and demonstrated that the bodies that have received his name were a constant feature in the nervous system of animals and man infected with the disorder. He mistakenly regarded them as parasitic protozoa. Other contributions included work on bacillary dysentery, and his demonstration that vaccinia virus passed through bacterial filters then in use. During the last years of his life he became particularly interested in malaria and took a very active role in endeavors to eliminate it from Lombardy.

NEISSERIA

Gram negative organisms causing gonorrhea.

Albert L.S. Neisser (1855–1916) German physician and bacteriologist, born in the Silesian town of Schweidnitz near Breslau (Wroclaw), the son of a well known Jewish physician. He studied at Breslau and Erlangen, gaining his M.D. in 1877, and becoming assistant to O. Simon in the dermatology clinic originally founded by Koebner (*v. supra*). He discovered the cause of gonorrhea in 1879 and three years later was appointed as director of the dermatology clinic, when Simon died of cancer of the stomach, and became Professor of Skin and Venereal Diseases, Breslau. He demonstrated that syphilis could be transmitted to lower apes in 1906 following an expedition to Java (which he personally financed) to study syphilis in monkeys, which had originally been described by Metchnikoff and Roux in 1903. He collaborated with Wassermann in the development of Wassermann reaction and was a close friend of Paul Ehrlich and collaborated with him in the testing of his organic arsenical preparations in the treatment of syphilis. He was publicly censored and fined in 1900 for injecting syphilitic serum into four healthy people and no useful observations were apparently obtained from this venture.

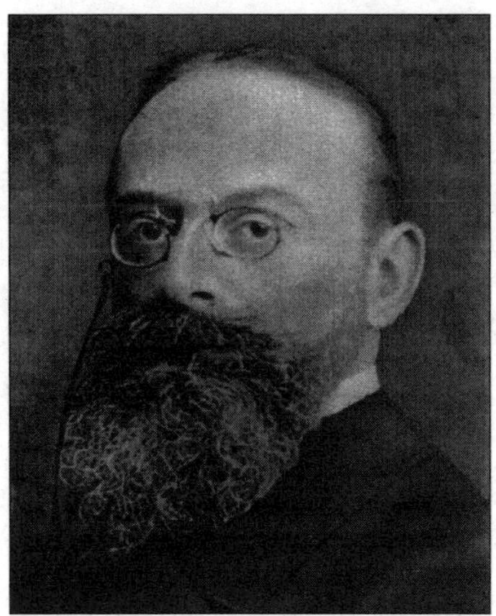

Albert L.S. Neisser (Courtesy of the Royal Society of Medicine, London, UK)

He was a diabetic and fell and broke his femur a few years before his death, never recovering his health completely. He suffered with renal calculi and after having colic and cystitis had the stone removed from his bladder in Berlin and returned to Breslau but developed septicemia and died.

NÉLATON LINE

A line drawn from the ischial tuberosity to the anterior superior iliac spine. In congenital dislocation of the hip the tip of the greater trochanter lies above this line.

Auguste Nélaton (1807–1873) French surgeon. He was born in Paris and graduated in medicine there in 1836. He was attached to the Hôpital St. Louis and became Professor of Surgery in 1851 and surgeon to Napoleon III in 1867. He had a remarkably fine reputation as a teacher and technical surgeon, and as a very modest and friendly person.

He invented a porcelain tipped probe for bullets, first used on Garibaldi, and invented a flexible rubber urethral catheter. He was a pioneer of ovariotomy in France and first described retro-uterine hematocele and improved the treatment of nasopharyngeal tumors.

NELSON SYNDROME

10% of patients with pituitary dependent adrenal hyperfunction develop pituitary tumors; most commonly after bilateral adrenalectomy. These are usually chromophobe adenomas which are rapidly growing and cause visual field defects. The most striking clinical feature is increasing cutaneous pigmentation.

Don H. Nelson (1925–) U.S. endocrinologist, born in Salt Lake City, Utah, graduated M.D. University of Utah 1947, interned at Milwaukee County Hospital and worked at Peter Bent Brigham Hospital, Boston, and held posts at the University of Southern California, returning as Professor of Medicine at University of Utah in 1966. His major research interests have been in the control and mechanisms of action of the corticosteroids.

NERI SIGN

1. With the patient lying down alternate raising of the legs results in flexion of the knee on the affected side in cerebral hemiplegia.
2. Arm sign – passive flexion of patient's elbow while lying down with the arms pronated causes supination of the affected arm in cerebral hemiplegia.
3. Sciatic nerve involvement – with the patient standing and flexing at the trunk, flexion of the knee on the affected side will result, to avoid stretching of the sciatic nerve.

Vincenzo Neri (1882–) Italian neurologist.

NERNST POTENTIAL

Potential across a membrane due to activities of ions on either side of the membrane.

Walter Nernst (1865–1941) German physicist. He was born in Briesen, West Prussia, and graduated Ph.D. from Würzburg University in 1887 and went to work as Ostwald's assistant in Graz. He became Professor of Physics at the University of Berlin in 1905 and won the Nobel Prize in Chemistry in 1921.

NETHERTON SYNDROME

Erythroderma ichthyosiforme congenitum.

Abnormality of the hair and frequent allergic reactions.

Earl W. Netherton (1893–) U.S. dermatologist.

NETTLESHIP DISEASE OR SYNDROME

Urticaria pigmentosa.

Edward Nettleship (1845–1913) English dermatologist and ophthalmic surgeon. He was born in Kettering, England. He studied at the Royal Agricultural College and King's College Medical School, London. He became Professor of Veterinary Surgery at the Royal Agricultural College in Cirencester in 1867, curator of the Moorfields Eye Hospital Museum in 1871, then in 1871 ophthalmic surgeon to St. Thomas's Hospital. He was inspector of the metropolitan poor schools and in this capacity he worked on incidence of eye disease and ophthalmia which led to parliamentary reforms. He wrote a book "Treasury of Human Inheritance" and his major research interest was in hereditary eye diseases. The Nettleship Medal of the Ophthalmological Society was established in his honor. He was elected F.R.S. in 1912.

NEUHAUSER SIGN

1. Sign of meconium ileus – bubbly appearance of inspissated meconium in X-rays of newborn's abdomen.
2. Absence of adenoid tissue in the nasopharynx in agammaglobulinemia.

NEUHAUSER-BERENBERG SYNDROME

Vomiting in infants due to a non-functioning cardioesophageal sphincter with dilation of the esophagus.

Edward B.D. Neuhauser (1908–) U.S. radiologist.

William Berenberg (1915–) U.S. radiologist.

NEWCASTLE BONE DISEASE

Form of renal osteodystrophy in dialysis patients associated with excessive deposition of aluminium.

NEWCASTLE DISEASE

Disease in fowls caused by Newcastle virus which results in pneumonia and encephalomyelitis and causes a mild conjunctivitis in man.

Newcastle City in the North of England.

NEWTONIAN

Relating to or described by the English mathematician and physicist, Newton.

Sir Isaac Newton (1642–1727) A graduate of Trinity College, Cambridge, in 1671, he invented calculus, discovered gravity (1665) and introduced the laws of motion and thermo-dynamics.

NEZELOF SYNDROME

Recurrent infections, absent delayed hypersensitivity, inability to reject skin allografts and reduced lymphocyte response to mitogens and specific antigens, strikingly reduced IgA and IgG levels and somewhat reduced IgM due to thymic deficiency. Inherited as an autosomal recessive.

C. Nezelof 20th century French pediatrician.

NICHOLAS-KULTSCHITZSKY CELLS

v. KULTSCHITZSKY CELLS

A. Nicholas French histologist.

NICOL PRISM

Prism for producing polarized light.

William A. Nicol (1768–1851) Scottish physicist.

NICOTIANA

A genus of plants including tobacco.

NICOTINE

An alkaloid from tobacco plants having stimulant and inhibitory effects on nervous tissue.

Jean Nicot (1530–1600) French diplomat who was ambassador to Portugal (1559–1561) and introduced tobacco to France in 1565. He had intended it for medical use rather than just for smoking.

NIEMANN-PICK DISEASE

Lipoidosis presenting in early life with anemia, hepatosplenomegaly, mental retardation, retinal degeneration and skin pigmentation due to accumulation of sphingomyelin secondary to a lack of the enzyme sphingomyelinase.

Albert Niemann (1880–1921) German pediatrician, described the condition in 1914 in a Jewish child with extensive central nervous system damage, who died aged 2. He isolated cocaine from the coca leaves.

Ludwig Pick (1868–1944) German pathologist in Berlin who proved histologically (1926) that it differed from Gaucher Disease, and drew attention to Niemann's original description. He reported a masculinizing ovarian tumor in 1905. He was described as very short and very fat and was a "workaholic" commencing at 6 a.m. and finishing at 7 or 8 p.m. He was a confirmed bachelor, commenting "love is an acute psychosis that may always be given a good prognosis." Imprisoned by the Nazis, he died in a concentration camp.

NIKOLSKY SIGN

A clinical sign of easy dislodgement of apparently normal epidermis under shearing stress, e.g. sliding pressure of a finger. It is related to lack of adhesion of epidermal cells in acantholysis. Nikolsky originally described this sign in relation to pemphigus vulgaris, but it also occurs in pemphigus foliaceus and toxic epidermal necrolysis and in porphyria cutanea tarda.

Pyotr V. Nikolsky (1858–1940) Russian dermatologist. He was born in Usman, Tambow, Russia, and studied at Kiev. He was assistant to Stoukowenkow in Kiev where he served in the skin clinic, commencing 1884. He became Professor of Dermatology in Warsaw in 1900 and later at Rostov. In 1896 he wrote "the skin shows a weakened coherence among its layers ... even in places between lesions on seemingly unaffected skin". He wrote a number of papers and books, the majority of which were written in Russian, but some appeared in French. These included articles on the treatment of syphilis and the incidence of syphilis amongst prostitutes in Kiev and dermatographism. He wrote books on syphilis and venereal disease as well as on skin diseases.

NISSL BODIES OR GRANULES

Chromophil granules in nerve cell cytoplasm.

NISSL DEGENERATION OR REACTION

Axonal degeneration.

NISSL STAIN

Stains to show extranuclear RNA in nerve cells.

Franz Nissl (1860–1919) German neuropathologist. He was born in Frankenthal, Bavaria. While still a medical student, in Munich, Ganser (von Gudden's assistant) suggested he write an essay on the pathology of cells of the cortex of the brain. This he undertook in 1884 and employed alcohol as a fixative and a staining technique which he improved upon but in which he demonstrated a number of previously unknown constituents of nerve cells and commenced a new era in neuropathology. Following his M.D. in 1885 he became an assistant to von Gudden and was in that position when his chief was killed by the mad King Ludwig (v. Kraepelin). In 1889 he went to Frankfurt-am-Main as second position under Sioli and here met Alzheimer for the first time. They became very close friends and collaborators. Invited by Kraepelin, he went to Heidelberg where he was Privatdozent in 1896 and Extraordinarius in 1901, and in 1904 he became Professor of Psychiatry and Director of the clinic in Heidelberg when Kraepelin went to Munich. In 1918 he joined Kraepelin in Munich to take up a research position in a new institute called the Deutsche Forschungsanstalt für Psychiatrie. After one year working with Spielmeyer and Brodmann he died of kidney disease.

Nissl was possibly the greatest neuropathologist of his day and also a fine clinician who popularized the use of spinal puncture introduced by Quincke. He was nicknamed "punctator maximus". Apart from his studies on the structure of the neurones, he examined connections between the cortex and thalamic nuclei. This work was still in progress when he died.

Nissl was described as a small man whose head was tilted to one side – perhaps to hide a large birthmark on the left side of his face. He was a bachelor who had a very keen sense of humor, but whose life revolved entirely around his work. The story is told that one morning he placed a row of empty beer bottles outside his laboratory and made sure a rumor reached his chief, Kraeplin, that he could be found lying under his desk, dead drunk. Kraeplin was a fierce campaigner against alcohol.

He was extremely fond of music, and a competent pianist.

NOBEL LAUREATE AND PRIZE

Annual award for outstanding contribution to medicine, chemistry, physics, literature and peace.

Alfred B. Nobel (1833–1896) Swedish inventor, manufacturer and philanthropist who endowed the above prize.

NOCARDIOSIS

An infection which usually occurs in patients with underlying ill-health, e.g. diabetes, carcinoma,

Hodgkin disease and leukemia, and often involves the maxillary sinus with a black eschar on the nasal surfaces.

Edmond I.E. Nocard (1850–1903) French veterinary pathologist and bacteriologist. He was born in Provins (Seine-et-Marne). His father was a wood merchant and he entered veterinary school at Alfort in 1868, but his work was interrupted by the Franco-German War in which he served as a volunteer in the 5th Lancers. In 1878 he held a clinical appointment in the Veterinary School of Alfort and became Professor of Pathology and Clinical Surgery. He became associated with the Pasteur group through his friendship with Professor Roux where he was highly regarded because of his knowledge of veterinary science.

In 1883 he went with members of the Pasteur Institute to Egypt to investigate a cholera outbreak, and Thuillier died of the disease. In 1887 he became Director of the Alfort School, but in 1891 he resigned this so that he could devote himself to his research. He became Chief of Service at the Pasteur Institute when it was established.

He discovered bovine pleuropneumonia with Roux and psittacosis in 1893. He worked on nocardiosis from 1888–1893 and again with Roux he first demonstrated the virulence of the saliva of dogs infected with rabies (1890). He was instrumental in the use of tuberculin in the diagnosis of tuberculosis in cattle and undertook studies on the prophylaxis of many of the disorders of horses and cattle and other farm animals which was of considerable economic importance. He published a book with Leclainche on the microbial illnesses of animals. He was highly regarded internationally and received decorations from Belgium and Italy for services rendered as an advisor on veterinary matters in those countries as well as being awarded the Cross of the Legion of Honour from his own country.

NONNE-MARIE SYNDROME

v. MARIE ATAXIA

NONNE-MILROY-MEIGE DISEASE

v. MILROY DISEASE, and MEIGE DISEASE

Max Nonne (1861–1959) German neurologist who worked in Hamburg and collaborated with Jakob. He described Milroy Disease in 1891 and studied proteins in the cerebrospinal fluid. He was a student of Erb and was one of the four German neurologists asked to examine Lenin during his final illness. He was one of the first to describe Adie syndrome and wrote a book on syphilis and its effect on the nervous system.

H. Meige (*v. supra*).

W.F. Milroy (*v. supra*).

NOONAN SYNDROME

cf. BONNEVIE-ULLRICH SYNDROME

These patients have a congenital heart defect, most commonly pulmonary stenosis, with a web neck and a chest deformity consisting of pectus carinatum superiorly and pectus excavatum inferiorly, together with hypertelorism and mild mental retardation and short stature. When males are affected they often exhibit cryptorchidism and then have elevated gonadotropin levels. The majority of females are fertile. Bleeding anomalies are common and are often associated with Factor XI deficiency or sometimes von Willebrand disease or platelet anomalies. Skin features include café au lait patches and sometimes hyperelasticity. There have been several reports of associated neurofibromatosis.

Jacqueline A. Noonan (1928–) U.S. pediatric cardiologist who graduated M.D. in 1954 from the University of Vermont College of Medicine. She works in the Department of Pediatrics at the University of Kentucky College of Medicine at Lexington, Kentucky.

NORDAUISM

Degeneracy.

Max S. Nordau (1849–1923) German author and physician.

NORRIE DISEASE

Sex linked hereditary blindness with non-malignant retinal tumors of both eyes and sometimes deafness and mental retardation.

Gordon Norrie (1855–1941) Danish ophthalmologist.

NORWALK AGENT

Viral gastroenteritis first reported in an institutional outbreak in Norwalk, Ohio, U.S.A.

NOTHNAGEL DISEASE

Acroparesthesia – numbness, pins and needles and pain, sometimes with stiffness in hands and feet, associated with pallor, cyanosis and edema.

NOTHNAGEL PARALYSIS

3rd nerve palsy and ipsilateral cerebellar ataxia or rubral tremor caused by a lesion of the 3rd nerve due to occlusion of the thalamo-perforating branches of the posterior cerebral artery or its nucleus and the superior cerebellar peduncle.

Carl W.H. Nothnagel (1841–1905) German physician and Head of University Clinic, Vienna. Von Economo was one of his students who worked with him for a year. He was a pupil of Traube and Virchow, and Leyden's assistant at Köningsberg (1865–68) and Professor of Medicine at Freiburg in 1872, Jena in 1874 and finally Vienna from 1882 until his death. He wrote a number of treatises on therapeutics and made many contributions to neurology. He was a very good speaker and a well-liked lecturer. His favorite clinical interests were in the diagnosis of cerebral diseases and diseases of the intestine and peritoneum. He edited an enormous book of 24 volumes on pathology and therapeutics. He suffered from angina pectoris and set down his own symptoms in great detail just before his death.

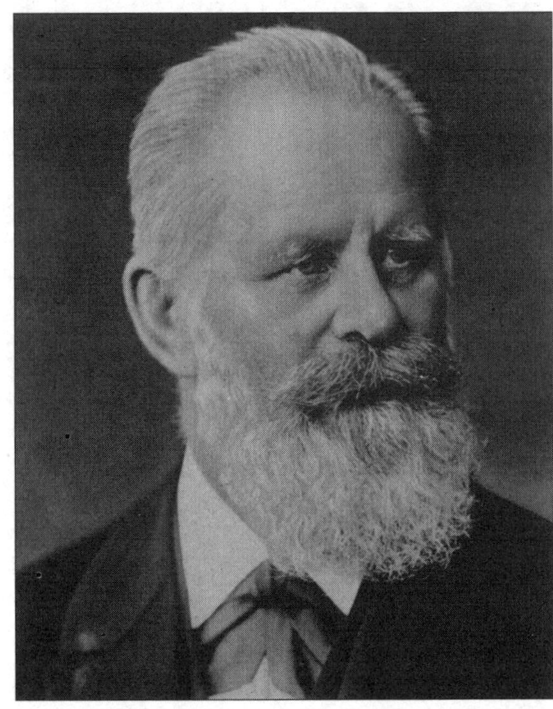

Carl W.H. Nothnagel (Courtesy of the Royal Society of Medicine, London, UK)

NOUGARET NIGHT BLINDNESS

Congenital night blindness due to absence of rods – transmitted as an autosomal dominant.

J. Nougaret (1637–1719) French physician.

NYSTEN LAW

Rigor mortis is first observed in the masticatory muscles, then facial, then cervical muscles and finally the lower extremities.

Pierre H. Nysten (1774–1817) French pediatrician who wrote one of the earliest medical dictionaries (1806). He was born in Liège, Belgium, but studied medicine in Paris and was a physician at the Hôpital des Enfants, Paris.

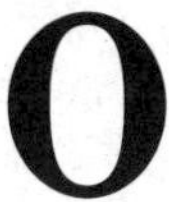

O

OCCAM RAZOR

This is the principle that assumptions introduced to explain something must not be unnecessarily multiplied.

William of Occam (1300–1341) English philosopher who founded a speculative sect reviving the doctrines of Nominalism, which means that universal or abstract concepts are mere names without any corresponding reality.

OCHSNER TEST

A test for median nerve injury distal to the antecubital fossa. The patient is asked to clasp the hands firmly together, and the index finger on the injured side cannot flex.

Alton Ochsner (1896–) U.S. surgeon, graduated M.D. Washington University, St. Louis in 1920, became Professor of Surgery at Tulane in 1927 and became interested in the possible relationship between cigarette smoking and lung cancer, and in 1941 published a study with Michael DeBakey concluding that the increase in lung cancer was due largely to increased tobacco smoking. He studied the use of bronchography in bronchiectasis.

OCHSNER-MAHORNER TEST

A modification of Perthes test (*v. infra*) in which the patient is disrobed and walks about; the tourniquet is then applied sequentially at the knee and mid-calf after observing the veins. If the veins collapse, the deep veins are patent and the communicating veins are competent. If they remain unchanged, deep and communicating veins are incompetent. If they increase in size and pain occurs the deep veins are occluded and the communicating veins are incompetent.

OCHSNER-SHERREN-TREATMENT

Conservative approach to appendicitis of more than 48 hours duration.

Albert J. Ochsner (1858–1925) He claimed to be related to Vesalius. He was born in Baraboo, Wisconsin, and graduated M.D. in 1886 from the Rush Medical College, Chicago. He studied in Vienna, Berlin, and London, and returned to Chicago in 1889. In 1900 he was appointed Professor of Clinical Surgery at the University of Illinois College of Medicine. He wrote a book on appendicitis in 1902 and contributed in many other clinical subjects. He died of coronary thrombosis.

Howard R. Mahorner (1903–) U.S. surgeon born in Mobile, Alabama, and graduated M.D. University of Pennsylvania in 1925 and was Fellow in Surgery at the Mayo Clinic 1926–1930. He went to Tulane University 1932–46 as Assistant Professor and then became Clinical Professor of Surgery at the Louisiana State University School of Medicine in 1950 and wrote a number of articles on varicose veins.

James Sherren (1872–1946) English surgeon. He was born in Weymouth, the son of a publisher, and initially served as an apprentice at sea, gaining his Master's certificate. During one of his voyages he became friendly with the ship's doctor and assisted him as an anesthetist and subsequently studied medicine, graduating from the London Hospital in 1899, obtaining his F.R.C.S. in 1900, and was appointed to the surgical staff of the London Hospital. He worked with Sir Henry Head and discovered the superficial hyperasthesia in the right inguinal region associated with early appendicitis, and published a book on injury of the nerves and treatment. He wrote numerous articles on abdominal surgery, in particular the management of gastric and duodenal ulcers. He retired abruptly when 54 years old and returned to sea as a ship's surgeon before retiring to the seaside.

ODDI, SPHINCTER OF

Bile duct sphincter at its entrance into the duodenum.

ODDI SYNDROME

Spasm of the sphincter of Oddi, causing pain and sometimes jaundice, mimicking a gallstone in the common duct.

Ruggero Oddi (1845–1906) Italian anatomist and surgeon in Rome. He re-introduced bedside teaching and one of his pupils, J. van Heurne, returned to Leyden and introduced it there. The sphincter had already been described by Glisson (*v. supra*) in 1654.

OEDIPUS COMPLEX

Sexual attraction of a son to his mother.

Oedipus was King of Thebes in Greek mythology, and unknowingly killed his father and married his mother.

OERTEL TREATMENT

Treatment of cardiovascular disease by weight reduction, diet and fluid restriction.

Max J. Oertel (1835–1897) German ear, nose and throat surgeon. He was born in Dilligen, Bavaria, and initially studied history at Munich before entering the Faculty of Medicine. He was appointed assistant to Professor Pfeuffer in 1860, and studied laryngology with Professor Czermak, being appointed Foundation Professor of Laryngology at Munich University in 1867.

He was the first after Bruns to undertake oral removal of a laryngeal polyp and wrote on this subject as well as circulatory problems. He was a fierce proponent of graded exercise as a means of treating cardiac failure ("Oertel Cure"). He wrote on the epidemiology and pathogenesis of diphtheria which followed a diphtheria epidemic in Munich and in which he set out a fine series of illustrations in great detail of the histology of diphtheria in many organs of the body. He believed he had discovered the bacillus of diphtheria, but this appears doubtful.

OFUJI DISEASE

This consists of recurrent itchy follicular papules and/or pustules which are most commonly seen on the face but also may appear on the palms and soles. Histological examination shows perifollicular eosinophil infiltration in the face whilst the eosinophils on the hands and soles are present in spongiotic vesicles. There may be peripheral extension with the residual lesions clearing but leaving pigmentation.

Shigeo Ofuji Japanese dermatologist who works in Kyoto, Japan.

OGILVIE SYNDROME

Abdominal distension and pseudo-obstruction due to an autonomic disturbance. This syndrome is now most commonly seen in patients on chemotherapeutic regimes containing neurotoxic drugs, e.g. vincristine. It is also used as a synonym for all forms of large bowel obstruction without a mechanical cause (pseudo-obstruction).

Sir Heneage Ogilvie (1887–1971) British surgeon at Guy's Hospital. He was born in Chile and studied medicine at Oxford University and Guy's Hospital graduating in 1913. The famous surgeon Arbuthnot Lane was his first role model and he gained more surgical experience by volunteering for the Balkan War of 1912–13, where his lifelong interest in war surgery commenced. He next served in the 1914–18 war in France and returned to Guy's Hospital where he was appointed to the staff in 1925. At the time Lord Moynihan was at the peak of British surgery and Ogilivie remarked "When in 1925, I stepped onto the stage, a humble follower of Lane, Moynihan bestrode the narrow world like a Colossus, and we petty men walked about under his huge legs, and peeped about to find ourselves dishonourable graves." He compared surgical advances with the progress of a barge up the Thames "the advance of knowledge must be wayward: the locks are periods of orthodoxy; the advances of heterodoxy." Always a keen traveller, in 1927 he founded the Surgical Traveller's Club which included visits to the major surgical centers in Europe. He was an enthusiastic yachtsman, although some said he spent more time in the water than on it because he was always experimenting with new gear and maneuvers. He held a number of yachting appointments including Commodore of the Oxford University Sailing Club and later of the Imperial Poona Yacht Club. He was much in demand as a postgraduate teacher and had wide command of written and spoken English which resulted in three books of biographical and philosophical nature as well as numerous contributions to the surgical literature. His literary interest and skill led him to be joint editor of The Practitioner 1946–1962. He was actively involved with the army again in World War II, serving in East Africa and the Middle East where he rose to the rank of Major General and published a text "Forward Surgery in Modern War". He was a charismatic teacher who emphasized the importance of a doctor's own shortcomings in dealing with patients illustrating this by saying the naturally timid should be wary of making a decision not to operate on a possible acute abdomen, whereas the naturally bold should be wary about operating too readily. He coined the expression that a patient "must earn his partial gastrectomy."

OGUCHI DISEASE

Hereditary night blindness.

Chuta Oguchi (1875–1945) Japanese ophthalmologist.

OHM

Unit of electrical resistance.

OHM LAW

Electric current varies inversely with the resistance.

Georg Ohm (1787–1854) German physicist. He was born in Erlangen, Bavaria, and taught maths and physics at a Jesuit school in Cologne. He was Professor of Physics at the University of Munich from 1849. He was elected F.R.S. in 1841.

OLIVER-CARDARELLI SIGN

(Also called OLIVER SIGN)

Tracheal pulsation synchronous with ventricular systole, best elicited by placing both fingers under the thyroid cartilage and lifting. It is seen in aortic aneurysm, mediastinal tumors – termed tracheal tug. Must be distinguished from tracheal tug of respiratory failure where it is synchronous with respiration.

William S. Oliver (1836–1906) English physician.

Antonio Cardarelli (1831–1927) Italian physician who was a member of the medical faculty in Naples and wrote on a wide range of topics ranging from functional disorders of the heart to aneurysms and mediastinal tumors and liver disease.

OLLIER DISEASE

Enchondromatosis.

Louis X.E.L. Ollier (1830–1900) French surgeon, born in Vans in Ardeche, he initially studied natural science at Montpellier and in 1849 was assistant in botany in the Faculty of Medicine. He was intern of Lyons Hospital in 1851 and became senior surgeon at the Hôtel Dieu in Lyons in 1860. When France was invaded by the Germans in 1870 he became head of the Lyons Ambulance. He was a pioneer of bone resection by operative techniques and studied the regeneration of bone by the periosteum after resection. He was one of the first surgeons to employ an audit on his operative procedures, stating "it is in the certification and criticism of old results that is to be found the true consecration of operative methods which are intended to be used for purposes of conservative surgery". Following a ceremony in which he was made a Commander of the Legion of Honour by President Carnot, the President was murdered and Ollier was called in an attempt to remedy his wounds surgically. It was the inability of the surgeons to deal with the President's wounds effectively which led Carrel (*v. supra*) to his initial studies on techniques of vessel anastomosis.

ONDINE CURSE

One form of sleep apnea with hypoventilation due to a central neurological mechanism – primary alveolar hypoventilation syndrome. The initial patient to whom this term was applied had an injury to the 9th and probably 10th nerve at surgery.

Ondine A water nymph who caused a human male who loved her to sleep forever.

ONYALAI

Acute thrombocytopenic purpura seen in Africa. Characterized by oral blood blisters.

Onyalai Term used by natives of what was formerly Portuguese West Africa. Its origin is uncertain.

OPALSKI CELLS

Large neural cells with a small nucleus whose cytoplasm is filled with PAS positive material thought to be degenerating cells and seen characteristically in basal ganglia of patients with Wilson Disease (*v. infra*).

Adam Opalski (1897–1963) Polish physician.

OPIE PARADOX

The host may be protected by the local tissue destruction resulting from anaphylaxis.

Eugene L. Opie (1873–1971) Born in Staunton, Virginia, son of a general practitioner, was in the first class at Johns Hopkins. He studied pathology under Welch and while still a medical student described lesions in the Islets of Langerhans in diabetes, and with W.G. MacCallum (also a student) demonstrated sexual conjugation of the flagellate forms of malaria in birds. They were both medical students at Johns Hopkins in 1896. He described pneumonia caused by influenza and investigated the pathogenesis of hemorrhagic pancreatitis, showing that it could be caused by obstruction of the Duct of Vater. In 1904 he moved to the Rockefeller Institute and in 1910 was invited as Professor of Pathology to Washington University, St. Louis. Here he discovered the importance of diet in influencing the onset of hepatic damage by chemicals and in 1923 he moved to the Chair of Pathology at the University of Pennsylvania and there carried out extensive pathological and epidemiological studies on tuberculosis. He was editor of the Journal of Experimental Medicine with Flexner, following Welch, and on retirement spent 30 years as "guest investigator" at the Rockefeller Institute.

OPPENHEIM DISEASE

Amyotonia congenita.

OPPENHEIM REFLEX

Stroking firmly down the medial side of the tibia may elicit dorsiflexion of the great toe in pyramidal tract lesions.

OPPENHEIM-ZIEHEN DISEASE

Dystonia musculorum deformans.

Herman Oppenheim (1858–1919) German neurologist who was born in Warburg, Westphalia, and studied medicine at Göttingen, Berlin and Bonn. He was a protégé of Westphal and whilst the latter was ill was in charge of his clinic but after he died, although unanimously nominated by the Berlin faculty to succeed Westphal, was vetoed by the Prussian secretary of education and was forced to leave the Charité, and in 1890 opened a private clinic. He was primarily a diagnostician and wrote extensively on numerous neurological disorders and produced a text book of neurology that was internationally famous. He was the first to emphasize the importance of bladder symptoms in disseminated sclerosis. In 1889 he published a treatise on traumatic neuroses which proposed that trauma caused organic changes which perpetuated psychic neuroses. This was fiercely opposed by Charcot, Nonne and others, especially with regard to malingering and hysteria. Oppenheim's diagnosis resulted in the first removal of a brain tumor by Koehler and he reported the first successful removal of a pineal tumor with F. Krause. In Oppenheim-Ziehen disease he emphasized the characteristic "dromedary gait" but this disorder was first described by Schwalbe.

Georg T. Ziehen (1862–1950) German psychiatrist, born in Frankfurt-am-Main. He worked with Edinger on the morphology of the brain (1892–9) and was appointed Professor at Jena in 1892 and investigated the psychopathology of children.

OPPENHEIM-URBACH DISEASE

Necrobiosis lipoidica.

Maurice Oppenheim (1876–1949) Austrian dermatologist, born in Vienna. He graduated from Vienna University in 1899 and after interning at the Allgemeines Krankenhaus joined the University of Vienna Dermatology Clinic in 1902, where he developed a complement fixation test for the gonococcus with R. Müller in 1906. He became Professor of Dermatology in 1927. He wrote several textbooks on venereal disease and skin disorders. He described necrobiosis lipoidica diabeticorum in 1932. He stressed the importance of occupation and cosmetics causing skin problems.

Eric Urbach (1893–1946) U.S. dermatologist. He was born in Prague, Czechoslovakia, and went to medical school at the University of Vienna for two years. When the 1st World War broke out he served in the Austrian army as a Lieutenant and a member of the surgical group of Professor A. von Eiselberg and was decorated for bravery. He graduated in 1919 from the University of Vienna under Professor W. Kerl, and in 1929 became an Associate Professor. From 1936 to 1938 he was Chief Physician of the Department of Dermatology and Allergy at the Merchant's Hospital, Vienna, but with the advent of Hitler migrated to the United States in 1938 and became an Associate of Dermatology at the University of Pennsylvania and from 1939 was Chief of the Allergy Department at the Jewish Hospital, Philadelphia. He was the author of many publications and published a very popular book "Allergy" with P.M. Gottlieb.

ORBELI EFFECT OR PHENOMENON

Stimulation of the nerve to a muscle together with its sympathetic supply results in increased contraction of fatigued muscles.

Leon A. Orbeli (1882–1958) Russian physiologist who was one of Pavlov's pupils. He was born in Yerevan, Armenia, and became Head of the Pavlov Institute and won the Stalin Prize.

OROYA FEVER

Fever caused by a *Bartonella* infestation.

La Oroya A town in the foothills of the Andes in Peru.

ORTNER SYNDROME

Left vocal cord paralysis associated with enlarged left atrium in mitral stenosis.

Norbert Ortner (1865–1935) Professor of Medicine, Vienna, at the same time as Wenckebach, and described the syndrome in 1897. A native of Linz he attracted Neusser's attention with two monographs on congenital disease of the aorta and mixed infection in pulmonary tuberculosis and became Neusser's assistant in 1893 in his clinic in Vienna. He remained in Vienna for his working life apart from 4 years as Professor of Medicine at Innsbruck. He returned to Vienna in 1911 to follow Strümpell as head of the most prestigious clinic in Vienna and became physician to the Emperor Franz Joseph. Apart from his studies on cardiac valvular disease he was best known for his book on pain and one on therapeutics of internal disease which was translated into many languages. He was a keen proponent of laboratory work and its application to bedside teaching and he said that the clinician's motto should be "Via the laboratory always to the clinic", "übers laboratorium dauernd zur Klinik". He died of motor neurone disease causing bulbar palsy.

OSGOOD-SCHLATTER DISEASE

Osteochondritis of the tibial tuberosity classically seen in adolescents.

Robert B. Osgood (1873–1956) U.S. orthopedic surgeon, Boston, U.S.A. Born in Salem, Massachusetts, graduated M.D. from Harvard in 1899. He described this disorder in 1903 and wrote extensively on all manner of orthopedic surgery, including a monograph on the history of orthopedic surgery, and became Head of the Department of Orthopedic Surgery at Harvard Medical School.

Carl Schlatter (1865–1934) Swiss Professor of Surgery at Zurich. He graduated in medicine in Zurich in 1888 after working as a student in Zurich and Heidelberg. In the winter of 1889 to 1890 he studied in Vienna with Billroth and E. Albert. He performed the first successful gastrectomy in 1897 and wrote his description of Osgood-Schlatter disease in 1908. He was invited by Professor U. Kronlein to join him at the University Clinic at Zurich. Here he remained until he became Professor of Surgery. His main interest was in casualties and trauma and he published a number of papers and books on this subject. In 1914–15 he worked in the German prisoner of war camps and in the Stuttgart Military Hospital. He was a very skilful surgeon and a fine teacher. He became ill shortly before his retirement was due and died suddenly of a pulmonary illness.

OSLER DISEASE

or

OSLER-RENDU-WEBER DISEASE OR SYNDROME

Hereditary hemorrhagic telangiectasia – an autosomal dominant disorder characterized by hemorrhages in the form of epistaxes or blood loss in the gastrointestinal tract, and sometimes associated with large arterio-venous anomalies in the lungs or elsewhere.

OSLER NODES

Painful indurated areas on the pads of the fingers seen in subacute bacterial endocarditis.

OSLER-VAQUEZ DISEASE

(Also called OSLER DISEASE)

Polycythemia rubra vera.

Sir William Osler (1849–1919) Born in the backwoods of Canada, the son of a missionary at Bond Head, Canada, into a large family, all of whom achieved success. He commenced study at Trinity College, Toronto, with the objective of joining the clergy, but switched to medicine and entered medical school at McGill University, Montreal. He graduated in 1872 and spent two years in London, Berlin, Leipzig and Vienna before returning to Montreal where, at the age of 26, he was appointed Professor of the Institute of Medicine (Physiology) at McGill University, Montreal, and pathologist to the Montreal General Hospital.

In 1884 he was appointed Professor of Clinical Medicine at the University of Pennsylvania, remaining there for 5 years before being recruited to Johns Hopkins as foundation Professor of Medicine in 1889. It was here that he established himself as the most outstanding medical educator of his time, and commenced the modern era of medicine as we know it today. He introduced bedside teaching to medicine, combined scientific knowledge with clinical skill and inspired all the students and housemen who came within his ambit. His book, "Principles and Practice of Medicine", first published in 1892, spread his fame throughout the English-speaking world. In 1904 he was appointed Regius Professor of Medicine at Oxford University and from the time of his arrival exerted a great influence on English medicine. He was largely responsible for the foundation of the Association of Physicians of Great Britain and Ireland, and the Quarterly Journal of Medicine. He presented evidence before the Haldane Commission which virtually assured the establishment of full time Chairs of Medicine in the University of London. He became a Fellow of Christ Church College which attracted him because of its association with Robert Burton, whose "Anatomy of Melancholy" he admired so much.

A man of immense personal charm, he epitomised Peabody's saying that "the secret of patient care is caring for patients". Osler himself was famous for many aphorisms which are still as cogent today as when he first introduced them: "To study medicine without reading textbooks is like going to sea without charts, but to study medicine without dealing with patients is not to go to sea at all". Many of his essays are classics which should be read by the modern medical undergraduate and graduate. Perhaps the two most famous are "A way of Life" and "Aequinimitas".

For a man who is held in such reverence by all the English-speaking medical profession, his scientific accomplishments were perhaps not great. However, his description of disease bordered on that of Hippocrates, and as he matured his writing became more and more succinct and easy to follow. He wrote some of the early descriptions of the platelets in morphology and wrote classical papers on hereditary telangiectasia, lupus erythematosus and polycythemia vera. His textbook was a goldmine of information and is still worth reading. His real strength however lay in his ability to inspire and influence his students and postgraduate fellows. Through these men and women he exerted an influence which had never been seen before and has never been equalled since. He was the example par excellence of his own saying that the future of a university or hospital "lies in the men who work in its halls and in the ideals which they cherish and teach". It is said that if he had a blind spot it was his inability to tell patients the reality of their disease and in consultation he sometimes caused the referring doctor problems since he would always leave the patient and relatives with the feeling that they could recover. However, perhaps this was one of the secrets of his success in a day when treatment was relatively ineffective.

He was a superb diagnostician who insisted on hospital patients being treated as human beings and not as "interesting cases". He had many personal ideals which he spelt out in his essays, but perhaps 3 recurring themes were:

1. Doing the day's work well and not bothering about tomorrow,
2. Always being courteous and considerate to professional colleagues and to patients, and
3. Cultivating a feeling of equanimity.

In many ways Osler was responsible for combining the best of German and English medicine, and was largely responsible for the ultimate shift of the center of progress in medical science to the United States. He was an outstanding teacher, a forceful speaker and a man with great personal charm and ready wit. He had a curiously impish side to his character which led him to use a pseudonym when involved with practical jokes – Egerton Yorrick Davis. Osler considered an editorial by Dr. Theophilus Parvin, a Professor of Obstetrics in Philadelphia, to be ridiculous. He wrote a fictitious tongue in cheek article about vaginismus and this was published in "The Medical News" and was reproduced in two books on sexual disorders!

It is said that his whole personality changed when his only child (Revere) died in an artillery barrage at the Ypres salient towards the end of the 1st World War. His son was named after Lady Osler's ancestor Paul Revere of the famous "ride" fame.

Osler died following bronchopneumonia and empyema on December 29th, 1919.

Henri J.L. Rendu (*v. infra*).

Frederick P. Weber (*v. infra*).

Henri Vaquez (*v. infra*).

P

PACINIAN CORPUSCLES

Lamellar structures which are sensory nerve end organs.

Filippo Pacini (1812–1883) Italian anatomist and physiologist who was born in Pistoia, Italy and graduated in medicine from Florence. He became Professor of Anatomy in Pisa and in 1849 was appointed Professor of Histology in Florence.

PAGE SYNDROME

Episodic hypertension with tachycardia, sweating, nausea, vomiting and glycosuria due to increased catecholamine secretion of pheochromocytoma or sometimes of a neuroblastoma or ganglioneuroma.

Irvine H. Page (1901–91) U.S. physician. Born in Indianapolis. He graduated M.D. from Cornell University, N.Y. in 1926. He interned at the Presbyterian Hospital, N.Y. in 1926–1928. He worked at the Kaiser Wilhelm Institute, Munich, 1928–31 and became an associate member Rockefeller Institute, N.Y. 1931–37. He was director of the Lilly Laboratory and Clinical Research 1937–45. His lifelong research was in hypertension and arteriosclerosis and he described tachyphylaxis (decreasing response to drugs or hormones if they are given repeatedly).

PAGET DISEASE

1. Of bone – osteitis deformans.
2. Of the nipple – carcinoma involving the areola and/or the nipple and characterized by large cells with a clear cytoplasm.
3. Of the skin – skin cancer involving the apocrine glands with the same cells seen in 2.

PAGET-SCHROETTER SYNDROME

Venous thrombosis of the axillary vein of unknown cause.

Sir James Paget (1814–1899) Born in Great Yarmouth, England. After apprenticeship with a surgeon he became a student at St. Bartholomew's Hospital, London, and was associated with that hospital throughout his life. He was a brilliant man

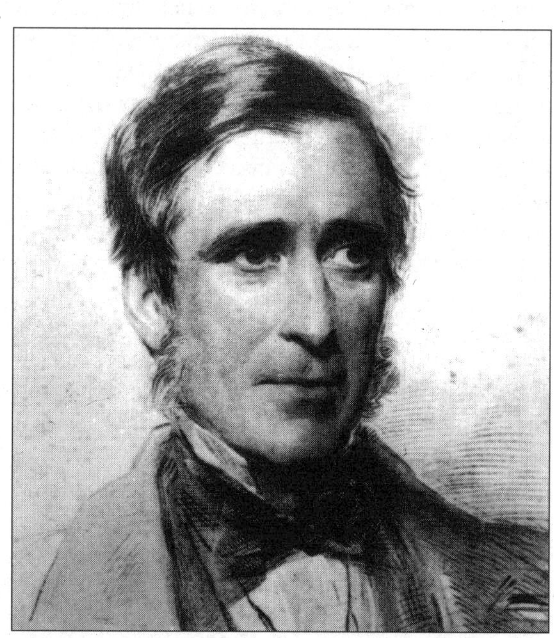

Sir James Paget (Reproduced from *"Memories of Sir James Paget"* edited by Stephen Paget [Published by Longman, Green & Co. Paternoster Row, London, 1901])

who stood head and shoulders above his contemporaries. He admired brevity and was famed for it; equally he disliked smart-Aleck cleverness, and had an antipathy towards epigrams and proverbs, although he used some himself! "To be brief is to be wise". During his first year at Barts as a student, he noted some white specks in the muscles of a cadaver he was dissecting and examined these with a microscope and found them to be small encapsulated worms. This was the first demonstration of trichinosis in man. He passed the College of Surgeons exams (1836) and then coached and was sub-editor of some medical journals and was appointed Curator of the College of Surgeons Anatomy Museum in 1837–43.

He became a demonstrator in anatomy and in 1847 became Professor of Surgery at the Royal College of Surgeons and in 1851 was elected F.R.S. In 1851 he commenced private practice and his success was phenomenal, resting on his charming personality as much as his anatomical pathological knowledge and surgical skill. He was created a baronet in 1877, the same year he described the bone disorder. Although his practice is alleged to have earned him 10 000 pounds a year he continued to make notable scientific contributions as well as to write important books on surgical pathology, tumors and surgery. His friends numbered Virchow, Ruskin, Cardinal Newman, Tennyson, George Eliot, Robert Browning, Pasteur, Hurley and Darwin (indeed, it seems most of the intelligentsia of the day). Gladstone is reputed to have said that he divided people into two classes – "those who had and those who had not heard James Paget". He was appointed Sargeant Surgeon to the Queen in 1877 and although he gave up operating when 64, continued to see patients in consultation, and in 1891 went to Rome to give his advice.

L. Schroetter von Kristelli (1837–1908) Austrian physician who described axillary vein thrombosis in Nothnagel's (*v. supra*) textbook in 1884. Born in Graz, he was the son of the chemist who discovered amorphous phosphorous. A favorite pupil of Skoda (*v. infra*) he was a pioneer of laryngology.

PAL-WEIGERT METHOD FOR STAINING NERVOUS TISSUE

Jacob Pal (1863–1936) Austrian physician who was the first physician in Vienna to introduce blood pressure measurement as routine in patient care.

Carl Weigert (1845–1904) German histopathologist. A cousin of Paul Ehrlich, he studied with Virchow and was Professor of Anatomical Pathology in Leipzig and Frankfurt.

PALTAUF DWARFISM

Pituitary dwarf.

PALTAUF-STERNBERG DISEASE

v. HODGKIN DISEASE

Richard Paltauf (1858–1924) Austrian pathologist and bacteriologist. He was born in Judenberg and went to medical school at Graz and Vienna where he was assistant to Kundrat. He established an institute and worked on agglutinin reactions and described status lymphaticus in 1889, Hodgkin disease in 1896 and mass produced diphtheria anti-toxin.

C. Sternberg

v. REED-STERNBERG CELLS

PANCOAST SYNDROME OR TUMOR

Usually epidermoid or adenocarcinoma of lung involving the superior pulmonary sulcus and involving the 8th cervical and 1st thoracic nerve, giving shoulder pain and pain in the ulnar distribution of the arm. Sometimes associated with lesions of 1st and 2nd ribs and Horner Syndrome (*v. supra*).

Henry K. Pancoast (1875–1939) U.S. radiologist, born in Philadelphia, son of a doctor, both parents were prominent Quakers, and he was educated at the Friends Central School. After a short period in a bank he entered the University of Pennsylvania Medical School and graduated in 1898. He interned at the hospital of the University of Pennsylvania and in 1900 commenced surgical training there, but was already attracted to radiology and when the hospital's first "skiagrapher" C.L. Leonard resigned in 1903, he was encouraged to apply by his chief, the Professor of Surgery, J.W. White.

He was a modest, hardworking and meticulous man who kept careful records. He soon was publishing papers on numerous aspects of radiology and rapidly became known nationally from his writing and presentations at meetings and by 1912 was elected President of the American Roentgen Ray Society and in the same year appointed Professor of Radiology at the University of Pennsylvania, the first such appointment in the U.S.A. He developed one of the best undergraduate and postgraduate training courses in the country. His principal publication concerned the pneumoconioses, but like all radiologists of his time he was a pioneer in radiotherapy, published on its use in hematological malignancies, and investigated the properties and effects of agents used in radiology such as bismuth. The esteem in which he was held by his colleagues is illustrated by his election as President of the 1st American Congress of Radiology in 1933 and in 1934 as President of the 1st American Board of Radiology.

PANETH CELLS

Secretory cells in the crypts of Lieberkühn (*v. supra*).

Joseph Paneth (1857–1890) Austrian physiologist who was born in Vienna and became Professor of Physiology there.

PANNER DISEASE

Osteochondrosis of the head of the humerus.

Hans J. Panner (1871–1930) Danish radiologist.

PAPANICOLOU SMEAR OR TEST

Test for cervical cancer.

George N. Papanicolou (1883–1962) U.S. pathologist. He was born in Coumi, Greece, and in 1904 graduated M.D. from the University of Athens and in 1910 gained a Ph.D. at the University of Munich.

He did not wish to study medicine but agreed to do so following the wishes of his father, but only on condition that after being qualified he could go to Vienna and study history and philosophy, but the ensuing wars determined otherwise. He fought in the Balkan War (1912–1913) against the Turks and was a 2nd Lieutenant in the Greek Army. At the end of the war he visited the United States and when the 1914–1918 war broke out he decided to remain there. He was first an assistant to the Professor of Anatomy at Cornell, New York, and became Professor and Chairman of the Department. In 1927 he obtained American citizenship. He worked with C.K. Stockard, a biochemist in New York, on the vaginal smear test for estrus and later with E. Shorr on its use in human females in the early 1930s. It was while he was doing the latter work that he noted cells which he had never seen before in his microscope specimens and identified them as being cancer of the cervix. One of the foremost pathologists of the day said to him "since the uterine cervix is accessible to diagnostic exploration by biopsy the use of cytologic examination is superfluous".

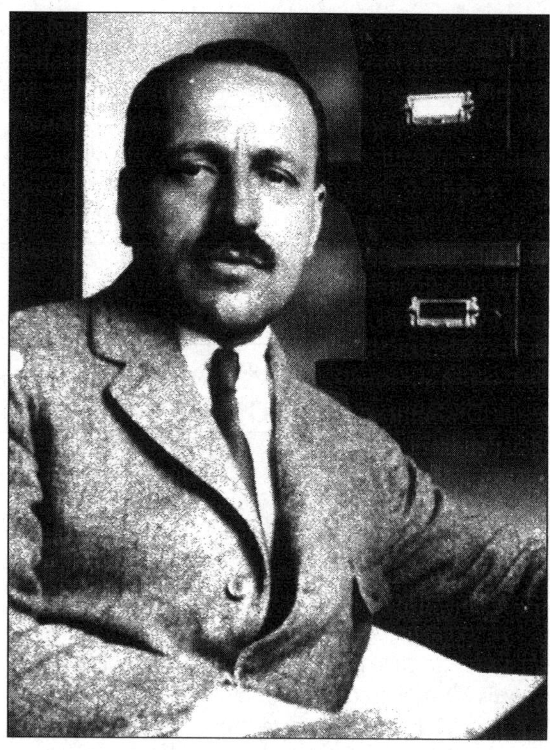

George N. Papanicolou (Courtesy of the Royal Society of Medicine, London, UK)

He was a modest man who was the last to claim that he originated the technique; indeed he always used to recount how in 1843 a London doctor called

Walsh published a book on diseases of the lung in which he drew attention to the fact that malignant cells could be seen under the microscope, in sputum from certain patients with cancer. He wrote numerous articles and three books including "Diagnosis of Uterine Cancer by the Vaginal Smear". He was quietly spoken, never lost his Greek accent, always welcomed discussion with those who disagreed with him, and often in this quiet way managed to convince people of the validity of his technique which was the forerunner of cytological testing for cancer.

PAPILLON-LEFÈVRE SYNDROME

Hyperkeratosis of hands and feet with periodontosis of the 2nd teeth and sometimes calcification of the choroid plexus and tentorium. Autosomal recessive.

M.M. Papillon French dermatologist.

Paul Lefèvre French dermatologist.

PAPPENHEIMER BODIES

Iron granules seen in erythrocytes in the peripheral blood, particularly after splenectomy.

Alwin M. Pappenheimer (1878–1955) U.S. pathologist. He was born in New York City and graduated M.D. from the Columbia University College of Physicians and Surgeons in 1902. He interned at Bellevue Hospital and after a brief period in private practice joined Dr. Charles Norris at the Bellevue Hospital Department of Pathology. A number of infective episodes including tuberculous lymphadenitis caused him to resign from his post and in 1910 he joined the Department of Pathology at Columbia which had just appointed W.G. MacCallum from Johns Hopkins. In 1907 he spent a year in Vienna studying pathology and another year with Professor F. Marchand in Leipzig and Professor L. Aschoff (*v. supra*) in Freiburg. He then returned to the Pathology Department in Columbia. He made an extensive study of the thymus and after numerous investigations came to the conclusion that "whatever its function, it is a rather superfluous organ". When the United States entered the 1st World War he joined up and was assigned as Head of the laboratory at Etretat, France, and he made a major contribution by showing that Trench Fever was transmitted by lice and was cited by General Pershing for exceptionally meritorious services as a member of the Trench Fever Commission. At the end of the war he returned to Columbia and commenced his work on experimental rickets, and together with Dr. A. Hess (*v. supra*) showed that cod liver oil was very active in both prevention and cure of the childhood disease, and that its dosage could be standardised in experimental animals. Using light filters he showed that it was ultraviolet rays which were responsible for prevention and cure of the disease. The experimental model that he established was used in laboratories in many parts of the world.

He was an outstanding teacher, but most at home in small groups and extremely well liked by the student body. He retired from Columbia in 1945 and moved to Harvard where he worked with an old friend, Dr. J.H. Muller, in the Department of Bacteriology and Immunology and continued to be productive, studying viral infections in animals. All in all he was a prototype for the modern experimental pathologist.

PARACELSIAN

Use of chemical agents in treatment.

Philippus Paracelsus or **A.T.B. von Hohenheim** (1493–1541) Swiss alchemist and physician. He was born in Einsiedeln, near Zurich, Switzerland. His father was a physician who graduated from Tübingen and became the town physician at Villach in Carinthia where Paracelsus grew up and perhaps went to the School of Mines. In 1510 he was at the University of Basel and is said to have got his doctor's degree with Leonicenus in Ferrara (1515). He went to many countries: Italy, Britain, Spain. He served as a surgeon in the Dutch army in 1518 and then with the Danish army when they unsuccessfully laid siege to Stockholm. He travelled through Russia, Poland and then joined the Venetian army fighting Charles V.

He returned to Strasburg (1525) and intended settling there when a grateful patient suggested he become physician to the City of Basel and the Professor of Medicine (1527). He campaigned against the traditional approach by lecturing in German, not Latin, and by publicly burning Avicenna's and Galen's works. This resulted in many disputes with his physician and faculty colleagues and he was forced to leave. From then on he led a wandering life, practicing here and there, and finally arrived in Salzburg in 1541; tired and ill, he wrote his will and died three days later. His tomb is in the Church of St. Sebastian. During his colorful life he first described occupational disease in the miners and disorders resulting from smelting fumes, mercury and arsenic. He noted the relationship between goitre and cretinism and introduced morphia for treatment, as well as alcoholic extracts, and used mercury for treating syphilis. He broke with the traditional four humors of Galen but his own theories were equally erroneous. He greatly respected Hippocrates. He was a popular physician who constantly seems to have been immersed in quarrels and controversy which persist till this day among historians.

PARDEE T WAVE

Downward deflection of the T wave characteristically seen in coronary disease.

Harold E.B. Pardee (1886–1973) U.S. cardiologist. He was born in New York, graduated from Columbia to enter medical school there and graduated from its College of Physicians and Surgeons. During his internship at New York Hospital he commenced research using an Einthoven electrocardiogram (ECG) imported from Holland. He was a captain in the U.S. army medical corps in World War I and worked with Sir Thomas Lewis on "Soldiers Heart" (v. DA COSTA SYNDROME). He was the first to describe the changes in the ECG in coronary occlusion in 1920 and wrote a book which gained him international renown, "Clinical Aspects of the Electrocardiogram". He was an associate Professor of Medicine at Cornell Medical College.

PARINAUD SYNDROME

1. Paralysis of conjugate gaze in a vertical direction usually up, sometimes down or both. There may be impairment of convergence. Upward or downward gaze may result in retractory nystagmus, due to contraction of all ocular muscles with the eyes moving backward and forward and sometimes spasming. There may also be pupillary paralysis, usually due to occlusion of the posterior cerebral artery or compression on the corpora quadrigemina by a pineal tumor or a metastasis, e.g. from carcinoma of the lung.
2. Conjunctivitis with palpable pre-auricular node.

Henri Parinaud (1844–1905) French ophthalmologist who was born in Bellac (Hte-Vienne), the son of a locksmith. He studied medicine at Limoges and came to Paris in 1869 where the war interrupted his studies and he went to work with the Red Cross ambulances at Metz under the direction of Lefort. After the war he returned to his medical studies in Paris and wrote a thesis, "A study on the optic nerve in meningitis of infants". This thesis attracted Charcot's attention and he became his collaborator at the Salpêtrière. In 1884 whilst in Charcot's clinic he described three forms of visual impairment in multiple sclerosis (M.S.)

1. Gradual impairment especially for color, affecting both eyes.
2. Rapid loss, sometimes with temporary blindness of both eyes with good recovery.
3. A unilateral loss of vision.

He contrasted the pale disc with relatively good vision in M.S. compared to the optic atrophy and blindness of tabes.

He rapidly became the founder of French ophthalmology, and although troubled throughout his life with ill health, he published extensively, especially in the general areas of stereoscopic vision and the projection of visual input in the cerebral cortex. He made many contributions on the control of eye movements and throughout his life published on various aspects of strabismus. He described infectious tubercular conjunctivitis transmitted from animals to man in 1889 and lacrymal pneumococcal conjunctivitis in newborn babies in 1894. He also wrote a number of musical works under the pseudonym of Pierre Erick. He developed bronchopneumonia and died a few weeks later.

PARKES WEBER SYNDROME

v. KLIPPEL-TRÉNAUNAY-WEBER SYNDROME

v. OSLER-RENDU-WEBER DISEASE

v. WEBER-KLIPPEL SYNDROME

PARKINSON CRISIS

Occulogyric crisis associated with acute anxiety. There is spontaneous and often sustained conjugate occular movement particularly in an upward direction. It is seen more commonly with Parkinsonism associated with previous encephalitis or drugs.

PARKINSON DISEASE

Paralysis agitans. Characterized by a tremor, muscle rigidity and passive facies with a shuffling gait and hypokinesia as well as dyskinesia.

James Parkinson (1755–1824) English physician and a pupil of John Hunter (*v. supra*). He was the son of a physician who practiced at Hoxton Square, London, and he himself practiced at Shoreditch. He published his now famous essay on the shaking palsy which he called paralysis agitans, in 1817. Charcot added one other feature to Parkinson's excellent clinical description, namely rigidity, and attached the eponym Parkinson Disease to the syndrome.

Although this is one of the best known eponyms in the world, Parkinson himself received little attention from his English-speaking colleagues until an article appeared by an American, J.G. Rowntree, in the bulletin of the Johns Hopkins Hospital (1912), volume 23, p.33, entitled, "English born, English bred, forgotten by the English and the world at large, such was the fate of James Parkinson". Perhaps one of the reasons for this was that he was an outspoken critic of the Pitt government and strong supporter for the under-privileged and probably also of the French Revolution. He published numerous political pamphlets under a pen-name of Old Hubert. He was a member of a number of secret societies including the London Corresponding Society which in 1794 was charged with complicity in an alleged plot to kill King George III*. Subsequently he confined himself to both medical and scientific work, including that of geology where his main interest was in the identification and collection of fossils. He was a founder of the London Geological Society.

Together with his son in 1812 he reported the first case of appendicitis in English, and the first instance in which perforation was shown to be the cause of death. He wrote pamphlets endeavoring to improve the lot of the insane and produced an excellent book on medical education. Like Sydenham he suffered from gout, and wrote on the subject. His essay on paralysis agitans is an excellent example of accurate clinical description of a case in the mould of Sydenham and Hippocrates.

* *"The popgun plot" as it was popularly called, because it was alleged that the plan was to fire a poison dart from a pop gun at the King.*

PARROT NODES

Nodes on the frontal and parietal bones of the skull seen in congenital syphilis.

Jules Parrot (1829–1883) He was born in Excideuil in the Dordogne. In 1852 he became interne des hôpitaux and by 1860 had obtained the title of Agrégé and was appointed Médecin des hôpitaux in 1862, but was forced, due to ill health, to spend two years in Algeria before returning to Paris. A student of Beau (*v. supra*) he initially studied cardiovascular disease and wrote a number of papers on cardiac vascular bruits, including those due to anemia and he also studied bruits in the neck. He combined clinical with pathological investigation and made careful measurements of the weights of organs. In 1867 he transferred to the Hospice des Enfants-Assistés and from here on devoted his studies to pediatrics and became one of the important pioneers in this discipline. He described and classified numerous disorders of the new born and devoted considerable attention to the development of the brain and the effects of hereditary syphilis both on the nervous system and other body organs including the bones, liver and lung. He wrote the first report of the pneumococcus in 1881 with Pasteur and also the Ghon lesion (*v. supra*) in 1876. Parrot described his nodes in the skull as resembling nates or buttocks; Treves (v. *infra*) commented "They have been termed natiform elevations by M. Parrot, from their supposed resemblence when viewed collectively, to the nates. To the English mind they would rather suggest the outlines of a hot cross bun!" An enthusiastic anthropologist, he was one of the founders of the French Society of Anthropology and was its President in 1881. He discovered the cave at Excideuil and explored it and wrote a description of it. He succeeded Lorain (*v. supra*) as the Professor of Medical History of the Paris Faculty from 1876–1879 when he was appointed Foundation Professor of Paediatrics. This Chair was established at his hospital, L'Hospice des Enfants-Assistés.

PARRY DISEASE

Hyperthyroidism.

v. GRAVES DISEASE

Caleb H. Parry (1775–1822) English physician. Born in Gloucestershire, England, he graduated in medicine in Edinburgh in 1777 and practiced for the rest of his life in Bath. He had a life-long habit of taking detailed notes and his "unpublished medical writings" which appeared 3 years after his death, contained the first recorded cases of congenital idiopathic dilation of the colon (Hirschsprung disease), and facial hemiatrophy, as well as a detailed account of exophthalmic goitre which he first noted in 1786. He gave excellent descriptions of angina pectoris which he related to coronary artery disease and first observed that slowing of the heart occurred following pressure on the carotid artery. Edward Jenner dedicated his work on smallpox "An Enquiry into Causes and Effects of the Variolae Vaccinae" to Parry, which shows that he exerted considerable influence on his colleagues of the day.

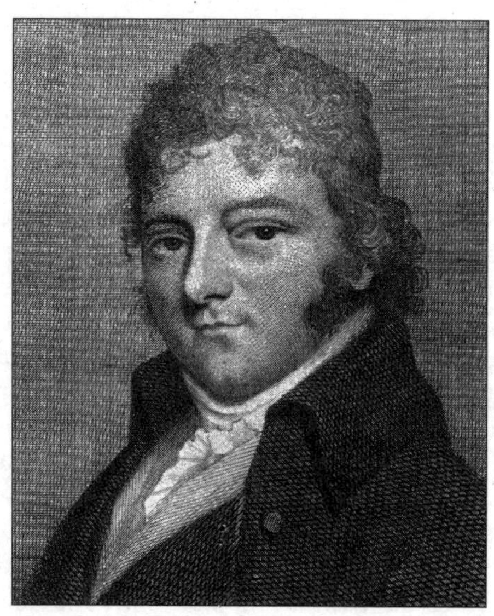

Caleb H. Parry (Courtesy of the Royal Society of Medicine, London, UK)

PASCHEN BODIES

Sometimes called elementary bodies which were found in the lesions of vaccinia and smallpox and represent aggregates of virus.

Enrique Paschen (1860–1936) German bacteriologist. He studied viral infections all his life but concentrated mainly on smallpox. Throughout his career he was convinced of the relationship between the inclusion bodies and the etiological agent of the infection but this was only proved towards the end of his life after he had retired as director of the Impfanstaldt at Hamburg. Although troubled by chronic cardiac failure he continued working until the end having a paper in press when he died.

PASSOVOY DEFECT

Mild hemorrhagic diathesis.

Passovoy was the name of the first patient in whom it was identified.

PASTEUR EFFECT

The inhibition of glucose consumption and lactic acid accumulation with the onset of oxygen consumption (aerobic versus anaerobic glycolysis).

PASTEUR PIPETTE

Tapered glass pipette in common laboratory use.

PASTEURELLA

Genus of Gram negative rods – one such, *Pasteurella pestis*, is responsible for bubonic plague.

PASTEURIZATION

Heat treatment to sterilize milk.

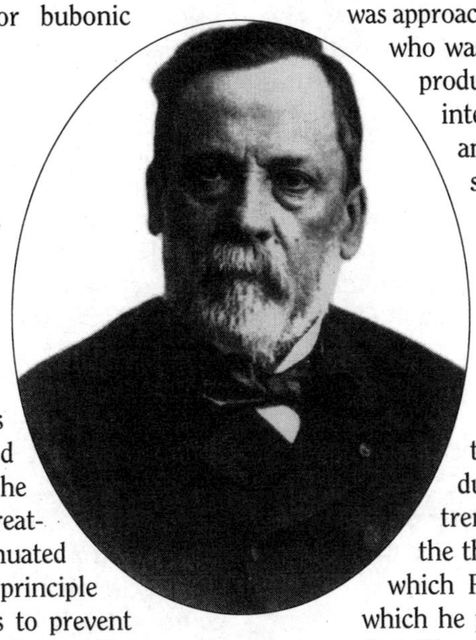

Louis Pasteur (1822–1895) French chemist and bacteriologist who made many contributions to establish the science of bacteriology and the principles of fermentation. His work saved the silk worm industry and he introduced the first successful treatment for rabies, using attenuated virus and thus establishing a principle used to develop other vaccines to prevent other viral infections, e.g. poliomyelitis. Pasteur's contributions to science were possibly the greatest in the history of mankind and frequently seemed to follow a statement he made in his inaugural address as Professor and Dean of the new Faculty of Sciences at Lille, "in the field of observation, chance favours only the prepared minds". (Dans les champs, le hasard ne favorise que les esprits préparés.) Pasteur was born in Dôle, Jura, the son of a tanner who was a sergeant in Napoleon's army. He attended school in Arbois and although not outstanding as a student, showed a talent for sketching and was an enthusiastic fisherman. He graduated from college at Besançon in 1840 and 2 years later gained a Bachelor of Science degree. In 1843 he went to Paris to the École Normale and attended lectures by Dumas at the Sorbonne. He became a laboratory assistant to the chemist, A.J. Ballard, and obtained his doctorate in 1848. With his revolutionary work on crystals he showed that the reaction of tartaric acid to polarize light depended on the composition and shape of the crystals in the preparations. Those that he showed on the microscope to be right-faced crystals rotated polarized light to the right while those that had left-faced crystals rotated them in the opposite direction. By mixing the two together, the solution became inactive. This founded the whole science of stereo-chemistry and gained him the Rumford Medal of the Royal Society of London in 1856. Whilst he was at Lille, he was approached by one of the manufacturers who was having problems with alcohol production. This commenced his interest in alcoholic fermentation and lactic acid fermentation in sour milk. He continued his studies on this when he was called back to Paris as Director of Scientific Studies at the École Normale in 1857 and concluded at that time that fermentation was caused by organisms and would not occur if these organisms were not introduced into the liquid. This aroused tremendous controversy because of the theory of spontaneous generation which Pasteur vigorously opposed and which he proved to be wrong by showing that if he placed liquid in a flask and boiled it, but left the flask open, putrefaction would occur, whereas if the neck of the flask was drawn to a fine point or sealed off, the solution would remain pure. As a result of such experiments he paved the way for the whole science of bacteriology and for the introduction of antisepsis by Lister.

Louis Pasteur (Courtesy of the Royal Society of Medicine, London, UK)

In 1849 the silkworm industry of France was crippled by a disease called pebrine. This was so called because the worms developed black pepper-like spots and Pasteur was asked by the French Government to attempt to overcome this menace. Pasteur, with his group, worked for 5 years near Alleis when microscopic examination convinced Pasteur that the disease was caused by bacteria and that the worms had to be bred from eggs which were healthy. Just as he had discovered this he found that there was another disease affecting the silkworm which initially caused him to be quite depressed after the years of work that he had put into the project. However, he finally realized that this disorder was due to the mulberry leaves being infected with a bacteria causing a very contagious intestinal disease. He showed that this could be prevented by using healthy mulberry leaves. These findings saved the French silk industry but prior to the successful termination of his studies, he had been subjected to a great deal of criticism, for his lack of success. Furthermore, the seed merchants themselves spread rumors about his lack of success because they greatly feared the financial loss that might be incurred.

In 1864 the wine industry in Jura was being injured by a disease which caused the wine to be sour. He showed that this was because of organisms in the wine and that this could be eliminated by heating it for a short period of time to 60°C. This process has since been used in many areas and is called "pasteurization".

In 1868 he had a cerebral hemorrhage which resulted in temporary loss of speech and for a while complete left hemiplegia, but after some months he made a complete recovery and continued with his work.

In 1870 the Franco-Prussian War broke out, and Pasteur, who was an intense nationalist, returned his honorary diploma of Doctor of Medicine sent to him 2 years earlier from the University of Bonn. Perhaps as a result he set out to improve French beer, which resulted in him showing that one of the problems with the industry was again micro-organisms which were different from the beer yeast. Again he showed that pasteurization could produce a much superior product. He then studied anthrax and chicken cholera and in the latter instance succeeded in isolating the organism involved and discovered that old cultures of this organism lost their virulence but could be used on injection to protect the animals from inoculation with a virulent culture. He applied a similar approach to anthrax and developed an attenuated culture which could be used to protect the animals against infection.

In 1880 he commenced his work on rabies. After studying the methods of transmission of the disease and the localization of the organism he developed a technique employing living rabbit brain for attenuating the organism. In 1885 he had shown that this technique could protect healthy dogs from the bite of rabid animals. However on July 6, 1885, a small Alsatian boy, Joseph Meister, was brought to Pasteur's laboratory by his mother with the history that her son had been bitten by a rabid dog 2 days earlier. He was hesitant about trying to treat the boy, but on seeing his state, and after consulting Dr. Vulpian (*v. infra*) and Dr. Grancher, he injected the boy with material from his rabbit experiments. The injections were continued daily and Pasteur went through a great deal of mental anguish so that he could not even sleep or work during the time he was treating the lad. The success of his treatment attracted enormous publicity and resulted in a fund being established which was contributed to by the Czar of Russia, the Emperor of Brazil and Sultan of Turkey as well as the people of France, and as a result the Pasteur Institute was founded. It was opened in 1888. By that time Pasteur was quite ill, and never in fact was able to work actively in the new laboratories. Pasteur was a very devout Catholic. He was a very sensitive man who suffered a great deal from criticisms levelled at him by people far his inferior. Single-handedly he altered the course of the history of medicine. His love for animals was a byword and his concern was such that it would have provoked amusement in his colleagues were it not that it was so patently real. He died with a crucifix in one hand and his wife's hand in the other.

PATAU SYNDROME

Trisomy 13 syndrome.

Failure to thrive, severe mental retardation, fits, sloping forehead, cleft palate, low set ears and rocker bottom feet as well as congenital heart defects.

Klaus Patau U.S. geneticist.

PATERSON-KELLY SYNDROME

v. PLUMMER-VINSON SYNDROME

Donald R. Paterson (1863–1939) British ear, nose and throat surgeon. He was born in Inverness and graduated in medicine from Edinburgh University in 1883. He went as a house surgeon in 1884 to the Cardiff Infirmary. Initially he practiced as a consulting physician but soon became interested in ear, nose and throat diseases, became the first person to be placed in charge of this speciality at Cardiff Infirmary, and remained there until his retirement from active duties. In 1919 he published a paper in the Journal of Laryngology "A clinical type of dysphagia" in which he described the glossitis, dysphagia and anemia.

He was a fine linguist and translated into English Killian's "Accessory sinuses of the nose". He was especially famed in his country and elsewhere for his pioneering work using esophagoscopy and bronchoscopy. Outside of medicine, he was an ardent archeologist and a keen golfer and fisherman. Most summers he spent trout fishing in Scandinavia, and he loved walking around the Welsh countryside, knowing by heart all the ancient monuments and historic homes. He had always been interested in nurse training. Following his retirement from Cardiff Infirmary he continued his association with the hospital. He had, just before his death, attended a meeting of the House Committee to consider a request concerning the allocation of facilities for training women as voluntary ambulance drivers, which most of his fellow members were not in favor of granting, but he said, "I think we should be sympathetic to this request". These were his last words, shortly afterwards he had a cerebral thrombosis and died 2 weeks later.

Adam Brown-Kelly (1865–1941) British ear, nose and throat surgeon. He graduated from Glasgow University in 1888 and studied in London, Berlin and Vienna. He concentrated his practice and research energy on the larynx and esophagus. He wrote on the neuroses of the larynx as well as neurological factors causing immobility of the vocal cords. He was especially interested in studies of the esophagus, and his most important contributions there were the description of congenital stenosis and shortening as well as nervous problems involving esophageal motility and his initial description in 1919 of the esophageal dysphagia associated with anemia and atrophy of the tongue. He was one of the pioneers of the use of the endoscope and wrote a number of papers on pharyngeal disease. A shy, retiring man, his only interest outside his speciality in medicine was music.

PATRICK TRIGGER AREA

Areas in the distribution of the 5th nerve which on stimulation precipitate an attack of trigeminal neuralgia (Tic doloreaux).

Hugh T. Patrick (1860–1938) U.S. neurologist and neuro-psychiatrist. He was born in New Philadelphia, Ohio. His father was a prosecuting attorney, later judge and eventually senator in the Ohio Legislature. He graduated from medical school at the Bellevue Hospital Medical College (New York University) in 1884 and after interning in New York went to practice in Chicago in 1886. From 1891 to 1894 he worked in medical centers in Germany, France and England and in 1895 he returned to be elected to the Faculty of Northwestern University Medical School as instructor and was appointed Professor of Nervous and Mental Diseases in 1902, retiring in 1919. He was the Founder and Editor of the Archives of Neurology and Psychiatry and founded the Chicago Neurological Society. He wrote on many aspects of neurology, in particular atherosclerosis and its effects, and syphilis as well as the factor of fear. Although in his fifties when America became involved in the 1st World War, he served as a consulting neurologist in the U.S. Army. Later in life he became interested in historical aspects of neurology. He died of cancer of the stomach.

PAUL SIGN

In pericarditis the apex beat may be difficult to feel although precordial activity is easily felt.

Constantin C.T. Paul (1833–1896) French physician, born in Paris and studied at the Louis-le-Grand, becoming interne des hôpitaux in 1857 and receiving his doctorate in 1861. He became an Agrégé in 1866 and worked successively at the Bicêtre, Saint-Antoine, Laribosière and La Charité. He was a student of Trousseau, Gubler and Pidaux and concentrated his life work on the study of disorders of the heart and therapeutics. He wrote a classical monograph on diagnosis and treatment of heart disease and contributed to the very successful book on therapeutics edited by Trousseau and Pidaux. Apart from his work on heart disease he wrote on a wide variety of subjects including lead poisoning, strontium salts and the advantages of a flexible stethoscope.

For his work with the ambulance at Val-de-Grace he was made a Chevalier of the Legion of Honour in 1871. He was adored by both his rich and poor patients and was a fine teacher of medical students. He was particularly interested in oriental art and had a fine collection which he gathered during trips to Bulgaria and Turkey.

PAUL-BUNNELL TEST

A test for infectious mononucleosis using red cells from different species to detect heterophile antibodies in the patient's serum.

John R. Paul (1893–1971) U.S. physician and pathologist. He was born in Philadelphia and after college in Princeton enrolled at Johns Hopkins in 1915. He spent his student vacation working at Dr. Greenfield's mission in Labrador. In 1917 he enlisted and worked in the 1st American Base Hospital with Walter Cannon who was working on shock and Hans Zinsser on wound infections. He graduated M.D. from Johns Hopkins in 1919 and then worked as assistant pathologist with W.J. McCallum and went with him to study Oroya fever (*v. supra*) in Peru. He wrote a book on the epidemiology of rheumatic fever in 1930 and clinical epidemiology in 1958 and spent a lifetime in research in infectious diseases. He was Professor of Preventative Medicine at Yale from 1940–1961. He described his observations with Bunnell in 1932.

Walls W. Bunnell (1902–1966) U.S. physician.

PAUTRIER MICROABSCESS

Seen in mycosis fungoides and reticulum cell sarcoma.

Lucien M. Pautrier (1876–1959) Born in South of France near Marseilles, he commenced his medical studies there, but transferred to Paris where he was influenced to become interested in dermatology by Leredde and in his thesis in 1903 on "A typical lesion of tuberculosis" attracted the attention of Darier with his demonstrations and clear patient presentation. He joined the army at the outbreak of the first World War and became a medical officer to a field artillery regiment. He was awarded the Croix de Guerre for bravery under fire and became a Chevalier of the Legion of Honour in 1916, finally becoming a Grand Officer. Towards the end of the war he established a centre for investigation of skin and venereal disease in Bourges. When the war ended and the Alsace once more became a part of France, he was appointed Professor of Dermatology at Strasburg and there rapidly built up a national and worldwide reputation which attracted students from all over the world. When the second World War commenced he was repatriated to Claivive in the Dordogne, but in 1942 he was invited to take the Chair of Dermatology in Switzerland in Lausanne when Professor Ramel died. At the end of the war he returned to Strasburg, but two years later retired. Here he occupied himself with his great loves of art and music. He was a close friend of Georges Enesco and he founded a society of the Friends of Music in Strasburg and was largely responsible for the 21st Festival of Music in that City. He founded the Society of Friends of the avant-garde cinema and finally whilst he was the President of the Friendly Society of the University of Strasburg he managed to find the necessary funds after much difficulty, to create a center for research in experimental surgery.

PAVLOVIAN CONDITIONING

The establishment of a conditioned reflex.

PAVLOV POUCH

Externalization of a portion of stomach separate from the rest but retaining vagal innervation.

Ivan P. Pavlov (1849–1936) Famous Russian experimental physiologist. He was born the son of a peasant priest in Rjazan, a village in Central Russia, and initially was educated to the priesthood. However, he began to study medicine at the University of St. Petersburg and won a two year Fellowship to study in Germany when he graduated. He worked with Carl Ludwig on the circulation in Leipzig and with Heidenhain (*v. supra*) at Breslau (Wroclaw) on pancreatic function and gastric secretion. Returning to St. Petersburg he eventually became Professor of Physiology at the Army Medical Academy and in 1890 was made Director of the Institute for Experimental Medicine. He modified the Heidenhain pouch so that it was a miniature stomach with an intact nerve supply opening to the outside of the body and this enabled him to study the process of digestion. He observed that the sight or smell of food caused copious secretions of both saliva and gastric guice in his animal even if the food never reached the stomach, and that this could be prevented by sectioning the vagus nerve. For his work on this experimental model Pavlov received a Nobel Prize in 1904. It is said that Pavlov always referred to his preparation as the Heidenhain-Pavlov pouch. Following this work Pavlov turned to an examination of so-called conditioned reflexes which won him acclaim throughout the world. He had noticed that decerebrate animals always acted the same way to a stimulus but that normal animals could modify their actions – he called the first inherited reflexes unconditional, and the second acquired responses conditional. The development of this theme not only produced important advances in the understanding of neurology but also introduced the subject of behavioral psychology.

He was one of the first – if not the first – physiologists to introduce modern operative techniques into the physiology laboratory. He was an extremely dexterous operator who was compulsive about his working hours and habits. He would sit down to lunch at exactly 12 o'clock, would play the same records on his phonograph on the same night of each week, month after month. He would go to bed at exactly the same hour each evening, and he would always leave Leningrad for Estonia on a summer vacation on the same day each year. This was only changed when his son Victor died in the White army and from that time on he had difficulty sleeping.

Pavlov's philosophy is perhaps best summed up by his own writing "First of all, be systematic, learn to do drudgery, second comes modesty; pride will deprive you of the ability to be objective, and the third thing necessary is passion – be passionate in your work and in your search for truth".

PAVY DISEASE

Recurrent proteinuria.

PAVY JOINT

Arthritis seen in typhoid fever.

Frederick W. Pavy (1829–1911) English physician who was a student at Guy's Hospital, he graduated M.B. in 1852 at the London University. After undertaking his residency at Guy's Hospital he went to Paris where he studied with Claude Bernard and returned to London, where in 1854 he was appointed lecturer in anatomy at Guy's Hospital. In 1856 he was appointed lecturer in physiology. He retained his post in anatomy until 1864 when he resigned but continued in physiology until 1877. He was elected physician to Guy's Hospital in 1858 and held many offices in the College of Physicians including that of censor and councillor. He received many honors and gave many named lectures and was elected F.R.S. in 1863. He had a large private practice to which he devoted his morning, but his afternoon he rigorously kept for research. He apparently taught little at the bedside, leaving it to the students to observe his techniques on a round in which the ward sister would always carry a tray with the implements he required for taking urine tests. A man of few words, he rarely bothered to explain his method of arrival at a particular diagnosis and the anecdote is told that he surprised his staff one afternoon by ordering a red hot iron to be applied later on in the day to the spine of a man who said he could not walk, and who all those attending believed had organic paraplegia. As soon as they left the ward, the patient fled the hospital, cured! Careful in his use of words, it is said that the only books he ever read were the dictionary and Roget's thesaurus.

He devoted his life as an investigator to diabetes, the digestion of food, dietetics and albuminuria. The majority of his views would not be entertained today and throughout his life he opposed those of Claude Bernard on glycogenesis. Nonetheless he contributed much as a teacher and added to medical knowledge with his studies on albuminuria, his dietetic treatment of diabetes, his development of a method of measuring blood glucose and his demonstration, perhaps the first, of a group of proteins in the body which contain carbohydrate. He also concluded that the degree of glucosemia is related to that of glycosuria. He was probably the first to recognize benign albuminuria and the importance of the presence of acetone in patients with diabetes. Apart from numerous papers he was the author of several books on diabetes and digestion.

PAYR DISEASE

Colonic obstruction due to kinking of the hepatic or splenic flexures of the colon.

Erwin Payr (1871–1947) German surgeon, born in Innsbruck and graduated there in 1894 and then went to work in Vienna and Graz. He was Professor of Surgery successively in Graz, Greifswald and Königsberg before Leipzig. He became Professor of Surgery at Leipzig (1911). He transplanted a portion of thyroid from a woman to the spleen of her myxedematous daughter with alleged success (1906) and worked on suture techniques for anastomosis of the intestine and blood vessels. He designed a colonic clamp which bears his name.

PEL CRISES

Ocular crises of tabes dorsalis.

PEL EBSTEIN FEVER

Febrile episodes at intervals of a few days to weeks characteristically seen with Hodgkin disease involving the thoracic nodes.

Pieter K. Pel (1852–1919) Dutch physician. He was born in Drachten and studied medicine at Leiden, enrolling in 1869 and graduating in 1876. After working as an assistant to Rosenstein at Leiden, he visited Paris, Berlin and Vienna and in 1877 became an assistant of Professor Stokvis at Amsterdam. He was appointed the latter's successor in 1883 becoming Professor of Pathology and Medicine and described the fever in 1885, two years before Ebstein. He was an excellent clinical teacher and very popular with students. He wrote textbooks on the heart, stomach and liver, but ill health forced him to retire in 1919 and he died shortly after.

Wilhelm Ebstein (1836–1912) (*v. supra*).

PELGER HÜET ANOMALY

A familial congenital anomaly of the granulocytes in which there is decreased segmentation of the nucleus, distinctive nuclear forms, and pyknosis of the nuclear chromatin out of proportion to the nuclear area. It is inherited as an autosomal dominant. It is also seen in rabbits. Acquired forms have been observed in chronic myeloid leukemia, viral illnesses and malaria. It may be seen associated with Fanconi anemia and mongolism.

Karel Pelger (1885–1931) Dutch physician who was born in Nijeveen and went to medical school in Groningen, commencing in 1904 and graduating in 1912 when he became a general practitioner in Amsterdam. He studied in Berlin with Schilling (*v. infra*) and learnt the hematological techniques which he applied and discovered the morphological feature to which his name is attached. Initially he thought this was a pathological feature, but with Hüet he finally concluded that it was a benign hereditary anomaly. He died at his farm in Havelte before completing a book he was writing on clinical hematology.

Gauthier J. Hüet (1879–1970) Dutch pediatrician. He entered medical school at Leiden in 1898 and graduated from there in 1904. In 1907 he commenced practice as a pediatrician at The Hague and was appointed medical superintendent of "Hoog Blaricum" Children's Hospital. He continued there until his 75th year in 1954. In 1934 he made the first description of mucoviscidosis. His other major interest was in asthma and he devoted much time to studying the psychogenic factors in asthmatic children.

PELIZAEUS-MERZBACHER DISEASE

An hereditary disorder of the nervous system characterized by rotary nystagmus, ataxia, intention tremor, spasticity and dementia. It begins in infancy and is slowly progressive.

Friedrich Pelizaeus (1850–1917) German neurologist who worked in Cassel.

Ludwig Merzbacher (1875–1942) German physician who practiced later in Buenos Aires, Argentina.

PELLIZI SYNDROME

Precocious puberty associated with a pineal tumor.

G.B. Pellizi Italian physician who worked in Pisa.

PEMBERTON SIGN

Raising the arms above the head causes venous congestion in the neck and/or face in patients with upper mediastinal obstruction secondary to lymphoma, tumor or retrosternal goitre.

John de J. Pemberton (1887–1967) U.S. surgeon. He was born in Wadesboro, North Carolina and graduated M.D. from the University of Pennsylvania in 1911. He joined the Mayo Clinic as a Fellow in Surgery in 1913 and remaining at the Mayo, became a Professor of Surgery in 1936. He was a pioneer in thyroid surgery but made a number of other contributions to general surgery including the use of blood transfusions in 1918. He died of carcinomatosis.

PEPPER SYNDROME

Neuroblastoma with hepatic metastases.

William Pepper (1874–1947) U.S. physician. Professor of Medicine at University of Pennsylvania, he followed his father and grandfather in that position and was succeeded by his son-in-law. It was said that to get into the faculty at the University of Pennsylvania you had to get out of or into a Pepper pelvis.

PERLS REACTION

Staining technique to demonstrate hemosiderin.

Max Perls (1843–1881) German pathologist.

PERTHES DISEASE

v. LEGG-CALVE-PERTHES-WALDENSTROM DISEASE OR SYNDROME

Osteochondritis of the head of the femur. It usually commences between 5–10 years of age. In a minority of cases it is bilateral.

PERTHES TEST

A test for varicose veins to determine patency of the deep veins and competence of the saphenous and communicating veins. With the patient standing and veins filled, a tourniquet is placed around the mid-thigh and the patient walks for 5 minutes. If the veins collapse below the tourniquet the deep veins are patent and the communicating veins are competent; if unchanged, both saphenous and communicating veins are incompetent and if the veins increase in prominence and pain occurs the deep veins are occluded.

Georg C. Perthes (1869–1927) German surgeon, Professor of Surgery at Tübingen, succeeding Bruns. Described osteochondritic hip deformity in 1910, one year after it was noted by A.T. Legg. He initiated deep X-ray therapy (1903) and was an early pioneer in the use of X-rays in cancer treatment.

PERUVIAN BARK

Cinchona alkaloids (quinine) first derived from trees in Peru.

PETRI DISH

One of the most universally used pieces of glassware in microbiology laboratories. A covered shallow dish for culturing and sub-culturing bacteria. The monument to Koch in Berlin shows him carrying a Petri dish.

Richard J. Petri (1852–1921) German bacteriologist. Born in Barmen and became a German army medical officer who was seconded to Koch as his assistant and was appointed head of the Goebersdorf Sanatorium, administered by the Imperial Board of Health. A Prussian disciplinarian, he ran the tuberculosis sanatorium on strictly disciplinary lines for both staff and patients. Prior to this appointment he had developed a technique for cloning bacterial strains using an agar slope and sub-culturing onto his dish, recognizing different bacterial colonies and again sub-culturing. He was in his later days a rather vain, overweight man, who dressed in the uniform of a chief army doctor whenever the opportunity presented itself. The sash around his protuberant abdomen reminded one observer of the equator around the globe.

PETTE-DÖRING DISEASE

Subacute sclerosing panencephalitis.

Heinrich Pette (1887–) German neuropathologist.

Gerhard Döring (1909–) German neuropathologist.

PEUTZ-JEGHERS SYNDROME

Benign intestinal hamartomatous polyposis associated with melanin deposits on the mucocutaneous junctions of the mouth and sometimes anus, and inherited as an autosomal dominant. The benign nature of these lesions contrasts with the polyps in Gardner syndrome and familial polyposis.

John L.A. Peutz (1886–1957) Dutch physician who worked in The Hague.

Harold J. Jeghers (1904–) U.S. physician who was Professor of Medicine at Tufts Medical School, Boston and later moved to the New Jersey College of Medicine and Dentistry.

PEYER PATCHES

Lymph follicles in the small intestine.

Johan C. Peyer (1653–1712) Swiss anatomist, born in Schaffhausen, Switzerland. He studied medicine in Basel. He noted these structures in patients who had died with typhoid fever. He did not realize they were lymphatic in origin but felt they were glands secreting digestive juices (1667). He wrote on the physiology of rumination (1685).

PEYRONIE DISEASE

Painless and slowly developing induration of penis with resultant deformity and, at times, inability to achieve an erection. Often associated with Dupuytren contracture (*v. supra*).

François de la Peyronie (1678–1747) French surgeon of Montpellier, and physician to Louis XIV. He influenced Louis to issue an ordinance banning barbers and wigmakers from practicing, so that to become a Master of Surgery one had first to become a Master of Arts. Together with G. Mareschal (1658–1736) he founded the Academy of Surgery. He personally funded a Chair of Surgery and obtained four professorships at Montpellier. In his will he left money to establish annual prizes in surgery and to build an amphitheater at St. Côme. He was a major force in establishing Paris as the world centre of surgery in the 18th century.

PFAUNDLER-HURLER SYNDROME

v. HURLER SYNDROME

Meinhard von Pfaundler (1872–1947) Austrian pediatrician who wrote a large textbook on pediatrics with A. Schlossmann. He was born in Innsbruck and trained with Hofmeister in Strasburg and with Escherich. He was appointed head of the Children's Hospital in Munich in 1939 and retired 2 years later. He moved to the Austrian Tyrol in 1944 when his house in Munich was destroyed in a bombing raid.

PFEIFFER BACILLUS

Haemophilus influenzae.

PFEIFFER DISEASE

Infectious mononucleosis.

Richard F.J. Pfeiffer (1858–1945) German bacteriologist. Born at Zduny, Posen, Poland. He graduated in 1880 in Berlin and served in the army as a bacteriologist until 1889. He worked with Koch at the Institute for Hygiene in Berlin and became Professor there in 1894. He moved to Königsberg in 1899 until 1909 and then to the Chair of Hygiene at Breslau (Wroclaw) until he retired in 1926. He discovered the *Haemophilus influenzae* in 1892 and was a pioneer in typhoid vaccination and described glandular fever in 1889. In 1894 he found that live cholera vibrios could be injected without ill effects into guinea pigs previously immunized against cholera and that plasma from these animals added to live vibrio caused them to become motionless and to lyse. This could be inhibited by previously heating the serum. He called this bacteriolysis and it became known as the Pfeiffer phenomenon.

PHOCAS DISEASE

Fibrous nodular dysplasia of the breast.

B. Gerasime Phocas (1861–1937) French surgeon. He was born in Greece but migrated to France when a child. He became Chirurgien des Hôpitaux de Lille in 1895 and worked on tuberculosis in children. He was appointed Professor of Surgery in Athens in 1902. He served in the war between Greece and Turkey in 1913 and returned to France in 1914 to serve in the French army in World War I.

PICK CELL

Foam cell. Histiocyte containing phagocytosed material giving its cytoplasm a foamy appearance.

Ludwig Pick

v. NIEMANN-PICK DISEASE

PICK DISEASE (1)

1. Cerebral atrophy of frontal and temporal lobes resulting in senile dementia.

v. ALZHEIMER DISEASE

Arnold Pick (1851–1924) Czech physician. He was born of German-Jewish parents in a village called Delkae Mezirici in Moravia. He studied medicine in Vienna and was student assistant to Meynert. He graduated in 1875 and became assistant to Westphal in Berlin, at the same time as Wernicke, who was also in that unit. All three influenced his work on aphasia. He became physician to the Landesirrenanstalt ("Katerinke") in Prague in 1877. He was made Director of a new mental hospital in Dobran in 1880. In 1886 he was appointed Professor of Psychiatry (Neurology) at the German University of Prague. This was a time of quite a deal of political and social upheaval – the University being in the Kingdom of Bohemia, whilst the academic teaching in both the German and Czech Universities was controlled by the Austro-Hungarian Empire. There was the problem of having German professors teaching German students in German, in the German part of the asylum, which had previously been a convent, St. Catherine's, while all the patients, or the majority of the patients, spoke only Czech. He commented "the surgeon has an easy life, all he has to do is ask 'does this hurt'? – to probe the patients' minds the way we are supposed to, we need quite a bit more". He discovered the disease named after him whilst investigating a patient's aphasia and described the disorder in 1892. He wrote a textbook on neuropathology and contributed greatly to the patho-anatomical basis of aphasia and wrote extensively on apraxia and agrammatism. These studies made him an acknowledged world authority on localization of cerebral function.

He engaged in correspondence with all the major figures of the day, Dejerine, Marie, Head and Hughlings Jackson. He was a close associate with the Professor of Medicine at the same University, Otto Kahler (*v. supra*). He had an extensive collection of books in German, French and English, and a great love of music. His skill in taking a history from patients who were psychotic and even mute was legendary. His secretary was a manic-depressive and an inmate of the asylum in which he worked. He had a great collection of friends, including the philosopher, F. Jodl, the philologist, Sauer, the physicist, Mark, and count Gleispach, the jurist.

He died from sepsis following an operation for a stone in the bladder.

PICK DISEASE (2)

1. Chronic constrictive pericarditis.
2. Polyserositis (v. CONCATO DISEASE and BAMBERGER DISEASE)

Friedel J. Pick (1867–1926) German physician. He described cirrhosis of the liver secondary to pericarditis in 1896.

PICKWICKIAN SYNDROME

Obesity, somnolence and hypoxia with CO_2 retention.

Mr Pickwick The term derived from a character, the fat boy, in Charles Dickens' "Pickwick Papers", and was first applied by Sir William Osler. It is one of the sleep apnea syndromes (v. ONDINE CURSE and PIERRE ROBIN SYNDROME).

PIERRE ROBIN SYNDROME

Congenital anomaly – micrognathia, cleft palate and prominent tongue. Detached retina and glaucoma sometimes occur. May be associated with sleep apnoea syndrome (v. ONDINE CURSE).

Pierre Robin (1867–1950) French dental surgeon. He was best known for his contributions to orthodontistry, but published on many aspects of dentistry and oral hygiene. He was Professor of the French School of Dentistry in Paris and in 1914 became the Editor-in-Chief with Nogue of the Journal La Revue de Stomatologie.

PIGBEL

Severe and sometimes fatal gastrointestinal syndrome due to ingestion of meat contaminated with bacterial toxin, caused by *Clostridium perfringens*. First described in New Guinea in natives eating pork stored after cooking. Pigbel is Pigeon English for pig's belly.

PILCZ REFLEX

Consensual light reflex in the pupil.

Alexander Pilcz (1871–1954) Austrian neurologist who was a student and assistant to Julius Wagner von Jauregg (*v. infra*). His principal interest was on hereditary factors in mental disease.

PINEL SYSTEM

The treatment of mental conditions in a humane fashion.

Phillipe Pinel (1745–1826) French physician. He was born near Laboise in France and initially was going to study theology but changed to medicine and graduated from the medical school at Toulouse in 1772. He then studied at Montpellier and finally came to Paris in 1788, where he supported himself by teaching mathematics. Work he undertook on the mechanics of bones and joints was widely acclaimed and he was appointed to a position at the Jardin des Plantes. A friend of his became insane and ran into the country where he was eaten by wolves. From that time he devoted his time to mental illness and was appointed in 1792 to the Bicêtre which was then a hospital for the insane. There he found appalling conditions, with patients being chained to the walls, treated like beasts, and put on display to the public, who paid admission to see them. He abolished the chains and introduced humane treatment for these people, which represented a landmark in the treatment of mental disease. Perhaps because of his interest in botany, he was greatly interested in systematic classification of disease and in 1789 published a treatise in which diseases were classified in a similar manner to plants and animals. This work was a great success and made him famous, and in 1794 he became physician to the Salpêtrière and in 1802 published "La Médecine Clinique" which was based on his experiences at the Salpêtrière and in which he extended his previous book on classification of disease. Pinel's system of classification was of course quite makeshift and grouped together many quite unrelated disorders; for example, under the classification of internal hemorrhage, he would have such diverse conditions as menorrhagia, hemoptysis, hematuria, hemorrhoids and aneurysms. He gave little attention to either autopsy findings or etiology, relating his classification to clinical symptoms rather than morbid anatomy. A statue in his honor stands outside the Salpêtrière in Paris.

PINS SIGN

Loss of pain in pericarditis when patient leans forward to the knee-chest position.

E. Pins (1845–1913) Austrian physician.

PIOTROWSKI ANTERIOR TIBIAL REFLEX OR SIGN

Tapping the anterior tibial muscle causes plantar flexion of the ankle and sometimes toes. This may be exaggerated in pyramidal tract disorders.

Aleksanda Piotrowski (1878–) German neurologist.

PIRIE SYNDROME

v. DEBRÉ-FIBIGER SYNDROME

George R. Pirie English physician.

PLUMMER DISEASE

Hyperthyroidism with a nodular goitre.

PLUMMER NAIL

Concave or ragged edge to the nail bed seen in early onycholysis occurring with thyrotoxicosis usually most prominent in the 4th and 5th fingers.

PLUMMER SIGN

Inability of patient to sit in a chair due to thyrotoxic myopathy.

PLUMMER TREATMENT

Use of iodine to treat thyrotoxicosis.

PLUMMER-VINSON SYNDROME

v. PATERSON-KELLY, WALDENSTRÖM KJELLBERG SYNDROMES

Sideropenic dysphagia. Koilonychia with glossitis and difficulty in swallowing due to iron deficiency. There is usually an associated iron deficiency anemia.

Henry S. Plummer (1874–1936) U.S. physician. Born in Hamilton, Minnesota he graduated M.D. in 1898 from North-western University and after practicing with his father in Racine, Minnesota, he joined the Mayo Clinic in 1901 and remained until he died. He was one of the first to investigate the therapeutic use of oxygen in respiratory disease. He was particularly interested in the diagnostic and investigative potential of bronchoscopy and esophagoscopy. This led to his interest in cardiospasm and esophageal stricture and in his development of hydrostatic dilators and esophageal sounds which he designed and made in his own workshop. He designed the medical record system which is still used at the Mayo as well as the examination couches which have become standard equipment of most doctors' offices and medical clinics throughout North America. He had wide interests in literature, music and the visual arts as well as being an authority on the cultivation of flowers. His death followed a cerebral thrombosis.

Porter P. Vinson (1890–1959) U.S. physician. Born in Davidson, North Carolina, he graduated M.D. from the University of Maryland in 1914. He came to the Mayo Clinic in 1916 as one of the first Fellows in Medicine and worked with Plummer (*v. supra*) on the techniques of esophagoscopy and bronchoscopy, becoming an authority on these maneuvers in diagnosis and in removal of foreign objects. He left the Mayo in 1936 to go into private practice in Richmond, Virginia with a particular interest in esophageal disorders and chest disease. He died two weeks after abdominal surgery, following a myocardial infarct.

POISE

Unit of measurement of viscosity.

POISEUILLE EQUATION

Mathematical expression to describe flow of water in a narrow bore glass tube.

POISEUILLE LAYER OR SPACE

The bloodstream close to vessel wall.

Jean L.M. Poiseuille (1799–1869) French physiologist, born in Paris and graduated in medicine there in 1828. He studied blood pressure and the viscosity of the blood. He showed that blood pressure rises on expiration and falls on inspiration.

POLAND ANOMALY OR SYNDROME

Microsyndactyly or lack of one hand with atrophy of the costal portion of the pectoralis major muscle. There may be associated costal cartilage defects, absence or hypoplasia of the nipple and breast, and genito-urinary abnormalities.

Alfred Poland (1820–1872) English surgeon who was apprenticed to Aston Key in 1839 and won several prizes as a student at Guy's Hospital. He was initially interested in eye surgery and worked at Moorfields' ophthalmic hospital for some years before he was appointed ophthalmic surgeon at Guy's and later full surgeon in 1861. He was a modest retiring man who was quite careless about his appearance and was warned by the Treasurer to dress more decently and cleanly but ignored this advice. He was known by his colleagues to be an excellent surgeon but would time his operations at unusual hours so that few observed him and perhaps for the above reasons, he had a small practice. Apart from his surgical dexterity he was renowned at the hospital for his encyclopedic knowledge and the excellence of his presentations, both oral and written. He was an extremely popular teacher but his career was punctuated by recurrent illness so that he remarked that he was like a cat and had nine lives. After one severe bout of hemoptysis his physician ordered him to bed only to see him the next day doing the rounds with his students. He died of consumption.

POMPE DISEASE

Glycogen storage disease due to a deficiency of α 1–4 glycosidase resulting in macroglossia, cardiomegaly and generalized weakness, due to excessive storage in skeletal muscle and hepatomegaly.

cf. GIERKE DISEASE and McARDLE SYNDROME

Also called glycogen storage disease type II.

Joannus C. Pompe (1901–1945) Dutch pathologist. He studied medicine at the University of Amsterdam and graduated M.D. with a thesis in 1936 which was on the disorder that bears his name. He was a very cultivated man who read Sophocles in Greek and could recite extensively from the works of the Dutch Vondel. He was a devout Catholic and interested in liturgy. In the 2nd World War a secret transmitter was found in his laboratory and he was imprisoned by the Germans in February 1945. After a railway line was blown up near St. Pancras he and nineteen others were shot as a retaliative measure.

PONCET DISEASE

Tuberculous polyarthritis.

Antonin Poncet (1864–1913) French surgeon.

PONFICK SHADOW

An erythrocyte which has lost its hemoglobin.

Emil Ponfick (1844–1913) German pathologist who was born in Frankfurt. He studied medicine in Tübingen, Freiburg and Heidelberg and for a while was assistant to the famous Heidelberg surgeon C.O. Weber. He worked with von Recklinghausen (*v. infra*) in Würzburg and then moved to work with Rudolph Virchow at the Pathological Institute in Berlin in 1868 and became a First Assistant there in 1873. Whilst there he published on pathology of the liver and spleen, as well as the blood and bone marrow, embolism of the mesenteric artery and in 1873 was appointed Professor of Pathology in Rostock.

In 1875 he accompanied the Grand Duke of Mecklenburg on an expedition to Egypt, Nubia and Palestine, and throughout his life was very interested in German colonial affairs. In 1876 he was appointed to a Foundation Chair of Pathology in Göttingen and there he continued his work on hematological topics such as myelogenous leukemia and hemoglobinemia. In 1878 he succeeded Cohnheim in Breslau (Wroclaw) and remained there until he died. It was here that he established the identity of aspergillosis and the animal and human forms of actinomycosis, writing a textbook on the subject in 1882. He made important contributions to myxedema and published a large topographical atlas of medical/surgical diagnosis. His last work was "Bright Disease" which commanded his attention when one of his sons died of chronic renal disease. He managed to finish his monograph just before he died.

PORTER SIGN

Tracheal tug.

v. OLIVER-CARDARELLI SIGN

William H. Porter (1790–1861) Irish surgeon who was Professor of Surgery at the Royal College of Surgeons in Ireland. Robert Graves (*v. supra*) enlisted his support for William Stokes' (*v. infra*) appointment at Meath Hospital to replace Stokes' father on his resignation. Porter was worried that the introduction of auscultation might reduce the study of pathology in the patient. When convinced by Graves that the reverse would be the case he threw his influence behind Stokes' appointment. He helped the surgeon Rynd who introduced the administration of drugs (morphine) subcutaneously by a hypodermic syringe. This was uncalibrated, as the first syringe capable of delivering specific quantities of drugs was designed and used by Pravaz in France in 1854.

POTAIN SIGN

Opening snap (Claquement d'ouverture).

This is a sharp, high-pitched sound which is often best heard along the left sternal edge in patients with mitral stenosis. It is made by the aortic cusp of the mitral valve being pushed into the left ventricle as the atrio-ventricular pressure is reversed at the end of isometric relaxation. The interval between this sound and the aortic 2nd sound is related to the left atrial pressure. The closer the opening snap to the 2nd heart sound, the higher the atrial pressure.

Pierre C. Potain (1825–1901) He was born in Paris. In 1849 whilst an intern at the Hôpital Salpêtrière he caught cholera during the epidemic. He gained his M.D. in 1853. His dissertation on graduation concerned the vascular bruits following hemorrhage, and showed his early interest in auscultation. He attracted Trousseau's attention and in 1856 became the Chief of the clinic of Boillard and in 1861 was appointed Professeur Agrégé. Although he was asked to take charge and join the Medical Corps in the 1870 war, he enlisted as an infantry man and took part in several battles. In 1882 he became physician at the Charité and remained there until his retirement in 1900.

He wrote extensively on cardiac murmurs and was the first to study gallop rhythms. He invented

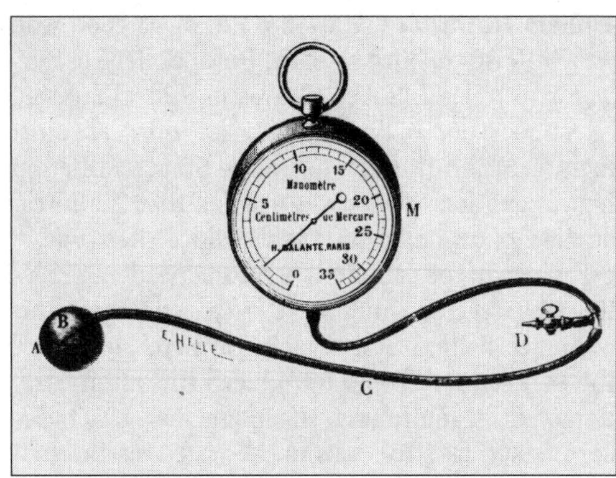

Close up of Potain's sphygmomanometer (Bibliothèque Interuniversitaire de Médicine, Paris)

a sphygmomanometer and an aspirator. He was a great clinician and pioneered and refined the use of auscultation in the diagnosis of cardiac disease. Potain's instrument for taking the blood pressure consisted of a compressible bulb filled with air which was attached by a rubber tube to an anaeroid manometer and the ball was then pressed on the arterial pulse till the beat disappeared, the point of disappearance being taken to be the systolic pressure. In 1875 he became Professor of Clinical Medicine. Reputed to be an extremely kindly examiner, it is said that if a candidate were asked a difficult question in a viva Potain would answer it himself if the candidate delayed the reply. He gave his last lecture in 1900 to a large audience, with tears in his eyes.

POTT CURVATURE

Angular kyphosis.

POTT DISEASE

Kyphosis secondary to tuberculosis.

POTT FRACTURE

Fracture of the fibula just above the ankle, sometimes associated with fracture of the tibia.

POTT GANGRENE

Vascular gangrene in the elderly.

POTT PECULIAR TUMOR OR PUFFY TUMOR

Swelling of scalp due to underlying osteomyelitis.

Percival Pott (1714–1788) English surgeon, born in London and at 16 apprenticed to Edward Nourse, a surgeon at St. Bartholomew's Hospital, London. He was a student of William Cheselden who was said to be the most rapid of pre-anesthetic operators, doing a lithotomy in about 4 minutes. A surgeon at St. Bartholomew's Hospital from 1744–1787, in his own words "man and boy, for half a century". He was thrown on to the street from a horse accident and sustained a fracture of the fibula which bears his name today, and wrote his first scientific paper whilst convalescing from the fractured ankle. This was followed by a succession of important papers on hernia, head injuries, an account of chimney sweep cancer (1775) which initiated one of the first epidemiological surveys of coal tar-induced cancer, and a paper on paralysis following spinal deformity. He had probably the largest surgical practice in London and was an extremely pleasant person who attracted many foreign students to St. Bartholomew's. He wrote on head injuries and made careful post mortem examinations, although some of his advice seems rather rough and ready. In head injuries the treatment was always "phlebotomy and an open belly"! He advocated trephine and removal of bone for suppuration beneath the bone and concluded that symptoms from head injuries were due to brain damage and not to a fracture of the skull *per se*. He died of pneumonia after visiting a patient some 20 miles away, and as he lay dying he said, "My life is almost extinguished. I hope it has burned for the benefit of others."

POTTER CLASSIFICATION OF POLYCYSTIC KIDNEY

Type I – Infantile polycystic disease of kidney.
Type II – Hypogenetic or dysgenetic cystic kidney, multi-cystic dysplastic kidney, unilateral multilocular cyst.

Type III – Adult polycystic disease of kidney with involvement of liver (43%), and less frequently cysts of pancreas, lung and spleen.

Edith L. Potter (1901–) U.S. pathologist. She graduated M.D. University of Minnesota in 1926, and became Professor of Pathology in the Department of Obstetrics and Gynecology in 1956. She described the association of a characteristic facies in babies with renal agenesis, consisting of prominent epicanthic folds, receding jaw and low set ears with less cartilage than usual.

POTTS ANASTOMOSIS OR OPERATION

Aortic-pulmonary artery anastomosis – early palliative procedure for Fallot tetralogy.

Willis J. Potts (1895–) U.S. surgeon, born in Sheboygan, Wisconsin, graduated M.D. in 1924 from Rush Medical College, Chicago, and commenced general practice in 1925 but then turned to surgery, spending 1930–31 in Frankfurt, Germany, and then returning to the U.S. to become Professor of Surgery at the Northwestern University Medical School. Apart from his research on congenital heart disease he wrote lay books and on his retirement in 1965 commenced a syndicated newspaper column. He served in the U.S. army in 1917 attached to a chemical warfare unit, and in the 2nd World War in the Southwest Pacific (1942–45).

POULET DISEASE

Rheumatoid osteoperiostitis.

Alfred Poulet (1848–1888) French physician.

POUPART LIGAMENT

Inguinal ligament.

François Poupart (1616–1708) French naturalist and anatomist in Paris. He was an entomologist – Fallopio first described the inguinal ligament in 1561. He was a surgeon at the Hôtel-Dieu.

POWASSAN VIRUS

Tick-borne arbovirus first isolated from a patient with encephalitis in Powassan, Ontario, Canada.

POZZI SYNDROME

Backache and leukorrhea sometimes associated with endometriosis.

Samuel J. Pozzi (1846–1918) French gynecologist. He was born in Bergerac, Dordogne, and went to school in Pau and Bordeaux. He entered medicine in Paris in 1869, became a favorite pupil of Paul Broca and was a brilliant student. He gained his Agrégé with a thesis on hysterotomy in the treatment of uterine fibroma. In 1883 he was appointed surgeon to the Hôpital de Lourcine, altered to de Broca after the latter's death.

He was a fine general surgeon but from the time of this appointment increasingly devoted himself to gynecology. He was a pioneer of this discipline in France. Apart from devising new technical approaches he wrote an important textbook on the subject "Clinical and Operative Gynaecology" which was translated into five different languages.

Interested in antiquity, he was a collector of coins and statuettes, and President in 1888 of the Society of Anthropology. He was keenly interested in medical history and suggested that the last illness of Princess Henrietta, King Charles I's daughter, was due to a ruptured extra-uterine pregnancy. He was a frequent traveller and was particularly impressed by Carrel's work at the Rockefeller Institute on organ transplantation and tissue culture. In 1898 he was elected a senator from his native district.

He had a worldwide reputation as a teacher where he was a striking figure on rounds, dressed in white overalls and wearing a black Florentine cap! He was murdered in his consulting room by a patient whom he had operated on two years previously and on whom he refused to operate again. The man shot him four times in the abdomen and although he was taken on his own demand to the Historia Hospital for a laparotomy, 12 perforations of the abdomen and a laceration of the kidney were found and he died shortly afterwards. The murderer committed suicide immediately after.

PRADER-WILLI SYNDROME

Obesity, sometimes diabetes mellitus, hypogonadism, hypotonia and mental retardation.

Andrea Prader (1919–) Swiss pediatrician.

Heinrich Willi (1900–1971) Swiss pediatrician.

PRAUSNITZ-KUSTNER REACTION OR TEST

Passive transfer test by hypodermic injection of serum from a sensitized to a nonsensitized person and subsequent exposure to the sensitizing agent.

Carl W. Prausnitz (1876–) German bacteriologist who worked in Breslau.

Heinz Kustner (1897–) German gynecologist.

PRICE-JONES CURVE

Distribution graph based on measurement of red cell diameter. Greatly distorted in situations such as severe megaloblastic anemia due to variations in the erythrocytes' size and shape.

Cecil Price-Jones (1863–1943) English hematologist. He was born in Surbiton, England, and graduated in 1889 from Guy's Hospital. For a while he worked in his father's practice at Surbiton and became the medical officer for health for Kingston-on-Thames and was appointed assistant bacteriologist to Guy's Hospital and as assistant pathologist in the Cancer Research Laboratory. When the 1st World War broke out he joined the British Expeditionary Force in the Royal Army Medical Corps. Following the war he worked with Professor Boycott at University College Hospital and applied statistical methods to hematological problems. It was here that he developed the Price-Jones curve which at the time became a standard form of investigation in hematology laboratories.

Throughout his life he was interested in normal variation of measurements of various parameters of the blood and this was emphasized by his work on red cell blood diameters, but the general importance of applying statistical methods to normal values was largely championed by him. He had a keen sense of humor and used to relate how, when there was argument concerning a normal level of hemoglobin in England and America, he went to Boston and although the discrepancies could not be resolved or explained, he used to chuckle at his own solution, viz "The effect of the exhaust of American cars upon the hemoglobin of the man in the street"! He was a cultured and talented person, who was at home playing the cello and piano, and was a skilful painter employing the media of watercolors, and had a fine palate for wines. He died after being bedridden for some time for a fracture of the femur.

PRINGLE ADENOMA SEBACEUM

Cutaneous abnormality seen in tuberous sclerosis or Pringle Disease. It can occur as a forme fruste but the complete syndrome consists of epilepsy, mental retardation and hamartomatous tumors in many tissues which may progress to malignancy.

PRINGLE DISEASE

Tuberous sclerosis.

John James Pringle (1855–1922) English dermatologist. As can be appreciated by his portrait, he was a flamboyant bon vivant who was a fine linguist and singer and who had a deep love for music. Loved by his students, who knew him affectionately as "Jimmy", he was a generous and caring person who treated the charity patients equally with those in private practice and whose kindliness to all was a byword. He used to pay a daily visit to a former senior colleague who had reached senility, and a Bohemian friend of earlier times who became poverty-stricken was put up in Pringle's house and looked after through his last illness. He was accurate and precise in everything that he did but this was moderated by his fine sense of humor and his fondness for embellishment. He had a life-long interest in the sebaceous glands but wrote sparingly and is perhaps best remembered for his editorship of the British Journal of Dermatology, and for his personal attractiveness which undoubtedly influenced many to become dermatologists.

No meeting was dull with Pringle as its Chairman, who was quick to cut down to size pompous and overloquacious speakers. He was dogged for the years of his later life with recurrent episodes of tuberculosis which commenced in 1903 when he dropped unconscious in the streets of London following a pulmonary hemorrhage. He spent 6 months in a sanatorium in 1903 but thereafter had recurrent episodes of the disease, and finally died in Christchurch, New Zealand, when he took a voyage following his retirement in an attempt to regain his health.

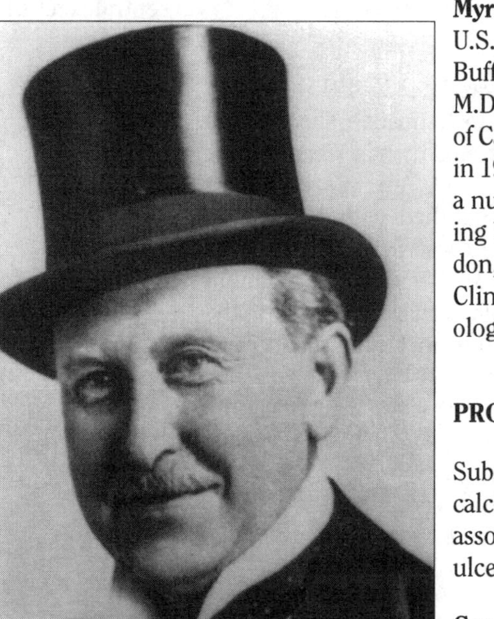

John James Pringle (Reproduced from the *British Journal of Dermatology,* 1923, Vol.35, p.39)

He was a relative of the famous John Pringle who wrote "Observations of disease of the army in camp and garrison" in 1752. He graduated from Edinburgh University in 1876 and then studied dermatology in Paris, Vienna and Berlin. He is said to have learned his French by attending the performances of the Comédie Francaise and his accent was so perfect that most Frenchmen took him for being French, and indeed when he went to Berlin he was known as "the Frenchman" due to his total adoption of French culture and French language. Indeed, his immaculate dress earned him the jingle in France "ce cher Pringle, toujours tirera quatre epingles". Whilst abroad he studied with Vidal and Fournier in Paris, and Hebra and Kaposi in Germany and Austria. He returned to London to take up a post as a medical registrar in 1883 at the Middlesex Hospital and was an assistant physician there for 10 years from 1885, so that he had an excellent grounding in general medicine as well as in dermatology, and became dermatologist to the Middlesex Hospital. During the 1st World War, although 60 years of age, and dogged by ill health, he directed the skin and venereal disease clinic of the No. 3 London General Hospital at Wandsworth.

PRINZMETAL ANGINA

Variant of angina characterized by ST elevation during an attack and associated with a poor prognosis.

Myron Prinzmetal (1908–) U.S. cardiologist, born in Buffalo, N.Y. and graduated M.D. from the University of California, San Francisco, in 1933 and after working in a number of centers including University College, London, in 1936–37, became Clinical Professor of Cardiology at U.C.L.A.

PROFICHET SYNDROME

Subcutaneous deposits of calcium around the joints associated with superficial ulceration.

Georges C. Profichet (1873–) French physician.

PROTEUS SYNDROME

Asymmetry of the arms and legs with some enlargement of the hands and feet. Plantar hyperplasia causing "moccasin" feet. Cranial hyperostoses with macrocephaly, lipomas, hemangiomas, varicosities and linear verrucous epidermal naevi. The condition must be distinguished from Maffucci Syndrome, Klippel-Trénaunay-Weber Syndrome (*v. supra*) and von Recklinghausen Disease (*v. infra*).

Proteus Greek mythology. Variously described as a prophet or King of the island of Pharos. He lived in a cave and could only be made to give his prophecies when caught asleep. When awake he could change his appearance at will and so not be recognized. It has recently been suggested that Joseph Merrick ("The Elephant Man") may have had this condition rather than von Recklinghausen disease (*v. infra*).

PROWAZEK-HALBERSTAETER BODIES

Cytoplasmic inclusion bodies near the nuclei of conjunctival epithelial cells in trachoma.

Stanislas J.M. von Prowazek (1876–1915) German zoologist. He was born in Neuhaus Bohemia, and studied initially at Prague and then in Vienna where he graduated Ph.D. in 1899. After working with Ehrlich in Frankfurt and then with Hertwig in Munich, he went to the Kaiserliches Gesundheitsant in Berlin and in 1907 followed Schaudinn as Director of the Zoological Department of the Tropical Medicine Institute in Hamburg. In 1913 he went to Belgrade and Constantinople to study typhus fever and found that it was caused by the same organism Ricketts (*v. infra*) had previously described, and the organism is now known as *Rickettsia prowazeki*. He also described the chlamydozoa and wrote a 3 volume text on protozoa. Like Ricketts he died of typhus at Kottvus in 1915.

L. Halberstaeter (1876–1949) German physician who, together with Prowazek first described the inclusion bodies in 1907. Born in Beuthen, upper Silesia, he initially studied surgery under Garre in Königsberg (now Kaliningrad, U.S.S.R.) and then dermatology with Neisser in Breslau, now Wroclaw, Poland. He demonstrated sensitivity of the ovary to irradiation in 1904. In 1907 he was a member of the research expedition on syphilis which went to Java under Neisser's direction. His interest in irradiation resulted in studies on its effects on lower forms of life and on tissues and cells. He became Director of the Radiation Department at the Institute for Cancer Research, Berlin-Dahlem and used thorium in an effort to treat cancer. He fled to Palestine in 1933 and became Director of Radiation Therapy at the Hadassar Hospital, Jerusalem.

PROWER FACTOR

(Also called STUART-PROWER FACTOR)

Factor X deficiency. Prower and Stuart were patients in whom this deficiency was first described and who presented with bruising tendencies.

PURKINJE CELLS

Cells of the cerebellar cortex whose axons run to the central cerebellar nuclei.

PURKINJE FIBRES

Special nerve conducting muscle cells of the heart.

PURKINJE IMAGES

Retinal perception of the shadows of blood vessels.

Johannes (Jan) E. Purkinje (1787–1869) Bohemian physiologist. He was born in Libochowitz, Bohemia, the son of Czech peasants. The German priest entered his name as Purkinje in the birth registry which was German phonetic spelling, which he used himself until 1850, from whence onwards he used the correct spelling Purkyne. He was educated by Piarist monks and as a novice taught school for 3 years, but left in 1808 protesting "against a continuous slavery to the superiors whose lives and dignity did not always come up to my expectations". He walked 200 miles to Prague and in 1810 was tutor to the house of Baron Hildprandt in Blatna. He entered medicine, graduating in 1819 and whilst a medical student already commenced to experiment on himself with a variety of drugs including belladonna, camphor and ipecac, and produced classic descriptions of acute poisoning with those agents! Influenced by Goethe's Farbenlehre, he wrote his thesis on the subjective aspects of vision and this commenced an interest which was to occupy him for some years. He made numerous studies on the physiology of sight and described the visual hallucinations produced by poisoning with digitalis and belladonna. His interest in the physiology of light led him to develop animated cartoons and therefore he was one of the early pioneers of the movies. In 1820 he made some fundamental studies on vertigo – the basic experiments of which were carried out on the swings and merry-go-rounds of the Prague amusement park. In 1823 he went to Breslau (Wroclaw) and established a physiological institute there, despite much opposition from the local faculty, who opposed the appointment of a Czech. When he introduced demonstrations and laboratory work to the teaching classes which were at that time new to biology, the faculty recommended his demotion but the Ministry of Education commended his methods. He married the daughter of the Professor of Anatomy, K.A. Rudolphi, in Berlin, and became friendly with Goethe who wrote regarding his series on vision "and should you fail to understand, let Purkinje give you a hand"!

In 1832 he commenced studies with a microscope and was the first to use a microtome, Canada balsam, glacial acetic acid and potassium dichromate in his pathological or anatomical preparations. With these techniques he described the sweat glands in the skin, the ganglionic cells in the cerebellum and ciliary motion. He was an extraordinarily innovative person who amongst other things first pointed to the individuality of finger-prints and wrote on the value of dreams as an index of personality. After years of waiting, he was appointed in 1850 to the Chair of Physiology in Prague, two years after the Czech uprising in 1848. Perhaps this delay was related to his own extreme nationalism. He had written "it is not right that one nation should rule another nation" and "where and how long God lets you stay, my friend, stay faithful both to him and to your land".

On his return to Prague, he was elected to the Czech provincial government and was an editor of one of the leading daily newspapers. This extraordinary man translated into Czech the works of Schiller, Shakespeare and Tasso.

PÜRTSCHER SYNDROME

Sudden blindness following severe trauma or prolonged exposure with exhaustion and shock in which edema and hemorrhages occur in the most posterior aspect of the retina.

Otmar Pürtscher (1852–1927) Austrian ophthalmologist. He was born in Schwaz in the Tyrol, and studied medicine in Innsbruck, graduating in 1876. He initially worked with Mauthner and attended Pfaundler's lectures on physiology of the optics and remained in the clinic as first assistant until it was taken over in 1877 by Schnabel. In 1879 he spent 6 months studying at various centers in Europe including a brief stay in London at the Moorfields Eye Hospital. He returned initially to Milan, but after a short stay decided to go to Carinthia (Austria) and to Klagenfurt because there were at the time no eye doctors in the country. Two years later (1882) he opened a small private hospital of 10 beds and by 1897 this had grown so that a new national hospital of 110 beds was established there.

PUTNAM ACROPARESTHESIA

Waking numbness. Vasomotor changes occurring in night or early morning characterized by tingling, numbness, anesthesia and discoloration of the hands.

PUTNAM-DANA SYNDROME

Subacute combined degeneration due to B_{12} deficiency.

James J. Putnam (1846–1918) U.S. neurologist. He was born in Boston, Massachusetts, and graduated M.D. from Harvard in 1866. He studied in Europe with Rokitansky, Meynert and Hughlings Jackson. He returned to the Massachusetts General Hospital and commenced a clinic which became the Department of Neurology at the Harvard Medical School. He was one of the 7 founders of the American Neurology Association and was its President in 1888. He became Professor of Diseases of the Nervous System at Harvard in 1893 and held that position until he retired in 1912. He was one of those instrumental in bringing Freud to the United States in 1907 and he became more and more interested in the treatment of psychoneurosis and the use of psycho-analysis. Apart from his many contributions to neuropathology and neurology he was one of the first to draw attention to the fact that hyperthyroidism may finish with myxedema. He was one of the earliest workers to study disorders of the basal ganglia. He was greatly concerned with social and ethical questions and published a book "Human Motives" in 1915.

Charles L. Dana (1852–1935) He was born in Woodstock, Vermont. Following graduation from Dartmouth College, New Hampshire, he became secretary to the U.S. senator for Vermont and so spent time in Washington, D.C. where he became interested in biology and after three years in politics became secretary to Professor Baird at the Smithsonian Institute and worked there and at Woods Hole, Massachusetts where he undertook zoological studies for the U.S. Fish Commissioners. These studies commenced his interest in medicine and in 1873 he became apprentice to Dr. Boyinton and gained an M.D. degree from the Columbia University Medical College in Washington in 1876 and the following year took a similar degree at the College of Physicians and Surgeons, New York. He interned at Bellevue, and Austin Flint senior and E.G. Janeway were his chiefs of service. It was here that he commenced his interest in neurology and was made a Professor of Physiology at the New York Women's College. Together with W.J. Morton he was involved in the trial and autopsy of C.J. Guiteau, which resulted in much publicity in the newspapers of the day, and was the beginning of an association with forensic medicine.

From 1884–1895 he was Professor of Diseases of the Mind and Nervous System at the Postgraduate Hospital and Medical School. Shortly after leaving that institution he became Professor of Nervous Diseases at the Cornell Medical School until 1902 when he retired. In 1892 the first edition of his book "Diseases of the Nervous System" was published. This was a most successful textbook which ran to several editions. He had quite a literary flare and published several books with the family publishing house "Elm Tree Press". These were mainly translations of Latin authors such as Horace. Together with Weir-Mitchell he was largely responsible for the improvement and development of American mental hospitals. He published quite extensively but his most important contribution was his clear description of subacute combined degeneration secondary to pernicious anemia, and he made a number of important contributions on topics such as arsenical neuritis and the effects of alcohol ("wet brain syndrome"). He made a number of notable contributions on the history of medicine and was a member of the Charaka Club of New York where many of his discussions on medical history and ancient physicians were presented and published in its proceedings.

PUUSSEP REFLEX

Slow abduction of little toe following light stroking of the outer sole of the foot seen in extra-pyramidal and pyramidal disorders.

Lyndoig M. Puussep (1879–1942) Estonian neurosurgeon who was a student of Bekhterev (*v. supra*) in Russia and with him a pioneer of psychosurgery.

Q

Q FEVER

Malaise, headache and pneumonia due to *Coxiella burnetii*.

Q is for query.

Frank M. Burnet (1899–1985) Sir Macfarlane Burnet, Nobel Laureate, graduated from medical school, University of Melbourne in 1921. His studies in virology led to his recognition as one of Australia's greatest scientists and he became director of the Walter and Eliza Hall Institute, Melbourne. He developed the clonal theory of antibody production and was awarded the Nobel Prize in 1960.

QUAIN FATTY DEGENERATION

Fatty degeneration of the heart.

Sir Richard Quain (1816–1898) Irish physician, born at Mallow-on-the-Blackwater, County Cork. He was apprenticed to a medical practitioner in Limerick when he was 15 years old. He went to London and enrolled in medicine at the University College in 1837, graduating M.B. in 1840. Later he was a resident medical officer on the staff of the University College Hospital and in 1848 was appointed Assistant Physician at the Brompton Hospital until 1875 when he became a consultant physician. He was elected F.R.S. in 1871. His article on fatty disease of the heart was published in 1850 but probably his major contribution was the multi-authored textbook of medicine "Quain's Dictionary of Medicine" which became the bible of all medical practitioners in the United Kingdom and was published in 1882.

He was very prominent in the affairs of medicine, being a censor and council member of the College of Physicians and was narrowly defeated in 1888 in the election for the position of president. He was active on many committees but probably the most important of these contributions was the Royal Commission to enquire into the nature and causes and methods of prevention of the rinderpest or cattle plague. This Commission included a number of famous people such as Dr. Henry Bence Jones and Dr. Edmond Parkes. Dr. Quain vehemently sided with the section who wanted the extermination of the plague at any price and was opposed in this by a number of the members of the commission, including Bence Jones. Quain's work and particularly letters he wrote to newspapers and other magazines turned the tide and the recommendations to exterminate were carried out with success.

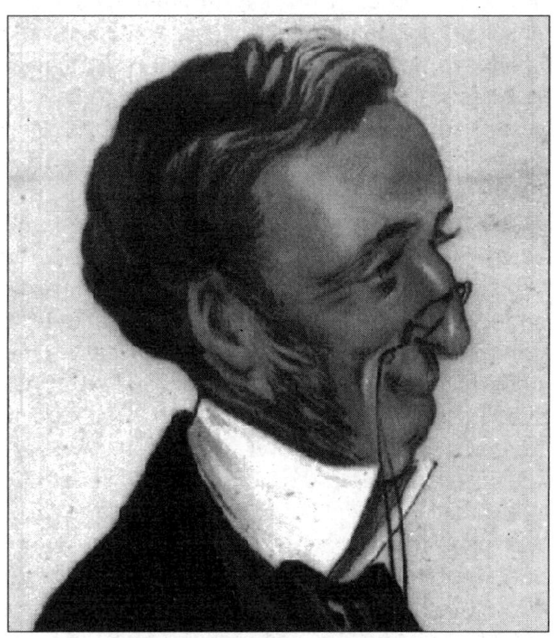

Sir Richard Quain
(From *Vanity Fair*, December 15, 1883 by Spy)

He was regarded universally as a fine physician, but apparently achieved his results by intuition and instinct rather than by analysis of the patient's problems. "Utility and progress" was his favourite motto and he was famous for his epigrammatic quotes, and regarded as a fine raconteur and club member of the Garrick and Athenaeum, his broad Irish accent adding color to the stories he told. In 1890 he was appointed physician extraordinary to Queen Victoria and in 1891 became a Baronet.

QUECKENSTEDT TEST

Compression of the internal jugular vein during a lumbar puncture to test patency of the subarachnoid space – normally this produces an immediate rise in cerebrospinal fluid pressure.

Hans H.G. Queckenstedt (1876–1918) German neurologist who was born in Leipzig-Reudnitz, the son of a poor schoolmaster. As a schoolboy he was very interested in the biological sciences and when he was roaming in the woods looking for specimens, would catch snakes which he sold to a local dealer to help earn his way through school and university. He went to the University of Leipzig and graduated from there in 1900, becoming a member of Professor S.J.M. Ganser's unit. Following a successful submission of his thesis in 1904 he went to Rostock to be assistant to Martius and in 1913 his work on iron metabolism in pernicious anemia enabled him to be promoted to Privatdozent. Queckenstedt became interested in dynamics of the cerebrospinal fluid and it was whilst he was investigating this that he noted that during a lumbar puncture there was a marked oscillation of the fluid in the manometer during respiration and that it was even more marked if the patient coughed or performed a Valsalva maneuver. This led him to study the effects of pressure on the jugular vein and he noted that if this did not cause a rise in fluid there was an obstruction between the foramen magnum and the site of lumbar puncture. He described his test in 1916 whilst he was in the German army. He became Chief of the Army Medical Service in Harburg near Hamburg. Two days prior to the armistice being signed, his horse reared, he fell and was run over by a passing munitions truck.

QUERVAIN

v. DE QUERVAIN DISEASE

QUEYRAT ERYTHROPLASIA

Circumscribed red velvety lesion at the mucocutaneous junction of the mouth, vulva, penis or prepuce, believed to prelude squamous cell carcinoma (cf. BOWEN DISEASE).

Louis Queyrat (1856–1933) French physician and venereologist. He was a hospital resident in 1881 and was first influenced by Grancher (*v. supra*) and Landouzy (*v. supra*). Both directed him towards the study of tuberculosis and his initial research was directed at tuberculosis occurring in babies. He was always interested in the social circumstances of his patients and later, when he changed directions and devoted himself to venereology, one of the aspects of this problem to which he gave a lot of time and attention were the social circumstances and the stigma and plight attached to patients who had these diseases. He fought particularly hard throughout his career to improve the hospital and support facilities for such patients. Whilst contributing to the study of bacterial causes of such disorders as balanitis and later syphilis, he devoted much of his time to improving public knowledge and understanding of these disease processes, emphasizing the importance of prophylaxis. He therefore made a major impact on public health initiatives, and greatly improved facilities at the hospitals to which he was attached, namely Ricord (*v. supra*) and later the Cochin. During the 1st World War, he served at Versailles, at the Dominique Larrey (*v. supra*) Hospital. He retired in 1922 but continued active participation in public health as well as taking part in a number of committees concerned with the development of prevention and treatment of venereal disease.

QUICK FACTOR

Factor V.

QUICK TEST

One stage prothrombin time. Platelet poor plasma is added to tissue thromboplastin and Ca^{++} and clotting time is measured. The coagulation factors measured by the test depend on vitamin K and normal hepatic synthesis, so the test may be employed to monitor anti-coagulants which act on this synthetic pathway as well as to detect severe liver disease and vitamin K deficiency.

Armand J. Quick (1894–1979) U.S. physiologist and physician. Professor of Biochemistry, Maquette University School of Medicine, Milwaukee, U.S.A. Born in Theresa, Wisconsin, he graduated Ph.D. in organic chemistry at the University of Illinois and M.D. in 1928 at Cornell, New York.

His test, developed in 1932 with F. Bancroft and Margaret Stanley-Brown, commenced a new era in coagulation and with it he defined a number of coagulation deficiencies for the first time, including Factor II, V and VII deficiencies. He also developed a test for liver function based on the synthesis of hippuric acid in 1933. He drew attention to the effects of aspirin on hemostasis and was the first to show that aspirin could prolong the skin bleeding time.

QUINCKE CAPILLARY PULSATIONS

Slight pressure on the fingernail results in visible pulsations in normal people. These are increased in aortic regurgitation and hyperthyroidism and hyperdynamic circulatory state.

QUINCKE MENINGITIS

Benign intracranial hypertension of uncertain etiology which may present with headache and papilledema.

QUINCKE EDEMA

Angioneurotic edema due to a defect in C1 esterase inhibitor.

Heinrich I. Quincke (1842–1922) German physician born in Frankfurt-an-der-Oder. He was the son of a distinguished physician and studied medicine in Berlin, Würzburg and Heidelberg with such teachers as Virchow and Helmholtz. He graduated in 1863 and in 1867 became assistant to Frerichs with whom he worked for 6 years on the anatomy and physiology of the cerebrospinal fluid (CSF) in dogs. In 1873 he was appointed Professor of Medicine at Berne and in 1878 moved to the Chair at Kiel where he remained until he retired in 1908. Besides his descriptions of capillary pulsations in aortic regurgitation and angio-neurotic edema (although others had described this earlier), he was the first to advocate surgical drainage of lung abscess and position patients to enable them to cough up sputum. He was also the first person to note poikilocytosis in pernicious anemia, and reported the association with gastric cancer in a patient in 1876. With E. Roos he first distinguished *Entamoeba histolytica* from *E. coli*. He investigated the mechanisms of body temperature control and postulated the existence of a heat center. He described anosmia in brain trauma and noted hyperthermia occurring in lesions of the upper cervical cord and first described a patient with aneurysm of the hepatic artery (1870).

His most notable contribution however was his introduction of the lumbar puncture as a diagnostic and therapeutic technique. He arrived at this in an interesting and logical fashion. Following his earlier work on the physiology of the CSF he reasoned that infants with hydrocephalus might be benefited by the removal of some of the spinal fluid and thus break the over-production and/or under-absorption of liquor. From the first he recognized its diagnostic potential (1891) and took accurate pressure measurements at the beginning and the end of the procedure. He also measured protein and sugar values and described the low sugar occurring in the CSF in purulent meningitis. He diagnosed tuberculous meningitis by demonstrating tubercle bacilli in the CSF and was the first person to puncture the lateral ventricle to obtain CSF in infants with hydrocephalus. When he first reported the technique at the Weisbaden Congress in 1891 it excited little comment, however over the years he had the satisfaction of seeing it become the premier diagnostic approach in neurological disorders. Quincke died at home surrounded by his books.

QUINQUAUD DISEASE

Folliculitis decalvans. Pustular eruption involving the hair follicles of the scalp and may lead to alopecia and scarring.

QUINQUAUD PHENOMENON OR SIGN

Sideways finger movement from the interossei seen in many tremors including that due to alcohol.

Charles E. Quinquaud (1842–1894) French physician born in Lafat in central France. He went to medical school at Limoges and in 1868 moved to Paris as an Interne des Hôpitaux de Paris and worked with Bazin (*v. supra*), being the latter's last interne, and here was influenced to study dermatology. He was made Agrégé in 1883 and in 1886 was Chief of Service at the Hospital Saint-Louis with Besnier, Fournier and E. Vidal as colleagues. He contributed to many areas of medicine, being a skilled bacteriologist as well as a clinician, and with N. Giehant he developed a method for measuring blood volume using carbon monoxide (1882). He gave popular courses in internal medicine and pathology as well as dermatology and unselfishly supported Louis Broq, enabling him to teach and see patients despite considerable opposition by some who were jealous of this young man's meteoric success and popularity.

R

RABSON-MENDENHALL SYNDROME

Insulin resistant diabetes, marked hirsutism and enlarged genitalia, acanthosis nigricans and pineal body hypertrophy.

Salem M. Rabson (1901–1984) U.S. pathologist. Born in New York City, he graduated M.D. from the New York University Medical School in 1926 and interned at the Harlem Hospital. He studied pathology with J. Erdheim (*v. supra*) at the Municipal Hospital in Vienna for a year in 1928 and spent another year there in 1933. He became Assistant Professor in Pathology at the New York Postgraduate School of Columbia University in 1939 and developed an interest in forensic pathology, specializing in legal medicine. In 1943, he left New York to become Director of Pathology at St. Joseph Hospital in Fort Wayne, Indiana until 1957. He then moved to California as Visiting Pathologist at the Harbor General Hospital in Torrance until 1980 when he retired.

Edgar N. Mendenhall (1891–1970) U.S. general practitioner. He was born in Indianapolis, Indiana and graduated M.D. from the Indiana University Medical School in 1913. He was in family practice from 1914 until 1960, and looked after the family first described. He followed and treated the 3 children from their birth to their deaths in 1934, 1939 and 1947 respectively.

RADOVICI SIGN

Palm-chin reflex. Vigorous scratching or pricking of the thenar eminence causes ipsilateral contraction of the muscles of the chin – occurs in pyramidal tract disease, increased intracranial pressure and latent tetany.

Jean Radovici (1868–) French-Romanian neurologist, a student of G. Marinesco.

RAEDER SYNDROME

Ptosis and meosis associated with ipsilateral headache often localized to the eye and occasionally with evidence of the 5th N. involvement, due to lesion at base of the skull or involving the carotid plexus.

Johan G. Raeder (1889–1956) Norwegian neuro-ophthalmologist.

RAIMIST SIGN

1. Of the hand – when a paralyzed upper limb is held vertical by the hand and this support is withdrawn, there is abrupt flexion of the wrist.
2. Of the leg – in upper motor neurone lesions abrupt adduction or abduction of the normal leg results in a similar movement in the affected limb.

J.M. Raimist German neuropsychiatrist.

RAMSAY HUNT SYNDROME

Involvement of geniculate ganglion with herpes zoster gives facial paresis, hyperacusis, loss of taste (unilateral), decrease in tear formation and salivation, and pain in the ear, with vesicles visible in the external auditory canal or on the ear drum.

James Ramsay Hunt (1874–1937) U.S. neurologist. Born in Philadelphia, he graduated M.D. from the University of Pennsylvania in 1893. He then studied in Paris, Vienna and Berlin and returned to practice neurology in New York, working at Cornell University Medical School from 1900–1910 with C.L. Dana, describing his syndrome in 1907. His other major research was on the anatomy and disorders of the corpus striatum and the extra-pyramidal system. He joined the Faculty of the College of Physicians and Surgeons at Columbia University, New York, becoming Professor in 1924.

RANVIER NODE

Area of local constriction in the myelin sheath of a nerve fibre.

Louis-Antoine Ranvier (1835–1922) French histologist and pathologist who became Professor of Histology at the College de France. He was born in Lyons, graduated in Paris in 1860. He commenced a private laboratory with his friend Cornil where they gave courses for students and Ranvier was soon noticed by Claude Bernard who appointed him the first director of a laboratory of histology which had just been established in the College de France in 1867. He became the first Professor of General Anatomy (1875). Always precise and accurate, he had the ideal personality and background for painstaking histological research for which he became famous. Together with Cornil, he wrote a book "Manuel d'Histologie Pathologique" which was widely read by students throughout Europe. He wrote a book on the technique of histology which was used by most laboratories of the time. He described the structures named after him in 1878 and published on the neuromuscular system and on the generation, degeneration and regeneration of nerves. His studies on the circulation and lymph led to better understanding of the role of the reticuloendothelial system in phagocytosis and these cells he called macrophage clasmatocytes. He described the histology and anatomy of the skin and the cornea. Although primarily a descriptive anatomist, he always kept the importance of experimental histology to the forefront, and the importance of learning the relation between structure and function. "Il faut étudier leurs properiétés et leurs fonctions à l'aide de l'expérimentation la plus delicate, il faut faire, en un mot, l'histologie expérimentale. Tel est le but suprême de nos recherches, telle est la base de la médecine future" – It is necessary to study their properties and their functions with the aid of the most delicate experimentation, it is necessary in a word to make histology experimental. Such is the supreme goal of our research, such is the basis of future medicine (translated).

He retired to his estate in Roanne in the Loire. When he died he left part of his fortune to the town to erect a sanatorium for tuberculosis.

RASCH SIGN

Amniotic fluid detected by ballotment in early pregnancy.

Herman Rasch (1873–) German obstetrician.

RASMUSSEN ANEURYSM

Mycotic aneurysm of a branch of the pulmonary artery in a tuberculous cavity.

Fritz W. Rasmussen (1834–1877) Danish physician who worked in Copenhagen.

RATHKE POUCH

Craniobuccal pouch.

RATHKE POUCH CYST

Craniopharyngioma.

Martin H. Rathke (1793–1860) German anatomist. Born in Danzig (Gdansk) and studied in Göttingen and Berlin, graduating there in 1818. He practiced in Danzig for 10 years and was then appointed Professor of Physiology at Dorpat and in 1835 Professor of Zoology and Anatomy at Königsberg. He discovered the avian and mammalian structures which were homologous to the fish's gill slits in 1832 and made one of the best and earliest descriptions of the pituitary gland in 1838.

RAY MANIA

Moral insanity.

Isaac Ray (1807–1881) U.S. physician and psychiatrist. Born in Beverley, Massachusetts, he commenced studying medicine as an apprentice to Dr. Hart of Beverley, completed his studies with Dr. Shattuck, the eminent Boston physician, and graduated from Harvard in 1827. He practiced in Portland,

Maine, where he delivered lectures on botany, a topic in which he maintained a life-long interest, but two years after he moved to Eastport and took up the problem of insanity and its treatment. Here he wrote the first book on legal aspects of the insane "The Jurisprudence on Insanity" (1839). In 1841 he was appointed as medical superintendent to the State Hospital for the Insane at Augusta, Maine. He moved to a similar position in Providence, Rhode Island, and remained in charge of the Butler Hospital, Rhode Island, from 1847–1867 when he resigned through ill health, moving to Philadelphia where he lived for the remaining years of his life. He was somewhat austere in appearance but a fine conversationalist, and friendly when the ice was broken. He wrote extensively in both the medical and lay press on most aspects of medical disease. Two years before his death his son died and this triggered a depression from which he never recovered.

RAYMOND SYNDROME

6th nerve palsy on the side of the lesion with contralateral hemiplegia.

RAYMOND-CESTAN SYNDROME

Tumor of the cerebral peduncles which involves the red nucleus and causes speech disorders, paralysis of lateral conjugate gaze, ipsilateral 6th nerve palsy, and anesthesia of the face and the remainder of the body, with contralateral hemiplegia.

Fulgence Raymond (1844–1910) French neurologist, born at St. Christophe (Indre-et-Loire), worked at the Salpêtrière and became Professor of Neurology there. His colleagues numbered Babinski, Marinesco and Marie, who succeeded him. Sicard was one of his more outstanding pupils. Initially a veterinary surgeon in the French army, he graduated in medicine in Paris in 1876 and was Charcot's chosen successor. Although his teaching was less dramatic, he gave excellent lectures, contributed to disorders of the cauda equina and spinal column and collaborated with Janet on neuroses and psychosomatic states. A monument was erected to his memory at St. Christophe.

Raymond Cestan (*v. supra*).

RAYNAUD DISEASE

Attacks of Raynaud Phenomenon.

RAYNAUD PHENOMENON

Sequential color changes in the fingers of the hand, usually following exposure to cold. The fingers become pale, then blue, and painful, and finally bright red at the end of the attack.

Maurice Raynaud (1834–1881) French physician. He was the son of a university professor and graduated from the medical school in Paris in 1862 and submitted a thesis which described his syndrome and established his name in medicine. He commenced his medical studies with the help of his uncle, A.G.M. Vernois, the well-known Parisian physician. He never achieved a senior appointment in any of the Parisian hospitals but he was attached to the Hôtel Dieu, Lariboisière and the Charité Hospitals on different occasions. He was made an officer of the Légion d'Honneur in 1871 and elected to the Académie de Médecine in 1879. He always wanted to hold a Chair of Medical History in Paris, but died before the International Medical Congress in London in 1881; his address on "Scepticism in Medicine, past and present" was read by one of his colleagues. He wrote a book "Medicine in Molière's Time" and an article on Asclepiades of Bathyinia. He was an excellent teacher and fine clinician. He died suddenly after some years of cardiac disease.

RÉAUMUR THERMOMETER

Freezing point is 0° and boiling point is 80°C.

René-Antoine F. Réaumur (1683–1757) French physiologist who was born in La Rochelle. He isolated the gastric juice from a pet bird and showed that it dissolved food (1752) and then showed similar findings with dogs. He wrote a 6 volume work on the natural history of insects and studied rivers, fossils and forests as well as developing a thermometer.

He was one of the outstanding scientists of his day, established the steel industry in France and was elected to the Academy of Sciences in 1708.

RECKLINGHAUSEN DISEASE

1. Neurofibromatosis – characterized by soft, sessile tumors in the skin and café au lait skin pigmentation.
2. Osteitis fibrosa cystica (hyperparathyroidism).
3. Hemochromatosis.

Friedrich D. von Recklinghausen (1833–1910) He was born in Gütersloh, Westphalia, and graduated in Berlin in 1855. He was assistant to Virchow for 6 years and then became Professor of Pathology, first at Königsberg, next Würzburg, and finally in 1872 at Strasburg, where he remained an active teacher and researcher until his death. He wrote one of the early descriptions of hemochromatosis and introduced this term into the medical literature. In 1862, while still Virchow's assistant, he published two important papers, one showing that connective tissue contained spaces which were drained by lymphatics and in which cells were present. He showed some of these cells had ameboid movements and identified them as leukocytes. He established the method of using silver to stain the lines of junction of cells and his work led to Cohnheim's studies on leukocyte migration and inflammation. Cohnheim was a young assistant in the laboratory at the time.

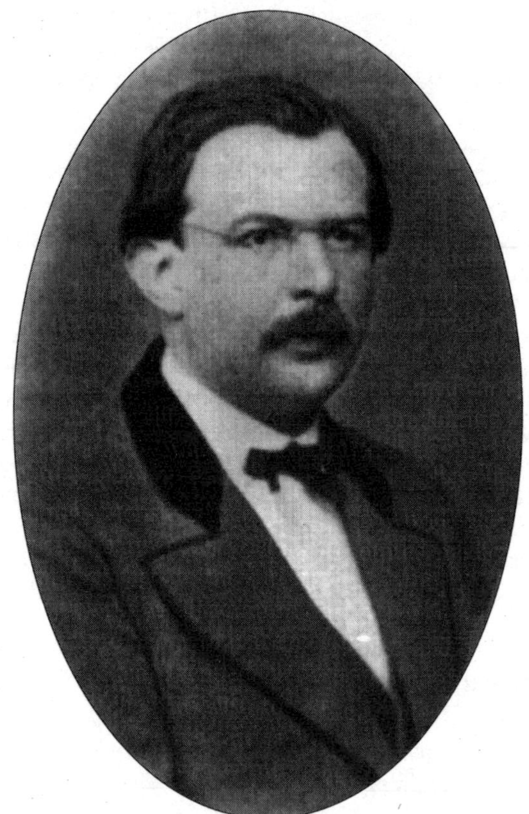

Friedrich D. von Recklinghausen (Bibliothèque Nationale et Universitaire, Strasburg, France)

Whilst in Würzburg, he demonstrated for the first time the relationship between metastatic foci of inflammation and bacterial infiltrates in blood vessels. Whilst in Strasburg, he helped recruit many of the famous names to the university, such as Waldeyer, and undertook a number of investigations on the heart and circulation, and published an authoritative book on the subject. In 1881 as a tribute to Rudolph Virchow's 25 year Jubilee he wrote his classical article on neurofibromatosis. He was the epitome of the traditional histopathologist of his time and was resistant to new changes such as the introduction of the microtome or the results of the new science of bacteriology, even though he made some of the outstanding contributions in the early understanding of inflammation and bacterial spread. He trained a host of people who became leaders in Germany including Friedländer, Zahn, Aschoff and many others.

He was quite a colorful personality and a pleasant colleague. He opposed Koch's concept that the tubercle bacillus was the cause of tuberculosis. He would argue that to say that tuberculous lesions contained Koch's bacillus and therefore the bacillus was the cause of tuberculosis was like saying that the pyramid-like piles of horse manure (a frequent sight in Strasburg streets before the advent of the motor car) were due to the sparrows which perched on top of them.

Von Recklinghausen described another disease to which his name has been attached, namely arthritis deformans neoplastica.

RÉCLUS DISEASE

1. Cystic dysplasia of the breast.
2. Intracystic papilliferous carcinoma.
3. Chronic cellulitis.

Paul Réclus (1847–1914) French surgeon – surgeon to the hospitals of Paris, and Professor of Surgery.

REDLICH ENCEPHALITIS

REDLICH-FLATEAU SYNDROME

A form of encephalomyelitis involving the brain and spinal cord. The scattered lesions result in mild symptoms, but the course is often chronic. They include paraesthesia and non-specific neurological signs.

Emil Redlich (1866–1930) Austrian neurologist. He was born in Brunn, Moravia and graduated in medicine from the University of Vienna in 1889. Following a few months in Paris with Marie and Dejerine, he returned to Vienna to become Wagner von Jauregg's assistant. He published on all aspects of neurology and advanced up the ranks of the University in Vienna. He was termed by his colleagues "the living conscience of neurology", which in part arose from his very intense and serious demeanor as well as his intellectual and scientific honesty. In 1914 he was appointed Director of a newly constructed and equipped hospital which the Rothschild Foundation funded and which he designed. In 1922 he became a full Professor at the University of Vienna. He was a keen art collector and naturalist and a very modest man who refused the title of Hofrat (Court Counsellor).

Edward Flateau (*v. supra*)

REED-STERNBERG CELL

Large cell with mirror image nuclei characteristically seen in Hodgkin disease.

Dorothy Reed (1874–1964) Dorothy Reed came from a wealthy, establishment family. Her initial education was by tutor. She entered Smith College, and whilst there she learned of a new medical school which was being started in Baltimore (Johns Hopkins). She wrote to Welch to ask whether women were allowed to be admitted there. She was accepted, and commenced her studies in 1896. Since there was a general prejudice against women in medicine in America in those days, she encountered quite a deal of unpleasantness, and indeed Osler initially tried to discourage her from becoming a medical student, although he later came to admire her greatly. One lecture which she remembered vividly almost decided her to abandon medicine – it was given by J.N. McKenzie, the Professor of Laryngology and Rhinology, who, during the lecture, compared the cavernous tissues present in the nasal spaces with the corpus spongiosum of the penis and told many risqué stories during the course of the lecture. Some things which he could not say in English he said in Latin, but Dorothy Reed was well versed in that language and understood all his quotations. She decided she would never object to a student or doctor who acted in the same manner as he would to another male, but if he discriminated against her as a female, or was offensive in a way he would not be to another of his male colleagues, she would take action either herself or bring it up to the Dean. She felt that she became a stronger, but not such a nice person, by undertaking the medical course.

In 1900 she graduated 5th in the class of 43, together with Florence Sabin. Only 12 students were given internships and both she and Florence Sabin were in the top 12 and both wanted to do internal medicine. This created problems as there had only previously been one intern allowed to do medicine who was a female, and if both were appointed, the roster demanded that one would be responsible for the white female ward and the other for the blacks. The hospital superintendent, H.M. Hird, thought it was impossible for a woman to serve the black males. Florence Sabin suggested that if there were only one internship then the appointment should go to Dorothy Reed, however Dr. Reed would not allow this to happen, and when this reached Dr. Hird's attention he interviewed her and indicated that he understood that she wanted to clerk on the colored wards and referred to experience with women physicians who had abnormal sex perversions. Dr. Reed stuck to her guns, stating that she had come to Baltimore to learn a profession, and that Dr. Osler had given her the appointment and that she would do her best until he returned.

Her major contribution to medicine was the accurate description of the cells that now bear her name, but more importantly her conclusion that the term Hodgkin Disease should be limited to histological findings in which these giant cells were present. She clearly separated this disorder from tuberculosis for the first time. This work she undertook whilst she was an assistant to Dr. Welch in 1902; later she worked in pediatrics at the Foundling Hospital in New York, and in 1906 married C.E. Mendelhall, a physicist, from Madison, Wisconsin, where she went to live. After raising her family, she lectured on nutrition, child care and contagious diseases, and campaigned to reduce the death rates of mothers and infants during childbirth. She visited Europe and in particular studied the Scandinavian countries which had the lowest maternal mortality rates, and published a report in 1929. This report dramatically improved the standards of maternal care in the United States.

Karl Sternberg (1872–1935) Austrian pathologist. Sternberg described the cells in 1898, however he never clearly separated Hodgkin Disease from active tuberculosis, since a number of his patients had both disorders.

REFSUM DISEASE OR SYNDROME

Heredopathia ataxia polyneuritiformis with retinitis pigmentosa, disturbances of cerebellar function (ataxia), polyneuritis and cardiac disabilities inherited as an autosomal recessive. The earliest symptom is night blindness. Failure to metabolize phytanic acid results in increased phytanic acid in the tissues and blood and can be modified by diet. This was the first example of a genetic disorder in fatty acid oxidation.

Sigvald Refsum (1907–) Norwegian physician. He was born in Telemark and graduated in medicine from the University of Oslo in 1932. He studied the family of the first patient with the above condition in 1937 and successfully submitted the study for his doctorate thesis in 1946 and established that it was inherited as an autosomal recessive. He became professor of Neurology in Bergen in 1952 and in 1954 was appointed to the Chair at Oslo.

REHBERG TEST

Creatinine clearance test for renal function.

P.B. Rehberg (1895–) Danish physiologist who was one of the first to attempt measurement of glomerular function.

REICHART MEMBRANE

v. BOWMAN MEMBRANE

Karl B. Reichart (1811–1883) German anatomist, born in Rastenburg, East Prussia, a pupil of von Baer (who some call "the father of embryology") at Königsberg. He then went to Berlin with Johannes Müller, and when Henle left he became prosector at the Anatomical Institute. He became Professor of Anatomy firstly at Dorpat (1843), then Breslau and, when Müller died in 1858, in Berlin. He was an excellent teacher, who introduced the cell theory into embryology and described visceral arches in the vertebrates (1837), but he opposed Darwin's theory of evolution and the doctrine of transmutation. He isolated oxyhemoglobin from guinea pig blood.

REICHMANN DISEASE

Continuous secretion of the gastric juice.

v. ZOLLINGER ELLISON SYNDROME

Mikola Reichmann (1851–1918) Polish physician who worked in Warsaw.

REICHSTEIN SUBSTANCE X

Hydrocortisone.

Tadeus Reichstein (1897–) Swiss chemist born in Wisclawck, Poland, but worked in Basel, Switzerland. Won the Nobel Prize (1950) with E.C. Kendall and P.S. Hench from the U.S. for work on ACTH and cortisone. Apart from his work on adrenal hormones he worked extensively on pregnane derivatives from plant cardiac glycosides, vitamin C and pantothenic acid.

REIFENSTEIN SYNDROME

Familial male pseudohermaphroditism with hypospadias, gynecomastia and incomplete virilization at puberty, together with infertility. Androgen levels have been found to be normal in many of these patients suggesting that it is due to defective response rather than lack of hormone production. The inheritance is due either to an X-linked recessive or autosomal dominant male limited trait.

Edward C. Reifenstein (1908–1975) U.S. physician and endocrinologist. He was born in Syracuse, New York and graduated M.D. from Syracuse University in 1934, while his father was Professor of Medicine. After initial clinical training in Syracuse he went to work with Fuller Albright (*v. supra*) in 1940 and remained there until 1946 and during this time was a co-author on the paper describing Klinefelter syndrome (*v. supra*) as well as his own syndrome and co-authored with Albright a classical textbook on bone metabolism and disease. He later moved to industry, working as Director of Research of a number of companies including Ayerst, Schering and Squibb, in which capacity he supported endocrine research and research conferences.

REILLY BODIES

(Also called ALDER-REILLY ANOMALY)

These are larger than usual basophilic and azurophilic granules in the granulocytes in the peripheral blood. The appearance resembles "toxic granulation" seen in sepsis etc. It is particularly associated with the mucopolysaccharidoses, e.g. Hunter, Hurler, Maroteaux-Lamy Syndromes (*v. supra*).

Albert Alder (1888–) Swiss physician.

William A. Reilly (1901–) U.S. pediatrician.

REINKE CRYSTALS

Rod-shaped inclusions in the interstitial cells of the testis (Leydig cells).

Friedrich B. Reinke (1862–1919) German pathologist.

REITER SYNDROME

This refers to a triad of symptoms of urethritis, arthritis and conjunctivitis. Other common associated features are cutaneous lesions, especially on the hands and feet, called keratoderma blenorrhagica and sometimes balanitis circinata. There is often a history of venereal contact or dysentery. There is a high association of HLA-B27 with this syndrome.

Hans C. Reiter (1881–1969) Reiter was born in Leipzig, the son of an industrialist. He studied medicine firstly at Leipzig then Breslau (Wroclaw) and finally Tübingen. He then spent some time in Paris, Berlin and London, where he worked with Sir Almroth Wright at St. Mary's Hospital, London, for 2 years. In 1913 he was Privatdozent at the Institute of Hygiene at Königsberg, and just before the 1st World War was appointed Deputy Director of the Institute of Hygiene in the University of Berlin. Whilst on the Balkan Front with the 1st Hungarian Army in 1916, he reported a young lieutenant who had had diarrhea and developed urethritis, arthritis and conjunctivitis. In fact this condition was first reported by Sir Benjamin Brodie (1783–1862) in a textbook entitled "Diseases of the Bones and Joints" (1818). Initially Reiter thought it was spirochetal in origin but revised this opinion later. Prior to this, whilst serving on the Western Front, he had identified for the first time the spirochete causing Weil Disease. He isolated a non-pathogenic variety of *Treponema pallidum* which provided the antigen for a test used in many laboratories throughout the world for the diagnosis of syphilis, namely the Reiter complement fixation test.

He was appointed Professor of Hygiene at Rostock University and in 1933 made Section Director of the Kaiser Wilhelm Institute of Experimental Therapy in Berlin-Dahlem.

He became a follower of Adolf Hitler, signed an oath of allegiance to him in 1932, and so received appointments under the Nazi government, and in 1936 was made Director of the Health Department of the State of Mecklenburg. Whilst it is difficult to reconcile a man of his abilities with his participation in Nazi political interests, he was accorded a number of honors overseas, including an affiliate membership of the Royal Society of London.

REMAK BAND

Axis cylinder of the nerve.

REMAK FIBRES

Non-myelinated peripheral nerve fibres.

REMAK GANGLION

Nerve ganglion where coronary sinus enters right atrium.

Robert Remak (1815–1865) German physiologist and neurologist. He was born in Posen of Jewish parents. He studied at the University of Berlin under J. Schönlein, at the Charité with J. Muller, and after graduation became assistant to Muller at the Charité and then Schönlein. He made major contributions to microscopic anatomy of nervous tissue, recognizing that sympathetic fibers were gray because they were non-myelinated and that the axons of nerves were continuous with cells in the spinal cord. He was one of the first to emphasize that proliferation of cells in tissue formation results from cell division and not endogenous formation as Schwann and Schleidin thought. He made important contributions in embryology, taught W. His, and described ascending neuritis (1861). He first described the three major tissue classifications, ectoderm, mesoderm, and endoderm (1845), and thus introduced the concept of three germinal layers, as well as discovering the autonomic nerve ganglia in the heart of the frog. He died suddenly aged 61. With Addison and Duchenne he pioneered electrotherapy with galvanic current.

REMAK REFLEX OR SIGN

Flexion of the toes following noxic stimulus to the anterior and proximal portion of the thigh in spinal cord lesions.

REMAK PARALYSIS

Lead poisoning causing wrist drop or other motor neuropathies.

Ernst J. Remak (1849–1911) German neurologist who was the son of R. Remak. His mother died when he was 14 and his father when 16, and he then lived with his father's sister in Breslau where he commenced schooling. In 1870 he graduated in Berlin, but did not present his thesis because of the outbreak of war. He participated in the siege of Strasburg and Belfort and after the war worked in Heidelberg and Strasburg with Erb and Hoppe-Seyler and went to Berlin where he was an assistant to Westphal (*v. infra*) at the Berlin Charité Hospital and submitted his thesis in 1875. He remained in Berlin and in 1902 became Professor and in 1910 Privy Councillor. His research concerned mainly neuropathology and especially peripheral nerve disorders. He first described the Babinski response, but did not appreciate its significance. It was said that he entered medicine with reluctance out of regard for his father and would have much preferred to have been a lawyer by profession.

RENDU-OSLER-WEBER DISEASE

v. OSLER DISEASE

RENDU TREMOR

Nervous tremor initiated or exaggerated by voluntary movement.

Henri J.L. Rendu (1844–1902) He was born in Paris, his mother the daughter of a distinguished painter and his father Inspector of Agriculture. Initially he studied agriculture for two years at Rennes and during this time developed a great interest in geology and botany and for the remainder of his life he wandered around France during the holidays obtaining specimens and classifying plants. He obtained a Doctor of Science degree for his work on the geological strata in the neighbourhood of Rennes. He had one of the finest private collections of plants in France and was keenly interested in the visual arts. He took his Doctor of Medicine degree in 1873, his thesis being concerned with the paralysis related to tuberculous meningitis.

In 1887 he became a physician to the Necker Hospital in Paris. He contributed many articles and collaborated with Potain in an article on the heart and wrote about liver disease and its inter-relationship with cardiac disorders. He wrote two volumes entitled "Clinical Lectures". He had a very large private practice and although he was offered the Chair of Pathology when Hanot died, he preferred to remain active clinically. He was an extremely tolerant, but deeply religious man, who was widely acclaimed for his teaching abilities.

RÉNON-DELILLE SYNDROME

Disorder of the pituitary resulting in hypotension, tachycardia, oliguria, hyperhidrosis and heat intolerance and insomnia.

Louis Rénon (1863–1922) French physician.

Arthur Delille (1876–1950) French physician.

RENSHAW CELL

Inhibitory interneuron cells modulating response of anterior horn cells.

B. Renshaw U.S. neurophysiologist.

RETT SYNDROME

The condition is believed to occur in 1:12 000 to 1:15 000 live female births. Following a normal pregnancy, the child develops normally and has a normal head circumference for the first 6–18 months. Skill development stops and the head circumference growth slows. The muscle tone is floppy. Non-purposeful movements commence and hand usage deteriorates and seizures occur. There is intellectual disability and scoliosis may develop with muscle wasting.

Andreus Rett (1924–) Austrian pediatrician. He was born in Fürth/Bayern and went to medical school at Innsbruck, graduating in 1949. He trained in pediatrics in Vienna and later with Professor Fanconi (*v. supra*) in Zurich. He first described the disorder in 1965.

REYE SYNDROME

Encephalopathy with fatty degeneration of viscera evidenced usually by hepatomegaly and raised liver enzymes in children 1–12 years. Hyperglycemia is frequently a feature in the under-five year olds. There is usually an antecedent viral type illness, most often chicken pox or influenza B and recently an association with aspirin administration has been reported.

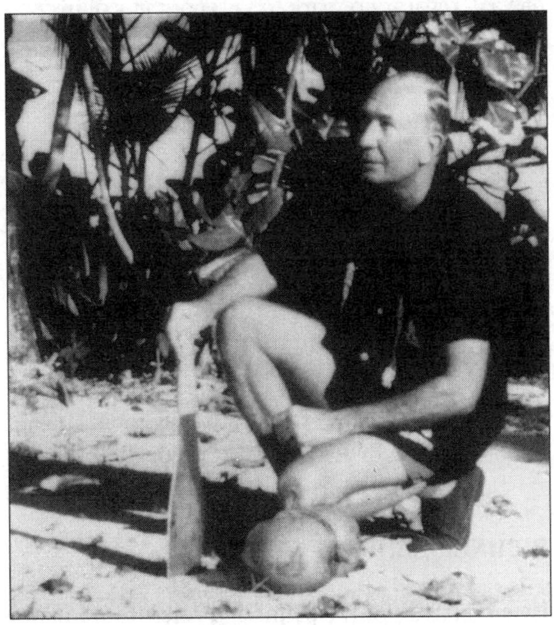

Ralph Douglas K. Reye
(Courtesy of Dr. Corrie Reye)

Ralph Douglas K. Reye (1912–1977) He was born in Townsville in the state of Queensland, Australia, the son of a migrant German family from the Schwarzwald. He spent most of life, however, in Sydney, New South Wales, and graduated from the Faculty of Medicine there in 1937, gaining his M.D. on histiocytic reticulosis in 1945. In 1946 he was appointed the Director of Pathology of the Royal Alexandra Hospital for Children in Sydney and, like all appointees of that day, he was supposed to encompass all areas of pathology, but Reye devoted himself almost entirely to histopathology. He was the first person to describe subdermal fibrous tumors in early childhood and to observe cytoplasmic inclusions in recurring fibromas. Locally these two tumors have been referred to as Reyeoma I and Reyeoma II. In 1963 he described the syndrome outlined above.

As a student one can remember his meticulously accurate lectures on inflammation; a tallish, lean figure, clutching the microphone rather like a crooner and earning himself the nickname by his students of "Dry Reye". For the postgraduate he had an extraordinary memory for details of patients whose disorders had not been categorized accurately and he was always very helpful to any who would call on him for advice. Unlike most he never had a derogatory remark to say about any of his colleagues who were at times critical of him. He died suddenly shortly after his retirement.

RIBBING SYNDROME

Osteosclerosis and hyperostosis occurring in a family.

cf. ENGELMANN SYNDROME

Seved Ribbing (1902–) Swedish radiologist who was born in Uppsala and worked at the Academic Hospital in Uppsala. Later he was appointed chief of radiology at St. Erik's Hospital in Stockholm.

RICHNER-HANHART SYNDROME

Hyperkeratosis of the palms and soles from infancy associated with pseudo-herpetic keratitis (often manifesting as photophobia) and mental retardation with high blood and urinary tyrosine levels. It is due to a deficiency of hepatic tyrosine aminotransferase and is an autosomal recessive disorder.

Herman Richner (1908–) Swiss dermatologist.

Ernst Hanhart (1891–1973) Swiss dermatologist.

RICHTER SYNDROME

Chronic lymphatic leukemia (CLL) terminating with localized lymphadenopathy and sometimes lymphopenia and dysglobulinemia, with some lymph nodes showing pleomorphic malignant lymphoma while other nodes may be consistent with CLL.

Maurice Richter (1897–) U.S. pathologist, Bellevue Hospital, New York.

RICKETTSIA

A genus of bacteria which multiply intracellularly in man and cause typhus and related disorders.

Howard T. Ricketts (1871–1910) Born in Findlay, Ohio, he graduated M.D. in 1897 from Northwestern University, Chicago. He interned for 2 years at the Cook County Hospital, Chicago, and then trained in pathology. In 1902 he was appointed Associate Professor of Pathology at the University of Chicago. In 1906 he demonstrated the transmission of Rocky Mountain Fever by infected ticks transmitting the disease to guinea pigs. In 1909 he reported the organism (a bipolar staining bacillus of minute size) in the blood of infected guinea pigs and monkeys as well as in the eggs of the infected ticks. In 1910 he went to Mexico with Russell Wilder to investigate a disease called Tabardillo, which was Mexican typhus. He found that this disease was caused by similar organisms to Rocky Mountain Spotted Fever, and was transmitted by the body louse. Unhappily, during this investigation, he himself contracted the disease and died of it.

Von Prowazek (*v. supra*) found that the same organisms were present in lice who had been obtained from typhus patients in an investigation in Serbia

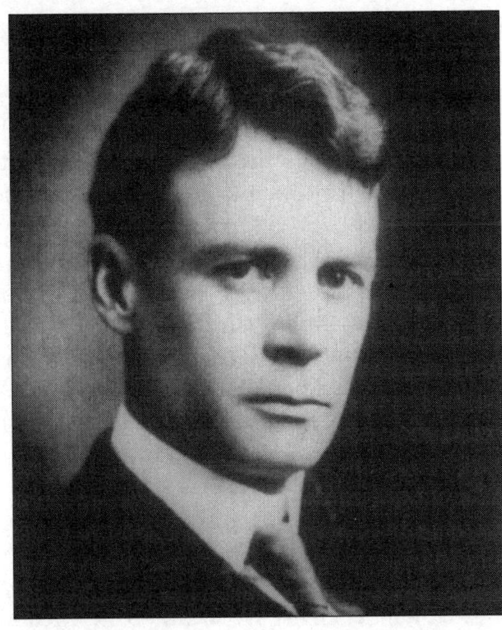

Howard T. Ricketts (Courtesy of the Royal Society of Medicine, London, UK)

in 1913. He also died of typhus in 1915, and this organism has been called *Rickettsia prowazeki*. There are at least 5 diseases caused by these organisms – typhus (*Rickettsia prowazeki*), Rocky Mountain Spotted Fever (*Rickettsia*), trench fever (*Rickettsia quintana*), Murine Typhus or Mexican Tabardillo (*Rickettsia muricolor*), tsutsugamushi, Japanese River Fever or Scrub Typhus (*Rickettsia orientalis*) and Q Fever (*Rickettsia burnetti*) (*v. supra*).

RICORD CHANCRE

The initial syphilitic chancre.

Phillipe Ricord (1799–1889) He was born in Baltimore, Maryland, of French parents, but studied medicine in Paris and graduated there. He discounted Hunter's (*v. supra*) concept that gonorrhea and syphilis were the same disease and clearly established them as two separate entities. He described the primary, secondary and tertiary stages of syphilis as well as vaginal, uterine and urethral chancres, and commented on the rarity of re-infection. He apparently had an immense fund of amusing anecdotes relating to venereal disease and indeed the word ricordiana was used in reference to this.

Oliver Wendell Holmes commented that he was "The Voltaire of pelvic literature – a sceptic as to the morality of the race in general, who would have submitted Diana to treatment with his mineral specifics, and ordered a course of blue pills for the vestal virgins". He was one of the first to popularize the use of the speculum for vaginal examination of women. One of his pupils was Ludwig Türck (*v. infra*), who worked with Ricord in 1844 in Paris, and who translated his lectures on syphilis into German.

Ricord always regarded himself as a surgeon despite the fame he gained for his studies in venereal disease. Indeed, his success in this regard was shown materially, by him purchasing a palatial mansion in Paris, close to the Luxembourg Gardens in Rue de Tournon. He also acquired a chateau at Versailles where he spent his summers. He commenced work at his office late and this would often go on into the night and at times, should he have a social engagement, such as attending the opera, he would return after the theater to continue his professional activities in his office. His rooms were quite luxurious, being lavishly decorated with objets d'art, and the patients were separated according to sex and social status. One of his patients was Marshall Niel, who was then the Minister of War. He had a large bladder stone, which caused him discomfort on horse riding, one of his favorite sports. Ricord advised him against an operation. However, one day he consulted Nélaton (*v. supra*) who had just been seeing the Emperor, Napoleon III. Nélaton said to the Marshall, "How are you? It seems to me that your trouble is lasting a long time. I believe that you can be more quickly relieved, so I shall call upon you tomorrow." Two to three days later, Nélaton operated, crushing and removing the large calculus. Ricord was not told of this by Nélaton, but was aware of what had taken place. On the day of the operation, both Nélaton and he were asked to consult on the Viceroy of Egypt in one of the spa towns. They both travelled together and at the various staging posts, news of the Marshall would be brought to Nélaton, who was obviously getting more and more disturbed, but did not mention anything to Ricord.

They both saw the Viceroy and received 7500 francs each. The next day the Marshall was much sicker and Ricord was summoned to his bedside. He pretended surprise at the news that the operation had been performed and unfortunately two days later the Marshall died!

Ricord is stated to be one of the first people to use mouth-to-mouth resuscitation to revive a patient, who had apparently died. He continued to apply this technique, although he had a mouthful of muco-purulent secretion, until the patient started to breath of his own accord and survived. Ricord remained very youthful in appearance and on one occasion was greeted by the President of the Royal College of Surgeons at a meeting, "Monsieur Ricord, permit me to salute you on behalf of my colleagues. We are indeed happy to pay our respects to the son of that man whose outstanding works we all admire so much and whom the English are happy to place along side of their great Hunter". Ricord replied, "I thank you indeed for the compliments you wish to address to my father, but my father in this case is myself." A man of many parts, Ricord even wrote poetry, composing a poem in honor of Edison's visit to Paris. In those latter years he suffered much from arthritic problems, but bore his illness well and had a remarkable reputation for never being malicious despite being involved in many heated arguments over the course of his career. One of his opponents at his hospital, the Midi, was Vidal de Cassis, also a surgeon, but it is said that Ricord wept openly when he heard that Cassis had died. He was known to be an easy mark for the children who lived nearby the hospital, who often approached him with minor bruises or scratchings with much crying and showmanship and were always rewarded by a coin. When an attendant tried to stop these gammons, Ricord would refer to the biblical quote, "Let the little children come unto me".

RIDDOCH MASS REFLEX

Noxic stimuli to the lower limbs result in flexion spasm of the legs and involuntary voiding of the urine and defecation when there is a spinal cord transection.

RIDDOCH SYNDROME

Inattention to objects often in one lateral half of the visual field, despite ability to recognize these objects when attention is directed to them. Seen with lesions between the thalamus and the occipital lobe.

George Riddoch (1889–1947) Scottish neurologist who spent virtually all his working life in London. He was born at Keith in Banffshire, Scotland, went to school at Gordon College, Aberdeen, and then entered medical school at the University of Aberdeen, graduating M.B.Ch.B. with 1st class honors in 1913.

In World War I he joined the R.A.M.C. and was appointed medical officer in charge of the Empire Hospital for injuries of the nervous system. It was here that he met Henry Head, who recognized his talents, and they worked in close collaboration. Head brought Riddoch to the newly formed unit at the London Hospital where he subsequently headed the neurology unit. He published on various aspects of spinal cord injury and also on phantom limb and body image. When Head became incapacitated with Parkinson Disease, Riddoch filled the role of physician and loyal friend. Known as "Wee Georgie" he was a very energetic person, who never spared himself, he had a very keen, but dry sense of humor, and loved fishing, books and especially music. He regularly performed the Highland fling at the pre-Christmas celebrations at the London Hospital on the billiard table. The Trustees of the hospital insisted that an annual fee of 40 pounds be paid to cover the damage to the table!

In World War II in 1941 he and Sir Hugh Cairns were largely responsible for the organization of the Army Neurological Service, although he was in poor health, and after some years of suffering he had a gastric operation undertaken and died postoperatively.

RIEDEL DISEASE OR STRUMA

Chronic thyroiditis with localized areas of stony hard fibromas.

RIEDEL LOBE

Normal hepatic variant in which there is an extension into the abdomen of the margin of the liver from the costal border of the right lobe.

Bernard M.C.L. Riedel (1846–1916) German surgeon and Professor of Surgery, Jena, Germany. He was born in Laage in the Grand Duchy of Mecklenburg, the son of a parson. In 1866 he studied medicine in Jena and in 1868 moved to Rostock. Just before the Franco-German War broke out he took an emergency degree and went to Glogau in military service as a corpsman with a rank of Corporal and he remained in the medical corps until the end of the war, during which he saw service both at the front and in military hospitals. He returned to Rostock and completed his medical examinations in 1872, topping his class. He became an assistant to F. König (*v. supra*) and spent two and a half years with the anatomist Merkel (*v. supra*). He said "anatomy and more anatomy is the essence of surgery". He studied with Langenbeck, Bardeleben and Fischer and again returned to work with F. Konig when the latter became Professor of Surgery at Göttingen. Whilst there he studied wound healing and joint effusions and commenced his interests in gastric surgery and cholelithiasis. He was appointed to the Chair of Surgery in Jena in 1888. He was one of the pioneers of the surgical approach for appendicitis and strongly advocated "the earliest early operation". Late in his life he developed a painful leg condition secondary to atherosclerosis which eventually led to him having his leg amputated at the knee and although he resigned from his Chair, he continued to be active and indeed resumed full activities when war broke out in 1914. In 1916 he became ill and diagnosed himself as having stomach cancer. When he died later that year, autopsy revealed that he had a primary lung cancer with metastases.

Apart from his work, Riedel was a keen hunter and loved the outdoors and forest regions of Germany. He was always an enthusiastic surgical advocate who looked down on the physician's approach to patients' problems, since he believed that they had little positive to offer the patient. He was a highly practical man who did not dwell much on theories and who emphasized the importance of treating common ailments such as finger infections, tenosynovitis, etc. This made him a very popular teacher both for undergraduates and general practitioners.

RIEDER CELL

Cells with a lobulated nucleus. Probably represent asymmetry of nuclear and cytoplasmic differentiation in lymphocytes, myeloblasts or monocytes. These cells are characteristically seen in leukemia but when few in numbers are of no significance.

Hermann Rieder (1858–1932) German physician, pathologist and radiologist. Born in Rosenheim, Germany, he was early in life interested in chemistry and botany, perhaps because his father was a pharmacist. He graduated in 1884 in Munich and joined Ziemssen's clinic in 1886. Whilst still an assistant there in 1892 he published a thesis "Contributions to the knowledge of leukocytosis and related states of the blood" and published two atlases "Atlas of Clinical Microscopy of the Blood" and "Atlas of the Urinary Sediment". In 1898 Ziemssen established an X-ray laboratory and put Rieder in charge as an Associate Professor. By 1900 Rieder had so developed the department, both for radiodiagnosis and for treatment, that an institute was built, of which he became director. In 1903 he published a book with Ziemssen "Radiology and Internal Medicine" and in particular he investigated the appearances of chest X-rays in patients with tuberculosis. The development of X-ray techniques was particularly helped by the X-ray physicist, Rosenthal, and they made great technical advances in X-ray radiography. In 1904 (independently of Cannon, *v. supra*) he published on the use of contrast media in examining stomach and bowel in man. Over the next years before the 1st World War he continued to study the physiology and pathology of the stomach by this technique and introduced the use of cinematography, working on these projects with Keastle and Rosenthal. He published a textbook on radiology with Rosenthal in 1913 and in 1928 another book on the examination of the small intestine, particularly emphasizing the use of cinematography X-ray. He was one of the first to recognize the dangers of radiation and in 1907 published a paper "On the usage of smaller dosage in X-ray therapy". He also studied the effects of radiotherapy on malignant tumors and disorders of the blood. He retained his interest in botany throughout his life and on his holidays would collect specimens and undertook studies which resulted in some publications such as "X-rays for the Visual Representation of Plants". He retired in 1924 after being one of the most influential pioneers of radiology.

RIEHL MELANOSIS

Idiopathic hyperpigmentation of the skin commonly involving the face.

Gustav Riehl (1855–1943) Austrian dermatologist in Vienna. He was an early protagonist of blood transfusion in the treatment of shock after burns.

RIESMAN MYOCARDOSIS

Degenerative fibrotic disease of the myocardium.

RIESMAN SIGN

1. Bruit over the eyeball in hyperthyroidism.
2. "Mushy" eyeball in diabetic coma.
3. Pain in the right hypochondrium on light percussion of tensed right rectus in cholecystitis.

David Riesman (1867–1940) U.S. physician, born in Saxe-Weimar, Germany, and graduated M.D. University of Pennsylvania in 1892. He was co-author of a textbook on pathology and he had a deep interest in the history of medicine and conveyed this in the clinics and talks to students in Philadelphia. He wrote an excellent book on Thomas Sydenham, other articles on the history of medicine, and inaugurated a course on the history of medicine at the University of Pennsylvania. He wrote a standard text "The Story of Medicine in the Middle Ages". He was Professor of Clinical Medicine at the University of Pennsylvania from 1912–1933 and then became Professor of the History of Medicine until he died.

RIFT VALLEY FEVER

Febrile illness with photophobia, myalgia, headache, anorexia and leukopenia. Viral illness with mosquito vector.

Rift Valley, Kenya.

RIGA-FEDE APHTHAE

Cachectic aphthae.

RIGA-FEDE DISEASE

v. FEDE-RIGA DISEASE

Antonio Riga (1832–1919) Italian physician.

RIGGS DISEASE

Periodontitis.

John M. Riggs (1810–1885) U.S. dentist who worked in Hartford, Connecticut. Periodontitis was first described by Pierre Fauchard in the 2nd edition of his textbook on dentistry 1746, but Riggs introduced the first effective treatment by scraping the tooth to the roots in 1876. He was the first person to insist that periodontal disease was due to local causes, when the remainder of the profession believed that it was a systemic problem. One of his best known patients was Mark Twain, who described him as follows: "He was gray and vulnerable and humane of aspect, but he had the composed surgical look, of a man who could endure pain on another person" ... "presently he laid the mirror aside, raked among his bodkins, selected one and gave it a pass or two over an Arkansas stone. Laid a rag over my chin, placed a couple of fingers where I could have closed on them, and approached my mouth with a bodkin, which he held in the grasp of his other hand. I began to shrink and curl together in a cold nightmare of expectance. Then he put the tool into my mouth, rooted it up under my gum and began to carve. If I had been honest enough to speak my mind, I would have said, "Oww!" to every dig and shouted it, but I was ashamed to do that and so I only said "Mmm" in a low voice and kept back the exclamation point." Despite claims of his aversion to the dentist he continued to consult Dr. Riggs and came to the conclusion that because of Dr. Riggs' help his teeth lasted 20 years longer than most peoples'.

RILEY-DAY SYNDROME

Dysautonomia and discoordination of swallowing. Very rare condition, autosomal recessive, occurring almost entirely in Ashkenazi Jews. Symptoms are dysphagia, emotional instability, lack of lacrimation, relative indifference to pain and lack of a flare response to skin scratch. Fungiform papillae are missing from the tongue and abnormal sweating and blotching and episodic fever are very common. Incoordination and unsteadiness are frequently present and 50% have a scoliosis.

Conrad M. Riley (1913–) U.S. pediatrician.

Richard L. Day (1905–) U.S. pediatrician.

RINGER SOLUTION

Physiological solution of NaCl, KCl and $CaCl_2$.

Sydney Ringer (1835–1910) He was born in Norwich into a Quaker family, whose father died whilst he was still very young. His elder brother, John Melanothon, went to Shanghai and amassed a vast fortune whilst his younger brother, Frederick, went to Japan, where he became so successful he was given the name "King of Nagasaki" and he was said to be well known in the commercial world from Cairo to San Francisco. Ringer showed his interest in science from a young age when a schoolmaster rashly offered a penny for every searching, scientific question the boys in the form could produce, and he is said to have made so many that the offer had to be withdrawn.

He entered the medical faculty of University College Hospital, London, in 1854, and graduated M.B. in 1860, being a resident medical officer at the University College Hospital from 1861–1862. He was influenced by the eminent physicians at that hospital, namely Fox, Russell Reynolds and Jenner. It is thought that Dr. Parkes, who made important contributions to public health, was the one who first suggested pharmacological investigations to him as being an interesting area for observation. In 1863 he gained his M.D. and that same year was appointed as assistant physician to the hospital, becoming a full physician in 1866. From 1865–69 he also held the position at the Children's Hospital, Great Ormond Street, as assistant physician and made the comment at the end of this time that "a man is a fool who holds two hospital appointments". He was an extremely able clinician, and a superb bedside teacher, although not in his element in set lectures.

He wrote a book on therapeutics which was a classic of its day. He was one of the early true clinical investigators, combining laboratory work with work in the wards, and by his example younger colleagues were similarly encouraged. In the 1880s his house physicians studied leukocytosis and its importance in diagnosis, as well as the significance of jugular vein pulsation. He was universally known for his punctuality and the fanatical way he would spend every spare moment in his laboratory. It is even recorded that he climbed the palings of the hospital wall one evening when he found the door locked, in order to get to his laboratory. Following his morning round he would always make an appearance in the physiological laboratory and make suggestions to the laboratory assistant, examine the traces and then depart for his rooms in Cavendish Place, where he would do his consultant work. He had a legion of devoted students, one of whom, in his obituary, made the following comments about what he had learned from his former tutor "first and foremost to be open-eyed and open-minded; then to be honest. He never confirmed his diagnosis by an avoidance of the postmortem room. On the contrary, he there sought confirmation of its correctness or conviction of its error ... but he never juggled with facts, never consciously strove to make things fit; facts were precious things to him. Further, he taught us by example to be strenuous; his life was full to the brim with energy, which he did not allow to remain potential, but forthwith made dynamic. Those who knew him more intimately – his house physicians and assistants – saw a great simplicity in his life; he hated display of all kinds and all affectations".

Although he was an F.R.S. his work really did not attract the attention that was its due when it is considered that he unveiled the importance of calcium and other salts in the physiological sustenance of tissue. It was his development of the solution which bears his name which enabled him to study frogs' hearts beating in tissue baths for a prolonged period. His work emphasized the role of calcium in tissue physiology, but also he performed numerous experiments related to the effects of digitalis and ionic composition which were of fundamental physiological importance. Both the obituaries which appeared in 1910 expressed the thought that he would have attained a far greater position in clinical medicine had he not devoted so much time to the laboratory, and indeed contrasted his attainments with the high place achieved in professional medicine by Sir William Jenner. It seems clear now that the pioneer investigations he undertook on salts and their effects on cardiac and other muscle contractility as well as blood coagulation far outweighed any of the attainments that he might have achieved in professional life.

Furthermore, there can be little doubt that he was an outstanding clinician and teacher; the mere fact that his handbook "Therapeutics" ran to 13 editions is a testimony of his skill and influence which he must have exerted on students of his day.

He died following a stroke, having had a preceding episode some 2 years earlier.

RINNE TEST

Normally air conduction of the sound of a tuning fork is longer than transmission of bone – if altered there is an abnormality of conduction, not perception. Tested by a tuning fork placed on the mastoid process and then when sound ceases held to the ear, normally it is then heard.

Heinrich A. Rinne (1819–1868) German ear, nose and throat surgeon.

RITTER DISEASE

Dermatitis exfoliativa neonatorum.

Gottfried Ritter von Rittershain (1820–1883) Austrian dermatologist in Vienna who described the disorder in 1878. Now known usually to be due to a staphylococcal infection and to cause a classical appearance called the scalded skin syndrome.

ROBIN

v. PIERRE ROBIN SYNDROME

v. VIRCHOW ROBIN SPACE

ROBINSON DISEASE

Group of clear vesicles composed of cystic sweat glands usually around the eyes – hydrocystoma.

Andrew R. Robinson (1845–1924) U.S. dermatologist, born in Claud, Ontario, Canada but subsequently became a U.S. citizen. He graduated M.D. at Bellevue Medical College in 1868 and studied in Edinburgh, London, Paris and Vienna. Always interested in pathology he at one time held an appointment as Professor of Histology and Pathology at the New York Medical College Hospital for women and became Professor of Dermatology at the New York Polyclinic Medical School Hospital. He wrote a manual of dermatology published in 1884. He was abrupt in manner and had few friends but was a keen member of the Robert Burns Society and the St. Andrew's Society.

ROCKY MOUNTAIN SPOTTED FEVER

Acute febrile illness due to *Rickettsia* – tick fever.

Rocky Mountains, U.S.A.

ROGER DISEASE

Ventricular septal defect (V.S.D.).

ROGER MURMUR

Bruit de Roger.

Pan-systolic murmur best heard para-sternally in 3rd and 4th left intercostal spaces and often accompanied by thrill due to a ventricular septal defect (V.S.D.).

Henri L. Roger (1809–1891) French physician who was born in Paris and became physician at Sainte-Eugene Hospital. He published his account on V.S.D. in 1879. He mainly worked in pediatrics and was the first to conduct systematic teaching of pediatrics in clinics.

ROGER REFLEX OR SYNDROME

Excessive salivation due to obstruction of the esophagus, e.g. with a tumor.

Georges H. Roger (1860–1946) French physiologist. He was born in Paris and graduated in medicine there. He was Professor of Experimental Pathology and Physiology and in 1930 became Dean of the medical faculty. He was an author of a very successful book entitled "Introduction to the Study of Medicine" which was translated into English. He wrote on diseases of the liver and the gastro-intestinal tract as well as the spinal cord. He was perhaps best known for his work in experimental pathology on cholelithiasis and hepatic disease, and was co-author with Widal and Teissier of "Nouveau Traité de Médecine" which was a work of 22 volumes! In the year of his death he published a paper in the Presse Medicale on Cheyne-Stokes breathing, recording observations he made on himself.

WILL ROGERS PHENOMENON

Stage migration or classification shift.

This term was introduced to describe a mechanism by which cancer survival statistics could be misleading because the introduction of new diagnostic techniques change a cancer's staging by detecting metastases earlier and therefore convert Stage I cancer to Stage III. Such an alteration would often improve the survival of both Stage I and III since it would transfer patients with asymptomatic metastasis and therefore less advanced disease improving Stage III groups but also improving Stage I since patients with metastasis would also be removed from this group. One of Will Rogers' quips about migrant workers during the Depression was that, "when the Okies migrated from Oklahoma to California the IQ was increased in both states".

Will Rogers (1879–1935) Widely acclaimed American comedian and folksy philosopher whose stage act became beloved by American audiences and consisted largely of his recitations of daily events, "what I see in the newspapers", whilst he performed some trick maneuvers with his lariat (lasso). He starred in a number of Ziegfield Follies as well as radio and movie pictures. He had a weekly and later a daily column on current affairs in the New York Times, which was syndicated to 350 other newspapers. He died in an aeroplane accident at Fort Barrow, Alaska, with his friend Wiley Post, the famous aviator who had been the first man to fly solo around the world.

ROKITANSKY DISEASE

Post-necrotic cirrhosis of the liver.

ROKITANSKY-CUSHING ULCER

Peptic ulcer associated with cerebral lesions.

Carl F. von Rokitansky (1804–1878) Austrian pathologist. Rokitansky was born in Königgratz in Bohemia. He studied medicine in Prague and Vienna where he graduated in 1828. He never practiced clinical medicine but went straight into a department of pathology and became the best descriptive pathologist of his day, and perhaps of all time. He performed his first autopsy in 1827 and when he retired 48 years later, it is said that he or an assistant directed by him had undertaken 59 786 autopsies. In addition there were 25 000 medico-legal autopsies or coroner's cases. He was the first person to show bacteria in lesions of bacterial endocarditis and to distinguish between lobar and bronchopneumonia. He gave an outstanding account of acute yellow atrophy of the liver, naming that disorder in 1843. He gave the first descriptions of spondylolithesis and the pelvic deformities which result therefrom in 1839, first described acute dilatation of the stomach in 1842, and differentiated Bright disease from amyloid degeneration of the kidney. He wrote an outstanding monograph on the diseases of arteries and on congenital defects of the heart. He wrote a book on pathological anatomy which attracted a great deal of criticism from Virchow because of many fanciful theories he advanced concerning "crases and stases" and it is said that following Virchow's criticism he could never look at his first edition of his textbook again, and in the 2nd edition all reference to "crases and stases" was eliminated.

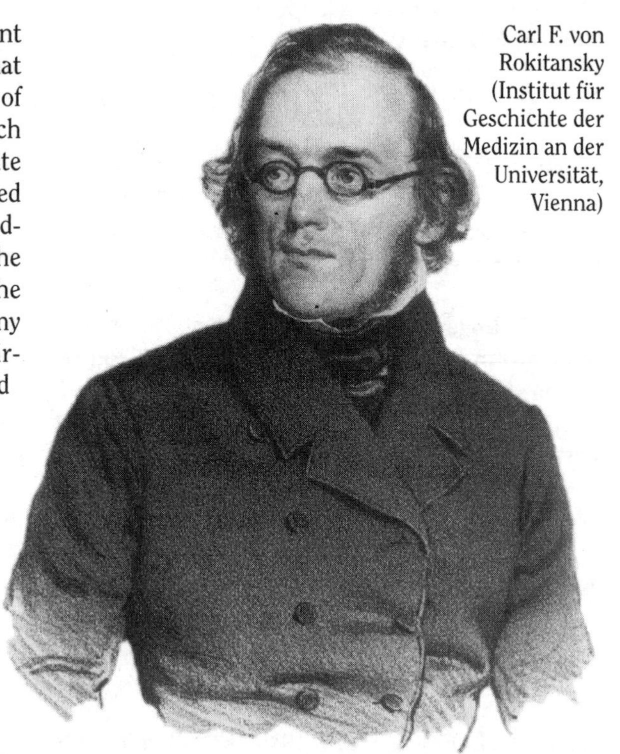
Carl F. von Rokitansky (Institut für Geschichte der Medizin an der Universität, Vienna)

Rokitansky had a reputation as an extraordinarily pleasant, happy-go-lucky and unassuming individual who was both charming and witty. He had four sons, two of whom were physicians and the other two singers, about whom he commented "die Einen heilen, die Anderen heulen". There is little doubt that he contributed a great deal to the strength and excitement of the Viennese school at that time. Rokitansky stood by Semmelweis during his persecution by his fellow clinicians. It was in fact the death of one of Rokitansky's assistants, Kolletschka, in 1847, from a dissection wound while Semmelweis was present at the autopsy, that convinced him about the transport of sepsis, since he noted that the pathological appearances of the body of his former instructor were similar to the puerperal sepsis he had seen in his own ward.

Harvey Cushing (*v. supra*).

ROLANDO AREA

Motor area of the cerebral cortex.

ROLANDO FISSURE

Central cerebral sulcus.

Luigi Rolando (1773–1831) This famous Italian anatomist first described the substansia gelatinosa in the spinal cord (Rolando gelatinous substance). He was born in Turin and when his father died was brought up by his maternal uncle who was a priest, Maffei. He entered medicine and showed an early liking for anatomy and became Cigna's favorite pupil. He proved to be very able in zoology and in clinical medicine. In 1802 he published a monograph on the structure and function of the lungs in numerous classes of animals. He continued his anatomy studies in Florence with Mascagni and met Fontana there. He was physician to the King of Savoy in Turin and spent some time in exile in Sardinia when Napoleon invaded Italy. In 1804 he was appointed Professor of Practical Medicine at the University of Sassari in Sardinia. In 1809 he wrote on the structure and function of the brain in man and animals and drew the illustrations and engravings himself. He did original work by damaging and extirpating the cerebellar tissue in animals and observed the resultant functional abnormalities. In 1814 he was appointed Professor of Anatomy in Turin. During the last years of his life he was physician to Maria Theresa of Austria and died of carcinoma of the pylorus.

ROLLESTON RULE

Upper limit of normal for systolic blood pressure is 100 + the patient's age in years.

Sir Humphrey D. Rolleston (1862–1944) English physician. He was born in Oxford and his father, George Rolleston, was physician to the Radcliffe Infirmary and subsequently Professor of Anatomy and Physiology. He graduated in 1888 from the University of Cambridge, and gained his M.D. in 1892. At Cambridge he became a close friend and collaborator with Sir Clifford Albut and helped him in preparing "The System of Medicine" which was one of the most successful textbooks of medicine of its day.

Initially an assistant physician at St. George's Hospital, he ultimately succeeded Albut as Regius Professor of Medicine at Cambridge. He is the only physician since Francis Glisson who was both Professor of Medicine at Cambridge and President of the Royal College of Physicians. He was also physician to George V. He wrote a book on liver disease and wrote a number of articles on the history of medicine, including articles on Thomas Willis, the endocrine organs and the cinchona bark.

ROMANA SIGN

In the first week of Chagas disease there may be painless unilateral swelling of the eyelids with conjunctivitis.

Cecilio Romana Brazilian physician.

ROMANOVSKY STAINS

Stains of peripheral blood films using eosin and methylene blue derivatives.

Dmitri L. Romanovsky (1861–1921) Russian physician, born in Pskoff and studied medicine in St. Petersburg. He extensively investigated malaria and devised his stain in 1891. He became Professor of Medicine. He died in Kislowdsk in the Caucasus.

ROMBERG DISEASE

Progressive facial hemiatrophy.

ROMBERG SIGN

Loss of position sense indicated by the patient's inability to remain standing immobile with his feet together and eyes closed.

Moritz H. Romberg (1795–1873) German neurologist. Born in Meiningen, Saxony and gained his M.D. in Berlin (1817) with a thesis in which he described achondroplasia. He became Professor of Medicine in 1838. He translated English texts into German, including that of Sir Charles Bell, and wrote his own text in 1840–46 when he was director of the University Hospital in Berlin. This was the first systematic book on neurology and in it he described his sign in tabes dorsalis and endeavored to advance rational treatment for the disease. He died of heart disease aged 78. He was renowned as a teacher and his clinic was always well attended, where he emphasized the importance of careful physical examination to ensure correct diagnosis. He worked unselfishly during the cholera epidemics in Berlin in 1831 and 1837 when he was in charge of the cholera hospitals.

RÖNTGEN

Unit of X-ray or irradiation.

Wilhelm K. Röntgen (1845–1923) German physicist. He was born in Lennep in the Rhineland, the son of a Dutch mother and a German father. When he was aged 3 the family moved to Holland. He went to school at Apeldorn and then at the technical school of Utrecht, from which he was expelled, because he admitted taking part in a schoolboy prank, but refused to name those involved. At the time he was an indifferent student, who hated

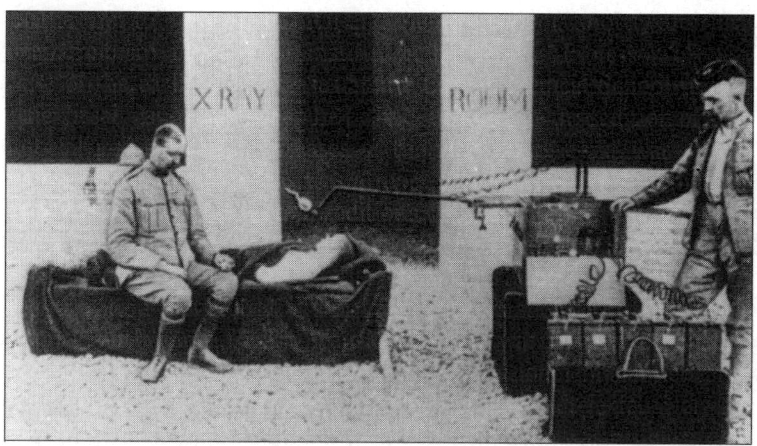

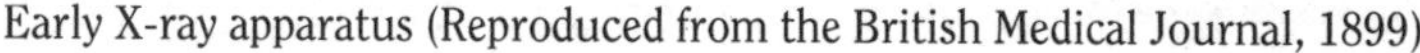
Early X-ray apparatus (Reproduced from the British Medical Journal, 1899)

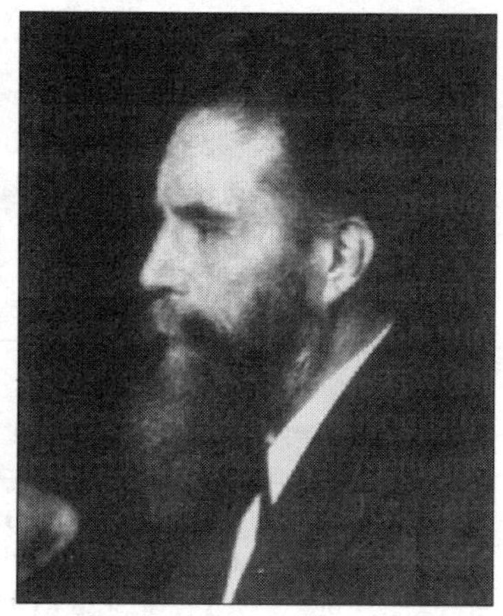
Wilhelm K. Röntgen
(Courtesy of the RSM, London, UK)

discipline and routine, and was a dreamer. He matriculated in 1865 from the University of Utrecht and then went to the Zurich Polytechnical School where he had his enthusiasm and imagination fired by Clausius who also taught Willard Gibbs (*v. supra*), and was the physicist who announced and proved the 2nd law of thermodynamics. His interest in physics was awakened by A.E.E. Kundt. He gained his Ph.D in 1869 on "States of Gases". He was then appointed assistant privatdozent in physics at the Agricultural Academy of Hohenhein, returning to Strasburg as Associate Professor in 1876 where he again worked with Kundt, and with whom he moved to Würzburg and became Professor of Physics and Director of the Institute of Physics there. In 1895 whilst experimenting with a Crooke's tube late at night in a darkened laboratory, he noted that although the tube was covered with black paper, some crystals of barium platinocyanide which were on the table began to fluoresce. He made a screen of this material and showed that fluorescence could be demonstrated on the screen, and if opaque objects were placed in front of the screen, a varying degree of intensity of fluorescence resulted. He noted that when he placed his hand in front of the screen he could see shadows of the bones. Substituting a photographic plate for the screen, the science of radiology was born. Few discoveries in science have attracted the worldwide publicity that his discovery made, the importance of which was rapidly recognized by the medical profession throughout the world. Shortly after Röntgen's initial announcement, the Journal of the American Medical Association recorded "the surgeons of Vienna and Berlin believe the Röntgen photograph is destined to render inestimable services to surgery ... the electric apparatus required is so expensive, a hundred dollars and upward, that few surgeons can use it yet in their private practice".

Röntgen was awarded the Nobel Prize in physics for his discovery in 1901. Röntgen was a very honest and straight-forward investigator who was not a great theoretical physicist but who was a fine experimentalist and an outstanding teacher of his students, to whom the term "midwife of the mind" has been given. He was meticulously tidy and said "apparatuses are cleverer than men and anyone who mishandles apparatus is my enemy". He disliked the publicity that resulted from his discovery. He became the victim of completely false rumors that it was really one of his assistants who had made the original findings. In 1900 he became Professor of Physics at the University of Munich where he remained until he retired in 1920. He was opposed to the 1st World War, became more and more withdrawn in his later years, and died of carcinoma of the rectum.

RORSCHACH TEST

Use of patterns of ink-blots to explore the psyche.

Hermann Rorschach (1884–1922) Swiss psychiatrist. He was born in Zurich, the son of a painter who earned his living as a drawing teacher in a boys' preparatory school. His nickname at school was klex, a word meaning ink blot! There has been much speculation as to the extraordinary coincidence of this nickname and the test for which his name is famous. Klecksographie was a game which was commonly played by Swiss children and consisted of spotting an ink blot on paper and folding it so that the forms of a butterfly or bird would be obtained. Towards the end of his schooling he wrote to Ernst Haeckel asking him whether he should go into further studies of art or natural science. Haeckel advised science so he entered medical school in Zurich, spending some time at Neuchatel, Berlin, and Berne, but spending the majority of his time in Zurich. During his time as a student he developed an intense interest in Russia and Russians and later in Zurich he met members of the Russian colony who included the famous neurologist C. von Monakow (*v. supra*). He commenced to learn Russian and in 1906 during his time in Berlin spent a short vacation in that country. At that time in Switzerland there was a considerable portion of the clinical course devoted to psychiatry and Zurich was a world center, having initially had A. Forel and his almost as famous successor, E. Bleuler, as teachers, and also C.J. Jung who had just worked out the association test to explore the unconscious mind. At this stage Freud's work was just beginning to gain in popularity. He graduated in 1909 and became engaged to a Russian girl in Switzerland and visited her family in Kazan. He decided to complete his training in Switzerland and then to move to Russia permanently. Since both he and his fiancee were poor, he elected to take a position in one of the asylums (Munsterlingen) because the salary was much better than he would have obtained in a university clinic. He married in 1910 and remained at the asylum until 1913, becoming very popular with the patients by organizing theatrical entertainment and keeping very close records of the patients including a photographic record which he himself took. At one time he bought a monkey and kept it to observe the patients' reactions to it, and also to entertain them. Here he interested himself in hallucinations and their mode of production and in 1911 together with a school teacher friend of his, K. Gehring, was already experimenting with ink blots and Jung's word association test on school children and patients, but he carried this no further because of his growing interest in psychoanalysis. He became interested in the interpretation of art works by psychotics and neurotics and their own abilities to paint. Like many psychiatrists of his day he was impressed by symbolic associations and in a paper "Clock and Time" he proposed that some neurotics' love of watches was related to a subconscious longing for the mother's breast with the ticking representing heart beats!

He obtained his doctorate in 1913 and left for Russia, but only stayed 7 months although he did obtain a well paid position in one of the fashionable asylums. It appears that he wished to continue in more scientific endeavors and could not do so in that position. He therefore returned to Switzerland but was forced to take a position at the Waldau Psychiatric Clinic. There was a saying amongst psychiatric residents of the day "if you want to eat well, go to Friedmatt; if you want to sleep well, go to Waldau; if you want to learn well, go to Burgholzli". The latter was the main university clinic in Zurich and was where Bleuler taught. Investigating some of the strange religious sects in Switzerland, he examined a gentleman called Binggeli who taught his disciples that his penis was sacred and that they should adore it; his urine was called "heaven's drops" or "heaven's balm" and he gave it to them as a medication or instead of the wine for the holy communion; one of his teachings was that the method of expelling demons from young women was to have sexual relations with him! Binggeli was imprisoned for incest with his daughter. When Rorschach examined the situation more fully he found that this sect was a similar one to the sect of Anton Unternahrer which had existed towards the end of the 18th century and which had also preached the holiness of incest. When he went back through the centuries he found that besides "normal" religious sects, similar aberrant sects which were identical or very similar to those of Binggeli's had been taking place in the same geographic regions back to the 12th century. When he examined the family tree of Binggeli, he found that over four centuries, 10 relations had played a leading role in these sects.

Towards the end of 1915 he was appointed Associate Director of the asylum at Herisau. Here he introduced a course of lectures for the nursing staff (the first of its kind in Switzerland) and continued his interest in psychoanalysis and psychopathology in religion. However, at this time a doctoral thesis was published in 1917 by S. Hens, working with Bleuler, and in it Hens employed a similar technique to the one that Rorschach had used in 1911. This led him to work frantically over the next few years and resulted in the publication of his book "Psykodiagnostik". In this book he outlines his new conceptions of psychology and also his tests exploring the subconscious with ink blots. This book represented his masterpiece, but was received coldly by critics and he himself became quite depressed. He was still exploring methods for improving the techniques that he published in his book and outlined this in a talk to the Psychoanalytic Society a month before his sudden death, which appears to have been the result of a perforated appendix. His work became widely respected and an institute was founded in his name in New York in 1939.

ROSENBACH DISEASE

v. HEBERDEN ARTHRITIS

ROSENBACH LAW

Lesions of the anterior horn cells on anterior spinal nerve trunks result in a paralysis of extensor before flexor muscles.

ROSENBACH SIGN

1. Fibrillation tremor in the closed eyelids in thyrotoxicosis.
2. Inability to close the eyes on command in hysteria.
3. Absence of ipsilateral abdominal reflexes in hemiplegia.

ROSENBACH TEST

Test for bile in urine using nitric acid (1876).

Ottomar Rosenbach (1851–1907) German physician. He described the abnormality of the vocal cords following partial or complete recurrent laryngeal nerve palsy and wrote a book on cardiovascular disorders. A fine clinician but a somewhat controversial figure in his day, since he emphasized psychosomatic causes and features of disease and opposed bacterial theory.

ROSE-WAALER TEST

The demonstration of rheumatoid factor using its properties to agglutinate red cells.

Harry M. Rose (1906–1986) U.S. physician who specialized in Infectious Disease. As a small child he had poliomyelitis and this left him with weakness in both his legs. He went to college at Yale and entered Cornell Medical School in 1928 where he graduated M.B. in 1932. That same year he developed pulmonary tuberculosis and was admitted to the New York State Hospital at Raybrook. After recovering from this he worked there as a physician until 1938 and then returned to the Presbyterian Hospital, New York, where he completed his internship in 1938 and entered a residency program in Bacteriology. He remained at Columbia, holding positions in the Department of Microbiology, including its Chairmanship from 1952 until he retired in 1974. During this period, he published extensively on a number of infectious diseases, including rickettsia and filariasis. He was one of the first to use ferritin conjugated antibodies to study events with the electron microscope. Depite his physical disabilities he was a very keen golfer and became club champion. He probably learnt to play while he was at the tuberculosis sanatorium in Raybrook since the Medical Director of that establishment was also a keen golfer who had constructed a 9-hole course for his and his patients' use. He was also an excellent pianist, playing in the band at Yale and was a church chorister. He died with progressive dementia over the last two years of his life.

Erik Waaler (1903–) He graduated in Medicine from the University of Oslo in 1927. After a year as an intern and another in general practice, he undertook Bacteriology training from 1930 to 1932 but had decided to specialize in Internal Medicine and, in particular, rheumatology, but in 1936 his former chief in Bacteriology, Professor Theodor Thjotta, encouraged him to return to Laboratory Medicine and to remain a Pathologist. During his subsequent training, he spent a year in the Department of Pathology at Columbia University in New York City, then returned to work at the Oslo City Hospital. It was here that he noted that some patients with rheumatoid arthritis caused agglutination of sheep red blood cells sensitized by rabbit anti-sheep red cell serum. He presented these results in view of the International Congress for Microbiology held in New York in 1939. Harry M. Rose, who was at that stage a resident of Bacteriology at the Presbyterian Hospital in New York was also present but the two men did not meet then or later. Waaler spent his war years in Bergen in the Pathology Department there and after the war organized a new medical faculty at Bergen becoming the Chairman of Pathology and Dean of the Faculty of Medicine in 1948. For a time, he was first violinist in the symphony orchestra at Bergen and enjoyed bushwalking in the nearby mountains.

ROSSBACH DISEASE

Hyperchlorhydria in the stomach.

Michael J. Rossbach (1842–1894) German physician. He was born in Heidingsfeld near Würzburg and studied medicine in Munich, Berlin and Prague and graduated in 1865 in Würzburg. His interests included pharmacology, laryngology and internal medicine as well as physical methods for treatment. When Nothnagel retired in 1882 he was appointed clinician in Jena. He died of renal failure and autopsy showed him to have granular atrophy of the kidneys with hypertrophy of the heart.

ROSSOLIMO REFLEX

Tapping of the plantar surface of the 2nd to 5th toes causes flexion which is exaggerated greatly in pyramidal tract lesions.

Gregory I. Rossolimo (1860–1928) Russian neurologist.

ROSTAN ASTHMA

Cardiac asthma.

Léon Rostan (1790–1866) French physician.

ROTCH SIGN

Obliteration of the cardio-hepatic angle in pericardial effusion. Dullness to percussion over right 5th intercostal space.

Thomas M. Rotch (1848–1914) U.S. physician. He was born in Philadelphia, graduated from Harvard in 1874, and spent 2 years in Germany before returning to Boston. He made the first scientific study of infant nutrition and was appointed in 1898 as Head of the first Department of Pediatrics at Harvard as an Assistant Professor. He established a research laboratory on milk, and rose to the rank of Professor. He wrote an important textbook on pediatrics and founded the Infants Hospital in Boston. He pioneered milk formulation for infant feeding and introduced X-rays into pediatrics.

ROTH-BERNHARDT *or* ROT-BERNHARDT DISEASE

(Also ROTH DISEASE and BERNHARDT ROTH DISEASE)

Meralgia paresthetica.

Vladimir K. Roth (Rot) (1848–1916) Russian neurologist.

Martin Bernhardt (1844–1915) German neurologist.

ROTH SPOTS

Oval retinal hemorrhages with a pale central area. Occur in 5% of patients with sub-acute bacterial endocarditis, but may also be seen in lupus and collagen disorders.

Moritz Roth (1839–1914) Swiss pathologist who was born in Basel and studied medicine in Basel,

Göttingen, Würzburg and Berlin, graduating in Basel in 1864. After working in Greifswald (1868–72) he returned to Basel as extraordinary Professor of Pathology, becoming Professor in 1874. He wrote a book on Andreas Vesalius in 1892 and this is a standard reference text.

ROTHERA TEST

Test for acetone in urine.

Arthur C.H. Rothera Australian biochemist at the University of Melbourne. Killed in the 1st World War.

ROTHMUND SYNDROME *or* ROTHMUND-THOMSON SYNDROME

Recessive hereditary oculocutaneous disorder with erythema, marble skin, pigmentation, telangiectasia, congenital cataracts, defective nails and teeth, partial to total alopecia, short stature and hypogonadism.

August Rothmund (1830–1906) German ophthalmologist who was born in Volkach, Bulgaria. He graduated in medicine at Munich in 1853 and went to work with V. Graefe (*v. supra*) in Berlin. He returned to Munich as a Professor of Ophthalmology in 1863 and became a renowned teacher.

Matthew S. Thomson (1894–1969) English dermatologist who was born in Earlsfield, Surrey and studied medicine at Cambridge and King's College Hospital, graduating in 1918. He became senior dermatologist at King's and was universally called Tommy. He would always open a door using his coat to cover the door handle.

ROTOR SYNDROME

Hyperbilirubinemia of the order of 80 mmol/l with increased conjugated bilirubin in the plasma. Primarily reported in patients from the Philippines. It is inherited as an autosomal recessive. Unlike Dubin-Johnson, the gall bladder is usually visualized on an oral cholecystogram and there is no secondary appearance of the dye during the performance of a bromsulphapthalien (B.S.P.) excretion test. May be the same condition as hepatic storage disease recently reported in Japan and France.

Arturo B. Rotor Physician from the Philippines.

ROUGET CELL

Branched contractile cell on the external wall of vessels in amphibia but not mammals.

Charles M.B. Rouget (1824–1904) French physiologist.

ROUGNON-HERBERDEN DISEASE

v. HEBERDEN DISEASE

Angina pectoris.

Nicolas F. Rougnon de Magny (1727–1799) French physician. Osler believed that he described angina in a pamphlet published in 1768 and this antedated the description by Heberden (*v. supra*).

ROUS SARCOMA

Transmissible fibrosarcoma in chickens.

Francis Peyton Rous (1879–1970) U.S. pathologist and virologist. He transferred sarcoma in Plymouth Rock chickens using transplants or cell free filtrates. He was born in Baltimore, Maryland, and graduated M.D. at Johns Hopkins in 1905, and after interning there went to the Pathology Department at the University of Michigan and then joined the Rockefeller Institute in 1909. He remained there until his retirement in 1945. He established the first blood banks in World War I and spent a lifetime in research on cancer viruses and liver pathology and physiology. He was editor of the Journal of Experimental Medicine. At one time he wrote a nature column in a newpaper. His expressive use of English is illustrated by his description of cancer, "Tumors destroy man in a unique and appalling way, as flesh of his own flesh, which has somehow been rendered proliferative, rampant, predatory and ungovernable".

In 1966, fifty years after his original work, he was awarded the Nobel Prize (shared with C. Huggins) for his work on cancer.

ROUSSY-DEJERINE SYNDROME

Thalamic syndrome. Over-reaction to painful stimuli to the side of the body opposite to the lesion.

ROUSSY-LÉVY DISEASE

Hereditary spinocerebellar degeneration with lower limb muscular atrophy with loss of deep reflexes and sometimes upgoing toes on examination of the plantar reflex. Cerebellar signs are often mild with truncal ataxia being the most prominent.

Gustave Roussy (1874–1948) French neuropathologist. He was born in Vevey in Switzerland. His first 3 years in medical school were at the University of Geneva and in 1897 he continued at the Faculty of Medicine in Paris. In 1902 he became Interne des Hôpitaux de Paris. He was in charge of the pathology laboratory at François-Franck's laboratory at the College de France from 1906–1908, and Chief of Medicine at the Hospital Paul Brousse in 1913. He was appointed Professor of Anatomical Pathology in 1925, made Director of the Institute of Cancer in 1930 and Dean of the Faculty of Medicine of the Institute of Cancer in 1930 and Dean of the Faculty of Medicine in 1933. Finally he was Rector of the University of Paris in 1937. As a resident medical officer his chiefs were Pierre Marie and Jules Dejerine, both of whom aroused Roussy's interest in neurology. He described the thalamic syndrome with Dejerine in 1906, and showed that it followed thrombosis of the thalamic branch of the posterior cerebral artery. In the 1st World War he wrote two books, one concerned with spinal cord injuries, in collaboration with J. Lhermitte, and the other on war psychoneuroses. He undertook experimental work on the production of syringomyelia in animals and studied the physiology of micturition and defecation. He made contributions to the understanding of the pituitary and tuber cinareum and was the first to show that damage to the hypothalamus on its own could cause polyuria, obesity, transient glycosuria and even gonadal atrophy.

Roussy was an extremely good organizer, and very highly cultured man. He was dismissed in November 1940 from his job by the Germans during the occupation, without any stated reason. He was reinstated to his position after the war.

J. Dejerine (*v. supra*).

G. Lévy (1881–) French neurologist.

ROUX SERUM

Tetanus antitoxin.

Pierre P.E. Roux (1853–1933) French bacteriologist, born in Confolens and went to medical school at Clermont-Ferrand; here he attracted the attention of the chemist Duclaux who took him to Paris and who introduced him to Pasteur. He worked with Pasteur on anthrax vaccination. He discovered filterable viruses and with Yersin (*v. infra*) the exotoxin of diphtheria, which led to Behring's work on diphtheria antitoxin. He introduced the latter treatment into France, developing the technique of using horses to provide the antitoxin and proving its effectiveness in clinical trials, and with Metchnikoff demonstrated the inoculability of syphilis into apes. Earlier, with Nocard (*v. supra*) he introduced glycerin agar as the medium for growing the tubercle bacillus. He was Director of the Pasteur Institute (1904–1933). Throughout his life he was plagued by ill health and pulmonary tuberculosis to which he finally succumbed.

ROVSING SIGN

Pressure over the left iliac fossa causes pain in the right iliac fossa in acute appendicitis.

Neils T. Rovsing (1862–1927) Danish surgeon. Professor of Surgery, University of Copenhagen. He graduated from the University of Copenhagen in medicine in 1885 and in 1899 was appointed Professor of Operative Surgery. Initially this appointment did not provide him with hospital beds and he therefore commenced a private surgical nursing home to overcome this problem. In 1904 he was put in charge of the Fredericks Hospital as senior surgeon and largely due to his advocation for better surgical accommodation, the Rigs hospital was commenced in 1905 and opened in 1910.

Always a forceful and imposing individual, he was in his element when questioning time honored principles and is said to have shattered the reputation of iodoform as an antiseptic with work that he did in conjunction with Heyn. Primarily famous as an abdominal surgeon, he wrote extensively on diseases of the bladder and gall bladder and became internationally recognized. He acquired a financial interest in a medical journal which he subsequently owned and finally presented to the Danish Medical Society which gives some idea of his entrepreneurial capacity. In 1926 he was forced to retire due to heart disease and later was diagnosed as having a malignancy of the larynx for which he received X-ray therapy without avail. Although time has shown his sign not to be of diagnostic value, he played a major role in promoting surgery in Denmark.

RUBINSTEIN-TAYBI SYNDROME

Congenital anomaly with small head, beaked nose, high arched palate, downward slant of the eyes, broad flat thumbs and big toes, mental and motor retardation and often small stature.

Jack H. Rubinstein (1925–) U.S. pediatrician who was born in New York and graduated M.D. from Harvard in 1952. He became Professor of Pediatrics at the University of Cincinnati in 1970.

Hooshang Taybi (1919–) U.S. pediatric radiologist born in Iran and graduated from the University of Teheran in 1944 and later moved to the U.S.A. and became clinical professor of radiology at the University of California (San Francisco).

RUBNER LAW

1. The law of constant energy production. The rapidity of growth is proportional to the metabolic rate.
2. The law of constant growth fraction. The same fractional part of total body energy is used for growth.

Max Rubner (1854–1932) German physiologist. Born in Munich, he studied with Ludwig and Voigt. He discovered that metabolism is proportional to the body's surface area (1883) and that protein exerts the greatest influence on the specific dynamic action of food on metabolism and carbohydrate the least. He was the first to use the calorimeter to measure metabolic changes in units of heat and energy. He also investigated the food requirements of infants with pediatrician Otto Heubner.

RUD SYNDROME

v. SJÖRGREN-LARSSON SYNDROME

Einar Rud (1892–) Danish physician.

RUFFINI CELL, CORPUSCLE OR END ORGAN

Sensory end organ in the subcutaneous layer made of branching nerve fibres.

Angelo Ruffini (1864–1929) Italian anatomist.

RUMPEL-LEEDE SIGN OR TEST

v. HESS TEST

Theodor Rumpel (1862–1923) German surgeon; with A. Kast wrote an atlas on pathological anatomy.

Carl S. Leede (1882–) U.S. physician who worked in Seattle.

RUSSELL BODIES

Hyaline eosinophilic inclusion bodies in the cytoplasm of plasma cells in conditions of chronic inflammation and multiple myeloma. They represent deposits of gamma globulin.

William Russell (1852–1940) Scottish pathologist and physician. He was born in Douglas on the Isle of Man where his father was stationed at the time, being an officer of Fisheries. Both sides of his family came from the Highland area of Scotland. He came to Edinburgh to enter medical school and graduated in 1876 and stayed there for the rest of his life. His first teaching appointment was a lectureship in pathology and later he gained a physician appointment and became a member of the staff of the Royal Infirmary, Edinburgh, for 30 years, becoming the first appointment to the Moncrieff-Arnott Chair of Clinical Medicine in 1913, a position he retained until he retired in 1919. His early research included investigations of the cancer cell and disorders of the circulation. His wife was forced to take her doctorate elsewhere after being a brilliant undergraduate and he became Dean of the Women's School and a champion for equal opportunity. He was the first editor of the Scottish Medical and Surgical Journal and was one of the most highly regarded clinical teachers of his day at a time when the Edinburgh Medical School possessed its greatest array of clinicians such as Byron Bramwell. As might be expected, he was a keen supporter of the physicians' cause and stated that the diagnosis of appendicitis required "the skilled palpation to which the physician is trained, and of which the surgeon may be capable". He was said to be a tall, handsome, bearded gentleman with a rather clerical manner which combined with his dogmatism made him well remembered by his students. He had a gift for succinct verbal expression and was widely read and an excellent conversationalist.

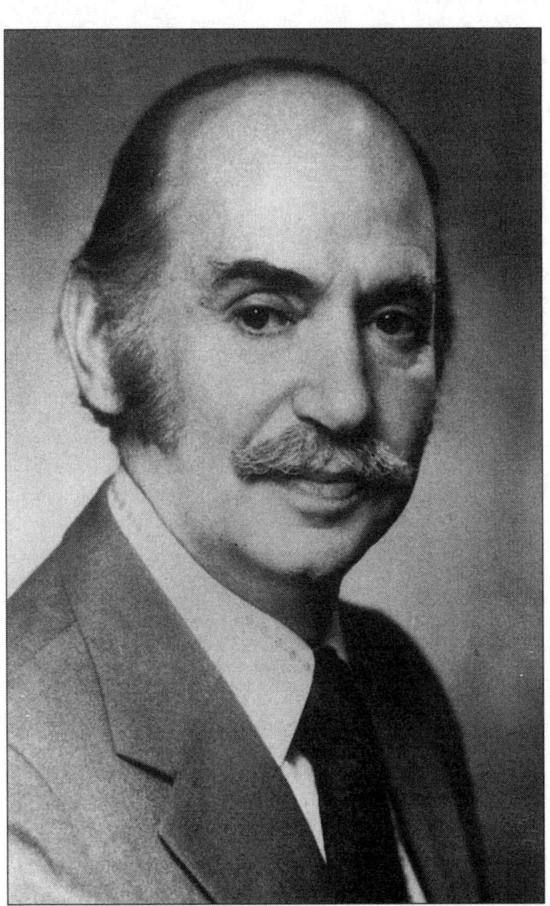

Alexander Russell (Courtesy of A. Russell)

RUSSELL DWARFISM

Intra-uterine dwarfism with low birth weight and short stature, skeletal changes resembling Silver Syndrome but not asymmetrical. Craniofacial dysostosis causes a triangular face with mandibular hypognathias and there are disproportionately short arms.

RUSSELL SYNDROME

1. Diencephalic syndrome – progressive weight loss, tremor, ataxia and sometimes nystagmus, and euphoric appearance usually due to a tumor in the diencephalon.
2. Dwarfism (*v. supra*).
3. Selective hypothalamo-hypophyseal thyroid stimulating hormone (TSH) deficiency – selective thyrotrophic hormone deficiency causing hypothyroidism.
4. Congenital hyperammonemia – an inborn enzymatic defect in biosynthesis of urea.

Alexander Russell English pediatrician. He was born in Newcastle, went to medical school at the University of Durham where he was greatly influenced by the innovative English pediatrician, J.M. Spense. He served in the R.A.F. during the 2nd

World War and studied the effect of carbon monoxide accumulation in bombers on the air crew, and became engaged in field research in malaria and kala azar whilst he was posted in the Middle East. After the war he returned to London, practiced as a pediatrician and by 1954 had become founder director of the first pediatric endocrine unit in the United Kingdom at the Queen Elizabeth Hospital in London. During this time he had worked in a number of areas of pediatrics and established a number of new and interesting metabolic syndromes in children. In 1966 he was invited to the new Chair of Paediatrics in child care at the Hebrew University of Jerusalem. Here he founded the Jerusalem Centre of Child and Family Developmental Rehabilitation which was aimed at a complete care in an educational and medical sense for handicapped children of all races and creeds. He followed this in 1970 by founding the first Arab Children's Hospital on the west bank at the town of Ramallah.

RUSSELL VIPER VENOM

Venom from Russell Viper – used in coagulation tests to activate factor X.

P. Russell (1727–1805) Born in Braidshaw, Scotland. Whilst medical officer with the British Army in India he wrote his four volume work "Account of Indian Serpents" (1896–1809) with the original description of Russell Viper (*Daboia russellii*). He also described the Aleppo Button (Endemic ulcer).

RUSSIAN AUTUMNAL ENCEPHALITIS

Japanese B encephalitis

RUSSIAN FAR EAST ENCEPHALITIS,

RUSSIAN FOREST SPRING ENCEPHALITIS,

RUSSIAN TICK BORNE COMPLEX

Characterized by gastro-intestinal features, hemorrhages, fever and neurological features.

RUSSIAN INTERMITTENT FEVER

Trench fever.

RUST DISEASE

Tuberculous spondylitis of the cervical region.

RUST PHENOMENON

Patient using hands to support head during movement with lesions of upper cervical vertebrae.

Johann N. Rust (1775–1840) German surgeon.

S

SABIN VACCINE

Live oral attenuated polio virus vaccine.

Albert B. Sabin (1906–1993) U.S. bacteriologist. He was born in Bialystock, then a part of Russia, but now in Poland. His family were poor Jews and were persecuted by anti-semitic attitudes at that time. They migrated to the United States in 1921, where he graduated from Pattison High School and went to New York initially to study dentistry. However the course did not excite him and partly from reading Paul de Kruif's "Microbe Hunters" he entered medicine. He worked his way through the New York

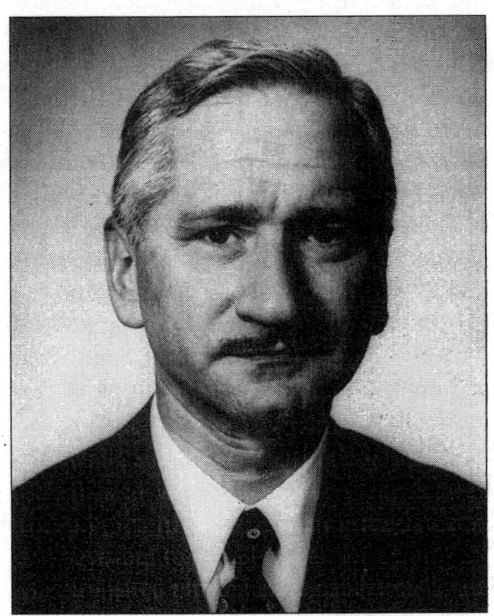

Albert B. Sabin (Courtesy of the Royal Society of Medicine, London, UK)

University's undergraduate college and School of Medicine and was taken under the wing of the Professor of Bacteriology, W.H. Park. He encouraged him to take up research into the causes of polio and in 1931 made his first contribution to this area by showing that a skin test then used to determine whether a person was liable to get polio or not was not valid. He graduated M.D. in 1931 and was a house physician in 1932–33 at the Bellevue Hospital. He worked at Lister Institute in London in 1934 and returned to the U.S.A. to take up a position with the Rockefeller Institute. He was appointed Professor of Research Pediatrics in 1946 and retired from that position in 1960. In 1974 he was appointed distinguished research Professor of Biochemistry at the University of South Carolina.

SABOURAUD AGAR

A liquid medium for culturing fungi.

Raymond J.A. Sabouraud (1864–1938) French dermatologist in Paris. In 1889 commenced training in dermatology with E. Vidal and E. Besnier at the Hôpital St. Louis where he maintained a life long association. He worked for a year at the Pasteur Institute and learnt the basics of bacteriology. He extensively investigated the role of fungal infections as a cause of diseases of the skin and published important papers on trichophyton (1894), eczema (1899), scalp diseases (1902) and pityriasis (1904). He developed a technique for monitoring the amount of radiation delivered. This enabled its safe use in epilation to treat ringworm of the scalp. He became famous for his knowledge of scalp diseases and had a "bald headed clinic" which attracted people from all over the world. R.L. Thompson is quoted, "It is said that Sabouraud can tell your moral character, the amount of your yearly income and what you have eaten for breakfast by looking at a root of one of your hairs." He was a fine musician with a deep knowledge of the arts and acknowledged as a gifted sculptor by critics of his day.

SACHS DISEASE

v. TAY-SACHS DISEASE

SAHLI METHOD

One of the original techniques for measuring hemoglobin calorimetrically.

Hermann Sahli (1856–1933) Swiss physician, who was the Director of the University Clinic at Berne, wrote books on methods of clinical investigation (1894) and introduced a number of instruments and techniques in that field including the hemoglobinometer (1902). He theorized on a number of topics such as hemophilia and antibodies, without making a major contribution.

SAINTS AND DISEASE

ST. AGATHA DISEASE

Any disease of female breast.

ST. ANTHONY FIRE

Ergotism.

ST. GILES DISEASE

Leprosy.

ST. LOUIS ENCEPHALITIS

Mosquito borne arbovirus.

cf. MURRAY VALLEY ENCEPHALITIS etc.

Named after an epidemic in St. Louis, U.S.A.

ST. MARTIN DISEASE

Dipsomania.

ST. VITUS DANCE

Sydenham chorea and the hysterical dancing mania in the middle ages.

ST. ZACHARY DISEASE

Mutism.

SAINT TRIAD

Association of hiatus hernia, gall bladder disease and diverticulosis.

Charles F.M. Saint (1886–1973) South African surgeon, Groote Schur Hospital, Capetown. He was born in Bedlington, Northumberland, and went to medical school at Durham University where he graduated in 1908. He became assistant to Professor Rutherford Morrison (who had trained with Berry) who was Professor of Surgery at Newcastle-upon-Tyne. He served in the 1st World War in France and was decorated for these services by the French and English governments, receiving the Commander of the British Empire and the Golden Medaille d'Honneur of the French Republic. In 1919 he was appointed to the Chair of Surgery in Capetown, South Africa, and remained there until his retirement in 1945. He was greatly influenced by Professor Morrison and published a book "An Introduction to Surgery" in 1925 in collaboration with him. Saint liked to emphasize the importance of considering multiple pathologies whenever the history and physical examination was atypical for any specific pathological condition. He frequently mentioned the association now called Saint Triad on ward rounds, but it was not until one of his students, C.J.B. Muller, wrote a paper on it and called it Saint's Triad that the eponym became attached. Indeed it is said that on one occasion Professor Saint asked one of his other protégés, J.H. Louw, "What the hell is Saint's Triad?" He himself did not write anything on the topic until 1966 when he described the story of its recognition in the "Review of Surgery". At that time he was 6 years into his retirement on the Channel island of Sark. He exerted a great influence on surgical training and teaching in South Africa and on his retirement his Chair was taken by one of his students, J.H. Louw. Another of his pupils was Christian Barnard. He bequeathed 75,000 pounds to the University of Capetown which was put towards establishing a Chair of Paediatric Surgery.

SALK VACCINE

Poliomyelitis vaccine.

Jonas E. Salk (1914–) U.S. bacteriologist. He graduated M.D. from the New York University in 1939 and interned at the Mt. Sinai Hospital, New York, 1940–42. He was a research associate in the University of Michigan in 1944–46 and assistant professor in 1946–47. He was Associate Research Professor in Bacteriology and subsequently Research Professor at the University of Pittsburgh from 1947–55 and Foundation Director of the Salk Institute in 1963. He developed his vaccine preventing poliomyelitis in 1954 and won the Nobel Prize for developing the first effective vaccine against poliomyelitis.

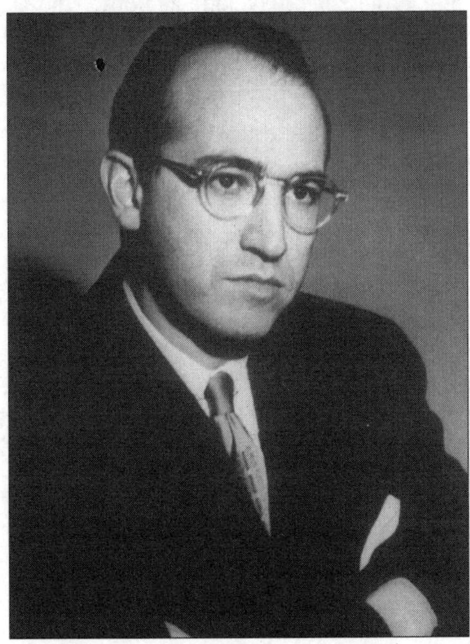

Jonas E. Salk (Courtesy of the Royal Society of Medicine, London, UK)

SALMONELLA

Gram negative rod shaped bacteria. It is a genus which includes the bacteria causing typhoid fever.

Daniel E. Salmon (1850–1914) U.S. veterinarian pathologist. He was born in New Jersey and studied at Cornell University, New York and at Alfort, France. He graduated in Veterinary Science from Cornell in 1872 and after practicing as a vet. in Newark, studied swine fever in 1878 at a veterinary division in the Department of Agriculture in Washington. In 1905 he was appointed Head of the Veterinary Department at the University of Montevideo, Uruguay, returning to the U.S. in 1910. He studied hog cholera and showed it to be due to a paratyphoid bacillus, and with T. Theobald Smith he showed that dead organisms could immunize animals against live organisms and this discovery was the basis for the development of typhoid and poliomyelitis (Salk) vaccines. He was appointed head of the section making anti-hog cholera vaccine in Butte, Montana, in 1910, remaining there until his death with pneumonia in 1914.

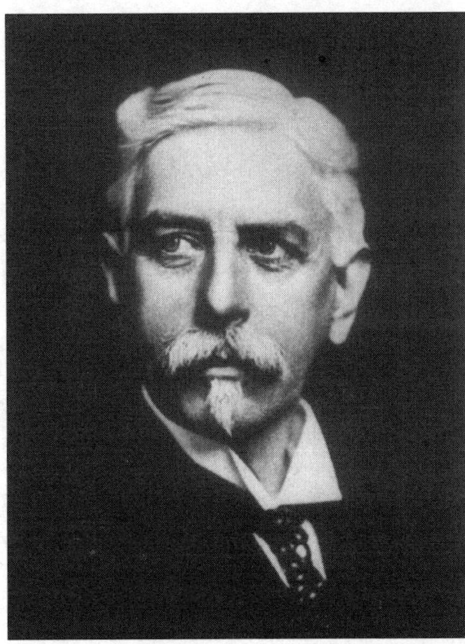

Daniel E. Salmon (Courtesy of the Royal Society of Medicine, London, UK)

SALZMANN NODULAR CORNEAL DYSTROPHY

Possibly the result of phlyctenular keratitis and causes one or more dense blue white nodules on the corneal surface – more frequently seen in women.

Maximilian Salzmann (1862–1954) Austrian ophthalmologist. He was born in Vienna and graduated in medicine there in 1887, a year later becoming assistant to Professor E. Fuchs (*v. supra*) in Vienna. He rose to Assistant Professor of Ophthalmology and was appointed Professor at Graz in 1911 where he remained. He wrote a classical book on the anatomy and histology of the eye and made many original observations and measurements of angles of the anterior chamber. He was an excellent painter and illustrated much of his work. Later in life retinal degeneration due to myopia caused considerable visual loss which he described in his last paper.

SAMPSON CYSTS

Cystic endometriosis of the ovary.

John A. Sampson (1873–1946) U.S. surgeon. Born in Troy, New York, he graduated at A.B. Williams College in 1895 and entered Johns Hopkins Medical School. His first paper in 1902 was on flat feet. In the four years he was resident and assistant resident under Kelly (1902–1905) he published 17 papers on gynecological subjects. In 1905 he went into private practice in Albany, New York, and became attached to the Albany Medical College until 1945 when he retired as Professor of Gynecology and Gynecologist-in-Chief of the Albany Hospital. While a resident of Kelly with Clark at Johns Hopkins, he worked on radical operations for cervical cancer with lymph node dissection and studied the blood supply to the uterus in an attempt to preserve this and lessen fistulae formation during lymph node resection.

In the early 1920s he began working on endometriosis and in all published 21 papers on this topic. He produced the theory of implantation, i.e. "that ovarian and other forms of peritoneal endometriosis arise from inflammation of bits of Müllerian mucosa, of either uterine or tubal origin, which, having been carried with menstrual blood escaping through patent tubes into the peritoneal cavity, have lodged on the surfaces of the various pelvic structures. The ectopic mucosa in these implants, regardless of their size or situation, may become additional foci for the spread of the endometriosis by direct extension and also by the implantation of bits of Müllerian tissue which escape from them during their reaction to menstruation. This latter phenomenon is most spectacular in the ovary where ectopic endometrial cavities may attain a much larger size than elsewhere, forming the well-known endometrial cyst of that organ."

SANARELLI VIRUS

Virus causing myxomatosis.

Giuseppe Sanarelli (1864–1940) Italian bacteriologist and Professor of Hygiene at Rome who extensively studied yellow fever (1897) but the etiological agent he proposed, *Bacillus icteroides*, was proven incorrect by Walter Reed. He believed he was the first person to discover the Schwartzman phenomenon.

SANDERS DISEASE OR SYNDROME

Epidemic keratoconjunctivitis.

Murray Sanders (1910–) U.S. bacteriologist who with C.W. Jungeblut first isolated an animal virus causing murine encephalomyocarditis.

SANDERS SIGN

Epigastric pulsation in constrictive pericarditis.

J. Sanders (1777–1843) English physician.

SANDHOFF-JATZKEWITZ DISEASE

Clinically similar to Tay-Sachs Disease but far more rare, and without a predilection for Ashkenazi Jews. Reduction in hexosaminidase A and hexosaminidase B.

K. Sandhoff German psychiatrist.

H. Jatzkewitz German psychiatrist.

SANFILIPPO SYNDROME

Gargoylism with progressive mental deterioration. It resembles Hurler syndrome but there is less hepatomegaly and no corneal or cardiac problems. It is inherited as an autosomal recessive. This is mucopolysaccharidosis Type III with increased amounts of heparitin sulphate in the urine. Abnormal granules present in the lymphocytes and occasionally in the neutrophils. Its incidence is 1:100 000.

Sylvester J. Sanfilippo U.S. pediatrician.

SANGER-BROWN ATAXIA

Hereditary spinocerebellar ataxia commencing in the 3rd decade or later, associated with optic atrophy.

Sanger Brown (1852–1928) U.S. neuropsychiatrist. He graduated M.D. from the Bellevue Hospital Medical College in 1880 and worked at the hospital for the insane, Ward's Island, N.Y. and then at the Bloomingdale Asylum where he became acting superintendent in 1886. He then went to London and worked with Professor E.A. Schafer at University College Hospital and showed for the first time conclusive proof that the occipital lobe was the center for vision in animals. Returning to the U.S. he worked in Chicago at the Rush Medical College and became Professor of Clinical Neurology at the College of Physicians and Surgeons, Illinois. He became owner and director of the Kenilworth Sanatorium and died of acute gastric dilatation following a prostatectomy.

SANSOM SIGN

1. Increased dullness to percussion parasternally in the 2nd and 3rd interspaces seen in pericardial effusion.
2. Murmur over the lips heard with thoracic aneurysm.

Arthur E. Sansom (1838–1907) English physician.

SANDSTRÖM BODIES

v. GLEY GLANDS

Parathyroid glands.

Ivor V. Sandström (1852–1889) Swedish anatomist. He was prosector in anatomy, Uppsala University, when he discovered and described these glands in detail. It was probably the last macroanatomical discovery of importance.

SAUNDERS DISEASE

Acute gastritis in infants due to excessive carbohydrate in the diet.

Edward W. Saunders (1854–1927) U.S. physician who worked in St. Louis.

SAUVINEAU OPHTHALMOPLEGIA

Ophthalmoplegia due to lesion in the medial longitudinal fasciculus. On lateral gaze, there is paresis of the medial rectus of the adducting eye and nystagmus of the abducting eye and often nystagmus on upward gaze but intact convergence when unilateral due to vascular or demyelinating lesion, when bilateral almost always due to demyelinisation.

Charles Sauvineau (1862–1924) French ophthalmologist who was an intern at the Salpêtrière and an assistant to Parinaud (*v. supra*). He contributed a number of studies on eye movements and nystagmus.

SCAGLIETTI-DAGNINI SYNDROME

v. ERDHEIM SYNDROME

Oscar Scaglietti (1906–) Italian orthopedic surgeon who was born in San José, Costa Rica, of Italian parents and studied medicine at the University of Bologna, graduating in 1930 and working in the orthopedic clinic there from 1932 to 1947, when he moved to the University of Florence, becoming the Professor of Orthopaedics there in 1956, retiring in 1977.

Guido Dagnini (1905–) Italian neurologist (*v. supra*).

SCARPA TRIANGLE

Femoral triangle.

Antonio Scarpa (1747–1832) Italian anatomist and surgeon. He was born in Motta, Italy, and studied anatomy with Morgagni in Padua, and surgery under Rivera at Bologna. In 1783 he was appointed Professor of Anatomy at Pavia and became Professor of Surgery. He illustrated his own textbooks and is said to have been the most artistic of all medical men to do so. He was a man of great wit who was a very able and interesting teacher, as well as being renowned for his sarcasm. He founded the subject of orthopedic surgery, first described the anatomy of the clubbed foot accurately and wrote a classic account of hernias. He wrote the first Italian text on eye diseases, recognized that atherosclerosis was a disease of the inner aspect of arteries and reported causalgia in 1832. He was also one of the first to give an accurate account of the nerve supply to the heart as well as the anatomy of the membranous labyrinth with its afferent nerves.

SCHÄFER SYNDROME

Congenital thickening of the nails.

Erich Schäfer (1897–) German dermatologist.

SCHAEFFER REFLEX

Extension of the great toe on pinching of the Achilles tendon. Seen in upper motor neurone lesions.

Max Schaeffer (1852–1923) German neurologist.

SCHAMBERG DISEASE

Progressive pigmentary dermatosis which often occurs on the lower limbs and must be distinguished from hemorrhagic manifestations since approximately half the patients have a positive Hess test (*v. supra*).

Jay F. Schamberg (1870–1934) U.S. dermatologist, who was born in Philadelphia and graduated from medical school at the University of Pennsylvania in 1893, interning at the University Hospital and being drawn into dermatology by Duhring, van Harlingen, Stelwagen and Hartzell, who had established a school in dermatology there. He spent a year studying in Vienna, Paris and Berlin, returning to Philadelphia and became Professor of Dermatology at the Temple Medical School, then at Jefferson Medical School and the Philadelphia Polyclinic, and when that affiliated with the University of Pennsylvania was appointed Professor at the graduate school of that university until his death.

He was particularly interested in the role of bacteria and with William Welsh published a book "The Acute Contagious Diseases". A good public speaker, he was a very effective opponent to the anti-vaccinationists. He described the disorder which bears his name in 1901 and in 1909 isolated the mite which was causing "grain itch". Realizing that arsphenamine would become unavailable to the United States should they enter the 1st World War, he worked in collaboration with others to develop and manufacture the drug and the profits established a research institute of cutaneous medicine of which he was director until he died. He published numerous books on skin disease and many papers on all aspects of dermatology.

SCHATSKI RING

Localized narrowing of the lower end of the esophagus, sometimes associated with dysphagia but probably of no singular significance, due to the insertion of the inferior esophago-phrenic ligament.

Richard Schatski (1901–) U.S. radiologist who migrated to the U.S.A. from Germany in the early 1930s. Three other brothers migrated at the same time; one became director of civil aviation in Israel, another the owner of a well known antique shop in New York and the third a physician in Melbourne. He received his training in radiology with H.H. Berg in Berlin and undertook experimental work on the effect of balloons in the esophagus of dogs, which resulted in a series of articles in the late 1920s which set out radiological principles for defining intra- and extra-mural lesions in the esophagus.

SCHAUMANN BODIES

Cytoplasmic calcium inclusion bodies in the giant cells seen in granulomatous conditions such as sarcoidosis and berylliosis.

Jörgen N. Schaumann (1879–1953) Swedish dermatologist whose work demonstrated that sarcoidosis was a systemic disease. Some call it BESNIER-BOECK-SCHAUMANN DISEASE (*v. supra*).

SCHEIE SYNDROME

Gargoylism with hypertrichosis, corneal clouding and opacity is often striking, and aortic valvular disease. Stature is usually near normal and there is little or no mental retardation. Abnormal granules are sometimes present in the white cells. It is inherited as an autosomal recessive and is compatible with a normal life span. Mucopolysaccharidosis Type I with excessive amounts of chondroitin B in the urine.

Harold G. Scheie (1909–) U.S. ophthalmologist. Born in Brookings County, South Dakota and graduated M.D. from the University of Minnesota in 1935. He became Professor of Ophthalmology at the University of Pennsylvania in 1956. His major research was in glaucoma.

SCHEUERMANN DISEASE

1. Osteochondrosis of the vertebrae associated with kyphosis.
2. Necrosis of the epiphyses of the vertebrae.

Holger W. Scheuermann (1877–1960) Danish radiologist. Born in Horsholm he was Director of Radiology, the Military Hospital and Sudby Hospital, Copenhagen.

SCHICK TEST

Test for immunity to diphtheria using diphtheria toxin.

Bela Schick (1877–1967) U.S. pediatrician, born in Boglar, Hungary, and studied medicine at Graz graduating in 1900. He introduced this test in 1910 and studied anaphylaxis. He worked in the Paediatric Clinic in Vienna (1902–1923) where he worked with von Pirquet on serum sickness and published his test for diphtheria in 1913. He migrated to the U.S.A. to join the staff of the Mt. Sinai Hospital, New York, in 1923. An oft quoted aphorism of his applied to the solution of medical problems was to use "a tincture of time".

SCHILDER DISEASE

A progressive demyelinating disorder in adult life associated with Sudan-positive phagocytes, also called encephalitis periaxialis diffusa. Visual impairment is an early symptom, with mental deterioration and progression until death.

SCHILDER-ADDISON COMPLEX

Melanodermic leukodystrophy.

Paul F. Schilder (1886–1940) Austrian neurologist who migrated to the U.S.A. Born in Vienna and graduated there in medicine in 1909 and then worked with G. Anton at Halle. Initially he studied choreic and athetoid movements and suggested athetoid movements in hemiplegia were due to a lesion in the dentate nucleus. He fought in World War I and later studied and published extensively on the body image. He moved to New York in 1930 as Director of the Psychiatric Division of Bellevue Hospital. He died after being struck by a motor car.

T. Addison (*v. supra*).

SCHILLING TEST

Test for vitamin B_{12} absorption. Radioactive B_{12} is taken orally and subsequently B_{12} is given parenterally and the amount of radioactivity secreted in the urine is measured in the next 24 hours. If abnormally low, intrinsic factor may then be given to see if this corrects the absorption as would be expected in pernicious anemia, but not small bowel disease causing malabsorption.

Robert F. Schilling (1919–) U.S. hematologist. He graduated M.D. from the University of Wisconsin in 1943 and interned at the Philadelphia General Hospital and saw military service as a battalion surgeon in the Marine Corps (1944–46). He was an N.I.H. post-doctoral fellow at the Thorndike Memorial Laboratory, Harvard Medical School, worked there with W. Castle and at this time commenced his studies on pernicious anemia. He returned to the University of Wisconsin, Medicine, in 1951, and became Chairman of the Department in 1964.

SCHILLING CLASSIFICATION

Method of neutrophil classification.

SCHILLING TYPE OF LEUKEMIA

Monocytic leukemia without any morphological components resembling a myelocytic origin.

Victor Schilling (1883–1960) Austrian hematologist who did much to popularize differential white cell counts in the peripheral blood. He was born in Torgan and became Professor of Medicine in Berlin.

SCHIMMELBUSCH DISEASE

Cystic dysplasia of the breast.

Curt Schimmelbusch (1860–1895) German pathologist and surgeon. He was born in West Prussia and studied medicine in Würzburg, Göttingen, Berlin and Halle where he was initially assistant to K.J. Eberth and with him wrote a classical article on thrombosis in 1888. He then turned to surgery and was assistant to von Bergman for a number of years. He published a number of papers on aseptic treatment of wounds and on bacteria found contaminating wounds. He described the disease which bears his name in 1892. He died with a thrombosis following a septic infection.

SCHIRMER TEST

A test for tear formation. A tape of filter paper 35 mm long, with J bend 5 mm is hooked into the inferior fournix at the junction of middle or outer third, and the absorption of tear fluid noted at the end of 5 minutes. Length of wetting should be 15 mm. If results are equivocal stimulate lacrimation by sniffing ammonia. Reduced in a number of conditions involving the lacrymal glands, e.g. rheumatoid arthritis, sarcoidosis, etc.

Otto W.A. Schirmer (1864–1917) German ophthalmologist.

SCHLATTER DISEASE

v. OSGOOD-SCHLATTER DISEASE

SCHLEMM CANAL

Irregular space at the sclerocorneal junction in the eye, draining the aqueous humor from the anterior chamber.

Friedrich S. Schlemm (1795–1858) German anatomist. Professor of Anatomy in Berlin.

SCHMIDT SYNDROME (1)

Ipsilateral paralysis of the 10th and 11th nerves due to a lesion of the nucleus or the nerve roots.

Johann F.M. Schmidt (1838–1907) German otolaryngologist who worked in Frankfurt.

SCHMIDT SYNDROME (2)

Addison disease with chronic thyroiditis and/or diabetes mellitus. Vitiligo is often present and the condition is thought to be auto-immune in origin.

Martin B. Schmidt (1863–1949) German physician.

SCHMINCKE TUMOR

Lymphoepithelioma.

Alexander Schmincke (1877–1953) German pathologist.

SCHMORL GROOVE

Grooves on emphysematous lungs due to pressure on ribs.

SCHMORL NODULE

1. Cartilaginous metaplasia in the vertebra.
2. Protrusion of the intervertebral disc into the vertebra in adolescent kyphosis.

Christian G. Schmorl (1861–1932) German pathologist. Professor of Pathology, Dresden. He attracted students from all over the world and he became known throughout the world for his book on histopathological methods which went through 15 editions and which was known locally as "Der kleine Schmorl". He wrote one of the early descriptions of myelofibrosis. He was particularly liked by students and trainees because of his kindliness towards them, and in this regard seems to be strikingly different from many of his colleagues of the same period. It is said that if he found it necessary to say that a section was too thick, he would add that after all the thicker a section the more there was to be seen in it! His weekly clinico-pathological conferences were attended not only by the clinical staff of the hospital, but also all the practitioners in the town.

SCHNABEL ATROPHY

Cavernous optic atrophy.

Isidor Schnabel (1842–1908) Austrian ophthalmologist. He was born in Neubydschow, Bohemia. A student and disciple of Jaeger, he was appointed Professor of Ophthalmology in Vienna in 1895.

SCHNEEBERG DISEASE

Occupational pulmonary cancer which developed in miners in the metal mines of Schneeberg, Saxony. The dust contained 0.5% arsenic as well as radioactivity and they developed pneumoconiosis with cancer occurring 10–12 years later. A similar disease was seen in the radium mines in Joachimsthal in Bohemia.

SCHOLZ-BIELSCHOWSKY-HENNEBERG DISEASE

Metachromic leukodystrophy. Cerebral sclerosis – subacute familial form of leukodystrophy, commencing in the teens with aphasia, progressive deafness, blindness, dementia and paralysis.

Willibald Scholz (1889–) German neuropathologist.

Max Bielschowsky (1869–1940) German neuropathologist. He was born in Breslau (Wroclaw) and studied at Breslau and Munich graduating M.D. in 1892. He worked with E. Mendel and later with O. Vogt (*v. infra* SPIELMEYER-VOGT DISEASE). He emigrated to England just before the 2nd World War.

Richard Henneberg (1868–1962) German neurologist.

SCHÖNLEIN DISEASE OR PURPURA

v. HENOCH-SCHÖNLEIN PURPURA

SCHOTTMÜLLER DISEASE

Paratyphoid fever.

Hugo Schottmüller (1867–1936) German bacteriologist and physician. He was Professor of Medicine at Hamburg. He showed that *Streptococcus irridans* could cause bacterial endocarditis and introduced pyramidon for treatment of rheumatoid arthritis. He isolated the organism causing rat bite fever in 1914.

SCHRIDDE CANCER HAIR

Thick dark hairs found in the beard and on the temple of cancerous or cachectic patients.

SCHRIDDE SYNDROME

Hydrops fetalis.

Hermann Schridde (1875–) German pathologist.

SCHÜFFNER DOTS, GRANULES OR STIPPLING

Pink/red/yellow granules seen in red cells stained by Romanovsky techniques due to malarial parasites.

Wilhelm A.P. Schüffner (1867–1949) German pathologist. He was born in Minde, Hannover, Germany, and was a medical student at Erlangen, Würzburg and Munich. When aged 30 he was appointed chief medical officer in Eastern Sumatra and it was in 1899 whilst there he described the stippling of red cells infected with *Plasmodium vivax* which became known as "Schüffner dots". In 1916 he was appointed medical adviser to the Dutch East Indies government where he introduced much public health reform and in 1922 to 1937 was Professor of Tropical Hygiene at the Royal Colonial Institute in Amsterdam and also Director of the Institute. In 1937–44 he was appointed Director of the Schüffner Laboratories of that same institute.

In 1900 he recognized the value of chenopodium oil in the treatment of ankylostomiasis. He became a world authority on leptospirosis and developed an agglutination test for its diagnosis. It was largely as a result of his work that leptospirosis was recognized as an important disorder in animals and man. He was a kindly, intelligent man, who was appalled at the rise of Nazism in Germany.

SCHÜLLER-CHRISTIAN DISEASE OR SYNDROME

v. HAND-SCHÜLLER-CHRISTIAN DISEASE

SCHULTZ SYNDROME

Agranulocytosis.

SCHULTZ-CHARLTON BLANCHING TEST

Subcutaneous injection of immune serum into erythematous region of a patient with scarlet fever results in blanching reaction.

SCHULTZ-DALE REACTION OR TEST

The contraction of isolated intestine (Schultz) or uterus (Dale) of an anaphylactic guinea pig when exposed to the agent causing anaphylaxis.

Werner Schultz (1878–1947) German physician who introduced the term agranulocytosis to describe the association of severe neutropenia with ulcerated infections of the throat (Schultz angina).

Willy Charlton (1889–) Berlin physician.

Sir Henry Dale (1875–1968) English physiologist and pharmacologist. He initially worked at Cambridge with Gaskell and Langley, then with Bayliss and Starling (*v. infra*) at the University College in London and with Paul Ehrlich (*v. supra*) in Frankfurt. He became Head of the Burroughs Wellcome Research Institute and the founder of modern pharmacology in England. In 1919 he reported the sympathomimetic action of amines. He introduced the concept of chemical transmitters and their role in nerve action, and first described the inhibitory activity of acetylcholine on the heart. For this work, with Loewi (*v. supra*) he was awarded the Nobel Prize in physiology and medicine in 1936. He coined the terms cholinergic and adrenergic nerves and was one of the early investigators of the action of histamine, oxytocin and ergotoxin.

SCHULTZE PARESTHESIA OR SYNDROME

Acroparesthesia: numbness, pins and needles and pains in hands and feet without vasomotor nerve abnormalities and increased electrical and nerve irritability.

Friedrich Schultze (1848–1934) German neurologist who worked in Bonn.

v. NOTHNAGEL DISEASE

SCHWABACH TEST

Compared duration of bone conduction of the impaired ear with that of the normal.

Dagobert Schwabach (1846–1920) German otologist who worked in Berlin.

SCHWANN CELL

Cells that surround the peripheral axons forming the myelin sheath.

SCHWANN SHEATH

Neurilemma.

SCHWANNOMA

Neurilemmoma.

Friedrich T. Schwann (1810–1882) German anatomist. He was born at Neuss near Düsseldorf. He was schooled at the Jesuit College in Cologne and entered the University of Bonn in 1829, and after graduating he worked in Würzburg and Berlin. He failed to get an academic appointment in Germany and finally accepted a Chair of Anatomy in the Catholic University of Louvain. He moved to Liège in 1848 and was Professor of Anatomy there until he retired in 1880.

He was a quiet, deeply religious man, who avoided controversies at all times, and perhaps it was this reticence which resulted in his failure to advance in German academic medicine, because he was one of the founders of neuro-histology, who by 1839 had made two major contributions to science.

He was one of the first to show that fermentation was associated with living organisms but this was not accepted until Pasteur's time, who wrote to him in 1878, "for 20 years I have been travelling along some of the paths opened up by you". In 1839 he published his monograph "Microscopic investigations on the accordance in the structure and growth in animals and plants", which was translated into English for the Sydenham Society in 1847 by Henry Smith. In this monograph he described cells to support the basic thesis that the cell nucleus and its protoplasm form a universal structure. In it he described and illustrated with beautiful drawings, the structure of nerve cells and muscle cells. Schwann was then founder of the cellular theory, although Schleiden, also working under Müller's influence, wrote a paper in 1838 in which he concluded that all plants are formed of cells and that they grow through changes which take place in the cell nuclei. As a result the cellular theory sometimes is referred to as the Schleiden-Schwann cell theory.

Schwann, apart from discovering the sheath of the axis cylinder of the nerves, which bears his name, also discovered the striped muscle in the upper part of the esophagus. He discovered pepsin in 1835, and in 1841, using an artificial biliary fistula in a dog, showed that bile is essential for digestion. He was one of the first to study muscular contraction, by physical and mathematical methods, and in 1837 made the classical experiment showing that the tension of a contracting muscle varies with its length.

He is said to have been a very amiable, pleasant person, of middle height, with lively eyes. He was a devout Catholic who submitted the manuscript of his work on cell theory to the Bishop of Malines for approval before publication. Subsequent to this he made no major contributions and it has been speculated that this was because of his relative isolation from his home land in Belgium. All of his productive work had occurred when he was with Johanns Müller, and where he had fellow students such as Henle, Bischoff and Remak. Only once was he involved in any controversy, and that concerned his faith, because the Catholic priest had quoted him as agreeing that the antics of a young woman pretending to be inspired by the Holy Ghost were genuine (the Louise-Lateau Affair). He refuted this in a pamphlet. He remained a bachelor and died while visiting his brother in Cologne in 1882.

SCHWARTZ-BARTTER SYNDROME

Inappropriate anti-diuretic hormone (ADH) secretion complicating oat cell bronchogenic carcinoma and resulting in a dilutional hyponatremia.

William B. Schwartz (1922–) U.S. physician.

Frederic C. Bartter (1914–) U.S. physician (*v. supra*).

SCHWARTZ-JAMPEL SYNDROME

Myotonia, hip dysplasia and short stature with blepharophimosis or spasm of the eyelids and irregular eyelashes. Presents in infancy with choking on cold fluids and may have hip dislocation. Muscles become increasingly stiff and may be hypertrophied as well as myotonic.

Oscar Schwartz (1919–) U.S. ophthalmologist.

Robert S. Jampel (1926–) U.S. ophthalmologist.

SCOMBROID-FISH POISONING

This results from the ingestion of bad fish, with symptoms of flushing, sweating, nausea, vomiting, diarrhea and palpitations with headache and sometimes swelling of the face and tongue. Respiratory distress and vasodilatory shock have occurred occasionally.

Scombroid Fish A fish derived from the families *Scombroidae* and *Scomberesocidae*. These include mackerel, tuna, skip-jack and bonito.

SECKEL SYNDROME

Bird-headed dwarfism.

Helmut P.G. Seckel (1900–) Swiss pediatrician.

SECRÉTAN DISEASE

Dorsal edema of hand or foot following trauma.

Henri Secrétan (1856–1916) Swiss surgeon.

SEELIGMUELLER NEURALGIA

Bilateral neuralgia of the auriculotemporal nerves with pain extending over the skull and seen characteristically in neurosyphilis.

SEELIGMUELLER SIGN

Ipsilateral dilated pupil in trigeminal neuralgia.

Otto L.G.A. Seeligmueller (1837–1912) German neurologist.

SÉGUIN SIGN OR SIGNAL

Involuntary muscle contraction anteceding a focal seizure.

Edouard Séguin (1812–1880) U.S. psychiatrist. He was a pupil of J.M.G. Itard, the otologist, who initiated the attempts to train mentally defective people commencing in 1840 on the wild boy found in the forest in France, "The Savage of Meyron" and also studied at Esquirol in France. In 1842 he was appointed instructor at the Bicêtre and the Academy of Sciences reported that his theories were sound. He returned to the U.S.A. establishing schools in several states and publishing a monograph on idiocy in 1846. His ideas were adopted throughout the U.S.A.

SEIP-LAWRENCE SYNDROME

Total lipoatrophic diabetes – a very rare condition characterized by gradual loss of subcutaneous fat, diabetes mellitus and high insulin levels. Often late in onset and associated with acanthosis nigricans, hypertrichosis, gigantism, penile or clitoral hypertrophy and hepatomegaly.

Martin Seip (1921–) Scandinavian (Norwegian) pediatrician and endocrinologist.

Robert D. Lawrence English physician. Endocrinologist at King's College Hospital, London.

SEITZ FILTER

Asbestos filter for removing bacteria.

Ernest Seitz (1885–) German bacteriologist.

SELDINGER TECHNIQUE

Method for introducing a catheter into a vessel via a needle puncture.

S.I. Seldinger (1921–) Swedish radiologist. In the early 1950s he catheterised arteries by introducing the catheter through a needle. He also designed catheters bent at the tip to enable their entry into renal arteries. He became head of radiology in Mora, Sweden.

SELTER DISEASE

Acrodynia, pink disease

v. SWIFT DISEASE.

Paul Selter (1866–1941) German pediatrician.

SELYE SYNDROME

General adaptation syndrome.

Hans Selye (1907–) French-Canadian physiologist and physician, who developed the concept that animals react to stress with a set pattern of responses and this could explain a number of conditions (e.g. the collagen disorders). He was born in Vienna, Austria, studied medicine in Paris and Rome and graduated M.D. from the German University of Prague in 1929. He migrated to North America and became Professor and Director of the Institute of Experimental Medicine and Surgery at the Université de Montreal.

SEMON LAW

In nerve lesions of the motor laryngeal nerves abductor muscles of the cord are first affected and the last to recover after paralysis.

SEMON SYMPTOM

Impaired vocal cord mobility with thyroid carcinoma.

Sir Felix Semon (1849–1921) British otolaryngologist. He was the son of a Berlin stockbroker and commenced his medical studies at Heidelberg, but these were interrupted by the Franco-Prussian War in which he served as a volunteer and whilst camped outside Paris (1870–71) he composed a military march which was used by his regiment of Uhlans when they marched in Berlin after peace had been declared. He then graduated in medicine M.D. from Berlin in 1873 and studied in Vienna and Paris, being attracted into the area of ear, nose and throat by the recent introduction of the laryngoscope. He came to London in 1875 becoming a clinical assistant at St. Thomas's Hospital and the Throat Hospital in Golden Square. He became a member of the Royal College of Physicians of London and in 1877 was appointed physician at the Throat Hospital, and in 1882 physician in charge of the Throat Department at St. Thomas's Hospital and in 1888 laryngologist to the National Hospital for Epilepsy, Queen Square. He worked in the Brown Institute with Victor Horsley and made a number of important contributions including evidence that cretinism, myxedema and post-thyroidectomy cachexia were one and the same. He and Horsley showed that it was difficult, if not impossible, to produce laryngeal paralysis from a one-sided cortical lesion. He showed that adductor paralysis of the larynx was usually due to either psychosomatic states, myasthenia or some other muscle disorder and that organic diseases of the nerves usually caused abductor paralysis although this was sometimes associated with adductor paresis as well. He worked and published extensively on malignant disorders of the cords and larynx and on methods of diagnosis and treatment of sepsis of the same area. He introduced the treatment of vocal rest for laryngeal tuberculosis which was soon used in most sanatoriums throughout the world. In 1893 he founded the Laryngological Society of London and in 1894 the German Emperor gave him the title of Royal Prussian Professor and in 1897 he was knighted and was appointed Physician Extraordinary to King Edward VII in 1901. His wife was a fine vocalist whom he used to accompany, and he also was a keen hunter and angler.

SENEAR-USHER SYNDROME

This syndrome describes the association of pemphigus foliaceus with clinical and immunological features of lupus erythematosus. The condition has been named pemphigus erythematosus.

Francis E. Senear (1889–1958) U.S. dermatologist.

Barney D. Usher (1899–1978) Canadian dermatologist. He was born in Montreal and graduated from medical school at McGill University in 1922. He became interested in dermatology during his internship and since there were, at the time, few trained dermatologists in Canada, he went to work with W.A. Pusey in Chicago and there he met Senear whom he credits with "putting it all together" for the publication of the disorder for which they are remembered. In 1926 he returned to Montreal to take up a post at the Montreal General Hospital and in 1931 he joined the McGill Faculty. His research interests were on the mechanisms of sweating and on the relationship of internal disease with eczema. His major contribution and interest, however, was to teaching, which he continued right till the end of his life. He trained many Canadian dermatologists and although he enjoyed spending time with patients, emphasized that no one could get fun out of running "a mill" i.e. seeing 60–70 patients per day.

SENGSTAKEN-BLAKEMORE TUBE

Tube with inflatable balloons used to control bleeding of esophageal varices.

R.W. Sengstaken (1923–) U.S. surgeon.

Arthur H. Blakemore (1897–1970) He was born in Lancaster County, Virginia, graduated from the William and Mary College in 1918, then went to Johns Hopkins where he graduated in 1922. He did his surgical training at Johns Hopkins, the Henry Ford Hospital, Detroit, and the Roosevelt Hospital, New York. In 1927 he became a U.S. marine surgeon at Cordova (Alaska) General Hospital and Territorial Commissioner of Health there.

He joined the Columbia Presbyterian Medical Centre in 1928 and maintained an active association until 1962 when he retired as Associate Professor of Clinical Surgery at the College of Physicians and Surgeons, Columbia University, and attending surgeon at the Columbia Presbyterian Medical Centre. In 1937 he published his first experimental paper on vascular surgery, and this was followed over the years with a number of articles on this topic. In 1954 the Sengstaken-Blakemore balloon was developed under his direction and used for the control of variceal hemorrhage in patients with portal hypertension. He pioneered the portocaval shunt as a procedure in this disorder. He was a past President of the Society for Vascular Surgery and a founder of the New York Society for cardiovascular surgery, the A.O. Whipple Surgical Society and the James IV Association of Surgeons. During the 2nd World War he served as the Director of the National Research Council Project on anastomosis of blood vessels for the wounded.

SENIOR-LOKEN SYNDROME

Hereditary nephronophthisis (medullary cystic kidney) with retinitis pigmentosa.

Boris Senior South African pediatrician who specialised in endocrinology and is head of pediatric endocrinology at the New England Center, Boston, U.S.A.

Aagot G. Løken Scandinavian pediatrician who worked in Oslo, Norway.

SEPHARDIC JEWS

Jews of Spanish or Portuguese descent.

Sephardim Hebrew word for Spain.

SERGENT LINE OR SIGN

White line of the skin of chest or abdomen after a light scratch seen in Addison disease.

Emile Sergent (1869–1943) French physician described the sign in 1903.

SERRATIA MARCESCENS

A nosocomial pathogen – probably a separate genus of the Enterobacteriaceae family. It often grows in foodstuffs and produces a pigment which looks like drops of blood and in the 6th century B.C. Pythagorus noted bloody discoloration of foodstuff. Its appearance on the bread of armies has been taken as an omen on a number of occasions. The starchy material used as sacrament in churches also provided evidence that it was the appearance of Christ's blood, thereby supporting the dogma of the Christian Church.

The organism was discovered by Bartolomeo Bizio, a young Italian pharmacist, who thought it was a fungus in 1819. His attention had been drawn to it by its appearance on an Italian foodstuff called polenta in a peasant household. Their neighbours believed it was divine retribution, for it was rumored they were hoarding the food and denying it to others during the famine of 1817.

Bizio named it after Serafino Serrati since he believed the latter to have priority in the discovery of the steamboat and felt he should be appropriately honored and remembered. Marcescens is from marcescere – to decay.

Serafino Serrati Italian physicist.

SERTOLI CELL

Cells of the seminiferous tubules.

SERTOLI-LEYDIG TUMOR

Arrhenoblastoma of the ovary.

Enrico Sertoli (1842–1910) Italian physiologist. Born in Sondrio, he became Professor of Experimental Physiology in Milan.

Franz von Leydig (*v. supra*).

SEVER DISEASE

Calcaneous apophysitis.

James W. Sever (1878–) U.S. orthopedic surgeon, based in Boston. He was primarily interested in children and described operations for neonatal palsies and recurrent shoulder dislocations.

SÉZARY SYNDROME

Exfoliative erythroderma (homme rouge) associated with lymphadenopathy and circulating lymphocytes usually large, with cerebriform or deeply folded nucleus "cellule monstreuse" which infiltrate the skin. These are helper T lymphocytes.

Albert Sézary (1880–1956) French dermatologist. He was born in Algiers and after an outstanding scholastic career he became an intern in Algiers and in 1903 moved to Paris. There he worked with Dejerine and Raymond, giving him a strong basis in neurology. He worked with Jacquet and Jenesele in dermatology and syphilology, and became the Chief of Service at the Hospital St. Louis from 1928–1945. He was Professor of the Faculty of Medicine at the University of Paris in 1927 and was appointed Emeritus Professor in 1942.

Initially he was interested in adrenal pathology and emphasized the role of endocrine glands in many of the skin diseases. His major investigational thrust was the study of syphilis and he introduced the combination therapy of arsenic and bismuth in 1921 and demonstrated that this could result in the cure of syphilis after re-infection in many of his patients. He introduced pentavalent arsenical (sodium acetarsone) in the treatment of general paralysis of the insane (GPI) and at the time this was hailed as a very important contribution to psychiatry.

He published a monograph on neurosyphilis (1927) and made contributions to many textbooks. He collected 150 cases of lymphogranulomatosis between 1932 and 1939 and it was in the course of this that he recorded the syndrome that bears his name. He was a very accurate observer and a kindly and polished teacher.

SHAVER DISEASE

Bauxite fume pneumoconiosis.

Cecil G. Shaver (1901–) Canadian chest physician.

SHEEHAN SYNDROME

Pituitary failure occurring postpartum characterized by lack of lactation and loss of menstruation. It often follows a serious obstetrical complication, e.g. severe post partum hemorrhage.

Harold L. Sheehan (1900–1988) Born in Carlisle, England, and graduated from Manchester University in 1921. He was in general practice in Carlisle for 6 years and then spent 7 years as a lecturer in Pathology at the University of Manchester. In 1934 he worked at Johns Hopkins for a year as a Rockefeller Fellow and in 1946 became Professor of Pathology at Liverpool. He was a classical morbid anatomist whose best teaching was in the autopsy room demonstrating the pathology of the fresh specimens to students. He was one of the first to recognize the liver damage associated with the use of chloroform in pregnancy and this was known in France as "Maladie de Sheehan".

SHERREN TRIANGLE

Area on the anterior abdominal wall defined by lines joining the umbilicus and the anterior superior iliac spine and the pubic tubercle.

James Sherren (1872–1945) English surgeon.

v. OCHSNER-SHERREN TREATMENT.

SHERRINGTON LAW

Each posterior spinal nerve supplies its own specific area of skin with some overlap of adjacent dermatomes.

Sir Charles S. Sherrington (1857–1952) English neurophysiologist. He was the son of a country physician who died when he was quite young and was brought up by his stepfather in Ipswich. He studied medicine at Cambridge University, commencing there in 1879 and there he was influenced by the "father of British physiology", Michael Forster, and also by two of his pupils who were already becoming world famous – Langley and Gaskell. After graduation he worked with Langley, studying the anatomical changes in the cord and brain stem of a decorticate dog which had first been exhibited by Goltz at the International Congress in 1881. Sherrington visited Goltz's laboratory in Strasburg on a number of occasions. Between 1884 and 1887 he turned his attention to bacteriology and studied cholera, and whilst in Spain studying the disorder, he met Cajal and was instrumental in the latter lecturing in England. He also went to Berlin where he met Robert Koch and spent a year at Virchow's laboratory. He was appointed lecturer in physiology at St. Thomas's medical school in London in 1887 and there continued to investigate the spinal tract and in 1891 was appointed Professor of Pathology at the Brown Institute, following Victor Horsley. This was a veterinary institute which many of the famous English neurologists and neurophysiologists and neurosurgeons attended, and here he was able to observe animals with chronic spinal lesions. Sherrington established the concept that the reflex arcs were co-ordinated and controlled and that there was a form of reciprocal innovation which by virtue of inhibiting antagonist muscles enabled smoothness of muscle action. He developed the theory of transmission at the synapse being in one direction, decerebrate rigidity was then a background in which the presence of reciprocal inhibition was lost and these findings and theories resulted in his publication in 1906 of a monograph entitled "Integrative action of the nervous system" which remains a classic. He established the nature of postural reflexes and their dependence on the anti-gravity stretch reflex and traced the afferent stimulus to the proprioceptive end organs which he had already shown to be sensory in nature. Most of this work occurred after he had been appointed Professor of Physiology at Liverpool in 1895.

In 1913 he was appointed to the Chair of Physiology at Oxford University where he stayed till his retirement in 1935. He was awarded the Nobel Prize for his fundamental investigations in the physiology of the nervous system and he shared this with Adrian in 1932.

He always had a love for classics and poetry and in 1925 published a volume of collected verse.

Following his retirement he had two interesting publications – one entitled "Man on his Nature" and a fascinating account "The Endeavour of Jean Fernel" which was published in 1946. From 1941 onwards he developed a painful arthritis which remained with him until he died. Right until the end he maintained his mental alertness and was an entertaining conversationalist.

SHIGA BACILLUS

Subgroup of *Shigella*.

SHIGELLA

Non-motile Gram-negative bacteria which are the causal organisms of some outbreaks of dysentery.

Kiyoshi Shiga (1870–1957) Japanese bacteriologist. He was born in Sendai, Japan, and studied in Tokyo from 1892–96 where he worked as an assistant to Kitasato. He then moved to Europe and worked with Paul Ehrlich (1900–1903). He returned to Japan to become the director of a department in the Institute for Infectious Diseases in Tokyo (1904–1920). He then became Dean of the medical faculty of the Keijo Imperial University, Chosen, Japan. He discovered the dysentery bacillus in 1897 and worked on numerous bacteriological and chemotherapeutic projects.

SHOPE PAPILLOMA

Virus induced papilloma of rabbit skin.

Richard E. Shope (1901–1966) U.S. pathologist who made fundamental research into influenza and its cause.

SHULMAN DISEASE

This is a scleroderma-like condition with diffuse fasciitis and eosinophilia, together with a polyclonal increase in gammaglobulins. Its onset is usually acute with tender symmetrical skin thickening, with the limbs being involved in the majority of cases but rarely including the face and also less commonly involving the trunk and neck. There is a 2:1 male to female preponderance. This condition is often responsive to steroid treatment.

Lawrence E. Shulman U.S. physician who worked in Baltimore.

SHWACHMAN SYNDROME

Syndrome of pancreatic insufficiency and bone marrow dysfunction. Seen in infants who failed to thrive and have evidence of pancreatic insufficiency and bone marrow hypoplasia which may result in any of the elements being diminished in number.

Harry Shwachman (1910–1986) U.S. pediatrician who graduated M.D. from Johns Hopkins and after training in pediatrics moved to the Boston Children's Hospital and became Professor of Pediatrics at Harvard. He started the cystic fibrosis clinic and became an international figure.

SHWARTZMANN PHENOMENON OR REACTION

1. Local:
   Hemorrhagic and necrotic lesion at the intradermal site of injected bacterial endotoxin when the same material is given intravenously 8–24 hours later.
2. Generalized:
   Bilateral cortical necrosis of the kidney, disseminated intravascular coagulation and other renal lesions seen when both injections are given intravenously.

Gregory Shwartzmann (1896–) U.S. immunologist.

SHY-DRAGER SYNDROME

Postural hypotension, dysphagia, cricopharyngeal crises, incontinence, with Parkinson-like features, believed to be due to a dopaminergic nerve lesion.

George M. Shy (1919–1967) U.S. neurologist. Born in Trinidad, Colorado, and graduated M.D. University of Oregon in 1943 and gained his London MRCP in 1947. Chairman of the Department of Neurology at the University of Pennsylvania 1962–7 and then at Columbia University, New York.

Glenn A. Drager (1917–1967) U.S. neurologist.

SIA TEST

A test for macroglobulins by dropping serum into distilled water. If positive a precipitate forms which resolubilizes on adding saline.

R.H.P. Sia (1895–1970) U.S. physician. The test is described in one of the few papers quoted from the Chinese Medical Journal.

SIAMESE TWINS

Living conjugated twins. Named after the Thailand twins Chang and Eng, who were exhibited in Europe in the 19th century.

SICARD SYNDROME

v. COLLETT SYNDROME

Jean A. Sicard (1872–1929) French physician and radiologist, born and educated in Marseilles and began to study medicine there but completed it in Paris where he undertook some studies in immunology with Widal. He was attached to Raymond in 1894 and a year later to Danlos, Widal, Troisier, Brissaud and Raymond. He was most influenced and helped by Brissaud and was Chef de Clinique in 1901, Médécin des Hôpitaux in 1903 and Agrégé in 1907, Chef de Service at the Hôpital Necker in 1910, and Professor of Internal Pathology in 1923. During World War I he directed the neurological centre of the 15th region. He was dubbed "The Healer of Pain" following his work on the mechanisms of pain and therapeutic strategies he evolved therefrom. He was very interested in diagnostic and therapeutic techniques involving direct injections. He introduced the injection of sclerosing solutions for varicose veins and alcohol injection for the relief of trigeminal neuralgia. With his student Jacques Forestier he introduced the use of radio-opaque iodized oil (Lipiodol). The use of this injection into the cerebrospinal fluid was a brilliant advance in diagnostic and localization techniques for intraspinal neoplasms. He recognized possibilities in its use in other situations such as sinus tracts and urethral disorders, bronchography and even the demonstration of intra-arterial thromboses. He was also one of the first to become interested in the possibilities of pneumo-encephalography (v. Dandy).

After a dinner that he hosted and in which he had been unusually effervescent, he developed angina pectoris and suggested the injection of the sympathetic ganglion with novocaine. He died before this could be undertaken.

SIDBURY SYNDROME

Enzyme deficiency causing a decrease in oxidation of butyric and n-hexanoic acids. This results in malodorous sweat, vomiting, acidosis, lethargy and coma, and there is sometimes an associated thrombocytopenia.

James B. Sidbury (1922–) Contemporary U.S. pediatrician. Born in Wilmington, North Carolina and graduated M.D. from Columbia University in 1947. He worked at Johns Hopkins and became Professor of Pediatrics at Duke University in 1965.

SIEGERT SIGN

The incurving of the little finger in Mongolism.

v. DOWN SYNDROME

Ferdinand Siegert (1865–1946) German pediatrician.

SIEMENS SYNDROME

1. Hereditary anhidrotic ectodermal dysplasia. There is deficient development of sweat glands, teeth and alopecia. Mild form dominant trait, and severe form a recessive.

2. Incontinentia pigmenti. Usually affects female infants with defects of teeth, eyes, brain and hair, and widespread pigmented macules of unusual shapes. Inherited as an autosomal dominant.

Herman W. Siemens (1891–1969) German dermatologist.

SILVER SYNDROME

Short stature, triangular shaped head, café au lait spots, incurved little fingers and asymmetrical development of part or one side of the body.

v. also RUSSELL DWARFISM

Henry K. Silver (1918–) U.S. pediatrician. Born in Philadelphia and graduated M.D. from the University of California in 1942. He became Professor of Pediatrics at the University of Colorado in Denver. He made an important contribution to the recognition of the "battered child syndrome".

SIMMONDS CACHEXIA OR DISEASE

Hypopituitarism.

Morris Simmonds (1855–1925) German physician, born on St. Thomas Island which then belonged to Denmark. He and his parents migrated to Hamburg in 1861 and he commenced medicine in 1879, attending Tübingen, Leipzig, Munich and Kiel and graduating in 1879. He went into general practice but persisted with his major interest, pathology, and in 1909 received a full time appointment and ceased practice. He was made an Honorary Professor of the University of Hamburg when it opened in 1919. He died with Parkinson disease.

SIMON FOCI

Caseous nodules going on to calcify at the apices of lungs in children with tuberculosis.

George Simon English radiologist.

SIMON SEPTIC FACTOR

Reduction or disappearance of eosinophils with associated neutrophilia with bacterial infections (now thought to be secondary to increased ACTH secretion).

Charles E. Simon (1866–1927) U.S. physician. Born in Baltimore the son of a well known merchant. He lived in Germany from 6–18 going to school at Baden Baden and to a gymnasium at Hannover. He returned to Baltimore and undertook a course in chemical biology which had been founded by the President of Johns Hopkins University, Gilman. After graduating from College (1888) he first studied medicine at the University of Pennsylvania and then the University of Maryland, graduating M.D. in 1890. Johns Hopkins Hospital had opened in 1889 and he was appointed as a resident with William Osler whom he greatly admired. Following Osler's advice he spent a year in Paris studying physiological chemistry with Gautier and then 3 months in Basel with Bunge where he met his wife. He returned to Baltimore in 1892 but a position to establish physiological chemistry at the Hospital failed to eventuate and with the help of a prominent Baltimore physician (Salza) he entered practice specializing in gastro-enterology. He wrote a book "Manual for Clinical Gastro-enterology". He wrote another "Manual for Clinical Diagnosis" in 1896 which became a standard text and had 10 editions. He had a mental breakdown described as a phobia and making it impossible for him to continue clinical practice. Osler was looking after him and suggested an ideal alternative: "There is a stable in the rear of your house. Get the landlord to fix it up and start a diagnostic laboratory." This he did and he soon established one of the first if not the first diagnostic pathology laboratory in the U.S. which attracted not only referrals for diagnostic reports but also people for training and research. He was eventually made Professor of Clinical Pathology at the College of Physicians and Surgeons in Baltimore and proceeded to publish several more books on this subject as well as research articles. His interest grew in the newly discovered filterable viruses and he eventually was appointed Professor of Filterable Viruses in the School of Hygiene and Public Health founded in 1918 at the Johns Hopkins

University. This institution established a journal "American Journal of Hygiene" and he was made managing editor. No hypocrite, he made no attempt to hide his pro-German sympathies during the 1st World War and this drew considerable criticism at the time. He spent his summers in Nova Scotia sailing and exploring places of historic interest. After a year of failing health with heart problems and a slight stroke he had another stroke and died.

SIMPSON SYNDROME

Prepubertal obesity resulting in female habitus in boys and accentuated secondary female traits in girls.

L.S. Simpson London endocrinologist.

SIMS POSITION

Lateral knee chest position with the patient lying on the left side.

SIMS SPECULUM

A vaginal speculum.

James M. Sims (1813–1883) American gynecologist who introduced his speculum for vaginal examination. He used silver wire sutures and devised one of the first successful operative approaches to vesicovaginal fistula. He was one of the most important pioneers of gynecology in the United States.

SINDING-LARSEN DISEASE

v. LARSEN-JOHANSSON DISEASE

SIPPLE SYNDROME

This is the occurrence of medullary carcinoma, parathyroid adenoma and phaeochromocytoma sometimes termed MEN 2A (Multiple Endocrine Neoplasia syndrome) to distinguish it from Wermer Syndrome (MEN1) and MEN 2B. The latter is the same syndrome but without parathyroid involvement. There have been no kindred of patients with MEN 2A that have MEN 2B. It is inherited as a Mendelian dominant.

John H. Sipple (1930–) U.S. respiratory physician born in Cleveland, Ohio, and graduated from Cornell Medical College in 1955. He interned at the Upstate Medical Center (SUNY), New York. The description of this syndrome was his only paper on an endocrinological topic. He was appointed clinical Professor of Medicine at SUNY Medical Center in 1977.

SIPPY DIET

Ulcer diet alternating alkali powders with milk-cream mixture with progressive introduction of bland foods until a normal diet was achieved.

SIPPY POWDER

Alkali powder.

Bertram W. Sippy (1866–1924) U.S. physician, who introduced his dietary management of ulcers in 1915, but which has now fallen from popularity.

SISTER MARY JOSEPH NODULE

A hard mass or nodule which can be seen or felt at the umbilicus. This is a sign of intra-abdominal malignancy which most commonly arises in the stomach or ovary, but may occur from any organ in the abdomen.

Sister Mary Joseph Dempsey (1856–1939) She was born Julia Dempsey in Salamanca, New York. In 1878 she entered the third order regular of St. Frances of the congregation of our Lady of Lourdes in Rochester. In 1889 she was assigned to St. Mary's Hospital and learnt nursing from Edith Graham, a graduate nurse who later became the wife of Dr. C.H. Mayo. From 1890 to 1915 she was the first surgical assistant to Dr. W.J. Mayo, became nursing superintendent of St. Mary's Hospital in 1892, a position she remained in until she died in 1939. She drew Dr. Mayo's attention to this sign and he published an article about it in 1928, referring to it as the pants button umbilicus.

SISTO SIGN

Constant crying as a sign of congenital syphilis in infants.

Genaro Sisto (–1923) Argentinian pediatrician.

SJÖGREN SYNDROME

Keratoconjunctivitis sicca xerostomia (dry eyes, dry mouth), enlarged parotid gland and polyarthritis. It has now been realized that the associated arthritis was rheumatoid arthritis. Other epithelial surfaces are often involved: nasal cavity, pharynx, trachea, vagina. Female: male incidence 9:1 – compare with Mikulicz Syndrome (*v. supra*).

Henrik S.C. Sjögren (1899–1989) Swedish ophthalmologist who was born at Köping on Lake Malaren. He entered medical school in 1918 at the Karolinska Institute, Stockholm. He described the syndrome in 1933. Whilst he was the head of the Eye Clinic in Jönköping in 1935, he developed the technique for corneal transplantation. In 1957 he moved to Gothenburg and in 1961 was appointed Professor.

SJÖGREN-LARSSON SYNDROME

Congenital ichthyosis associated with mental deficiency and spastic paralysis. Retinal degeneration and dysplasia of the enamel of the teeth and epilepsy may occur. It is inherited as an autosomal recessive.

Karl G.T. Sjögren (1896–) Swedish Professor of Psychiatry.

Tage Larsson (1905-) Swedish physician.

SKENE DUCT

Para-urethral duct.

SKENE GLANDS

Para-urethral glands.

Alexander J.C. Skene (1838–1900) U.S. gynecologist. He was born in Aberdeenshire, Scotland, and migrated to North America when he was 19, commencing medicine at Toronto in 1860 and graduating from Long Island College Hospital M.D. in 1863. The following year he joined the U.S. army and planned an army ambulance corps. He returned to private practice working as an assistant to Austin Flint Senior. He then specialized in gynecology and was appointed Professor of Gynaecology at Long Island College Hospital in 1870. He was a founding member of the American Gynecological Society, being President in 1886–7. He wrote five textbooks as well as many scientific papers including his description of his glands in 1880. These had earlier been described in 1672 by Reiner de Graaf who also had noted that they were involved in gonorrheal infection but this had been forgotten.

SKLOWSKY SIGN

Light pressure of the finger near or over a vesicle will rupture it when it is varicella but not with smallpox or herpes.

E.L. Sklowsky German physician.

SKODIAC RESONANCE

Increased resonance heard on percussion over the chest above the level of the pleural effusion or in the upper portion of the lung whose lower lobe has been affected by pneumonic consolidation.

Josef Skoda (1805–1881) He was born in Pilsen, Bohemia. He was the Professor of Medicine in Vienna at the same time as Rokitansky was Professor of Pathology. He taught all his life at the Allegemeines Krankenhaus. In 1839 he wrote his monograph on percussion and auscultation in which he classified the various sounds heard in the chest. As a student he used to walk from Pilsen to Vienna to study medicine, graduating in 1831. After two years' practice

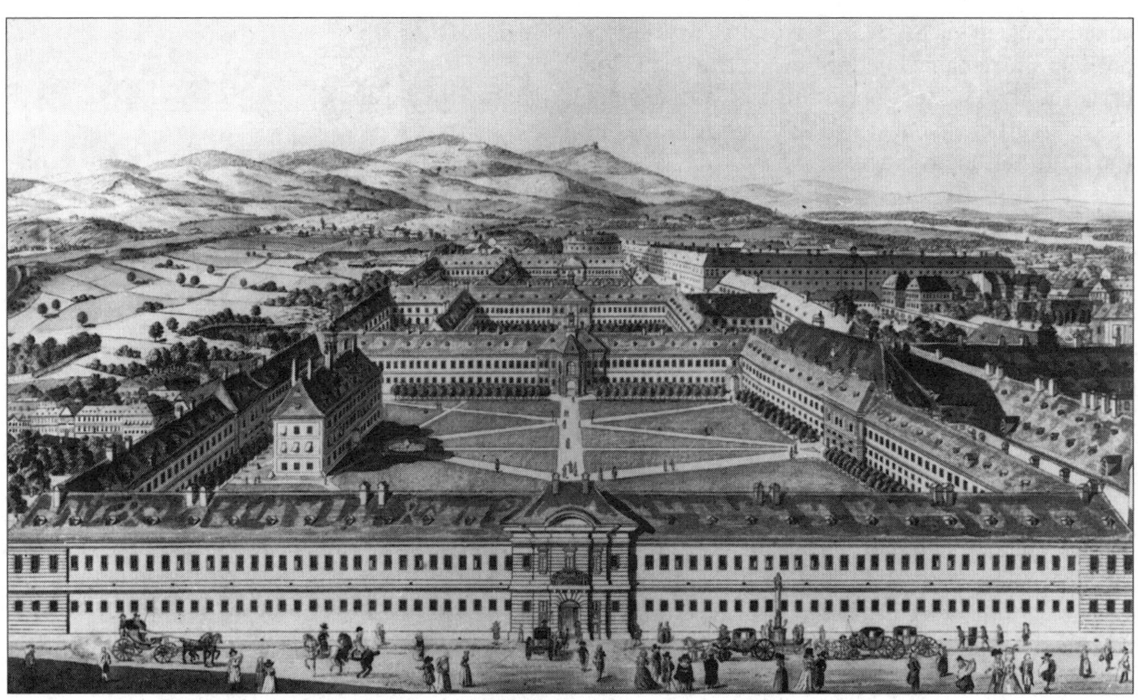

The Allegemienes Krankenhaus. Institut für Geschichte der Medizin an der Universität, Vienna (Courtesy of *Institut für Geschichte der Medizin an der Universität, Vienna*)

in Bohemia he returned to Vienna to the Allegemeines Krankenhaus as a second physician, with no pay, and lived simply on his practice, and at the time attended the hospital and autopsy room where he was greatly influenced by Rokitansky's teaching. It was during this time that he undertook his study on percussion and auscultation, verifying his diagnoses. He was asked by Baron von Turkheim of the Imperial Chancellory to give another opinion on the French Minister, le Duc de Blacas, in whom other doctors had made the diagnosis of liver disease, but after examining the patient, Skoda diagnosed an aneurysm of the abdominal aorta. At autopsy Skoda's diagnosis was proven to be correct and Turkheim created a Department of Chest Diseases for him at the Allegemeines Krankenhaus. In 1841 Skoda was appointed first physician and in 1846 he was appointed Professor of Medicine. He was an excellent teacher, but said to be much more reserved and pedantic than Rokitansky although he had an eccentric charm. All his life he wore odd clothes, allegedly for fear of offending a personal friend of his who was his tailor. On the other hand, he once sued a clergyman for not paying his bill. He completely neglected the humane and psychosomatic side of disease and treated the patient virtually as an experimental animal. He was the first person in Vienna to teach in German. Thus in this respect and in the way he treated his patients, he resembled Schönlein, and whereas he himself had initiated careful study of the patient and subsequent autopsy investigation, his approach led to the snap diagnoses which became the fashion in Vienna. He championed the approach of therapeutic nihilism and said, "whilst a disease can be described and diagnosed, we can dare not to suspect to cure it by any manner of means". Nonetheless he was one of the leading lights of the "New Vienna School" which numbered among them many of the great clinicians who were to influence medicine for years to come.

SLUDER NEURALGIA OR SYNDROME

Infection of nasal sinuses gives referred pain to root of the nose, upper teeth, eyes and sometimes ears, mastoid region and occiput.

Greenfield Sluder (1865–1928) U.S. ear, nose and throat surgeon who worked in St. Louis and developed the snare technique for tonsillectomy.

SLY SYNDROME

The original patient had a short stature with hepatosplenomegaly and frequent pulmonary infections. Others have been reported with hepatosplenomegaly and sometimes slow development and including a coarse facies and clouded corneas but there has been considerable phenotypic variation. The condition is a mucopolysaccharidosis which may be indicated by metachromatic granules in the lymphocytes in the peripheral blood film. The condition is due to a Beta-glucuronidase deficiency.

William S. Sly Contemporary U.S. pediatrician. He graduated M.D. from St. Louis University in 1957. He worked at the National Heart Institute in Washington, U.S.A. and later at the University of Wisconsin. In 1984, he became Chairman of the Department of Biochemistry at St. Louis University.

SMITH-LEMLI-OPITZ SYNDROME

Autosomal recessive. Broad upturned nares and broad maxillary alveolar ridges with cryptorchidism and hypospadias in the male. Severe mental deficiency and frequent vomiting and failure to thrive as an infant.

David W. Smith (1926–1981) U.S. pediatrician. He was born in Oakland, California and went to medical school at Johns Hopkins, graduating in 1950. After two years in the army, he trained in pediatrics at Johns Hopkins and then moved to the University of Wisconsin Medical School, where he became Professor of Pediatrics in 1966, until he moved to a similar position at the University of Washington, Seattle and remained there, thereafter. He was well known to enliven specialty medical meetings with a rendition on his mouth organ as part of the closing ceremonies!

Luc Lemli U.S. pediatrician.

John M. Opitz (1935–) U.S. geneticist. He was born in Germany but moved to the United States in 1950 and graduated M.D. from the University of Iowa in 1959. He became Chairman of the Department of Medical Genetics at the Children's Hospital, Helena, Montana.

SMITH-PETERSEN NAIL OR PIN

Nail used in repair of fractured neck of femur.

Marius N. Smith-Petersen (1886–1953) U.S. orthopedic surgeon. He was born in Grimstead, Norway, but attended school in the United States from the age of 17 and graduated M.D. from Harvard Medical School in 1914, then worked for a time in orthopedic surgery in Boston with Dr. E.G. Bracett. He joined the faculty of Harvard Medical School in orthopedic surgery in 1920 and was a Clinical Professor from 1935–1946 when he retired. At the same time he retired as chief of the orthopedic service of the Massachusetts General Hospital, a post to which he was appointed in 1929. He remained a citizen of Norway until 1924 when he became a naturalized American citizen.

SMITH PHENOMENON

Anaphylaxis.

Theobald Smith (1859–1934) U.S. pathologist. Born in Albany, New York. He was appointed Professor of Comparative Pathology at Harvard University in 1896. In 1886 with D.E. Salmon he showed that filtered products of hog cholera organisms could produce immunity in animals to hog cholera. This was the first work in this type of immunization and was soon followed by similar work by von Behring and Roux. In 1889 he discovered the parasite causing Texas fever (a protozoan *Pyrasoma bigeminum*) and showed it was transmitted by the cattle tick. He demonstrated the phenomenon of anaphylaxis in 1903, employing the products of diphtheria bacilli. His discovery was termed the Theobald Smith phenomenon by Paul Ehrlich. He made the first clear cut distinction between human and bovine forms of tuberculosis which was confirmed by Koch and others and made the first observations on pleomorphism in bacteria. In 1915 he was appointed director of a Department of Animal Pathology of the Rockefeller Institute at Princetown, New Jersey.

SNEDDON SYNDROME

This is the association of prominent livedo reticularis usually over the upper lower limbs and buttocks of a patient who also develops cerebrovascular lesions which are often transient. Other conditions known to be related to both livedo reticularis and cerebrovascular problems such as disseminated lupus erythematosus, essential thrombocythemia, and the antiphospholipid syndrome, polyarteritis nodosa and other immune complex disorders are not present. Sometimes the livedo reticularis becomes more evident during the neurological episode.

I.B. Sneddon Contemporary British dermatologist, who works in Sheffield, England.

SNELLEN CHART

Visual acuity chart.

SNELLEN REFLEX

Hyperemia of the ear when the auriculo-temporal nerve is stimulated.

Hermann Snellen (1834–1908) Dutch ophthalmologist: born in Zeijst and graduated M.D. from Utrecht in 1858. He described his chart in 1862 which was the first attempt to standardize visual acuity. He became Professor of Ophthalmology at the University of Utrecht in 1877. He considered that the cones were the end organs of vision and that if two points were identified the cones had to be stimulated and the ones between not.

SODERBERGH PRESSURE REFLEX

Firm downward stroking of the ulna may result in flexion of the 3 medial fingers, firm downward stroking of the radius may give flexion of the thumb. Seen in pyramidal tract lesions.

G. Soderbergh (1878–) Swedish physician who became a Professor of Medicine in 1938 and published on alcaptonuria and many neurological subjects. He was a pianist and composer.

SÖMMERING RING CATARACT

Doughnut shaped ring behind the pupil.

SÖMMERING SPOT

Macula lutea.

Samuel T. Sömmering (1755–1830) German anatomist who was particularly interested in neuroanatomy and one of the first to draw attention to the white matter of the brain, seen on macroscopic cross sectioning. He was born in Thorn, Poland, the son of a doctor. He commenced studying medicine at the University of Göttingen in 1774. He studied the art of engraving and languages at the same time. In 1778 he graduated with a doctoral thesis which consisted of a discussion of the cranial nerves and produced a classification which superseded that of Willis. He worked with John and William Hunter in England, Munro in Scotland and Pieter Camper in Holland. In 1784 he was appointed Professor of Anatomy at Mainz and remained there for 11 years. Afterwards he practiced medicine in Frankfurt-am-Main. He moved to Munich where he became interested in physics, astronomy and the study of fossils. He investigated sun spots, meteors and also invented an electric telegraph. He was one of the first to record and describe a case of achondroplasia.

SONNE DYSENTERY

One of the common forms of epidemic dysentery due to *Shigella sonnei*.

Carl Sonne (1882–1948) Danish bacteriologist who was born in Allinge, Bornholm, but grew up in Svaneke. He graduated in medicine from the University of Copenhagen in 1907 and then worked in the State Serum Institute where he identified the dysentery bacillus for which he is known, and this was published in his dissertation for his doctorate in 1914. From 1913–17 he was a resident physician at the University Clinic at the Rigshospitalet in Copenhagen and was appointed chief of the experimental laboratory at the Finsen institute in 1918 remaining in that post until 1929. Here he was one of the first to show that sunlight formed vitamin D in skin and explained its value in the treatment of rickets and perhaps for the success of light-bath treatment for lupus vulgaris. He raised the question of which part of the spectum was important for this. When Gram (*v. supra*) retired in 1923 he was one of the short listed candidates for the chair of medicine but was unsuccessful (C. Lumdsgaerd being appointed); other unsuccessful candidates were E. Meulengracht and E.H. Thaysen. One of his major research interests was respiratory physiology and he championed the cause of non-homogeneity of distribution of lung air which brought him into conflict with the views of Krogh. He developed a technique for sampling alveolar air and anticipated much of modern thinking by emphasizing the abnormalities of air distribution in pathological states, e.g. emphysema and asthma and in cardiac disease and the complementary importance of the pulmonary circulation. From studies on himself he correctly predicted a constriction of one of his main bronchi shown at autopsy which he had requested after his death from a coronary thrombosis. An affectionate and likeable man he was always prominent in the students' end of term celebrations where he would join in with the speech making and singing and again become a carefree student.

SOUQUES SIGN

1. Elevation and extension of paretic arm results in involuntary extension and spreading of the fingers.
2. In Parkinsonism suddenly throwing a seated patient off balance by tipping the chair backwards does not result in extension of the legs to maintain balance due to loss of associated movement.
3. In Parkinsonism there may be sudden and violent over-exertion when the patient attempts to walk or run due to generalised rigidity.

Achille A. Souques (1860–1944) French neurologist who was one of the founding members of the Societé de Neurologie de Paris with Babinski and others. A student of Charcot, he confirmed Schiller's observation that deep sensibility of the face is conveyed centrally by the facial nerve. He was regarded by the pioneer French neuro-surgeon Clovis Vincent as the finest teacher and clinician – praise indeed in that school at that time.

SOUTHEY TUBE

A small cannula inserted subcutaneously to drain off edema of limbs.

Reginald S. Southey (1835–1899) English physician. He was the son of Dr. H.H. Southey, and nephew of Robert Southey, the poet. He went to school at Westminster and later to Christ Church College, Oxford. He graduated B.A. in natural science with 1st class honors in 1855 and M.A. in 1857. He studied medicine at St. Bartholomew's Hospital and graduated in 1858. He won the Radcliffe Travelling Fellowship, visited Berlin and Vienna, and wrote on tuberculosis and Bright disease. He translated from German some of the articles on structural diseases of the kidney and general symptoms of renal disease. He became assistant physician at St. Bartholomew's Hospital in 1863 and physician in 1868, and that year was appointed lecturer in Forensic Medicine and Hygiene. He resigned in 1883 when he was appointed as Commissioner in Lunacy, which he held until his ill health forced him to retire in 1898. He was a quiet, sympathetic man who was painstakingly diligent at the bedside. He had a keen interest in clocks and watches, which he collected and repaired.

SOUTTAR TUBE

Prosthetic device to replace esophagus.

Sir Henry S. Souttar (1875–1964) English surgeon. He studied medicine at Oxford and later at the London Hospital and whilst he was at Oxford also studied engineering. He graduated in 1906 and undertook his residency at the London Hospital, gaining his F.R.C.S. in 1909. At the outbreak of the First World War, he was appointed Surgeon-in-Chief to the Belgian Field Hospital at Antwerp and wrote a book on his experiences there, "A Surgeon in Belgium". After the war he returned to civilian practice and continued his association with the

London Hospital which remained until he retired. He successfully operated on a 15 year old girl with mitral stenosis in 1925, an operation which was not repeated for 22 years. He designed a number of surgical instruments, one of which was a metal spiral tube, which was a useful palliative measure in overcoming obstruction of the esophagus secondary to cancer and stricture. He was always interested in the physics of radium, in part stimulated by his early education and interest, and by his father-in-law who was Professor of Physics at Oxford. One of the instruments he developed was an introducer for inserting radon seeds. He was a skilled draftsman and illustrated one of his textbooks, "The Art of Surgery", with his own line drawings. In 1933, he flew to India with his anesthetist, J.H.T. Challis, and his nurse, Miss M.A. Bradford, as well as an Australian Registrar, Konrad Hirschfield, to undertake an operation on a woman relative of the Maharaja of Nepal. This journey lasted five or six days in each direction and the apocryphal story is told that only palliation was possible by the use of his "Souttar tube" which was inserted for a reputed fee of 10 000 guineas.

He was a keen musician, regularly playing his piano in the morning and occasionally the violin, and in his early days was extremely athletic and a keen member of the London rowing club.

SPALDING SIGN

Overlapping of fetus' skull bones on X-ray – sign of fetal death.

Alfred B. Spalding (1874–) U.S. radiologist.

SPENGLER FRAGMENTS

Small discoid bodies seen in tuberculous sputum.

Carl Spengler (1861–1937) Swiss physician who directed one of the best known tuberculous sanatoria in Davos founded by his father Alexander. He was born in Chur and studied medicine at Heidelberg and Zurich and worked as an assistant physician at Strasburg from 1886–9 and then went to Davos to work with his father on the treatment of tuberculosis. His work was noted by R. Koch (*v. supra*) who collaborated with him on the best method of using tuberculin therapeutically – one of Koch's few scientific errors. Spengler like others was unhappy with the efficiency of tuberculin and introduced other forms of immunotherapy of equal or even more dubious efficacy. He believed he had identified immune antibodies in red cells, which has never been verified.

SPENS SYNDROME

v. STOKES-ADAMS SYNDROME

Thomas Spens (1764–1842) Scottish physician in Edinburgh who reported his patient in 1792 but the syndrome was originally described by Morgani in 1700 (*v. supra*).

SPIEGLER TUMOR

Cylindroma.

SPIEGLER-FENDT SARCOID

Lymphocytoma cutis.

Eduard Spiegler (1860–1908) Austrian dermatologist, Vienna.

Heinrich Fendt German dermatologist.

SPIELMEYER-VOGT DISEASE

Juvenile amaurotic familial idiocy (sometimes called BATTEN DISEASE) (*v. supra*).

Walther Spielmeyer (1879–1935) German neurologist. He was born in Dessau. He nearly failed school and was made to give up his piano lessons as a punishment. He studied medicine at Halle and was especially attracted to the pathologist Eberth and the physiologists Hitzig and Heilbronner. In 1906 he was appointed Privatdozent at Freiburg where he studied psychiatry under Hoche and set up a laboratory on histopathology. He showed that amaurotic family idiocy was the result of a disturbed lipid metabolism and demonstrated primary degeneration of the posterior columns and cerebral changes in experimental trypanosomiasis. In 1911 he published his book on microscopic studies of the nervous system which became an important manual and Kraepelin asked him to come to Munich to succeed Alzheimer as the head of the anatomical laboratories for the psychiatric and nervous disease clinic. He became Extraordinarius in 1913 and Director of the histology section of the newly founded German Institute for Psychiatry in 1917 and Honorary Professor in 1918. He wrote important monographs on peripheral nerve injuries which occurred in World War I and when Nissl came to Munich to head a second histopathology section, they had a very close and happy relationship. In 1922 he wrote an important book on histopathology of the nervous system which was the first text-book of general histopathology. Later on, Spielmeyer began to explore the possibility that disordered cerebral function could follow temporary circulation disturbances. In 1928 the Rockefeller Foundation financed the Kaiser Wilhelm Institute with Spielmeyer as director of the histopathology institute and here he remained until he died of pulmonary tuberculosis.

Spielmeyer was a modest person who had a great interest in music and often would have musicians from the National Theatre in Munich at his home after a performance. He could be very outspoken in his dislike for pomposity and would be very sarcastic with regard to hypotheses which were not founded on solid scientific evidence. His open denunciation of the Nazi regime brought him into great personal danger and he was said to have been tireless in his efforts to help Germans who had been displaced from Nazi Germany to enable them to get started in other countries.

Oskar Vogt (1870–1959) He was half Danish, half German (Schleisweig-Holstein). He studied anatomy at Jena and with Flechzig at Leipzig. He also studied with the Swiss neurologist, Auguste Forel, and then moved to the Salpêtrière to study clinical neurology with Dejerine in 1898. In Paris he met his future wife, Mademoiselle Mugnier, who at that stage was working with Pierre Marie at the Bicêtre. They married in Berlin in 1899 and set up a neurological laboratory which they supported from private practice. Many brains were sent to them by Pierre Marie who, following a heated argument on a point of anatomy, said "Monsieur Vogt, you need some brains to study!" As their work became better known, they were successful in establishing a neurological institute in 1915 and in 1931 an imposing institute was opened for them in Buch, a suburb of Berlin. Brodmann and Bielschowsky were assistants to them. They studied the anatomy and pathology of the cerebral cortex, investigated extra-pyramidal diseases and made numerous contributions. They undertook physiological mapping of monkey brains which set the stage for Foerster's electrical stimulation of the human brain. His wife made a number of important contributions to athetosis and they both published important works on the connections between the thalamus and corpus striatum. Vogt was one of the neurologists asked to consult on Lenin's illness and obtained his brain for histological study after Lenin's death. Because of opposition to the Nazis he was forced to retire from the directorship of his institute in 1937 but he and his wife had already anticipated this and built a small private institute in the Schwarzwald – near Neustadt. This was financed by the Krupps family because Vogt had defended a family member in court. Initially the Nazis left them alone but at the outbreak of war he was drafted into the army as a private and made to organize a military hospital in the area. Before directing the medical officers to their duties, he would cover his private's uniform with a white gown. After six weeks he was discharged. He was then aged 69! Their work continued, and cytology became more and more their interest. Together they studied genetic mutations occurring in insects. Vogt was a compelling speaker and a well-versed conversationalist.

SPIGELIA

Plant of the family Loganiaceae. *Spigelia marilandica* rhizome and roots once were used as a worm cure.

A. van der Spieghel (also called Spigelius) (1578–1625) Belgian botanist and anatomist. He was born in Brussels and studied medicine at Louvain and Padua. In Padua he was influenced by Fabrizio. After graduating he went to Moravia but on Casserio's death (1616) became Professor of Anatomy and Surgery at Padua where he taught for 20 years. He wrote books on botany, helminths and anatomy.

SPOONERISM

Inappropriate or misuse of words or transposition of syllables.

William A. Spooner (1844–1930) Church of England clergyman. Warden of New College in Oxford.

SPRENGEL DEFORMITY

Congenital elevation of the scapulae.

Otto G.K. Sprengel (1852–1915) German surgeon. He was born in Waren, Mecklenburg. He studied at Tübingen, Rostock, and Munich, graduating in medicine in 1877 from Marburg. He then worked in Halle with Volkmann (*v. infra*) and in 1896 was appointed Professor of Surgery at Braunschweig. He described congenital dislocation of the shoulder joint but he was mostly renowned as an abdominal surgeon. He died in Berlin following an operation on a gunshot wound, whereby he contracted septicemia.

STAEHLI PIGMENT LINE

Horizontal brown line in the lower part of the cornea in senile degeneration.

Jean Staehli Swiss ophthalmologist who worked in Zurich.

STAHL EAR

Congenital deformity where the helix is broad and the fossa of the antihelix and the upper part of the scaphoid fossa are missing.

Friedrich K. Stahl (1811–1879) German physician and psychiatrist who was at Würzburg.

STAMEY TEST

Test designed to detect unilateral renal disease.

Thomas A. Stamey U.S. surgeon, Stanford University, San Francisco.

STARGARDT DISEASE

Juvenile macular degeneration.

Karl B. Stargardt (1875–1927) German ophthalmologist.

STARLING LAW OF THE HEART

The force of contraction of the cardiac muscle is proportional to its initial length.

Ernest H. Starling (1866–1927) British physiologist. "Science has but one language, that of quantity and but one argument, that of experiment." He was born in Bombay, India, and studied medicine at Guy's Hospital and worked with W. Kuhne in Heidelberg in 1885.

In 1892 he demonstrated that serum proteins induced an osmotic pressure and produced his famous concept of events at the capillary beds concerning the filtration and re-absorption of fluid.

In 1899 he was appointed demonstrator of physiology at Guy's Hospital and in 1899–1923 was Professor of Physiology at University College, London, where he succeeded E. Sharpey-Schaefer. With Bayliss he discovered secretin, the product of the mucosa of the duodenum which causes bile and pancreatic juice secretion, and he introduced the term "hormone". His heart-lung preparation was a major advance in physiological studies of the heart and attracted world-wide attention. In 1924 he showed that the renal tubules re-absorbed water as well as glucose and electrolytes from the glomerular filtrate. Starling's laboratory became a world centre in physiology.

STARR-EDWARDS PROSTHESIS

Prosthetic cardiac valve consisting of a ball in a cage.

A. Starr U.S. physician.

M.L. Edwards U.S. physician.

STAUB-TRAUGOTT EFFECT

A second dose of glucose one hour after the initial one will not raise the blood sugar in a normal person.

Hans Staub (1890–) Swiss physician in Basel.

Karl Traugott (1885–) German physician who was based in Frankfurt.

STAUFFER SYNDROME

Hepatomegaly and splenomegaly with a raised alkaline phosphatase secondary to non-metastatic hypernephroma, Grawitz tumour (*v. supra*).

Maurice H. Stauffer U.S. gastroenterologist, who was born in Hymer, Kansas and graduated M.D. from the University of Kansas in 1941, interning at the University of Kansas Hospital and then joining the Medical Corps in the U.S. Navy from 1942–46. He saw active service at Iwo Jima and was, for a while, with the U.S. occupation forces at Fukuoka in Japan. He went to the Mayo Clinic in 1946, initially in surgery, but he transferred to become a first assistant in medicine in 1947. There he developed an interest in gastroenterological diseases and became an Associate Professor of Clinical Medicine.

STEELE-RICHARDSON-OLSZEWSKI SYNDROME

Progressive supranuclear paralysis. It is characterized by loss of downward gaze, neck rigidity, pseudobulbar palsy and lack of tremor.

John C. Steele Canadian neurologist.

John C. Richardson (1909–) Canadian neurologist.

Jerzy Olszewski (1913–1966) Canadian neurologist who was born in Poland.

STEIN-LEVENTHAL SYNDROME

Hirsutism, amenorrhea, enlarged polycystic ovaries.

Irving F. Stein (1887–) U.S. gynecologist.

Michael L. Leventhal (1901–1971) U.S. obstetrician.

STEINER TUMOR

Juxta auricular nodule.

L. Steiner German physician.

STEINERT DISEASE

Myotonic dystrophy which involves both smooth and striated muscle and may present with limb weakness. There may be gastrointestinal problems such as dysphagia, anosphinctal abnormalities and poor gall bladder contractibility and cholelithiasis as well as anicteric cholestasis. Cardiac involvement usually is due to abnormalities of the Bundle of His and Purkinje but cardiac muscular dystrophy can cause supra ventricular and ventricular arrhythmias.

Hans Steinert German physician in Leipzig.

STEINMANN PIN OR NAIL

Orthopedic bone pin for applying traction.

Fritz Steinmann (1872–1932) Swiss surgeon born in Berne and became Professor of Surgery there in 1899.

STELLWAG SIGN

Infrequent blinking in hyperthyroidism, and in Parkinson disease.

Carl Stellwag von Carion (1823–1904) Austrian ophthalmologist who noticed the pupillary changes in tabes (Argyll Robertson pupil), and was one of the early ophthalmologists to introduce test types to test visual acuity.

STENSEN DUCT

Parotid duct.

Niels Stensen (1638–1686) Danish anatomist (also called Steno). He was born in Copenhagen (his father was the court jeweller) and he studied medicine in Copenhagen with Bartholin, at Leyden with Sylvius and finally in Amsterdam with Blasius, and here he discovered the excretory duct of the parotid gland in sheep in 1661. In 1664 he investigated the glands of the eye and made observations on muscles and identified the muscular nature of the heart. In 1667 he postulated that the ovary in the female was not, as had been previously thought, a female testis, but was in fact an organ which corresponded to the egg-producing organs of birds and reptiles. He named the ovary and his views were proven by de Graaf (*v. supra*). He described muscles as being parallel strips of bundles of structural units and argued that the total response of the muscle was the summation of the tensile force developed by each unit, opposing the view of other anatomists of the time (Birilli) that the apparent increase in size of a muscle during contraction was due to the inflow of hypothetical fluid. He was led to his study on geology by a dissection of a shark in which he recognized that its teeth resembled the fossil teeth found in fossil remnants in Tuscany.

In 1666 he went to Italy as court physician to Ferdinand II in Florence and continued in this position with Cosimo III. It was here that he was converted to the Catholic faith by a nun and entered the priesthood. In 1672 he was appointed Professor of Anatomy at Copenhagen and remained there until Pope Innocent XI named him Bishop of Titiopolis in 1677. In 1672 he described the tetralogy of Fallot (*v. supra*) and spent the remainder of his life in Hannover and Hamburg.

STERNBERG CELL

v. REED-STERNBERG CELL

STERNBERG LYMPHOMA OR SYNDROME

Mediastinal mass progressing to a picture resembling acute lymphatic leukemia – leukosarcoma.

Karl Sternberg (1872–1935) Austrian pathologist. He was born in Vienna and graduated in medicine at the University of Vienna in 1896. After training in general medicine he worked in the Rudolph Foundation as a pathologist and was influenced by Professor R. Paltauf. Sternberg lymphoma was first described by Ehrlich in 1862 and next by Grawitz (1890); his report appeared in 1905. In 1908 he moved to Brünn and was made Associate Professor. In 1914 he was mobilized and spent the entire war with the combat troops and earned a great reputation for fighting for the soldiers' rights and well being. He became one of the most decorated doctors of his military rank in Austria. After the war he returned to Brünn, but in 1920 moved back to Vienna where he became head of the pathology department of the general hospital there. In 1922 he became Professor of Pathology, but never achieved his ambition of becoming the head of an academic unit. Apart from the war years when he worked largely on bowel infections and typhoid fever, his main research concerned tuberculosis and leukemia. He died suddenly of a coronary occlusion.

STEVENS-JOHNSON SYNDROME

Mucosal ulceration involving mouth and conjunctivae with erythema multiforme and pyrexia.

Albert M. Stevens (1884–1945) U.S. pediatrician.

Frank C. Johnson (1894–1934) U.S. pediatrician.

STEWART MID LINE GRANULOMA

A very rare condition involving the maxillary sinus with progressive bone destruction which was universally fatal until the introduction of megavoltage radiotherapy for its management.

J.P. Stewart Scottish ear, nose and throat surgeon who worked at the Royal Infirmary, Edinburgh.

STEWART-HOLMES PHENOMENON

Rebound phenomenon in cerebellar disease.

STEWART-MOREL-MORGAGNI SYNDROME

Hyperostosis frontalis interna associated with obesity, headache, hypertension.

(Also called STEWART-MOREL SYNDROME.)

Sir James P. Stewart (1869–1949) English neurologist.

Sir Gordon M. Holmes (1876–1966) English neurologist (*v. supra*).

Bénédict A. Morel (1809–1873) French psychiatrist in Paris.

Giovanni B. Morgagni (*v. supra*).

STICKLER SYNDROME

Arachnodactyly with abnormal epiphyseal development and mild joint hypermobility. There is an associated progressive myopia with a tendency to retinal detachment.

Gunnar B. Stickler (1925–) U.S. pediatrician. He was born in Peterskirchen, Bavaria. He went to school at the Wilhelmsgymnasium at Munich and graduated in medicine from Munich in 1949. He commenced training in pathology there, but migrated to the United States in 1951 and became a resident in pediatrics at the Mayo Clinic in 1953. After finishing his training he was appointed Chief of Pediatrics with the Second Field Hospital of the U.S. Army in Munich, returning to work at Roswell Park Memorial Institute in Buffalo, New York until 1957, when he moved back to the Mayo Clinic, remaining there and becoming Chairman of the Department of Pediatrics in 1974. He retired in 1989.

STILL DISEASE

Juvenile rheumatoid arthritis often with hepatomegaly, lymphadenopathy and splenomegaly occurring before the second dentition.

STILL MURMUR

Early systolic murmur heard near the left sternal edge in children and usually disappears at puberty.

Sir Frederick Still (1868–1941) He was born in Holloway, London, the son of a surveyor of customs. He went to school at Merchant Taylors and then Caius College, Cambridge. He did his clinical training at Guy's Hospital and graduated from there in 1893, becoming a house physician in 1894 and the same year won the Murchison Scholarship of the Royal College of Physicians. Whilst at Guy's he was influenced by James Goodhart who had an interest in childhood disease. He therefore became a house physician at the Hospital for Sick Children, Great Ormond Street, and he retained an association with that institution for the remainder of his days. In 1896 he was awarded his Cambridge M.D. for a thesis entitled "A special form of joint disease met with in children". Thus he shares with Maurice Raynaud and Tooth the distinction of having an eponym named after an M.D. thesis. A shortened form of this thesis appeared in Albutt's "The System of Medicine" in 1897.

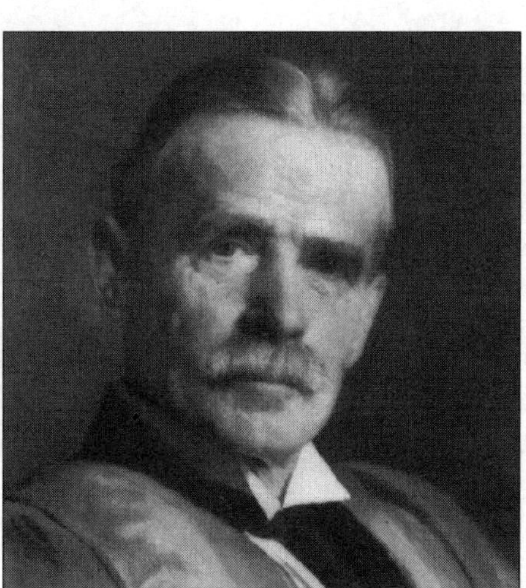

Sir Frederick Still (Courtesy of the King's College Hospital Medical School, Department of Child Health, London, UK)

In 1899 he was appointed as Physician of the Diseases of Children to King's College Hospital, the first hospital with a medical school to establish a section for children and in 1906 he became its first Professor of Diseases of Children. In 1905 he collaborated with Sir James Goodhart, his previous chief, as editor of "Diseases of Children". In 1909 he published his own textbook "Common Diseases of Children" which was based on the lecture series he gave at Great Ormond Street and King's College. This book was one of the most popular pediatric textbooks of its day. He wrote an account of congenital hypertrophy of the pylorus for Albutt and Rolleston's "System of Medicine". Although first described by Samuel Gee, it was his description and lectures which brought it to the attention of the English medical profession. In 1919 he contributed to the Osler birthday volumes an article entitled "Some 17th century writings on diseases of children". This work aroused his interest in medical history so that he gave a series of lectures on the topic and finally wrote a book entitled "A History of Paediatrics".

He was a bachelor who lived for nothing but his work, and in his early days took no interest in social aspects of life or sporting activities, devoting himself entirely to medicine. As he grew older, he returned more to his early love of the classics and on the centenary of King's College Medical School wrote a Latin verse entitled "Carmen Scholae Medicinae" which was set to music and sung during the commemoration. He was given innumerable honors and was knighted in 1937 when he retired. He had been Chairman of the National Society for the Prevention of Infant Mortality for 20 years. He was an extremely good-looking man, although somewhat slight of build, and of a retiring but courteous manner. He was very close to his widowed mother with whom he lived until she died, taking her to church every Sunday. His waiting room in an old house in Queen Anne Street had a great number of toys to help amuse the young people waiting their turn to see him. He was probably one of the most popular pediatricians in London, so that almost every sick child of well-to-do parents had seen him at one time or another.

STOKES-ADAMS ATTACKS, SYNCOPE OR SYNDROME

Syncope or epileptic convulsions occurring in complete heart block.

William Stokes (1804–1878) Irish physician. Stokes received no formal education. His grandfather was a Professor of Mathematics and his father was a respected physician and a senior Fellow of Trinity College, but he left the established church to follow the teachings of the Rev. John Walker, the so-called "Walkerite" sect. As a result, his father resigned from his fellowship of Trinity College and would not expose his son to a society which he believed did not follow the scriptures accurately. So although born

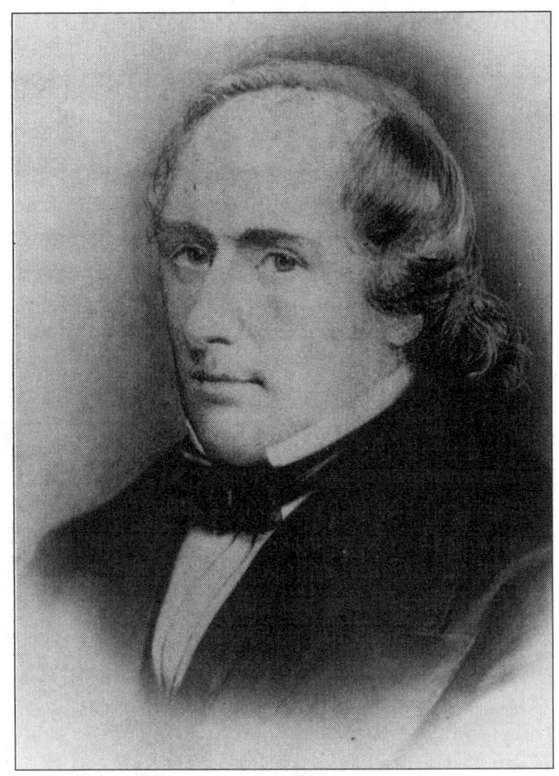

Sir William Stokes
(Courtesy of the Royal Society of Medicine, London, UK)

in Dublin he spent most of his early life at his father's country house in Ballinteer in the Dublin hills and learnt the ballads of Sir Walter Scott by heart, the latter remaining one of his favorite authors. As he grew older he helped his father in the laboratory and rambled with him through the countryside and saw patients with him. His father had initiated teaching in the natural sciences at Trinity College and lectured on these subjects there from 1806 onwards. Furthermore, his father's Dublin household was visited by numerous intellectuals such as George Petrie, an artist, archeologist and musician, whose biography he was to write; Henry Grattan, James Martineau, the Unitarian Pastor and scholar, and O'Connor, the Irish landscape painter. The Rev. John Walker acted as a private tutor and from him he learned the classics and mathematics. Stokes enrolled in the College of Surgeons School in Ireland in 1822 in a course of anatomy where his father had succeeded John Cheyne as Professor of

Medicine. Initially he was interested in chemistry, and went to Glasgow University to study this under the Professor of Chemistry there, Thomas Thompson. After two years, however, he decided to switch to medicine and he went to Edinburgh where he graduated M.D. in 1825. Whilst there he heard of Laennec's teachings on auscultation and wrote a book entitled "An Introduction to the Use of the Stethoscope" which was the first on this topic in English.

His father resigned from Meath Hospital in 1826 and he was elected in his place. He introduced the stethoscope to the medical school and this innovation caused much comment, often sarcastic, rather than laudatory. He wrote a monograph entitled "Treatise on the diagnosis and treatment of the chest" which was enthusiastically endorsed by Corrigan.

Although he was by this time a well established and well-liked physician, the College of Physicians could not make him a Fellow because he had not graduated in Arts, and his medical degree had been obtained in Edinburgh and not Dublin. This was finally circumvented by Trinity College awarding him an honorary M.D. and Stokes was admitted to Fellowship. He was President from 1849–50. In 1854 his monograph entitled "Diseases of the heart and aorta" contained a description of Stokes-Adams Syndrome. This syndrome had first been described by R. Adams, a surgeon at the Richmond Hospital, in a Dublin Hospital Report in 1827. Stokes was one of the few physicians who ever received the Prussian Order Pour le Mérite. During the Dublin epidemic of typhus in 1826 he worked amongst the poor, and in fact developed the disease himself in 1827. He also recorded the first case of cholera in the Dublin epidemic of 1832. He became Regius Professor of Medicine in Dublin, succeeding his father, in 1845. He was a colleague and close friend of Robert Graves. Stokes is said to have commented "my father left me but one legacy, the blessed gift of rising early".

Robert Adams (1791–1875) Irish surgeon. Born in Dublin and studied medicine in Dublin and later in Europe. He was surgeon to the Richmond Hospital and was appointed surgeon to the Queen in Ireland in 1861 and Professor of Surgery in Dublin the same year. He was an authority on arthritis and gout.

STOKVIS DISEASE

Enterogenous cyanosis.

Barend J.E. Stokvis (1834–1902) Dutch physician and physiologist. Born in Amsterdam obtaining his M.D. at Utrecht in 1856. He was Professor of Medicine at the University of Amsterdam.

STOOKEY REFLEX

Tapping of semimembranous and semitendinosus tendons results in flexion of the leg while the leg is semiflexed.

Byron P. Stookey (1887–1966) U.S. neurosurgeon.

STRACHAN SYNDROME

Polyneuritis seen in Jamaica secondary to dietary deprivation. It was also observed in prisoners of war and characterized by sensory symptomatology with painful paresthesia. Amblyopia with 8th nerve involvement leading to "camp dizziness" and deafness. It is probably due to a deficiency of the vitamin B group. There are associated mucocutaneous lesions – glossitis, stomatitis and skin desquamation of face and genital regions. This is probably secondary to riboflavin deficiency.

William H.W. Strachan (1857–1921) British physician who described the condition in Jamaican natives in 1888.

STRASSMAN PHENOMENON

Engorgement of umbilical vein following pressure on fundus of uterus showing the placenta has not separated.

Paul F. Strassman (1866–1938) German obstetrician.

STRAUSS PHENOMENON

Eating fatty foods results in increase in fats in chylous ascites.

Hermann Strauss (1868–1944) German physician.

STRÜMPELL REFLEX OR SIGN

Spastic paralysis in the leg. Flexion of the thigh causes marked dorsiflexion in the foot.

STRÜMPELL-MARIE DISEASE

Rheumatoid spondylosis.

STRÜMPELL-WESTPHAL PSEUDOSCLEROSIS

v. WILSON DISEASE

Ernst A.G.G. von Strümpell (*v. supra*, MARIE-STRÜMPELL DISEASE).

Pierre Marie (*v. supra*).

Carl F.D. Westphal (*v. supra*, EDINGER-WESTPHAL NUCLEUS).

STUART-PROWER FACTOR

Factor X. Factor X deficiency in a rare hereditary bleeding disorder first described in patients named Stuart and Prower, respectively.

STUDENT'S *t* TEST

A test to determine mean error.

Student was a pseudonym used by William S. Gossett (1876–1937) in his statistical publications. His paper, "The probable error of a mean" (*Biometrica* 6, 1–25, 1908) gave a clear description of what is now known as the *t* distribution, though this was developed further by R.A. Fisher into the *t* test for comparing two means from populations of unknown variants. Gossett worked for Guinness as a research chemist. He published his statistical papers pseudonymously because the Guinness Company forbade employees to disclose discoveries.

STURGE-WEBER DISEASE OR SYNDROME

Port wine naevus on upper part of the scalp and other vascular abnormalities both intracranially and in other parts of the body.

William A. Sturge (1850–1919) English physician. He was born of Quaker parents in Bristol and commenced his medical studies at Bristol Medical School and completed them at University College, London. He was an intern and registrar at the National Hospital for Paralysis and Epilepsy and here commenced his interest in neurology. In 1876 he went to Paris to study with Charcot, but besides neurology he had experience in general pathology and medicine with Fournier at the St. Louis Hospital. In 1887 he returned to London and was appointed physician and pathologist at the Royal Free Hospital and one of the lecturers at the Women's Medical School. He was strongly liberal and was one of the keenest supporters of women's medical education, marrying doctor Emily Bovell, and they commenced practice together in Wimpole Street. He was a fine speaker, an excellent teacher and extremely interested in the welfare of his patients. He had a very large practice of patients with organic conditions and also of patients with psychosomatic problems.

In 1880 his wife became ill and he decided to move to Nice, where he lived for the next 27 years during the autumn, winter and spring. He gradually became very well known and socially prominent as a physician in the Riviera and looked after Queen Victoria during her four visits to Cimez. He had rheumatic fever in 1894 which recurred in 1899 and in 1907 he decided to give up practice and return to England. During his holidays he studied early Greek art and was a collector of Etruscan vases and during his leisure time devoted most of it to studying archeology.

When he settled in England he chose to live at Icklingham Hall in Suffolk which was near the diggings where the Piltdown skull was found. There he established one of the finest private museums of flint implements in the world, carefully classified and catalogued.

He was one of the founders and first President of the Society of Prehistoric Archaeology of East Anglia, bequeathing his collection of more than 100 000 pieces to the nation. His second wife was a keen archeologist whom he married in 1886. He only wrote four papers on medical matters. One concerned progressive muscular atrophy for which he was awarded a Silver Medal by the Medical Society of London, and the others related to erythromelalgia, spondylitis, and nerve stretching. Towards the end of his life, he had recurrent bouts of tachycardia.

F.P. Weber (*v. infra*).

SUDECK ATROPHY

Aseptic necrosis of bone following injury.

Paul H.M. Sudeck (1866–1945) German surgeon who was Professor of Surgery in Hamburg.

SULTZBERGER-GARBE DERMATOSIS OR SYNDROME

An extraordinarily itchy skin eruption which may resemble mycosis fungoides or contact dermatitis, but may be distinguished from them by its predilection for middle-aged Jewish males and a high incidence of penile lesions with rapid changes of the skin lesions from lichenoid to exudative to edematous hive-like. Patch tests are normal and spontaneous cure occurs without removal of contactants. It does appear to respond to steroids but not irradiation and runs a non-fatal self-limited course.

Marion B. Sulzberger (1895–) American dermatologist. Born in New York. He studied medicine in Europe graduating M.D. in Zurich in 1926. Returning to the U.S.A. he became Professor of Dermatology at the New York University Bellevue Medical Center.

William Garbe (1908–) Canadian dermatologist from Toronto.

SUTTON LAW

Always perform at the outset the diagnostic test or therapeutic maneuver most likely to establish the diagnosis.

Willy Sutton (1901–1980) American bank robber. Born in Brooklyn, he began his career at the School of Hard Knocks, commencing with shoplifting in the late 1920s and graduating from a number of the leading penitentiaries including Sing Sing. His career ended in 1952 when he was sentenced to 30 years to life, but was paroled and retired to Florida. Regarded at his peak as America's most successful bank robber, his robberies are said to have netted approximately $2,000,000. He once said he felt "more alive when I was inside a bank robbing it than at any other time in my life". When he was asked why he robbed banks, he replied "because that's where the money is" (Sutton Law). He was in and out of State penitentiaries throughout his life and had a penchant for adopting disguises. The term was proposed by Petersdorf and Beeson in an article on pyrexia of unknown origin published in Medicine (1961).

SVEDBERG UNIT

Unit used in ultracentrifuge measurement of the molecular size of organic materials.

Theodor Svedberg (1884–1971) Swedish chemist. Together with his fellow Swede,Tiselius, was one of the foremost chemists to advance the understanding of protein chemistry. He invented the high speed centrifuge (ultracentrifuge) which enabled him to study the behavior of serum and plasma proteins. This instrument has proved to be of extreme value both in the analysis of serum plasma proteins and lipids and in isolation of components both from plasma and from cells which have been appropriately treated to release their organelles. It is said that in the development of the centrifuge, the area was like a World War I battlefield with trenches and sandbags and with members of the staff wearing tin helmets because the centrifuges would explode unexpectedly.

SWAN-GANZ CATHETER

Cardiac catheter with terminal inflatable balloon inserted through right atrium and ventricle into pulmonary artery to measure pulmonary artery and pulmonary wedge pressures to measure end diastolic pressure.

Harold J.C. Swan (1922–) U.S. cardiologist, Cedars of Lebanon Hospital, Los Angeles.

William Ganz (1919–) U.S. engineer, Cedars of Lebanon Hospital, Los Angeles.

SWEDIAUR DISEASE

Achillodynia (pain in the calcaneous tendon or its bursa).

François X. Swediaur (1748–1824) Austrian physician.

SWEET SYNDROME

Dark red plaques occur on face, arms and legs which resemble erythema multiforme in appearance but there is an associated neutrophil leukocytosis and infiltrate into the lesion.

Robert D. Sweet British dermatologist.

SWIFT DISEASE

v. FEER DISEASE

Acrodynia or Pink disease. Characterized by painful swollen and reddened hands and feet in young children. Insomnia and hypotonia were common. The child would constantly complain of pain and adopt various postures in bed in attempts to obtain relief. Thought to have been due to mercurial salts used in teething powders. Their elimination has resulted in the disappearance of this disorder.

Harry Swift (1858–1937) Australian pediatrician who described the condition in 1914. Born in Ely, England, he went to medical school at Cambridge, graduating in 1883. He migrated to Australia in 1887 and became a visiting physician at the Adelaide Children's Hospital in 1890. In 1912 he was appointed the first clinical lecturer in medical diseases of children at Adelaide University. The first description was by P. Selter in 1903 (*v. supra*).

SWISS TYPE OF AGAMMAGLOBULINEMIA

Absence of humoral and cellular immune responses with little lymphoid development. Autosomal recessive. Also called Glanzmann-Riniker (*v. supra*) lymphocytophthisis.

SWYER-JAMES SYNDROME

v. MACLEOD SYNDROME

Unilateral hyperlucency of the lung. It is due to decreased vascular perfusion to the affected side and is associated with diminished ventilation and its cause is unknown.

Paul R. Swyer (1921–) English-born Canadian physician.

G.C.W. James U.S. physician.

SYDENHAM CHOREA

Infectious chorea (St. Vitus Dance). This is a movement disorder encountered in childhood between the ages of 5 and 15. Females are affected twice as commonly as males and rheumatic valvular disease may develop later. It may be associated with emotional lability and inappropriate behavior. Its onset may occur with pregnancy although usually such patients have had a previous attack. Apart from rheumatic fever, it has been reported in other situations such as hyperthyroidism, systemic lupus erythematosus and some of the other commoner exanthemata.

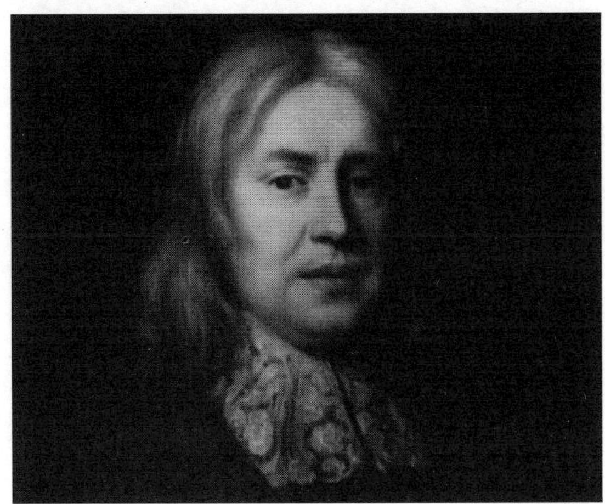

Thomas Sydenham (Courtesy of the Royal College of Physicians of London Portraits, by G. Wolstenholme and D. Piper (J & A Churchill Ltd, London))

Thomas Sydenham (1624–1689) He was born in Winford Eagle and entered Oxford in 1642, but left it to fight for Cromwell against Charles I. He then returned to Oxford and entered Wadham College. In 1649 he became a Bachelor of Medicine and was appointed Fellow of All Souls College. He moved to London and although becoming a close friend of Robert Boyle, appeared to distrust all recent discoveries in anatomy, botany and physiology and seemed to have no knowledge of William Harvey's discovery of the circulation.

In 1656 he married and took a house in London and commenced practice. In 1659 he studied for a while at Montpellier with Barbeyrac. Charles II became King in 1660 and since Sydenham had fought for the Cromwellian army and his brother had been one of the well known commanders, he was not in favour in court. In 1663 he became a Licentiate of the College of Physicians and in 1666 published his first work on fevers which he dedicated to Robert Boyle. His favorite books were Hippocrates, Cicero, Bacon and Don Quixote, and he revived Hippocrates' technique and in particular his methods of accurate description of disease process at the patient's bedside. He himself suffered with renal stones and gout, and apart from his accurate descriptions of these disorders he described a number of other disorders accurately for the first time. These included malaria, measles (which he distinguished from scarlet fever), bronchopneumonia, hysteria and of course chorea. He preached that a doctor must rely on his own observation and clinical experience and he appears to have practiced largely common sense medicine. Although he advocated bleeding, he did this in relative moderation compared with that of his contemporaries and followers. He noted the link between fleas and typhus fever.

SYLVIAN AQUEDUCT

Cerebral aqueduct.

SYLVIAN AQUEDUCT SYNDROME

Retraction nystagmus, paresis of upward gaze, lid retraction due to tumor of, or vascular lesion in the peri-aqueductal tissues.

Franciscus Sylvius (1614–1672) Dutch physician. This was the Latinised version of Francois de Boë, born in Hanau, Germany. His ancestors were French (Dubois) altered to de la Boë. He studied in Sedan, Leyden, Paris and Basel, where he graduated in 1637 and practiced first at Hanau and then Amsterdam. In 1658 he became Professor of Medicine at the University of Leyden. He had studied as a chemist as well as a physician and physiologist and therefore established what was probably the first chemical laboratory in a university. He introduced bedside teaching, stressed the importance of autopsy study, and taught Harvey's theory on circulation. He was not a brilliant investigator but was an outstanding teacher and students from all over Europe came to attend his lectures, including de Graaf, Stensen, Swamerdam and van Horne, all of whom were greatly influenced by him. He considered digestion to be a chemical fermentation and felt that saliva and the pancreatic juice played an important role.

SZABO SIGN

Sensory loss along lateral aspect of foot in sciatica.

Diorys Szabo (1856–1918) Hungarian physician who worked in Budapest.

T

TAKAHARA DISEASE

Acatalasemia – manifest clinically as oral ulcerations around the neck of the teeth which may give progressive loosening and also ulcers in the tonsillar fossa – autosomal recessive.

Shigeo Takahara Professor of Otorhinolaryngology at Okayama Medical School, Japan who during an operation noted that the blood of the patient turned black on exposure to air which he initially thought was due to the erroneous use of silver nitrate and then investigated and found the true cause.

TAKATA-ARA TEST

Test for globulin in cerebrospinal fluid.

Maki Takata (1892–) Japanese pathologist.

Kiyosha Ara Japanese pathologist.

TAKAYASU DISEASE OR SYNDROME

v. MARTORELL SYNDROME

Pulseless disease – an arteritis of unknown origin which classically involves the aortic arch with narrowing of the major branches with a predilection for young women, causing headache, syncope and muscle wasting.

Michishigie Takayasu (1860–1938) Japanese ophthalmologist.

TAMM-HORSFALL GLYCOPROTEIN

A glycoprotein found in urine thought to be derived from cells of the proximal tubules. It is present in the matrix of renal casts.

Igor Tamm (1922–1971) U.S. investigator at the Rockefeller Institute, New York.

Frank L. Horsfall (1906–1971) U.S. virologist, born in Seattle and graduated M.D. McGill University in 1932. Professor of Microbiology, Sloan Kettering Institute and Cornell University, New York.

TANGIER DISEASE

Lipid abnormality causing enlarged yellow tonsils, lymphadenopathy, splenomegaly and eventually vascular complications. Due to reduced serum lipoproteins and depositions of cholesterol esters in reticulo-endothelial system.

Tangier Island Located in the Virginian section of Chesapeake Bay and home of the first patient described with this disorder.

TAPIA SYNDROME

Unilateral paralysis of motor 10th and 12th nerves, giving paresis of pharynx and larynx and unilateral atrophy of the tongue. Sometimes the 9th nerve is involved.

Antonio G. Tapia (1875–1950) Spanish physician. He was born in Ayllon, Segovia, and graduated in medicine when he was 20. For the next three years he worked in a number of European universities studying otolaryngology. He joined the Spanish forces in 1898 and went to the Philippines. When his term of military duty was over he returned to Spain, married, commenced teaching and practicing as an otolaryngologist in Madrid. In 1912 he established what became one of the most important institutes for ear, nose and throat specialists in the Spanish world attracting students from both Spain and Latin America and commonly called "The Villa Sur". He was a brilliant lecturer who appreciated the importance of health care in rural areas and established a foundation to enable special tuition for rural doctors called "Fundacion de Riraza". Dejerine and Tilney's work placed this lesion in the medulla.

TARDIEU ECCHYMOSES OR SPOTS

Hemorrhagic areas beneath the pleura after death by suffocation or strangulation.

Auguste A. Tardieu (1818–1879) Born and died in Paris. French physician who was interested in jurisprudence and toxicology, and wrote a review of the recognizable characteristics (alterations of the bodies) of people following various trades (48 in all) and wrote a book on medico-legal and clinical aspects of imprisonment. He was Médecin des Hôpitaux in 1850, Professor of Legal Medicine in 1861 and Dean of School of Medicine in 1864.

TARUI DISEASE

Myopathy with compensated hemolysis with a normal or even slightly increased hemoglobin level with an elevated reticulocyte count due to a phosphofructokinase deficiency.

S. Tarui Japanese investigator.

TASHKENT ULCER

Oriental sore.

Tashkent, Uzbekistan.

TAUSSIG-BING MALFORMATION

Congenital malformation in which the aorta arises from the right ventricle posteriorly to the pulmonary artery which arises from both ventricles.

TAUSSIG-BLALOCK OPERATION

v. BLALOCK-TAUSSIG OPERATION

Helen B. Taussig (1898–) U.S. pediatrician who classified and described many of the cardiac malformations. Daughter of F.W. Taussig, a well known economist and adviser to Woodrow Wilson, she schooled at Radcliff College and gained an A.B. at the University of California, Berkeley. She attempted to enter Harvard but at the time this University would not admit women. She then took a course of anatomy at Boston University and greatly impressed Professor Alexander Begg, Dean and Professor of Anatomy, who advised her to apply to Johns Hopkins. This she did with a letter of support from Walter Cannon, and she commenced at Johns Hopkins in 1923, gaining her M.D. in 1927. She did not succeed in obtaining an internship in medicine and entered pediatrics. Professor E.A. Park, at the time, was initiating specialty clinics, and in 1930 she was appointed Physician in Charge at the Harriet Lane Home. Fluoroscopy had just been introduced and she studied its use in following rheumatic fever and at Park's insistence congenital heart disease. This soon led her to appreciate that most cyanotic heart babies had an enlarged right ventricle. She connected the downward march of cyanotic heart disease and death with anoxemia and first recognized that patients with a patent ductus and cyanotic heart disease did far better than those without, and that closure of the ductus in such circumstances was followed by a worsening of the condition. When Blalock came to Johns Hopkins in 1941, Taussig suggested to him that the construction of a patent ductus might provide a solution to the anoxia of children with Fallot's tetralogy. After much work on laboratory animals, the Blalock-Taussig procedure was successfully performed (*v. supra*). She was appointed Professor of Pediatrics in 1959. She also was largely responsible for the prevention of thalidomide being marketed in the U.S.A. when one of her German students drew her attention to the congenital malformations occurring in Germany. She investigated the problem in Germany and England and campaigned successfully against the introduction of thalidomide into the U.S.A.

Richard R. Bing (1909–) One of the pioneers in the use of cardiac catheterization in the investigation of heart disease. Graduated from the University of Munich and the University of Berne. In 1935 he worked with Alexis Carrel and Charles Lindbergh on whole organ perfusion at the Rockefeller Institute, New York. He then worked on hypertension, suggesting that it might be linked to breakdown of amino acids to pressor amines. In 1943 he was appointed to Johns Hopkins to set up a diagnostic laboratory employing cardiac catheterization and rapidly developed this technique to make it a major investigative procedure for patients with cardiovascular disease. He wrote a number of important papers on the pathophysiology of congenital heart deformities and introduced a technique to measure myocardial blood flow using nitrous oxide. In 1951 he was appointed Professor of Clinical Physiology at the University of Alabama and then was Chairman of Medicine at the Veterans Administration Hospital, Washington University, St. Louis and in 1959 moved as Chairman of the Department of Medicine, Wayne State University. In 1969 he was appointed Professor of Medicine at the University of Southern California.

Alfred Blalock (1899–1964) U.S. surgeon (*v. supra*).

TAWARA NODE

The atrioventricular node.

Sunao Tawara (1873–1952) Japanese pathologist.

TAY CHOROIDITIS

Choroiditis guttata.

TAY-SACHS DISEASE

Amaurotic familial idiocy.

Autosomal recessive disease due to accumulation of ganglioside in the brain due to a deficiency of hexosamidase A. Appears at 5 months of age with progressive paralysis, dementia and blindness with a cherry red spot in the retina.

Warren Tay (1843–1927) British ophthalmologist and surgeon. He was a Yorkshireman and was a student at London Hospital, graduating in 1866. He was greatly influenced at the London Hospital by Sir Jonathan Hutchinson of whom he was a disciple and whose habits and mannerisms he adopted, even to the degree of being a "Universal specialist" as Hutchinson was often called. The relationship between these two Yorkshiremen as master and pupil soon progressed to friendship. In 1868 he was appointed Assistant Surgeon to the Hospital for Diseases of the Skin and held a post there until 1907. In 1869 he was appointed as Assistant Surgeon and Ophthalmologist to London Hospital, retiring from that hospital in 1902. He became Clinical Assistant with Edward Nettleship to Jonathan Hutchinson at Moorfields Eye Hospital, and it was here in 1874–1875 that he discovered "Tay Choroiditis" which consists of minute yellow to white dots in the choroid around the macula occurring in elderly people. When Bowman (*v. supra*) retired in 1877 from Moorfields, Tay was appointed in his place. He was a foundation member of the Ophthalmological Society and in Volume I of its transactions he reported "symmetrical changes in the region of the yellow spot in each eye of an infant". This was the first description of the cherry red spot of "Amaurotic familial idiocy" or Tay-Sachs Disease. In 1894 in Volume 4 of the same journal he gave a complete description of the clinical symptoms of this disorder, recording a second patient from the same family. A quiet, kindly man, he was extremely dexterous as an operator and was very keen to show young men the techniques he had learned and because of his expertise and this willingness to teach he attracted many people to work with him. Apart from his contributions to ophthalmology, he translated one of the volumes of Hebra's "Diseases of the Skin" for the new Sydenham Society. He continued at Moorfields until his retiring age, but unlike most people as they got older he became less dogmatic and self-assertive and in fact is said to have been unduly deferent to the opinion of younger and less experienced people.

He was a keen walker and an enthusiastic cyclist, riding a tricycle, being a familiar figure at all the cycle shows and incorporating any new feature on his tricycle. He was a bachelor and later in life became fearful that his sight might be lost since he was an avid reader, particularly of thrillers, and like Jonathan Hutchinson he had chronic glaucoma. As with the latter, only one eye was seriously involved and sight was preserved in the other eye by using miotics. One obituary said, "Tay was one of the hewers of wood and drawers of water in medicine. Such men accumulate the material with which others build. He was a walking dictionary at the London in the 90s. No-one knew more about skin or tumors, or syphilis or eyes, and he had seen more outpatients there and at Blackfriars and Moorfields than any living man. He had a prodigious zeal for knowledge, without the desire and perhaps without the power of exploiting it. Tay owed his appointment on the staff to Jonathan Hutchinson, but Hutchinson owed very much to Tay, whose industry was ever at his call." The younger surgeon was indeed overshadowed by the great clinical teacher, even it seems at times weakening his own initiative and judgement. Later on he became senior surgeon to the hospital at the time when Hughlings Jackson was senior physician, and had to treat surgically the complicated brain cases which only Jackson, at that time, could diagnose. Possibly Tay knew too much to be a great practitioner. He considered every possibility, and knew how surgery could go in pre-antiseptic days. He was quietly independent in a small way and was fond of cycling out to a simple lodging out on the Brighton Road. When a colleague pressed him to join in a holiday, Tay always declined. "My landlady would be so disappointed if I did not go as usual for Whitsun."

Bernard P. Sachs (1858–1944) His father was a teacher and he was raised in a small town in Bavaria near Schweinfurt. Whilst studying in Würzburg, he eloped with a girlfriend to Hamburg in 1857 and boarded a ship to the U.S.A. Bernard was born in Baltimore and studied at Harvard in 1874–1878. One of the teachers, William James, was having trouble with his eyes and asked a member of the class to read a chapter from Wundt's "Psychology". Sachs undertook this task and this influenced his career. He graduated B.A. from Harvard in 1878 and returned to Europe where he studied medicine in Strasburg. He chose Strasburg because of the strong medical faculty there at the time. He was most impressed by Kussmaul but also found von Recklinghausen an inspiring teacher and quoted a comment of Waldeyer who did not like any of the textbooks of anatomy except Josef Hyrtl's because "it contains anecdotes: you will remember the anecdotes and promptly forget the anatomy".

While working with Galtz he wrote his first paper which appeared in Virchow's Archives in 1882. He visited and worked with Westphal and Virchow in Berlin, Meynert and Freud in Vienna, Charcot in Paris and Hughlings Jackson in London. He then sailed back to the U.S.A. in 1884 to New York, where his parents had settled. In 1887 he became an Instructor at the New York Polyclinic and translated into English Meynert's "Psychiatrie". At this stage he wrote his article on arrested cerebral development with special reference to its cortical pathology in which a cherry red macula had been noted clinically by his associate Knapp. Later on recognizing the familial nature of the condition, he called the disorder "amaurotic familial idiocy". He was unaware that Tay had already published an account of a brownish-red circular spot in each macula surrounded by a white halo in an infant. Tay considered the change to be similar to the picture of embolism of the central artery of the retina. Hughlings Jackson had been called in as a consultant and was unable to find any evidence of cerebral problems. Later it was recognized that Tay and Sachs were seeing different facets of the same condition. Sachs' principal hospital affiliations were the Mt. Sinai, Montefiore and Bellevue Hospitals. He had a lucrative private practice but he lost most of his money in the depression. He was outspoken and could be very sharp in repartee, but he was also a very generous man. As a neuro-psychiatrist he was often called in to court cases and in his autobiography tells the story of a lady who was suffering from senile dementia and who had left most of her money to the lawyer who had drawn up her will. "'I suppose' asked the cross-examining lawyer, 'that it is very easy for you, Dr. Sachs, to tell whether a person is sane or insane. I presume you can tell by looking at me whether I am sane or insane.' Very promptly I answered 'Not by looking, but possibly by listening to you.' That settled him."

He wrote a number of books including "The Normal Child" (1926) wherein he largely advocated that parents should be guided by common sense and not psychological theories, and in which he particularly attacked Freudian psychology. This followed an earlier work directed at the medical profession rather than the lay public, "Nervous and Mental Disorders From Birth Through Adolescence".

He was a leading figure in arranging aid for displaced German medical scholars and scientists and helped find positions for them in the U.S.A.

TAYLOR BRACE

Orthopedic steel brace for support of the back.

Charles F. Taylor (1827–1899) U.S. orthopedic surgeon who was born in Williston, Vermont, and graduated M.D. at the University of Vermont in 1856. Initially introduced the brace as part of the treatment of tuberculosis of the spine.

TERRY NAILS

The nail lunules are red in color, usually associated with cardiac failure.

R. Terry British physician.

TERRY SYNDROME

1. Angioid streaks associated with Paget disease.
2. Retrolental fibroplasia.

Theodore L. Terry (1899–1946) U.S. ophthalmologist. He was born in Ennis, Texas, and graduated M.D. from the University of Texas in 1922. After his internship in the Henry Ford Hospital, Detroit, he returned to the University of Texas where he trained in general pathology and then moved to the Massachusetts Eye and Ear Hospital, working both as a clinician and a pathologist. He was eventually appointed ophthalmic surgeon to that hospital in 1937 and acted as the Head of the Ophthalmology Department at Harvard University during the war years. He was extremely enthusiastic and with a keen sense of humor he was an excellent teacher. In the last years of his life his research concentrated primarily on retrolental fibroplasia and he documented that this was one of the most prevalent causes of infant blindness and proceeded to build a research team devoted to discovering its cause and prevention. An avid reader, he was a good story teller and in particular enjoyed car travel. Throughout his life he suffered from recurrent peptic ulcer hemorrhages and had many operations for this problem. He died suddenly of cardiac failure.

THIERSCH GRAFT

Split skin graft.

Karl Thiersch (1822–1895) Born in Munich and studied medicine in Berlin, Vienna and Paris and graduated in 1843 in Munich. He served as an army surgeon in 1850 in the campaign against Denmark and after was a Prosector in Pathology and Anatomy in Munich for 6 years, and a pupil of Stromeyer (an orthopedic surgeon). He went to Erlangen in 1854 as Professor of Surgery. He moved to Leipzig in 1857 and remained Professor of Surgery there until his death. He was a consultant surgeon in the Franco-Prussian War and returned to become a vigorous supporter for Lister's antiseptic technique and was the first continental surgeon to introduce this method as standard practice. He made contributions to epithelial cancer (1865), healing wounds (1867) and phosphorus necrosis of the jaw (1867). He introduced split skin grafting in 1874. He disproved Virchow's theory of the connective tissue origin of carcinoma but so great was the latter's authority that it was only after two further confirmatory papers by Waldeyer (*v. infra*) that it was accepted.

THOMA-ZEISS CELL OR COUNTING CHAMBER

Early graduated chamber to count blood cells.

Richard Thoma (1847–1923) German histologist.

Carl Zeiss (1816–1888) German optician and lensmaker.

THOMAS SIGN

Test for fixation of hip in flexion.

THOMAS SPLINT

Splint used for hip and knee fractures.

Hugh O. Thomas (1834–1891) Son of a famous "bone-setter" he was a founder of orthopedic surgery in Liverpool although he was a general practitioner in the Liverpool slums throughout his life. He introduced the splint in 1886, which found universal use later. He devised a technique of active and passive congestion to aid healing of fractures which were slow to unite. This technique was later advocated by the German A. Bier (1904). His major contribution was the advocacy of complete rest for which he employed his splints which he designed himself and which were made in his own workshop. The use of his methods and his splint reduced the mortality of compound fracture of the femur in World War I from 80% in 1916 to 7.3% in 1918.

THOMSEN DISEASE

Myotonia congenita.

Autosomal dominant. Early onset, present at birth, but symptoms may not develop until first or second decade, with falls and painless stiffness, made worse by cold and improved by repeated movement.

Asmus J.T. Thomsen (1815–1896) Danish physician, who described the condition in himself and his family in 1876.

THROCKMORTON REFLEX

Percussion over the metatarso-phalangeal joint medial to the extensor hallucis longus results in dorsiflexion of the great toe in pyramidal tract lesions.

Tom B. Throckmorton (1885–1961) U.S. neurologist who worked in Philadelphia.

TIETZE SYNDROME

Costochondritis giving pain in chest and costochondral junctions; it often resolves after a few days of anti-inflammatory therapy. This may be mistaken for coronary disease – (female:male ratio 2:1) and is usually unilateral on the left side with a high incidence of anxiety state and previous cardiac problems.

Alexander Tietze (1864–1927) German surgeon, Professor of Surgery at Breslau (Wroclaw). He wrote an excellent textbook on emergency surgery which was published in 1927 and contributed numerous papers on surgical topics.

TILLAUX DISEASE

v. PHOCAS DISEASE

Paul J. Tillaux (1834–1904) French surgeon and Professor of Surgery in Paris.

TINEL SIGN 1

Tapping over regenerating nerve trunk causes tingling in its distribution up to the site of regeneration.

TINEL SIGN 2

Tapping over the carpal tunnel results in tingling sensation in the distribution of the median nerve in carpal tunnel syndrome.

Jules Tinel (1879–1952) French neurologist. He was born in Rouen to a family which for five generations had had members who were in the medical profession. He was a brilliant student and commenced his studies in Rouen, but soon moved to Paris where he was Externe des Hôpitaux in 1901 and became an intern in 1906. He was a student of Troisier, Dejerine, Landouzy and Netter. He was most influenced by Netter, who introduced him to the importance of infective organisms, viruses, anatomical pathology, and Dejerine, who made him decide to become a neurologist. His thesis published in 1910 on nerve involvement of tabes resulted from work done with Dejerine at the Salpêtrière and with Landouzy and Laennec. He was Chef de Clinique in 1911 and Chief of the Laboratory at the

Salpêtrière in 1913, but was called up in 1914 and headed the neurological centre at Mans. Here he studied wounds involving the nerves and their regeneration. He was demobilized in 1919 and commenced work on psychosomatic aspects of medicine, an interest which he had first acquired with Dejerine. He was particularly interested in the sympathetic nervous manifestations which seemed to accompany some of the psychosomatic problems such as depression. In 1922 he was associated with the first description of a chromaffin cell tumor of the adrenal medulla. Initially as Médecin des Hôpitaux at La Rochefoucauld from 1922–1936 he moved to Beaujon where he worked until 1940 and finally at Boucicaut until he retired in 1945. He became ill in 1939 with heart trouble, but returned to work after some months rest. He was greatly upset by the occupation and took an active part in the French resistance, hiding many allied flyers whom his son, Jacques, would smuggle across France to Spain. One day Jacques did not return, and Tinel went to Bayonne to locate his son and learnt that he had been arrested. He himself was put in prison in Bordeaux at the Fort de Ha. Some days later his wife and second son were also arrested and imprisoned in Fresnes. After several months they were freed, but Jacques was deported and it was only in 1945 that Tinel learnt that he had died in the death camp of Dora.

He was a very modest man and as secretive about his work for the French resistance after the war as he had been during the occupation. In 1947 he had a transient aphasic attack but after some weeks recovered and returned to work. His cardiac problems continued and he died of heart failure.

TISELIUS ELECTROPHORESIS

Free boundary electrophoresis – a technique which first enabled the electrophoretic separation of plasma proteins and resulted in the designation of $\alpha 1$, $\alpha 2$, β, fibrinogen (φ) and γ globulins according to their speed of migration.

Arne Tiselius (1902–) Swedish biochemist and physical chemist who won the Nobel Prize for his analytical techniques of separating plasma proteins and other particles and proteins by charge. He showed antibodies to be gamma globulins.

TOBEY-AYER TEST

A test for occlusion of the lateral sinus by measuring rise in cerebro-spinal fluid pressure following compression of one or both internal jugular veins.

George L. Tobey (1881–1947) U.S. ear, nose and throat surgeon, born in Lancaster, Massachusetts and graduated M.D. Harvard 1903 and trained at the Massachusetts Eye and Ear Infirmary as well as in Berlin, returning to Boston to enter practice in 1905. He served with the U.S. Medical Corps in World War I and was President of the American Otological Society in 1933.

James B. Ayer (1882–) U.S. neurologist. Born in Boston and graduated M.D. Harvard in 1907. He described aseptic meningitis and introduced cisternal puncture to obtain cerebro-spinal fluid. He was a Professor of Neurology at Harvard and worked at the Massachusetts General Hospital.

TODD PARALYSIS

Localized paralysis that may follow a focal epileptic seizure such as dysphasia, sensory disturbances, monoparesis or hemiparesis which may last for minutes or rarely hours after a seizure.

Robert B. Todd (1809–1860) Irish anatomist and physician. He was born in Dublin. Initially studying at Trinity College, Dublin, he moved to Pembroke College, Oxford, and graduated in medicine in 1833. He was Professor of Physiology at King's College, London, from 1836–1853, became a Fellow of the Royal Society in 1838 and a Founder of King's College Hospital in 1840. He was a practicing physician and wrote on numerous medical topics including gout and rheumatic fever as well as a five volume textbook of anatomy with William Bowman (*v. supra*). An enthusiastic supporter of alcohol, he probably over-indulged since his liver was found to be cirrhotic at autopsy.

TOLOSA HUNT SYNDROME

Painful ophthalmoplegia secondary to granulomatous vasculitis of the carotid syphon due to polyarteritis or Wegener granulomatosis giving a 3rd, 4th and 6th nerve palsy, and often involvement of the 1st division of the 5th nerve with a raised ESR and usually responsive to steroids.

Eduardo Tolosa Spanish neurosurgeon in Barcelona, Spain.

William E. Hunt (1921–) U.S. neurosurgeon, Columbus, Ohio.

TOMMASELLI SYNDROME

Hematuria and pyrexia due to a quinine overdose.

Salvatore Tommaselli (1830–1902) Italian physician at Catania, who studied the effects of quinine on malaria.

TOOTH MUSCULAR ATROPHY

v. CHARCOT-MARIE-TOOTH DISEASE

Howard H. Tooth (*v. supra*).

TORKILDSEN PROCEDURE

Establishment of a communication between the cisterna magna and the lateral ventricle.

Arne Torkildsen Norwegian neurosurgeon.

TORNWALDT ABSCESS

Abscess in the pharyngeal tonsil caused by an infection in the pharyngeal bursa.

TORNWALDT BURSITIS

Pharyngeal bursitis. A cystic condition of the tonsil with mucopurulent discharge.

Gustav L. Tornwaldt (1843–1910) German physician.

TORRICELLIAN VACUUM

Vacuum above the mercury in a barometer tube.

Evangelista Torricelli (1608–1647) Italian physicist and mathematician who invented the barometer in 1643. He invented a primitive microscope and made improvements to the telescope.

TOULOUSE-LAUTREC DISEASE

Autosomal recessive disease of bone, resulting in short stature, a large skull with persistent anterior fontanelle, receding chin and short fingers and toes with increased bony fragility – also terminal pyknodysostosis.

Henri de Toulouse-Lautrec (1864–1901) French painter and lithographer.

TOURETTE DISEASE OR SYNDROME

v. GILLES DE LA TOURETTE DISEASE

TOURNAY SIGN

Dilatation of the pupil of the abducted eye in extreme lateral fixation.

Auguste Tournay (1878–) French ophthalmologist.

TOUTON CELLS

Multinucleated giant cells with a foamy fat containing cytoplasm.

Karl Touton (1858–1934) German dermatologist.

TOWNE PROJECTION OR POSITION

Positioning of the head for X-ray to demonstrate the foramen magnum, posterior fossa and long axis of the calvaria without overlap of the facial bones.

Edward B. Towne (1883–1957) U.S. neurosurgeon. Born in West Newton, Massachusetts, he graduated M.D. Harvard in 1913 and trained at the Peter Bent Brigham Hospital and later the Mayo Clinic. In the 1st World War he served firstly with the British Expeditionary Forces and then with the U.S. Army, rising to the rank of Major. On discharge he entered practice in California and became Clinical Associate Professor of Surgery at the Stanford Medical School.. Before retiring he published widely on neurosurgical subjects especially pituitary tumors.

TRAUBE SEMILUNAR SPACE

Variable tympanic area to percussion present below the left 6th rib anteriorly due to gas in the stomach.

TRAUBE SIGN

Pistol shot heard over femoral vessels in aortic incompetence.

TRAUBE-HERING CURVES OR TRAUBE WAVES

High deflection of sphygmograph seen in complete respiratory arrest – arrhythmic variations in blood pressure due to the vasoconstrictor centre (1865).

Ludwig Traube (1818–1876) German physician. He was born in Ratibor, Silesia, to Jewish parents. He studied medicine in Breslau (Wroclaw) with Purkinje and in Berlin under Johannes Müller and Schönlein where he received his degree in 1840. He then went to Vienna where he worked with Rokitansky and Skoda. He investigated the results of section of the vagus nerve on pulmonary function in 1846 and also studied suffocation in 1847. He next studied the pathology of fever, and introduced the thermometer routinely in the examination of his patients in 1850. In 1849 he became Schönlein's assistant and was one of the first Jewish physicians to receive official recognition after the problems of 1848, which resulted in so many Germans migrating to the United States and even as far as Australia (the 48'ers). He was in constant dispute with Frerichs, who was the Physician-in-Chief and therefore had the lion's share of the clinical material at the Charité. His clinics at the Charité were extremely popular and he was kindly and sincere in his handling of patients.

In 1872 he first described pulsus bigeminus and he investigated the relationship between cardiac and renal disease. He was an extremely fine teacher and had a number of famous students, including Hitzig, and his monograph on experimental pathology gave him a world-wide reputation. He advised Billroth in the writing of his thesis. Virchow liked Traube but hated Frerichs. Traube was far more interested in his patients than Frerichs and therefore had a bigger private practice, but he was not as sound in chemistry and was almost servile in his following of Virchow in pathology, and in an attempt to make clinical medicine related and explicable by physiology sometimes drew superfine distinctions. When Traube and Frerichs were taking their classes in the Charité, they would not take the slightest notice of each other and each assumed that their pupils would not associate in public!

Karl E.K. Hering (*v. supra*).

TREACHER COLLINS SYNDROME

Mandibulofacial dysostosis.

Edward Treacher Collins (1862–1932) English ophthalmologist. He was the son of Dr. W.J. Collins, a London physician, and a Miss Treacher who came from an old Huguenot family. He went to school at University College and entered Middlesex Hospital in 1879, graduating in 1883. He interned at Moorfields (The Royal London Ophthalmic Hospital) in 1884 and in 1887 was appointed pathologist and curator of the hospital's museum. He remained in this position until 1895 when he was appointed surgeon to the hospital and remained there for 27 years when he was appointed as a consultant. His work as a pathologist at the hospital formed the basis of his lectures and a book which he published in 1896 called "Researches into the Anatomy and Pathology of the Eye". His publication attracted people from America and Europe as well as the United Kingdom to the hospital to work with him. In 1895 he was married to a New Zealander and spent a romantic honeymoon in Persia in Isfahan where he had been asked to treat the elder son of the reigning Shah, Prince Izel A'Sultan and was awarded the Lion and the Sun decoration in appreciation of his services. He wrote a book about his experiences entitled "In the Kingdom of the Shah". He wrote another book entitled "Pathology and Bacteriology of the Eye" in 1911, and another, "Arboreal Life and the Evolution of the Human Eye" which dealt with changes and adaptations of the eye during evolution and the adoption of erect posture. Finally, in 1929, he wrote a book "The History of Moorfields Eye Hospital" which traced the development of this famous hospital from 1805, giving interesting sketches of the personalities involved in its development.

Apart from his diverse scientific interests, in his early days he had been an excellent rugby player and was an outstanding horse rider, following the Queen's Buck Hounds, just as his father had done and was a skilful sketcher and painter and illustrated much of his work. He is said to have preferred investigation for its possible application and utility rather than purely for the love of discovery. He applied his mind to each problem in a careful and methodical manner, but once he had worked it out and decided upon a hypothesis based upon his facts, he was said to be very difficult to shift, even when evidence was produced which seemed to make his explanation unlikely. His dogmatism, although perhaps a drawback for scientific advancement, was an advantage in his teaching. He was said to be somewhat dour in appearance but had a fine sense of humor and was a witty after-dinner speaker. He did much both on the national and international scene in development of ophthalmology. He was a leading figure in the organisation of the British Ophthalmological Society as well as the International Society of Ophthalmology.

TREITZ FOSSA

Inferior duodenal fossa.

TREITZ HERNIA

Hernia through Treitz fossa.

Wenzel Treitz (1819–1872) Austrian physician born in Hovernic, Bohemia. He worked with Hyrtl and was appointed Professor of Anatomy and Pathology in Cracow, Poland, in 1852, returning to Prague as Head of the Pathology/Anatomy Institution in 1855.

TRENDELENBURG POSITION

Patient supine on a table tilted 45° downwards with legs and feet over the edge of the table.

TRENDELENBURG TEST

1. For varicose veins – patient lies on his back and raises his leg to empty the veins. A tourniquet is applied just below the saphenous opening. The patient is then stood up if the veins fill rapidly with the tourniquet *in situ*, there are incompetent communicating valves. If on release the veins fill rapidly from above it is due to incompetent sapheno-femoral valves.*
2. For congenital dislocations of the hip. If the child stands on the leg of the affected side, the pelvis tilts downwards towards the sound side and the buttock sags down, normally the pelvis tilts upward and the buttock therefore rises.

In addition to congenital dislocation of the hip, this sign may be seen in late Perthes disease, infantile paralysis of the gluteal muscles, old fractures of the neck of the femur and advanced osteo-arthritis.

Friedrich Trendelenburg (1844–1924) German surgeon, Professor of Surgery, Leipzig. He was born in Berlin and studied in Glasgow and Berlin, graduating M.D. in Berlin in 1866. He was a very innovative surgeon and initially was assistant to Langenbeck (1868–1874). It was during this time that he worked on stricture of the trachea and went to Rostock as Professor of Surgery in 1875. Here he introduced gastrostomy in the treatment of esophageal stricture and was the first surgeon to suture the patella in Germany in 1878. He used his position for operating on viscera in 1881. In 1882 he was appointed Professor of Surgery at Bonn and afterwards went to Leipzig in 1895, where he remained until his retirement in 1911. He introduced an operation for varicose veins and made an attempt at surgical removal of a thrombosis in a patient with pulmonary embolism in 1908, and lived to see his pupil, Kirschner, perform the first successful embolectomy in 1924. He was founder of the German Surgical Society in 1872, and was greatly interested in surgical history, writing an account of ancient Indian surgery as well as an autobiography. He died with a carcinoma of the mandible.

* *First described by Sir Benjamin Brodie (v. supra).*

TRESILIAN SIGN

Bright red appearance of opening of parotid duct seen in mumps.

Frederick J. Tresilian (1862–1926) English physician, who was born in London to an old Cornish family. Both his parents died when he was young and he was brought up by his grandmother in Cloyne in County Cork, Ireland. He graduated from Queens College, Cork, in 1885, and obtained his M.R.C.P. Edinburgh in 1887. He practiced in Enfield from 1890 until he died. He worked as a clinical assistant in the Ear, Nose and Throat Department of two London hospitals. Apart from his description of mumps he wrote a number of articles on nervous disorders.

TREVES FOLD

Ileocecal fold.

Sir Frederick Treves (1853–1923) English surgeon who drained the appendicael abscess of King Edward VII in 1902. He was born in Dorchester, Dorset, and wrote a textbook of surgery in 1895 and a dictionary of German medical terms in 1890. He made original contributions to surgical anatomy, peritonitis, intestinal obstruction and appendicitis. He fought in the Transvaal in the Boer War. He studied medicine in London and was lecturer in anatomy and assistant surgeon at the London Hospital and appointed surgeon there in 1883. He was a brilliant lecturer and a very able surgeon and an ardent supporter of aseptic as opposed to antiseptic surgery.

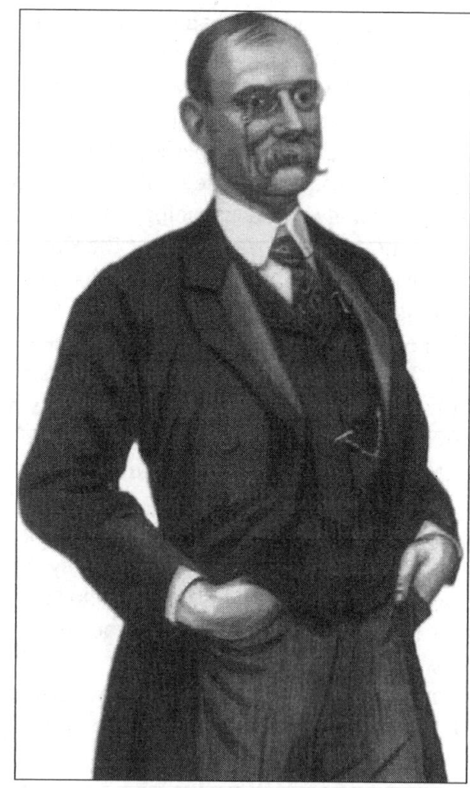

Sir Frederick Treves
(From *Vanity Fair,* 1900, and labelled "Freddie")

He proposed that Hirschsprung's disease was due to a congenital spasm of a distal segment of the large bowel (1898). He has recently become famous because of his association and help to the "Elephant Man", an autobiographical account of which appeared in some of his clinical experiences, called "The elephant man and other reminiscences". He wrote a number of interesting books on travel and a textbook, "Surgical Applied Anatomy", which continued a number of editions after his death.

TROISIER NODE OR SIGN

Enlargement of left supraclavicular nodes due to carcinomatous deposits from carcinoma of stomach or lung.

TROISIER SYNDROME

Bronzed diabetes or hemochromatosis.

Charles E. Troisier (1844–1919) French pathologist, who graduated from the University of Paris in 1869 and gained his Agrégé in 1880. He was an excellent clinician as well as a first class pathologist whose main work was concerned with the spread of cancer. This commenced with his doctorate of medicine where he studied the lymphatic spread of pulmonary carcinoma and emphasized both its lymphatic spread in a contiguous manner as well as by embolization. He called particular attention to the lymph nodes which were behind the clavicle and which are frequently involved in cancers of the esophagus and stomach, intestine, liver, kidneys, etc. He wrote on other topics including rheumatoid nodules, meningitis, and deep vein thrombosis. He became Professor of Pathology in Paris.

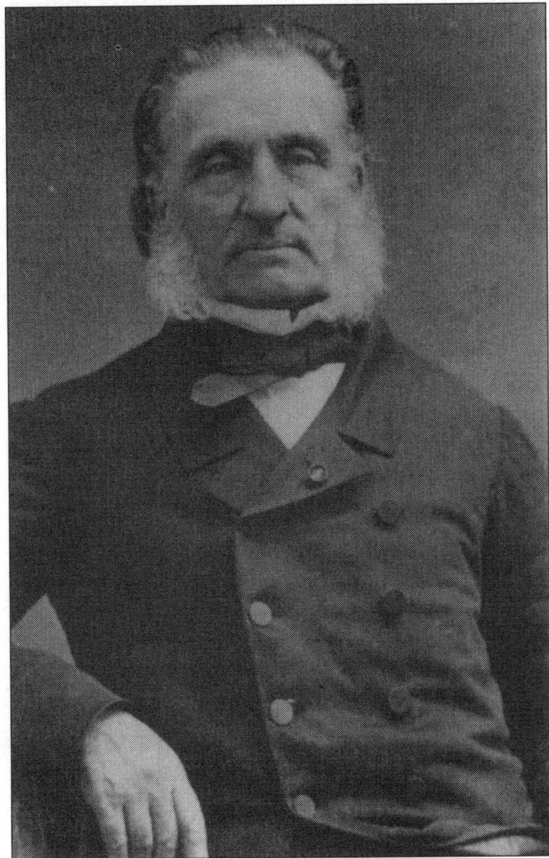

Armand Trousseau (Courtesy of the Royal Society of Medicine, London, UK))

TROUSSEAU SIGN OR PHENOMENON

1. Elevate sphygmomanometer cuff to occlude arterial pulse for 5 minutes. In patients with tetany, carpal spasm will occur (main d'accoucheur).
2. Tache cérébrale – streak produced by lightly scratching the skin.
3. Superficial thrombophlebitis due to visceral carcinoma.

Armand Trousseau (1801–1867) French physician who noted (3) as his own death warrant. Coined the term "aphasia" and popularized the eponyms such as Addison, Graves and Hodgkin Disease.

He was born in Tours and was a pupil of Bretonneau there, graduating in medicine in Paris in 1825. He became one of the outstanding personalities and figures in Parisian medicine. He became Agrégé in 1826 and worked on Yellow Fever which, together with a monograph on laryngeal pthisis, led to his early recognition in Paris. He was appointed as a physician at the Hôpital Ste. Antoine in 1839 and at the Hôtel Dieu in 1850. He was the first person in France to perform a tracheotomy, (1831) and wrote a monograph on this as well as intubation in 1851. He wrote a textbook on therapeutics and one on clinical medicine, both of which were extremely popular and translated into English. He introduced the use of thoracocentesis in 1843. He was above all an outstanding clinician and a superb teacher who was adored by his students and colleagues alike, due to his astuteness, integrity and generosity. Numerous students of his achieved fame – they included Dieulafoy, Da Costa, Brown-Séquard and Lasègue. Always ready to acknowledge the work of others, he did much to publicize French clinicians such as Duchenne and Charcot, who were making such major contributions to the clinical sciences at that time. He was one of the greatest of French teachers, and through his books their accurate description of clinical problems became world renowned.

TRUETA SHUNT

Blood bypasses the cortex of the kidney through the juxta-medullary glomeruli during shock and in its extreme can cause cortical anoxia and aseptic necrosis.

Joseph Trueta (1897–) Spanish surgeon, subsequently worked at Oxford. He was Chief Surgeon of the Military Hospital in Barcelona during the Spanish Civil War and re-introduced the use of plaster splints to treat compound fractures. In England he studied the effect of shock and postulated a shunting mechanism in the kidney to explain cortical necrosis.

TULAREMIA

Infectious disease caused by *Pasteurella tularenis*, prevalent in wild animals and birds, and transmitted by direct contact or ingested, or by insect vectors.

Tulare County, California.

TÜRCK BUNDLE

Temporopontine tract.

TÜRCK COLUMN

Anterior corticospinal tract.

Ludwig Türck (1810–1868) Austrian neurologist and ear, nose and throat specialist. He was born in Vienna where he went to medical school graduating in 1837. In 1840 he was appointed physician to the Allgemeines Krankenhaus. In 1844 he went to Paris and was most impressed by Ricord's lectures which he translated into German. In 1847 he was put in charge of a newly established sub-department of neurology in Vienna. He established the principle that the direction of degeneration of a neuronal tract corresponds to the direction of conduction. Using this approach he was able to outline six tracts, one of which, the anterior corticospinal tract, was given his name. He was one of the first to describe the mechanism for papilloedema and to equate petechial retinal hemorrhage with cerebral tumors. He was the first to describe the segmental arrangement in the cutaneous supply of the sensory nerve roots (1856). Towards the end of the 1850s he left neurology to develop laryngology.

Türck had been stimulated to develop a laryngoscope by Carl Ludwig and the Spanish singing teacher Manuel Garcia, and Czermak borrowed the first instrument from Türck himself and used it extensively in exploring the physiology of speech and phonetics, whereas Türck had confined himself to purely clinical application – a feud ensued between the two, termed "Türckenkreig". He was a very quiet and shy person and his rival Czermak used to say "Herr Türck was always a bit too late". He described laryngitis sicca sometimes called "Türck trachoma". He died suddenly from typhus.

TÜRCK CELL, IRRITATION CELL OR LEUKOCYTE

Stimulated lymphocyte with morphological appearance between that of a lymphocyte and plasma cell.

Wilhelm Türck (1871–1916) Austrian physician who first reported agranulocytosis.

TURCOT SYNDROME

Intestinal polyposis with intra-cranial neoplasia.

Jacques Turcot (1914–) Canadian surgeon who worked at the Hôtel Dieu de Quebec Hospital, and Laval University.

TURNER SIGN

Local discoloration of the skin seen in the loin, unilateral or bilaterally 2–3 days after an attack of acute pancreatitis.

George Grey Turner (1877–1951) Graduated from the University of Durham and a protégé of Rutherford Morrison, Professor of Surgery at Newcastle upon Tyne. Turner was appointed Professor of Surgery at the Postgraduate Medical School, London, where he remained until he retired.

TURNER SYNDROME

Ovarian dysgenesis – characterized by short stature, webbed neck, shield chest, wide carrying angle of arms, congenital heart defect, especially coarctation and female appearance, café au lait spots, black freckles, double layered eye lashes. Characteristically they have XO karyotype with reduced numbers of Barr bodies in the buccal smears.

Henry H. Turner (1892–1970) U.S. physician. He was born in Harrisburg, Illinois and graduated M.D. in 1921 from the University of Louisville. He studied in Vienna and London and became Professor of Medicine at the University of Oklahoma. He was one of the founders of the Endocrine Society, becoming its President. He died of cancer of the lung.

TYNDALL EFFECT OR PHENOMENON

Small particles suspended in liquid or gas may cause a beam of light to be luminous.

John Tyndall (1820–1893) British physicist, born in Leighlin Bridge, County Carlow, Ireland. He recorded the effect of penicillium inhibiting bacterial growth and that it did not effect *Pseudomonas pyocanea*. He studied dust and bacteria in the atmosphere and published his findings in a book "Essay on the Floating Matter in the Air in Relation to Putrefaction and Infection" in 1881. He pioneered the technique of heat sterilization and together with Pasteur destroyed the doctrine of spontaneous generation (v. BASTIAN). He was a friend of Faraday. A keen mountaineer, he wrote on practical aspects of the sport as well as scientifically on the Alps and the glaciers. He died of accidental poisoning.

TYRODE SOLUTION

Salt solution used in physiological experiment containing NaCl, $CaCl_2$, KCl, $NaHCO_3$, $MgCl_2$ and $Na_3(PO_4)_2$ + glucose.

Maurice V. Tyrode (1878–1930) U.S. pharmacologist.

U

UHL ANOMALY

Aplasia or hypoplasia of the right ventricle.

Henry S.M. Uhl (1921–) U.S. physician at Johns Hopkins.

ULLRICH-TURNER SYNDROME

Webbing of neck, short stature, wide carrying angle of arms and hypogonadism in a male, also called male TURNER SYNDROME.

Otto Ullrich (1894–1957) German pediatrician who described a number of other congenital abnormalities, including a variant of Oppenheim disease (*v. supra*) and another with a conglomeration of skeletal and soft tissue abnormalities (v. BONNEVIE-ULLRICH SYNDROME).

Henry H. Turner (*v. supra*).

ULYSSES SYNDROME

This is the excessive use of diagnostic investigations which fail to benefit and may even harm the patient following the chance observation of an abnormal test.

Ulysses Greek mythology. King of Ithaca who after the Trojan War returned home by a most circuitous route and became involved in a series of disastrous adventures. He was the hero of Homer's "Odyssey".

UNDERWOOD DISEASE

A disorder of lipid metabolism. In the mildest forms it may present at birth or shortly after, with some hardening of the subcutaneous fat and the appearance of firm nodules in the buttocks, trunk, thighs, cheeks and arms. It may regress as the child grows. In the more severe form, the subcutaneous fat imposes a generalized waxy appearance, with a cold, tight skin. This is often fatal. Histology shows an inflammatory reaction in the fatty tissue with lymphocytes, and Langerhans giant cells, calcification and necrosis.

Michael Underwood (1736–1820) English obstetrician, surgeon and pediatrician. Born in Surrey, he trained at St. George's Hospital, London. He attended the Princess of Wales for the birth of Princess Charlotte in 1796. He wrote a treatise on leg ulcers and a book "Treatise on the Diseases of Children" first published in 1784 with further editions later. Underwood virtually founded the subject of modern pediatrics and apart from sclerema neonatorum (Underwood disease), the earlier editions gave a classical description of congenital heart disease in childhood, thrush and infantile paralysis.

UNNA BODIES OR CELLS

v. RUSSELL BODIES

UNNA PASTE

Treatment of varicose ulcers by a bandage placed over zinc oxide and gelatine paste.

UNNA-THOST SYNDROME

Hyperkeratosis of hands and feet either congenital or in acquired form preceding hyperhidrosis.

Paul G. Unna (1850–1929) German dermatologist born in Hamburg. He was the son of one of the most prominent local physicians with a long family tradition of medicine. He commenced medicine at Heidelberg but joined the army and was badly wounded in the Franco-Prussian War. After the war he completed medicine at Strasburg being influenced by Waldeyer but had problems with his thesis which contained original and contentious proposals which drew intense criticism from von Recklinghausen. As a result it was rewritten and accepted despite continued opposition from von Recklinghausen. This was the harbinger of his continual unconventional and original approaches. After studying in Vienna he initially joined his father's private practice in general medicine but then founded a private clinic and hospital for skin disease in Hamburg in 1884. He described a number of skin conditions including seborrheic dermatitis and wrote extensively on anatomy, histopathology and treatment of skin disease, including the classical book on histopathology in 1894 which established him as one of the foremost dermatologists in the world. He described the plasma cell. Harshly described as a pompous little man who seldom smiled he had as many admirers as detractors but his ability and standing cannot be doubted since he held his own with German academics who would have been rated as possibly the most competitive of all time and he himself held no academic post until he was appointed the first Professor of Dermatology at the age of 68 at the University of Hamburg. He founded journals of skin disease and edited international atlases of skin disease. He introduced the use of ichthyol and resorcin (1886).

Arthur Thost (1856–   ) German physician.

UNVERRICHT-LUNDBORG DISEASE

Progressive familial myoclonic epilepsy, also termed Unverricht Disease or Syndrome. Fits and myoclonus occur in childhood and there is a slowly increasing ataxia and dysarthria. Spasticity ultimately occurs but dementia is slight or not present – autosomal recessive.

Heinrich Unverricht (1853–1912) German physician who worked in Magdeburg.

Hermann B. Lundborg (1868–1943) Swedish physician. He described this disorder in 1901 when it was the first human disease reported with a clear genetic pattern of autosomal recessive. He became Professor and Head of Department for Human Genetics at the University of Uppsala in 1921.

UPSHAW-SCHULMAN SYNDROME

Congenital thrombocytopenia and microangiopathic hemolytic anemia without clotting abnormalities and corrected by plasma infusions.

Jefferson D. Upshaw U.S. hematologist, Memphis, Tennessee.

Irving Schulman U.S. pediatrician, Chicago, Illinois.

UROV DISEASE

v. KASHIN-BECK DISEASE

USHER SYNDROME

Co-existent deafness and blindness. Initially the visual fields constrict and night blindness is a feature and retinitis pigmentosa is seen on fundoscopy. Visual deterioration may continue to give total blindness. It is inherited as an autosomal recessive.

Charles H. Usher (1865–1942) Scottish ophthalmologist who was born in Edinburgh but studied medicine at Cambridge University and St. Thomas's Hospital, London, graduating in 1891. He was greatly impressed by the famous ophthalmologist Edward Nettleship and later co-authored a book on albinism with him. After his training in ophthalmology he worked in Aberdeen apart from the 1st World War when he served in Salonika. He was a keen bird watcher and fisherman as well as being a cellist.

V

VALSALVA ANTRUM

Mastoid antrum.

VALSALVA MANEUVRE

Forced expiration against a closed glottis and nose results in increased intrathoracic pressure and raised venous pressure.

VALSALVA SINUS

Aortic sinus.

VALSALVA TEST

When Valsalva maneuvre is performed air passes into the tympanic cavity if the auditory tubes are patent.

Antonio M. Valsalva (1666–1723) Italian anatomist. He was born in Imola and went to medical school at Bologna where he was taught by Malpighi and graduated in 1687. In 1697 he became Professor of Anatomy at Bologna where he remained until he died. In 1704 he published a book on the ear in which he included his method for inflating the Eustachian tube (*v. supra*) and described the tympanic antrum. He noted that motor paralysis is on the opposite side to the cerebral lesion both in stroke and in cases of cranial injury.

His greatest pupil was Morgagni who confirmed the above observation in numerous autopsies.

VAN BOGAERT SUBACUTE SCLEROSING LEUKOENCEPHALITIS

Subacute sclerosing panencephalitis.

VAN BOGAERT-BERTRAND SPONGY DEGENERATION

v. CANAVAN DISEASE

VAN BOGAERT-DIVRY SYNDROME

Corticomeningeal diffuse angiomatosis. A recessive sex linked disorder which may have associated skin pigmentation together with telangiectasia, and widespread neurological involvement with pyramidal and extra-pyramidal features, epilepsy and mental deficiency.

VAN BOGAERT-NYSSEN DISEASE

Familial form of Schilder diffuse sclerosis (*v. supra*) occurring in late adult life.

Ludo van Bogaert (1897–) Belgian neuropathologist who trained with the famous French surgeon Clovis Vincent.

Ivan G. Bertrand (1863–1965) French neuropathologist.

Paul Divry (1889–) Belgian neuropathologist.

René Nyssen Belgian neuropathologist.

VAN BUCHEM SYNDROME

Thickening of the base of the skull, calvarium, mandible and other bones associated with a raised alkaline phosphatase. Stenosis of exit foramina of the skull may lead to optic atrophy, deafness and facial palsy.

Francis S.P. van Buchem (1898–1979) Dutch physician. He was born in Wognum and went to medical school in Leiden, graduating in 1921. He became Professor of Medicine in Gröningen, the Netherlands.

VAN CREVELD-VON GIERKE DISEASE

v. GIERKE DISEASE

Simon van Creveld (1894–1971) Dutch physician, born in Amsterdam where he graduated M.D., in 1922. He worked with Finkelstein in Berlin and commenced pediatric practice in Amsterdam in 1926, becoming the head of the Baby Clinic at the University Hospital. He founded a clinic for convalescent children and for hemophilia and wrote his clinical description of von Gierke disease in 1927. He and his wife were imprisoned by the Germans during the war. After the war he returned to be Professor of Paediatrics at the University of Amsterdam.

VAN DEN BERGH METHOD (TEST)

Test for bilirubin. Positive direct van den Bergh reaction reflects conjugated bilirubin, indirect, unconjugated bilirubin.

Albert A.H. van den Bergh (1869–1943) Dutch physician born in Rotterdam and graduated in 1896 from Leiden where he interned. In 1900 he went to the Prussian (now Polish) city of Breslau (Wroclaw) visiting with the famous pediatrician Czerny and afterwards returning to Holland to practice in Rotterdam. In 1912 he succeeded Wenckebach (*v. infra*) as Professor of Medicine at Gröningen. In 1918 he was appointed Professor at Utrecht, retiring in 1938. In 1918 he became personal physician to the German Emperor, Kaiser Wilhelm II, and remained in that capacity during the German occupation, although he was a Jew. The Germans did not deport him to a concentration camp when the ex-Kaiser died in 1942, but held him under house arrest. He suffered with diabetes and angina. Apart from his discovery of the two forms of bilirubin, he made significant contributions to the porphyrias and paroxysmal hemoglobinemia. An avenue in Utrecht is named after him.

VAN GIESON STAIN

Connective tissue stain.

Ira van Gieson (1865–1913) U.S. neuropathologist. His picric acid stain was initially introduced to study nerve tissue but then applied to liver, bone marrow and other sections. He directed the pathological studies on Bernard Sachs' initial studies on the brains of his patients with amaurotic familial idiocy and he drafted the illustrations for Sachs' paper.

VAN SLYKE APPARATUS OR TECHNIQUE

Manometric method for measuring blood gases.

Donald D. van Slyke (1883–1971) Born in Pike, New York, he was a biochemist and graduated Ph.D. University of Michigan in 1905. He introduced techniques for measuring amino acids and conversion of protein into urea in the liver, and made major advances in the understanding of acid base and electrolyte problems, including measurement of blood urea which pointed the way to fluid and electrolyte therapy. He introduced techniques for measuring blood gases, leading to a better understanding of respiratory physiology.

VAQUEZ DISEASE

(Sometimes called VAQUEZ-OSLER DISEASE)

Polycythemia rubra vera.

Louis H. Vaquez (1860–1936) French physician. Born in Paris he did his medical training there, graduating in 1890 just ahead of Widal (*v. infra*). He was appointed Professor Agrégé in 1898 and a Professor in 1918. Initially he investigated hematological disorders, including the leukemias, polycythemia, hemolytic anemia and the role and indications for splenectomy. Influenced by Potain, he specialized in diseases of the heart, and rapidly became one of France's leading physicians. He described polycythemia vera in 1892 (Osler published his classical description of the disorder in

1903 and at first thought it was a new clinical entity but learnt of Vaquez's report and acknowledged his priority).

He was one of the first to recognize that Stokes-Adams attacks were related to interference to the Bundle of His resulting in a discordant beating of the auricle vis-à-vis the ventricle. He introduced recording of the jugular venous pulse and the electrocardiogram to France, and pursued Potain's work on hypertension. He wrote a book on the cardiac arrhythmias in 1911 and another on cardiac disorders in 1920 and was the founder and editor of a journal on disorders of the heart, vessels and of blood (Archives des Maladies du Coeur, Vasseaux et du Sang). His close friends included Babinski, Widal, and the poet André Rivoire.

VATER, AMPULLA OF

Entrance of the bile duct into the second part of the duodenum.

Abraham Vater (1684–1751) German anatomist. He was born in Wittenberg and became Professor of Medicine there.

VEDDER SIGN

Beriberi causes pain on calf pressure, loss of the knee jerk, anesthesia of the lower leg anteriorly and difficulty in rising from the squatting position.

Edward B. Vedder (1878–1952) Born in New York, he graduated from the University of Pennsylvania Medical School in 1902. In 1903 he worked with Simon Flexner on the etiology of bacillary dysentery. That same year, 1903, he joined the U.S. army and took part in attempts to improve typhoid vaccination. He was posted to the Philippines from 1904–1919. Whilst there he studied beriberi and observed that it followed the eating of polished rice. He substituted half polished rice and found that this corrected the vitamin deficiency (later shown to be vitamin B_1). He made valuable contributions to other dietetic deficiencies such as scurvy. In 1911 he introduced emetine for the treatment of amebic dysentery. From 1913–19 he was Assistant Professor of Pathology at the Army Medical School in Washington, and became Chief of the Medical Research Division on Chemical Warfare and published articles on this and on the epidemiology of syphilis

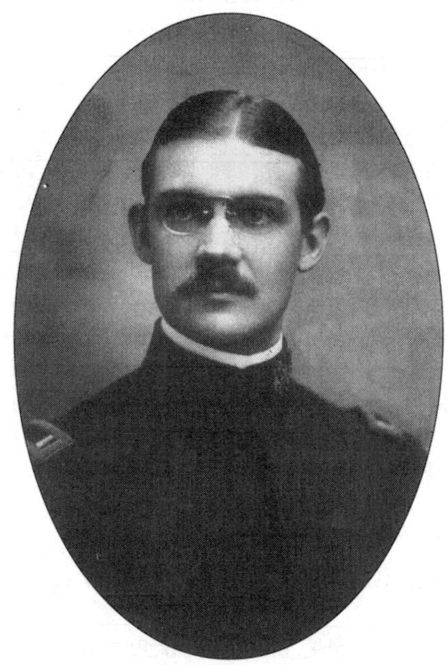

Edward B. Vedder (Courtesy of the Royal Society of Medicine, London, UK)

in the army. He was a Colonel on his retirement from the army in 1933 and became Professor of Experimental Medicine in the George Washington University until 1942, then Director of Medical Education at Alameda County Hospital until his retirement in 1947. He died in the Walter Reed Hospital in Washington.

VEILLONELLA

Species of bacteria, anaerobic Gram negative cocci.

André Veillon (1864–1931) French bacteriologist. He undertook his internship with Professor I. Strauss who visited the Pasteur Laboratories and who initially interested him in bacteriology. He next went to Grancher's laboratory at L'Hôpital des Enfants-Malades and with his friend Zuber commenced his research into micro-organisms. He was particularly interested in the saprophytic bacteria in the mouth and intestine, his name being associated with the discovery of anaerobic organisms and also a tube for bacterial cultures, one end of which was stoppered with a rubber bung and the other plugged with cotton-wool. Veillon was interested in dermatology and collaborated on many occasions with Brocq. A bon vivant and wit, he was the life of the party at social gatherings, and had a wide interest in literature and the arts, and many friends amongst the Bohemian population of Paris.

VERNER-MORRISON SYNDROME

Non B cell tumor of the pancreas associated with hypokalemia, watery diarrhea and sometimes achlorhydria and a high V.I.P. (vasopressor intestinal peptide).

John V. Verner (1927–) U.S. physician.

Ashton B. Morrison (1921–) U.S. physician.

VERNET RIDEAU PHENOMENON

Movement of posterior wall of pharynx like the drawing of a curtain when the patient says "Ah"; absent in 5th nerve palsy.

VERNET SYNDROME

Paresis of 9th, 10th and 11th cranial nerves due to extension of tumor into the jugular foramen.

Maurice Vernet (1887–) French neurologist who described his syndrome in 1916.

VEROCAY BODIES

Whorls of fibrils surrounded by radially arranged cells in neurofibromas.

José Verocay (1876–1927) Uruguayan pathologist.

VESALIUS LIGAMENT

Inguinal ligament.

Andreas Vesalius (1514–1564) Flemish anatomist, born in Brussels. His family came from Wessel in the Duchy of Cleves and initially had been called Witting, but changed their name to Wessel after the town. There were many outstanding medical practitioners in his family and his great-grandfather Johannes was physician to Maria, the wife of Emperor Maximilian I. His grandfather, Eberhardt, also attended court as a physician and wrote a paper on Hippocrates. His father, Andreas, was a pharmacist to Charles V and accompanied him on his army campaigns. Vesalius was always interested in anatomy and as a child dissected mice, rats and other animals. He went to Paris for his medical schooling (1533–35) and with the outbreak of war he moved to Louvain where he graduated in 1537. He studied there under the direction of Jacobus Sylvius and Johann Guinterius. Sylvius in particular was a world renowned teacher who attracted people from all over Europe with classes of 400 students. He was convinced of the infallability of Galen and therefore opposed the views of Vesalius.

Vesalius was the leading figure in European medicine after Galen and before the advent of Harvey. It was his investigation and teaching which made anatomy a scientific subject, and his major work, "De Humani Corporis Fabrica", in 1543, was a landmark which broke with the previous tradition of Galen and was regarded as heresy by the establishment of the day. When he had finished his work in Paris, Vesalius returned to Louvain where he renewed public dissection for medical students. Shortly thereafter he moved to Venice where he met a fellow countryman, J.S. van Calcar, a painter who was studying with Titian. Calcar illustrated his works and these illustrations added greatly to the "De Humani Corporis Fabrica", which was published in Basel. This work was completed when he was 28 and Professor of Surgery and Anatomy at Padua. Osler commented: "In itself for what it contains but still more for what it did the "De Humani Corporis Fabrica" is one of the great books of the world with which in the literature of medicine only "De Motu Cordis" of Harvey is to be compared ... The Fabrica remains a monumental human effort, one of the greatest in the history of our profession." Vesalius was reputedly so distressed by the acrimony following the publication of his work (he was bitterly attacked by his old teacher Sylvius, and even by some of his own students), that he burnt his manuscripts and left Padua to accept the lucrative post with Charles as Court Physician in 1544.

Vesalius performed many post-mortems and noted senile changes in joints, that the omentum could prolapse into the inguinal hernia, and was the first to diagnose and describe abdominal and thoracic aortic aneurysms. He operated successfully on Don Carlos of Arragon for empyema and is said to have excised breast cancers. He remained as court physician and surgeon to Charles' army for the remainder of his life. He died on the island of Zante returning from a pilgrimage to Jerusalem. His five years in Padua had produced his masterpeice but his later life was relatively unproductive.

VILLARET SYNDROME

Unilateral paralysis of cervical sympathetic 9th, 10th, 11th and 12th nerves due to a lesion in the retropharyngeal or retroparotid space

v. COLLET SYNDROME

Maurice Villaret (1877–1946) French physician and neurologist. Born in Paris, his mother was a well known pianist and his father a physician who was an amateur painter and had an interest in history. He grew up with a passionate fondness for literature and history and appreciation for painting, enjoying visits to the museums in Italy with his father. He was very keen on outdoor activities, was an alpinist as well as a keen sailor and bicycled all over Corsica as well as most parts of Europe.

He graduated in medicine in 1902 and as a student worked with Bouchard, Roger and D'Hallopeau, but his major influence was Gilbert. He became Agrégé in 1913 and following the war in 1919 became Médecin des Hôpitaux. He was interested in the therapeutic effects of spas and rehabilitation medicine and in 1927 was made Professor "d'Hydrologie et de Climatologie". In 1938 he was appointed a Clinical Professor at the Broussais Hospital.

His major research involvement was in the physiology of the circulation, with an especial interest in the portal circulation and the causes of portal hypertension which he investigated extensively with Gilbert (*v. supra*). He undertook pathological studies on cirrhosis in man, and that produced experimentally in animals. He was especially interested in vascular lesions of the brain and followed the traditional clinical investigator's path of first a clinical observation, then the precise anatomical localization of the lesion, next the application of experimental techniques to reproduce it in animals, thus allowing a better clinical interpretation of a defined problem. He described his syndrome in 1918. He recognized the social aspects of the sick and established a rehabilitation centre for patients under his care, as well as organizing social workers to help patients in their re-adaptation to life following their illness. He was an ideal combination of the clinician and the experimental physiologist.

VINCENT ANGINA

Infection of pharyngeal and tonsillar space.

VINCENT GINGIVITIS

Necrotizing ulcerative gingivitis.

Jean H. Vincent (1862–1950) French bacteriologist. Born in Bordeaux he studied medicine there and in Paris. He became a member of the staff of the Val de Grace Military Hospital in 1896 and was appointed Professor of Epidemiology there in 1912. In 1894 he discovered Nocardia madurae (Actinomysis madurae), an etiological factor in Madura Foot. In 1896 he isolated *Borrelia vincenti* and *Fusobacterium*, and showed that these two organisms were involved in ulceromembranous stomatitis (Vincent Angina). He worked on tetanus and typhoid vaccination and prepared a paratyphoid vaccine which was of value to the French army in the 1st World War and used chlorine to clean infected wounds.

VINSON-PLUMMER SYNDROME

v. PLUMMER-VINSON SYNDROME

VIRCHOW CELL

Lepra cell.

VIRCHOW NODE

Enlarged left supraclavicular lymph node with cancer of stomach.

VIRCHOW SPACE

Perivascular space of Virchow-Robin.

VIRCHOW TRIAD

Factors concerned in the pathogenesis of thrombosis are:

1. Changes in the vessel wall.
2. Changes in the pattern of blood flow.
3. Changes in the constituents of blood.

Rudolf L.K. Virchow (1821–1902) Born in Pomerania in the small town of Schievelbein, the son of an official. Initially he considered entering theology, but chose medicine because he felt his voice was not sufficiently strong to be effective from the pulpit. After finishing school at Köslin, he went to Berlin to enter the Friedrich-Wilhelm Institute for training as an army doctor. He graduated in 1843, receiving his degree, as he wrote to his parents, from "the Dean of the Medical Faculty, the most famous physiologist in the world, Johannes Müller". He was appointed as Frosieps' Prosector at the Charité Hospital in 1845. In that year he presented his work on thrombosis and hemostasis which enunciated his triad and afterwards wrote to his uncle that his voice had not been strong enough at several points in his address. He was released from military service in 1847 to become Privatdozent and following dissatisfaction with editors of journals which refused some of his papers, founded a new journal called "Archiv für pathologische Anatomie" which became known as Virchow's Archiv. He wrote that the aim of the journal was a close union of clinical medicine, pathological anatomy and physiology and this remained his lifetime objective. He strongly propounded the concept that unproved hypothesis is an anathema for the practice of medicine and that no man could be regarded as infallible with regard to knowledge, judgement or supposition.

In 1848 he was sent by the Prussian government to investigate a typhus epidemic prevalent in the weavers of Upper Silesia. He quickly appreciated that the epidemic was largely due to the dreadful living conditions. His report and its severe indictment of the government for allowing this type of misery to occur and his emphasis on social injustices and poor hygienic regulations which were currently operative made him very unpopular with the government. The report was in part politically motivated; it stated inter alia "the proletariat is the result, principally, of the introduction and improvement of machinery" ... "shall the triumph of human genius lead to nothing more than to make the human race miserable?".

Virchow continued to be very active politically, helping construct some of the barricades during the Berlin uprising in 1848 and participating in a movement by doctors to appoint a Minister for Health and secure greater rights. As a result of these activities, he was relieved of his official duties in 1849. With the help of the obstetrician Scanzani, he was appointed to the Chair of Pathology at Würzburg, where he remained until 1856 and established for himself a brilliant reputation both as a teacher and as an investigator. He had already defined leukocytosis and described leukemia and then set about the investigation of thrombosis showing that thrombosis may be an essential primary condition in phlebitis and result in embolism. He was the first to recognize pulmonary and cerebral embolism. He recognized the special lymphatic sheaths on the cerebral arteries in 1851. His fame became such that when the Chair of Pathology at the University of Berlin became vacant he was appointed despite stiff competition (v. Billroth), and intense political opposition. The King told the Faculty of Medicine to ignore Virchow's political views.

In 1858 he published his book "Cellulare Pathologie", one of the most influential and important books in medicine. In it he looked upon the body "as a cell-state, in which every cell is a citizen". Disease he regarded as "merely a conflict of the citizens in the state, brought about by the action of external forces". Although there were important errors in some concepts Virchow put forward, e.g. "there could be no diapedesis of blood cells", he encouraged research and the latter idea was disproved with his encouragement by one of his principal students and pupils, Cohnheim.

His dictums "every cell is derived from a cell" ("omnis cellula a cellula") and "pathological form has its physiological prototype" became the basis of future investigational approach and scientific research. He demolished the older views of humors and crases and was especially virulent in his attack of Rokitansky's first textbook which had otherwise presented an excellent morphological account. In the second edition of this book Rokitansky eliminated and omitted all reference to this type of theoretical thinking! Apart from excellent texts on morphological studies of tumors, Virchow described a number of pathological entities including endocarditis. In neuropathology, he first described neuroglia and also the phagocytic actions of certain of the neural cells in areas of encephalomalacia. He wrote descriptions of subdural hematoma, cerebral hemorrhage, meningitis, as well as tumors of the central nervous system and congenital anomalies of the skull, vertebra and brain and spinal cord.

He was described as a small, mobile figure with a quick wit and somewhat of a martinet in the autopsy or lecture room. He would often be extremely sarcastic in dealing with incompetence, foolishness or inattention; on the other hand he could be extremely generous and helpful and always remembered those who had made contributions. For example, despite his virulent attack on Rokitansky, he highly praised the best features of his work. The clinics and those of his colleagues in Berlin must have been entertaining to visit because he, Remak and others often hurled abuse at the speaker during the lecture courses. He was particularly virulent with the clinician Frerich (many would say unjustly so), whereas he was kindly disposed towards Traube, who many felt was over-respectful to Virchow, fearing that he might come under the great man's ire. It was said of Virchow in later life that he remained a liberal in politics but became a reactionary in science. He certainly maintained his strong political interest and convictions and was a member of the Reichstag from 1880–1893, where he espoused liberal policies and was a constant and bitter political opponent of Bismarck, and leader of the radical party in the Reichstag (he had joined the Prussian Lower House in 1862). His strength of conviction and character is perhaps best illustrated by his consistent political activity in a society which was at the pinnacle of authoritarianism. He nonetheless was an extreme patriot and during the Franco-Prussian War organized the Prussian ambulance corps and superintended the erection of an army hospital on the Tempelhof. Indeed when he heard of a pamphlet of Quatrefages written following the accidental shelling of the museum of natural history in Paris, stating that Prussians were not a Germanic, but were a barbaric Mongolian destructive race, Virchow organized a colossal public census of the color of the hair and eyes of 6 million German school children!

He opposed Darwin's concept of the origin of species and could not accept the views of Koch and Behring concerning toxins and antitoxins. Later in life he became increasingly interested in anthropology and archeology. He secured the good sanitation system of Berlin by his efforts in the Reichstag and his knowledge of public health, and preventive medicine. He wrote a number of interesting historical and biographical essays on Schönlein, Morgagni and Müller, the latter whom he greatly admired and regarded as one of his inspirations in science. This extraordinarily active and at times controversial man died of a road accident. He leapt at the age of 81 from a moving tram and fractured his hip.

Charles P. Robin (1821–1885) French anatomist who was co-author of a medical dictionary. Born in Jameson. Appointed Professor of Histology, Faculty of Medicine in Paris 1862. He described osteoclasts and wrote on many subjects ranging from cataracts to inflammation and cardiac movement. He was elected to the French Senate from Ain in 1876.

VOGT-KOYANAGI SYNDROME

Severe headache with meningeal features and illness precedes uveitis associated with vitiligo, deafness and poliosis (whitening of the ends of the hairs).

VOGT-KOYANAGI-HARADA SYNDROME

Here there is retinal detachment rather than uveitis.

Alfred Vogt (1879–1943) Swiss ophthalmologist who worked in Zurich and published an important book on biomicroscopy of the eye in 1921 and introduced cyclodiathermy for the treatment of glaucoma. Some believe Goya suffered from this syndrome and that the sudden onset of deafness resulted in the dramatic change of his style from paintings which were colorful and gay to scenes depicting devastation and death characteristic of his "black period".

Yoshizo Koyanagi (1880–1954) Japanese ophthalmologist.

Einosuke Harada (1892–1947) Japanese ophthalmologist.

VOGT SYNDROME

Congenital chorea or choreo-athetosis. There are marked choreiform and athetoid movements which begin in the first year of life and cause walking problems and speech disorders and there may be associated spasmodic laughing or crying, and mental deficiency. Pathologically, there is an abnormality in the corpus striatum.

Cecile Vogt (1875–1962) Mademoiselle Mugnier met her husband Oskar Vogt while she was studying with Pierre Marie at the Bicêtre. She moved with her husband to Berlin in 1899 and established herself as one of the leading women scientists, her contemporaries being Madame Curie, Madame Dejerine-Klumpke and Madame Nageotte. She did much of the pioneering work on the neuro-anatomy of the thalamus and together with Oppenheim (*v. supra*) published on hereditary (pseudo-bulbar) palsy, athetose double, in which she noted the mottled appearance of the striatum which was acknowledged by Kinnier Wilson. She made early and most important contributions to disease states of the basal ganglia and her husband remarked "It is marvellous! When my wife looks down the microscope she always finds something new".

VOLHARD AND FAHR TEST

1. Specific gravity of urine should reach 1.025 after fluids are withheld for 24 hours.
2. After 1½ litres of water the specific gravity should fall to < 1.003.

Franz von Volhard (1872–1950) German physician, born in Munich and educated in medicine at the University of Bonn and Strasburg. His first appointment after graduation was as a Lecturer at Giessen University in 1901. Three years later he was the acting director of the Medical Clinic there and moved to become Chief of the Medical Department at the Dortmund Municipal Hospital. Eventually he was appointed Professor of Medicine at the University of Halle in 1918 and in 1927 moved to Frankfurt-am-Main to be Professor of Medicine.

Although he was mainly clinically orientated he realized the importance of the application of pathology and physiology to medical study and in collaboration with the pathologist Fahr wrote the monograph on Bright Disease which became a classic and made Volhard's clinic the centre of world nephrology. Although principally interested in renal disease he made a number of important contributions in other areas, discovering lipase in the heart and kidney and describing the digestion of fat as well as developing a method for studying enzyme content in gastric juices in 1903. He collaborated with Schmieden in 1923 in investigations which led to the first pericardectomy for constrictive pericarditis. He died following an accident.

K.T. Fahr (1877–1945) German pathologist who studied medicine in Munich, Berlin and Kiel, graduating M.D. from Giessen in 1903. He became director of Pathology at Mannheim and moved to Hamburg as Professor of Pathology in 1924.

VOLKMANN CANALS

Vascular canals in compact bone.

Alfred W. Volkmann (1800–1877) German physiologist and Professor of Physiology at Halle, who in 1842 showed that the sympathetic nerves were largely made up of small medullated fibres arising from sympathetic and spinal ganglia.

VOLKMANN CONTRACTURE

Ischemic muscular contracture due to external pressure causing death of muscle and fibrosis with a resultant claw hand.

Richard von Volkmann (1830–1889) He was born in Leipzig, the son of A.W. Volkmann who was a Privat-dozent at the time. Richard entered medical school and graduated from Berlin in 1854 and in 1867 became Professor of Surgery and Director of the Surgical Clinic at Halle where he remained until his retirement. He was a consulting surgeon in the Franco-Prussian War and one of Lister's major champions in Europe. He performed the first excision of carcinoma of the rectum in 1878 and described his contracture in 1881. He devised a splint and spoon which bear his name. He tried to treat tuberculosis in bones and joints by iodine, cod liver oil and diet which heralded attempts at preventive surgery. In 1894 he reported three patients with scrotal cancer who worked with paraffin and tar.

He possessed a great literary ability and under the pen name Richard Leander wrote poetry and a book entitled "Dreams by French Firesides" which has a permanent place in German literature. He was one of Lister's most ardent admirers and it was his support which resulted in the early introduction of antiseptic surgery throughout Germany and undoubtedly helped Lister's triumphal tour in 1875.

VOLTOLINI DISEASE

Chronic infective otitis media.

Friedrich E.R. Voltolini (1819–1889) German ear, nose and throat surgeon who worked in Breslau. He first employed galvano-cautery in surgery of the larynx, performed the first operation on the larynx through the mouth (1889) and wrote a textbook on rhino-laryngology.

VON ECONOMO DISEASE

v. ECONOMO DISEASE

VON GIERKE DISEASE

v. GIERKE DISEASE

VON HIPPEL-LINDAU DISEASE

v. HIPPEL-LINDAU DISEASE

VON JAKSCH ANEMIA

Acute hemolytic anemia in childhood.

Rudolf von Jaksch (1855–1947) Czech physician in Prague.

VON PIRQUET TEST

One of the earlier tests for tuberculosis in which tuberculin was applied to an abrasion on the skin. It was soon replaced by the Mantoux Test (*v. supra*).

Clemens P. von Pirquet (1874–1929) Austrian physician born in Vienna and became Professor of Pediatrics at Johns Hopkins in 1908 then moved to Breslau (Wroclaw) and finally Vienna in 1911. In 1911 he described the glomerulonephritis associated with serum sickness and coined the term allergy.

VON RECKLINGHAUSEN DISEASE

v. RECKLINGHAUSEN DISEASE

VON WILLEBRAND DISEASE

The first hereditary bleeding disorder distinguished from hemophilia, characterized by a prolonged bleeding time, a low von Willebrand factor and an autosomal dominant family inheritance, although in some instances it may be recessive.

VON WILLEBRAND FACTOR

The plasma protein absent in the severe forms of von Willebrand disease.

Erik A. von Willebrand (1870–1939) He was born in Vasa, the son of the district engineer and graduated in medicine in Helsinki. He became the doctor in Mariehamn, the capital of the Åland Islands, where he was registrar at the Mariehamn spa in 1894 and 1895 and learnt about "Alandic hemorrhagic disease". In 1899 he gained his Ph.D. with the thesis "Blood changes after venesection". He was lecturer in anatomy from 1901–1903 and then worked in the Department of Physiology at Helsinki University where he described blood changes during muscular exercise, metabolism and obesity and CO_2 and water exchange through the human skin. He published two papers on "Physiology and Clinical Management in Treatment with Hot Air" (the Finnish sauna)! Throughout his lifetime he maintained his interest in the latter form of treatment as well as in metabolic disorders and hematological problems.

In 1903 he gained his "Docent" in physical therapy and in 1908 in internal medicine. From 1908 to 1935 when he retired he was a member of the Department of Medicine at the "Diakonissanstaltens" Hospital in Helsinki (Helsingfors) and was Director of this hospital between 1922 and 1931. He was appointed Honorary Professor in 1930. He wrote extensively on obesity, gout and diabetes, published a method for assessing the ketone bodies in the urine in 1912, and in 1913 wrote on dietetic management of diabetes. He was one of the first to employ insulin and in 1922 wrote a paper on its use in the treatment of diabetic coma. His principal papers in hematology included one in 1899 "Regeneration of the Blood in Chlorosis" and in 1918 "Knowledge of Aplastic Anaemia".

In 1925 a five year old child from the Åland Islands came to Helsinki for investigation. Both the mother and father belonged to families with histories of bleeding, and three other siblings died from hemorrhage. Von Willebrand mapped the pedigree and found among 23 bleeders of the 66 members of the family, 16 were women and 7 were men. He discussed these findings with a geneticist, who concluded from von Willebrand's family history that this disease was dominant in inheritance pattern in contrast to that of genuine hemophilia and that there was an equal distribution in both sexes. In 1926 von Willebrand first gave a detailed account of this particular family and compared it with other known hemorrhagic diatheses described at the time by Glanzmann in Berne and Frank in Breslau (Wroclaw). He concluded that this was a previously unknown form of hemophilia and termed it pseudohemophilia with a prolonged bleeding time as its most prominent sign. His findings were noted by Minot in Boston, who described similar families in 1928. The picture was somewhat muddied by joint investigations he undertook with the German authority Jurgens who felt that the disorder was primarily a problem of platelet function abnormalities rather than an abnormality in a plasma factor. Von Willebrand was a very modest man and bowed to the dominating forces from the renowned medical schools of central Europe. Jurgens was the German leader of an organisation called the "Pathfinders" which was ordered to join a Nazi organization. He refused, was forced to leave Germany and went to Switzerland where Glanzmann and Fornier helped him, until von Willebrand wrote to George Minot in Boston who agreed to provide a position in his clinic for Jurgens.

VOORHEES BAG

Bag inserted into the cervix and inflated with water to induce labour.

James D. Voorhees (1869–1929) U.S. obstetrician born in Morristown, New Jersey, a direct descendant of one of the first settlers on Long Island from Holland (Albert Cooke van Voorhees). He graduated in 1893 from the College of Physicians and Surgeons, Columbia University, New York, and became an Associate Professor of Obstetrics there. He became one of New York's most fashionable obstetricians. He died following a stroke after holidays in California some years after retiring.

VULPIAN ATROPHY

Progressive muscular atrophy of muscles in the scapulo-humeral region.

VULPIAN-HEIDENHAIN-SHERRINGTON PHENOMENON

Stimulation of sensory nerves supplying paralyzed atrophic muscles may result in slow contraction due to antidromic impulses.

Edmé F.A. Vulpian (1826–1887) He was born in Paris where his father wrote successfully for the stage, but died of smallpox after refusing vaccination, leaving four children in poverty. To make a living, Vulpian obtained a technician's job with Flourens, the discoverer of the respiratory centre of the medulla oblongata. The latter work had shown that the cerebellum and the semicircular canal were important for the co-ordination of movement in pigeons. Through Flourens' influence, Vulpian was entered into medical school and his doctoral thesis in 1853 was regarded as being of the highest standard. He was appointed Médecin des Hôpitaux in 1857 and Agrégé in 1860, but continued to teach neuro-physiology until 1866 when he succeeded Cruveilhier despite a great deal of opposition from the Bishops on the Senate because of the paper Vulpian had written on the higher functions of the brain. In 1862, together with Charcot, he took over the Salpêtrière.

Vulpian was an experimenter as well as a fine teacher but he was somewhat retiring and therefore greatly overshadowed by Charcot. He confirmed Flourens' observations concerning the functions of the semicircular canal and the cerebellum and established principles of regeneration of nerves as well as investigating the vasomotor functions. Using chromium salts he discovered the chromaffin system of the adrenal gland and demonstrated that curare caused paralysis by affecting a point between nerve and muscle. He recognized the lack of the use of the microscope in French investigative medicine, and with it showed that tabes dorsalis was not primarily a dorsal column disease, and demonstrated the retrograde changes in the spinal columns after amputation or nerve sectioning.

He was a prodigious worker who started his day at 4 a.m. and was much admired by his students as an outstanding teacher. Madame Dejerine was impressed by his intelligence, gentleness and good looks, and has recorded how he pointed out to her the extension of the big toe in paraplegics long before Babinski's demonstration. Together with Charcot he founded the journal "Archives de Physiologie Normale et Pathologique". He was permanent secretary of the Academy of Sciences and undoubtedly was one of the great influences on French medicine. The achievements of both his colleague, Charcot, and his students, the Dejerines, perhaps kept him from the international recognition that might normally have been expected.

Rudolf P.H. Heidenhain (*v. supra*).

Charles S. Sherrington (*v. supra*).

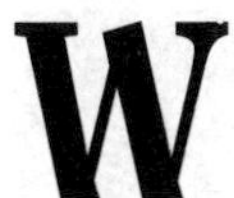

WAARDENBURG SYNDROME

White forelock, deafness, broadbased nose and heavy eyebrows. It is inherited as an autosomal dominant.

Petrus J. Waardenburg (1886–1979). Dutch ophthalmologist. He was born in Nijeveen and graduated in medicine from the University of Utrecht. He maintained a lifelong interest in hereditary eye disease and genetics and wrote a book in 1932 and then collaborated with Klein and Franceschetti to produce a two volume classic "Genetics in Ophthalmology".

WAGNER CORPUSCLES

Tactile corpuscles.

Rudolf Wagner (1805–1864) German anatomist and physiologist in Göttingen who re-issued Goennery's treatise on anatomy (1791–6) in 1839–45 with Henle's assistance. He showed that the Bell law of spinal nerve roots applied to fish in 1846, and with von Baer organised the first congress of anthropologists. He discovered the germinal spot and wrote a treatise on physiology.

WAGNER-JAUREGG TREATMENT

Treatment of syphilis involving the central nervous system by infecting the patients with malaria.

Julius Wagner von Jauregg (1857–1940) He was born in Wells, Austria. His father was a state official from Silesia and was born plain Wagner but was granted the right of a noble title in 1883 and added his mother's name, von Jauregg (her real name was Jauernigg). At the end of the World War I Austrians were deprived by law of their titles but he was granted permission to use the hyphenated name Wagner-Jauregg.

Following typhoid as a child he became quite athletic, but whilst a student developed tuberculosis with hemoptysis. Not having the money to go to a sanatorium he continued his studies. He maintained a lifelong interest in athletics, performing regular calisthenics and weight lifting.

He studied medicine at Vienna, graduating in 1880 and then worked at the Stricker Pathology Institute in Vienna. Initially he was unsuccessful in obtaining a post in internal medicine, so he went to a psychiatric clinic with Leidsdorf, and in 1885 became a Privatdozent. He was appointed Head of Psychiatry at Graz in 1889 and in 1892 returned to Vienna, taking charge of Psychiatry at the Allgemeines Krankenhaus. He became Professor of Neurology and Psychiatry in 1902 following Krafft-Ebing. In 1887 he developed the idea that fever might be of value in the treatment of psychosis since he noted "not rarely psychoses were healed through intercurrent infectious disease" and he suggested that "one should intentionally imitate this experiment of nature". He initially tried typhoid vaccines, tuberculin and erysipelis but in 1917 tried an inoculation of malaria. The blood was obtained from wounded and sometimes shell shocked troops with malaria admitted to his clinic. Of 9 patients with general paralysis of the insane so treated, 6 were benefited and 3 were still working 4 years later. For this work he won the Nobel Prize in 1927, the first psychiatrist to do so. These studies led to all the methods of stress therapy, electric shock, insulin, etc. used in psychiatry.

He was a pioneer in attempts to prevent cretinism by the addition of iodide to table salt in areas which were endemic for goitre. He attracted many people to his clinic who became famous, von Economo, Pilcz, Gertsmann and Poetzl, the latter succeeding him. He slept poorly and would get up and play chess with an imaginary opponent. On a winter's night he would often play with a friend by telephone. He was a complete conservative and his dress did not change throughout his life, which made him a readily recognizable figure in Viennese society.

WALDENSTRÖM DISEASE (1)

Acute thyrotoxic encephalopathy. Characteristically seen in the elderly and consists of a goitre, exophthalmos and thyrotoxic crisis with vomiting, diarrhea, auricular fibrillation and fever, and often associated with bulbar paralysis with 6th, 7th and 12th nerve palsies which may be combined with psychotic manifestations.

WALDENSTRÖM HEPATITIS

Chronic active hepatitis.

WALDENSTRÖM HYPERGLOBULINEMIA

or

WALDENSTRÖM HYPERGLOBULINEMIC PURPURA

A polyclonal increase in gamma globulin which characteristically occurs in women and runs a benign protracted course with recurrent purpuric eruptions over the lower limbs, leaving brown pigmentation. Hepatosplenomegaly may be associated.

WALDENSTRÖM MACROGLOBULINEMIA

A dysproteinemia characterized by a monoclonal increase in IgM. Clinically the patient often presents with mucosal bleeding such as epistaxis, visual disorders and hepatosplenomegaly. The clinical symptoms are caused by hyperviscosity. Sometimes a widespread polyneuropathy occurs due to antibody activity to neural components in the IgM (v. Bing Neel Syndrome).

WALDENSTRÖM UVEOPAROTITIS

v. HEERFORDT SYNDROME

WALDENSTRÖM-KJELLBERG SYNDROME

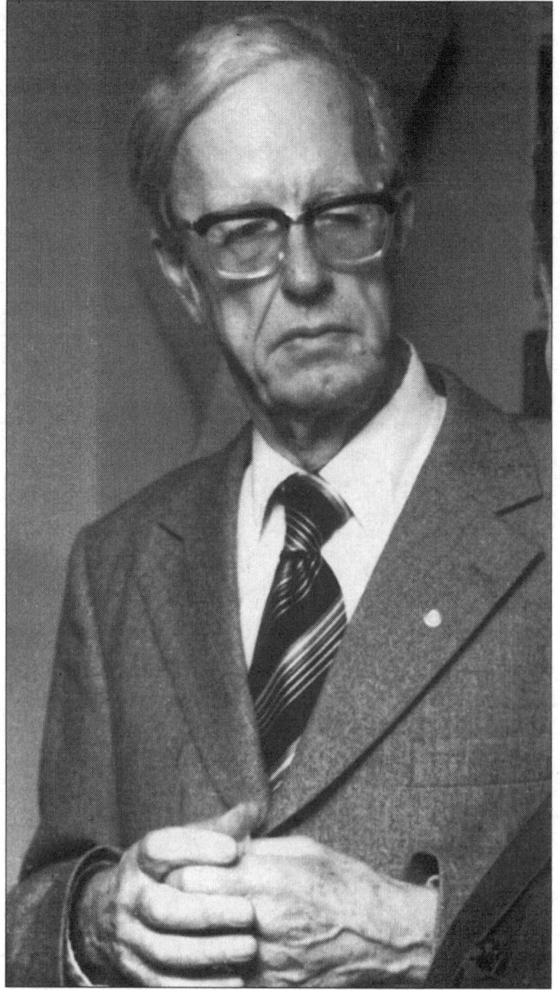

Jan G. Waldenström (Courtesy of Jan Waldenström)

v. PLUMMER-VINSON SYNDROME

Jan G. Waldenström (1906–) Swedish physician, son of Johann Waldenström (*v. infra*). He was Professor of Theoretical Medicine at Uppsala University in 1947 and in 1950 became Professor of Medicine at Lund University and head of the department of medicine in Malmö General Hospital. He wrote his thesis on acute porphyria which contained the first report on the heredity aspects of this disease. He introduced the term porphyria cutanea tarda. Later he worked with Vahlquist on the colorless chromagen which was named porphobilinogen. Another subject of continued interest was dysproteinemia which he studied with Kai Pedersen in Uppsala and

C-B. Laurell in Malmö. The monoclonality (M component) of the immunoglobulin present in large quantities in myeloma and macroglobulinemia was established. He also described a non-progressive form of paraproteinemia which he called benign monoclonal gammopathy. He discovered the carcinoid syndrome which consisted of flushing attacks and diarrhea and investigated the metabolic reasons for these symptoms. His interest in paraneoplastic mechanisms resulted in the book "Paraneoplasia" which was published in 1978.

Waldenström travelled extensively and was a visiting Professor at many world centres. He stressed that medicine is a part of biology and was quoted by one of his colleagues as saying "A professor of medicine had to travel widely before the Second World War to hear the latest developments and after the war to see if they were correct!" For many years he was editor of the Acta Medica Scandinavica (now The Journal of Internal Medicine). Three of his sons are doctors making them the fifth successive generation of medical practitioners in his family.

WALDENSTRÖM DISEASE (2)

Osteochrondritis deformans juvenilis.

v. LEGG-CALVÉ-PERTHES DISEASE

Johann Henning Waldenström (1877–1972) Swedish surgeon. Professor of Orthopaedic Surgery and head of orthopaedics at the Karolinska Hospital in Stockholm. The father of Jan Waldenström (*v. supra*). He established by liver biopsy that amyloid disease of the liver secondary to bone tuberculosis disappeared when the bone lesion was healed.

WALDEYER RING

Ring of lymphatic tissue consisting of the lingual, pharyngeal and the palatine tonsils as well as other collections of lymph tissue in the area.

Heinrich W. Waldeyer (1837–1921) He was born in Hehlen, Brunswick. He was a pupil of Henle and became an inspiring teacher himself. Whilst at Breslau (Wroclaw, Poland), Carl Weigert was his assistant in 1868. He moved to Strasburg as Professor of Anatomy to make that school a very exciting one, with other great teachers such as von Recklinghausen and Kussmaul. Whilst there in 1877 he directed Ludwig Edinger (*v. supra*) in his initial studies and he influenced Bernard Sachs (v. TAY-SACHS DISEASE). He made many important contributions, coining the term neurone to describe the cellular function unit of the nervous system and enunciating and clarifying that concept in 1891. He described the plasma cell in 1875 and the ring of lymphoid tissue in 1884. He studied the anatomy of the pelvic viscera and the pregnant uterus. He became Professor of Anatomy in Berlin in 1883. Waldeyer conducted important studies in embryology and discovered the germinal epithelium in the ovary (1870). He investigated the development of cancer (1867–1872). He introduced the term chromosome in 1888.

WALKER SARCOMA

Tumor of the rat.

George Walker (1869–) U.S. pathologist.

WALLENBERG SYNDROME

Syndrome of posterior inferior cerebellar artery thrombosis. Ipsilateral cerebellar signs, hemiataxia, hemianesthesia, contralateral loss of pain and temperature sensibility in the arm, trunk, leg, ipsilateral paralysis of larynx and palate leading to difficulty in swallowing, Horner syndrome and facial anesthesia.

Adolf Wallenberg (1862–1949) German neurologist who described the avian brain while working with Edinger and examined the role of the olfactory system in the assessment, recognition, and ingestion of food. He elucidated the trigeminal lemniscus and described his syndrome in 1895.

WALLERIAN DEGENERATION

Secondary degeneration of nerve fiber when continuity with the cell of origin is interrupted.

Augustus V. Waller (1816–1870) He was born on Elverton Farm in Faversham, England, but spent his youth in the south of France, returning to school in England when he was 14 years old. He was a student in Paris and graduated in medicine in 1840. Whilst there he became interested in the histology of the frog's tongue. He practiced in Kensington, London, for 10 years from 1842 but whenever he could spare the time he undertook histological studies and during this time published papers in the Transactions of the Royal Society. One concerned the diapedesis of red cells which had already been described by Addison. The second dealt with the section of the glosso-pharyngeal and hyperglossal nerves of the frog in which he showed that the distal segment cut off from the cells underwent degeneration, whilst the proximal segment remained intact for a long period of time. He concluded that nerve fibers were simply prolongations of the cells from which they derived their nourishment and from this arose the term Wallerian degeneration. He severed the anterior spinal nerve root and the resultant degeneration showed that the main part of the cell was in the spinal cord, whereas when the posterior root was sectioned they were in the posterior root ganglia. In 1851 he gave up practice and went to Bonn where he worked with an ophthalmologist J.L. Budge, and worked on the control of the size of the pupil. Together they described the vasodilator activity of the cervical sympathetic, confirming the findings of Claude Bernard and Brown-Séquard. He won the Monthyon prize twice, once for this work with Budge and then for the work on the pathway of degeneration. In 1856 he moved from Bonn to Paris but became ill possibly with rheumatic fever. He spent two years in England in an effort to regain his health and became Professor of Physiology at Birmingham till illness forced him to retire to Bruges. In 1868 he resumed medical practice in Geneva but was troubled with angina pectoris and died shortly after. His son A.D. Waller was also a distinguished physiologist and in 1887 demonstrated an electric current in the human heart by placing electrodes on the surface of the body, the forerunner of the electrocardiogram. On one occasion when his father's name was mentioned the younger Waller remarked "I am *the* Wallerian degeneration!"

WANGENSTEEN TUBE

Tube for continuous drainage of stomach or duodenum.

Owen H. Wangensteen (1898–) U.S. surgeon, Professor of Surgery, University of Minnesota, who worked with F. de Quervain (*v. supra*) in Berne (1927–28) and wrote extensively on etiology and management of peptic ulcer and bowel obstruction.

WARBURG APPARATUS

Method for measuring respiration of tissues or gaseous products of chemical reactions.

Otto H. Warburg (1883–1970) He came to Berlin in 1896 when his father Emil Warburg was appointed as Professor of Physics and later elected President of the Imperial Institute of Physics. Visitors to his parents' home influenced his future. Engelmann (a famous German physiologist who was interested in muscle) discussed the effects of light on marine plant cells and Emil Fischer raised his interest in enzymes whilst van Hoff discussed the problems of transformation of energy in chemical reactions. He was trained by Emil Fischer as well as other notables including his father. After working with Fischer he spent some time at the zoological research station in Naples where he investigated the eggs of the sea urchin. During the First World War he served as an officer at the front and after the war recommenced his studies in biochemistry.

In 1904–5 whilst working with Fischer he studied the effects of pancreatin in splitting racemic leucine ethyl ester. From 1910–1914 he studied the red cells and the respiration of sea urchin eggs, and in 1918–20 developed the biochemical manometry techniques which made him world famous. From 1923–1925 he employed tissue slice methods and investigated tumor metabolism. In 1924 he discovered the iron oxygen transferring constituent of the respiratory enzymes and in the next couple of years examined the effects of carbon monoxide on inhibition of cell respiration. He discovered the yellow enzymes (1922–27) and elaborated the role of nicotinic acid amide in the transfer of hydrogen. He isolated several glycolytic enzymes and discovered anaerobic and aerobic glycolysis in tumor cells. He established the quantum requirement for photosynthesis which possibly derived from his father's ideas in physics. He purified many enzymes in crystalline form and continued working in biochemistry during the 2nd World War holding himself aloof from the politics of the day. He won the Nobel Prize in 1933 and attracted many students, three of whom won the Nobel Prize in 1953 (Lynen, Krebs and Theorell). He was a confirmed bachelor with a passion for dogs and horses. A relative, G.S. Plant, comments that the dogs always made a visit to his house a perilous undertaking. His butler and assistant was a soldier who had been his orderly in World War I. Although Jewish his fame was such that the Nazis let him continue his scientific work. Few, if any, biochemists made so many important discoveries in half a century.

WARDROP DISEASE

Ulcer in the matrix of the nail with resultant sloughing of the nail seen in very debilitated patients. Also called onychia maligna.

James Wardrop (1782–1869) Born in Torbane Hill, Scotland, he graduated in medicine from Edinburgh but settled in London in 1809. He treated aneurysm by ligation at the distal end of the tumor and performed this operation successfully on two occasions on the carotid artery and once on the subclavian in the case of an innominate aneurysm. He wrote an important monograph on the morbid anatomy of the human eye in 1808 and introduced the term keratitis. He wrote some very sarcastic and venomous papers in The Lancet in 1826–27 and in the same journal in 1834 in some correspondence called "intercepted letters" he abused some of the leading names of the London medical profession.

WARTENBERG DISEASE

Numbness and pain in the hand supplied by the superficial branch of the radial nerve.

WARTENBERG SIGN

1. Diminution of the palpebral vibration of the upper lid on the affected side when both eyelids are closed in 7th nerve palsy.
2. Diminished abduction of the thumb in median nerve palsy. Also called Wartenberg oriental prayer sign – the patient is asked to hold his hands palms away in front of the face with index fingers touching and thumbs fully extended – paralysis of the median nerve prevents the thumb touching its mate.
3. Little finger in a position of abduction in ulnar paralysis.
4. Pyramidal sign of the upper limb—flexion of fingers against resistance causes flexion and opposition of the thumb on the affected side (v. HOFFMAN SIGN).
5. In Parkinson disease there is a decrease in free swinging of the legs hanging passively over the edge of the bed, and caused to swing.

Robert Wartenberg (1887–1956) U.S. neurologist. He was born in Grodno in Germany and graduated from the University of Rostock in 1919. He worked with Nonne in Hamburg and Forster in Breslau (Wroclaw, Poland) and became head of the nerve clinic at Freiburg and Privatdozent (Associate Professor) in neurology in 1933. He left Germany in 1935, migrating to San Francisco and was finally appointed in 1952 as Clinical Professor of Neurology at the University of California. He was a dynamic teacher who enthused his students and combined his thoroughness with a keen sense of humor, always kind and helpful and impressed them with expressions such as "by the great Babinski, no!" He could be very caustic with his colleagues but here too he mainly had admirers. In Germany he had been very impressed by Bing's work and translated the first edition of Bing's textbook on neurology into English. This book has been updated by his colleagues. Although persecuted by the Nazis he staunchly defended his German colleagues who had remained in Germany and whom he thought were wrongly accused during the post-war period.

WARTHIN SIGN

Exaggeration of pulmonary sounds in acute pericarditis.

WARTHIN TUMOR

Benign salivary gland tumor with lymphoid tissue covered by epithelium.

WARTHIN-FINKELDEY GIANT CELLS

Multinucleated giant cells seen in the lymphoid tissues of patients with measles.

Aldred S. Warthin (1866–1931) U.S. pathologist, born in Greensberg, Indiana; worked on the pathology of lymph nodes and the hemopoietic system as well as the effects of mustard gas poisoning. He developed a technique for identifying spirochetes in tissue and in 1913 wrote a classic description of fat embolism. He was Professor of Pathology at Ann Arbor, Michigan.

Wilhelm Finkeldey German pathologist who worked in Augsburg.

WASSERMANN TEST

Complement fixation test for syphilis using sensitized lipid extracts of beef heart as antigen.

August P. von Wassermann (1866–1925) He was born in Bamberg, the son of a wealthy banker, and graduated in medicine from Strasburg in 1888. Some felt he carried on his investigations as a hobby and he certainly did not need to earn a living. He joined the Robert Koch Institute for Infectious Disease in 1890 and remained there until 1906. He was short and hunch backed but always dressed with extreme elegance as if trying to hide his deformity.

He was a superb speaker, expressing his conclusions openly without scientific inhibitions. It was said that his theoretical knowledge was rather weak and that his practical application was not all that good either but that he relied on a number of technicians to do his bidding in the laboratory. These were dubbed his scientific "coolies". He recognized the importance of Bordet's and Genou's discovery concerning complement and initially endeavored to develop this as a test for tuberculosis. This led him to give a talk and conclude that the complement reaction was a valuable method in the diagnosis of tuberculosis. He later disproved everything he had said in that particular talk, and when he came to talk on the subject again the audience arrived expecting to hear quite a deal of acrimonious discussion. However he dealt with each discussant extremely well, admitting immediately without any attempt at dodging the issue, that they were right, congratulating them on the pains they had taken to check his statements and show that the complement reaction was not a suitable method for the diagnosis of tuberculosis. The audience was rather disappointed at the tameness of the lecture up until this stage. At this point he stopped, turned towards the audience, raised his finger and said that the complement reaction was however of superlative value in the diagnosis of syphilis and was 100% successful even in the oldest of cases. In view of his previous claims for tuberculosis, this was greeted with somewhat lukewarm applause and people such as Julius Citroen left to undertake the test on patients of their own and showed conclusively that Wassermann was right. The Wassermann reaction soon became a worldwide test and an invaluable method in the diagnosis of syphilis. This was only a year after Schaudin's demonstration of the causative organism (the spirochaete *Treponema pallidum*) which had also received a lukewarm reception. Wassermann attributed the development of his test to the findings of Bordet and Genou and the theoretical hypotheses put forward by Ehrlich in his explanation of antibody formation. Wassermann received numerous honors, but he never became a Professor at Berlin University and was never awarded the Nobel Prize, to which he is said to have aspired.

WATERHOUSE-FRIDERICHSEN SYNDROME

Association of bacteremia (usually meningococcemia) with extensive skin hemorrhage, shock, acute adrenal hemorrhage and adrenal insufficiency.

Rupert Waterhouse (1873–1958) English physician born in Sheffield and studied medicine at St. Bartholomew's Hospital, qualifying in 1897. He moved to Bath in 1901 and became a physician at the Royal United Hospital and the Royal National Hospital for

Rheumatic Diseases. He wrote a number of papers which were mainly related to rheumatology and published his description of acute adrenal deficiency in 1911. After he retired as a physician he practiced as a consultant pathologist. In the 1914–1918 war he served first as a soldier in the North Somerset Yeomanry and later with the Royal Medical Army Corps in Gallipoli, Egypt and France. He was well known for his sense of humor and wit, and was regarded as one of the finest after-dinner speakers in the west country. Towards the end of his life he became very deaf and had increasing disabilities due to osteo-arthritis and Paget disease of his hip.

Carl Friderichsen (1886–) Danish pediatrician who published his report in 1918. He wrote on vitamin A deficiency and acidosis in babies.

WATSON-SCHWARTZ TEST

Test for porphobilinogen in urine using Ehrlich reagent.

Cecil J. Watson (1901–) U.S. physician born in Minneapolis and graduated M.D. University of Minneapolis in 1925. He was the son of a physician but, influenced by the Professor of Pathology E.T. Bell, he initially trained as a pathologist and wrote a Ph.D. thesis on splenic disorders. He developed hepatitis and this commenced his interest in bile pigments which in turn led to him going to Germany to study basic pyrrole chemistry with Hans Fischer in 1930, returning to the U.S. in 1932. He became Professor and Chairman of Medicine in 1942 until 1966. He made major contributions in liver disease and porphyria.

S. Schwartz (1916–) U.S. physician born in Minneapolis and graduated M.D. University of Minneapolis in 1943 and became Research Professor of Medicine there in 1961.

WEBER-CHRISTIAN DISEASE

Febrile relapsing nodular non-suppurative panniculitis.

Frederick Parkes Weber (1863–1962) British physician who wrote many fascinating articles including one on death in art (1910). He had a life-long interest in rare disorders, writing two books on this subject as well as others on medical philosophy. He was the son of H.D. Weber (*v. infra*) and educated at Cambridge and St. Bartholomew's Hospital. He studied in Vienna and Paris. Like his father he was a keen alpinist and collector of coins and vases which towards the end of his life he gave to museums.

Henry A. Christian

v. HAND-SCHÜLLER-CHRISTIAN DISEASE

WEBER-KLIPPEL SYNDROME

v. KLIPPEL-TRÉNAUNAY-WEBER SYNDROME

WEBER SYNDROME

Ipsilateral ophthalmoplegia and ptosis with contralateral hemiplegia due to a midbrain lesion at the 3rd nucleus and cerebral peduncle.

Sir Herman D. Weber (1823–1918) He was the son of a German father and Italian mother and lived on his father's farm in Bavaria and then in Hesse-Cassel. He entered medical school in Marburg and graduated in Bonn. There he met a number of Englishmen including the Waterloo veterans, Sir Peregrine Maitland and Sir Henry Havelock, as well as Sir James Simpson. Whilst at Marburg he met Carlyle and had frequent walks and talks with that philosopher and this, together with his love of Shakespeare and his desire to read the plays in their native language, led him to learn English. He obtained a position at the German Hospital in Dalston, England, and married an Englishwoman in 1854. He went to Guy's Hospital and became a member of the Royal College of Physicians in 1855. He was an extremely charming and companionable man who gathered a circle around him at any soiree and rapidly had them in his spell. In his early days his friends included Addison, Henry Parkes, Wilson Fox and Hilton Fagg. He became especially interested in the treatment of tuberculosis and was the English founder of "Climato-Therapy". He advised his patients to go to Switzerland for the winter, where he himself was in the habit of spending his holidays in either the Swiss Tyrolese or the Italian Alps. He was a member of the Alpine Club and when he was 68 climbed both the Wetterhorn and the Jungfrau and when he was 73 crossed the Capuchin from Pontresina to Sils, and on his 80th birthday crossed the Diarolezza. He was a great advocate of healthy exercise and walked between 40–50 miles per week. He wrote numerous papers on the importance of climate in the treatment of tuberculosis. In his later years he collected coins and became an authority on Greek coins. He travelled extensively visiting Greece, Sicily, Tunis and Palestine. Although retired from practice, he continued to enjoy life and gave a lecture to the Royal College of Physicians entitled "Prolongation of Life" wherein he attributed longevity to muscular exercise. He thus antedated Dr. Paul White by some years! He influenced several Prime Ministers to undertake climatotherapy, viz. Lord Darby, Earl Russell, Lord Salisbury, Lord Roseberry and Sir H. Campbell-Bannerman, and particularly advised climatotherapy in the high valleys of the Engadine.

WEBER TEST

This is a hearing test. Vibrations from a tuning fork placed centrally on the forehead are better heard in the diseased ear in middle ear deafness but in the normal ear in nerve deafness.

Friedrich E. Weber-Liel (1832–1891) German otologist.

WEGENER GRANULOMATOSIS

Necrotising respiratory granulomas, angiitis, glomerulonephritis and frequent involvement of the sinuses and sometimes peripheral neuritis.

Friedrich Wegener (1907–1990) German pathologist who was born in Varel Oldenburg. His father was a physician and his mother was a Swedish gymnastic director. He was a fine athlete who became the German hammer-throwing champion in 1931 whilst a medical student. He graduated at Kiel in 1932 and commenced training in pathology at the University of Kiel under the direction of Professors L. Jores, R. Huckel and Martin Staemmler. The latter was appointed as director of the Pathology Institute at Breslau (Wroclaw) University in 1935 and took Wegener with him as an assistant. In Breslau he studied two patients with granulomatosis who were similar to one he had already studied in 1934 and presented the three to the German Pathological Society meeting in 1936 as a variant of periarteritis nodosa. The paper was widely acclaimed and Ludwig Aschoff (*v. supra*) hailed it as reporting a previously undescribed entity. Wegener continued his studies until the outbreak of the war in 1939, when he became a German army pathologist to be captured by the British and after the war was a farmer for two years and then became a public health officer, joining the medical academy in Lubeck and eventually was appointed as a professor there (1966–1970). A torchlight procession was held for him on his retirement and this was led by the medical students and doctors of Lubeck.

WEGNER DISEASE

The separation of orthochondritic epiphyses in congenital syphilis.

Friedrich R.G. Wegner (1843–1917) German pathologist.

WEIL DISEASE

Leptospirosis. This may present with jaundice, fever, oliguria, hemorrhagic tendencies and circulatory collapse.

Adolf Weil (1848–1916) German physician who worked with Aberhalden and isolated norleucine in 1913. Professor of Medicine in Tartu, Estonia and in Berlin.

WEIL-FELIX REACTION

Agglutination of strains of *Proteus vulgaris* by sera from patients with rickettsial infection.

Edmund Weil (1880–1922) Austrian bacteriologist.

A. Felix (1887–1956) British bacteriologist who was born in Silesia and studied chemistry in Vienna, spending two years working with Lafar in mycology. He was called up in 1914 and worked in a field ambulance near Cracow. It was there that he met Weil, who was an Associate Professor of Bacteriology at Prague. They developed the test and adapted it for the diagnosis of typhus in troops on the Eastern front. At the end of the 1st World War he worked with Weil in Prague, but in 1921 strong Zionist leanings led him to migrate to Palestine. In 1927 he moved to the Lister Institute in London. Here he discovered the Vi antigen in the typhoid bacillus and developed techniques for Vi-phage typing. In 1939 he was appointed to the Emergency Public Health Laboratory Service which became the central enteric reference laboratory and he remained as its Director until his retirement in 1954 when he returned to the Lister Institute.

WEINGARTEN SYNDROME

Tropical pulmonary eosinophilia – thought to be an allergic response to a filarial infestation. Occurs most commonly in Indians living in Singapore. Characterized by cough and nocturnal bronchospasm with eosinophilia and diffuse small pulmonary infiltrates.

R.J. Weingarten German physician who worked in India.

WEINSTEIN SYNDROME

One of the primary gonadal failure syndromes in the male. Small testes with germinal hypoplasia and hyalinised tubules but normal Leydig cells. Associated features are retinal degeneration causing blindness, neurosensory deafness, cataract, obesity and short stature. There is hyperuricemia and hypertriglyceridemia and low testosterone levels with no response to human chorionic gonadotrophins (H.C.G.).

Richard L. Weinstein U.S. physician.

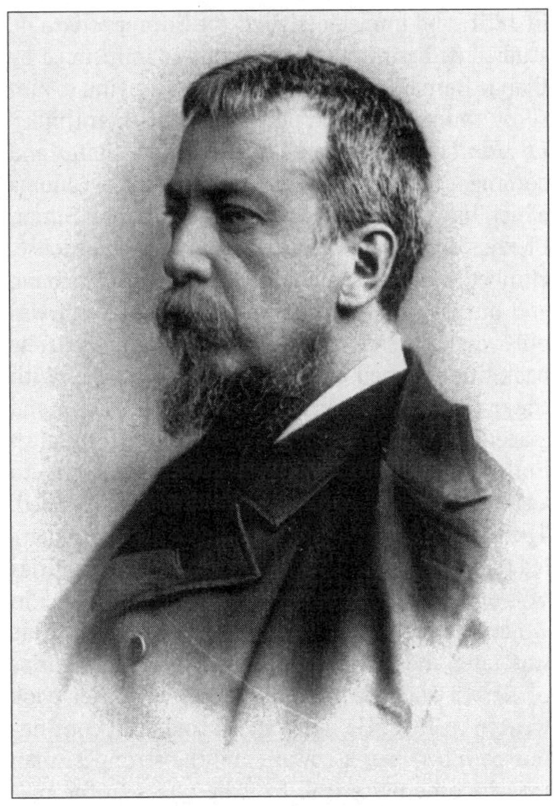

Silas W. Weir-Mitchell (Courtesy of the Royal Society of Medicine, London, UK)

WEIR-MITCHELL THERAPY

Treatment of neurotic conditions by isolation and diet.

Silas W. Weir-Mitchell (1829–1914) He was born in Philadelphia to a family that had 3 generations of physicians, was accustomed to wealth and cultural pursuits, and was deeply religious. He was required to read a daily bible text and to attend church twice on Sundays where he wiled away his time reading novels such as "Midshipman Easy". When he first joined the University of Pennsylvania he had a poor record, preferring to play billiards, write poetry, and play truant rather than to deal with subjects such as mathematics which he cordially disliked. His father, a distinguished physician, J.K. Mitchell, said to him "you are wanting in nearly all the qualities that go to make a success in medicine". He enrolled at the Jefferson Medical College in 1848, graduated M.D.

in 1851, and immediately left for Europe where he studied in Paris and there was most influenced by Claude Bernard who impressed him by saying to him "Why think? Exhaustively experiment then think." (*v. Hunter*). He returned to the United States and commenced work with Hammond on snake venoms which he later extended with W.W. Keen and Simon Flexner. It is said that once a rattlesnake got loose, climbed the back of a chair on which he was sitting and put its swaying head over his shoulder. It was only when the snake touched the hot lamp and drew back that Mitchell could leap back to escape! With the outbreak of the American Civil War, Hammond placed him in charge of Turner's Lane Hospital in Philadelphia and with W.W. Keen he went to Gettysberg and brought back cartloads of wounded. Their records and studies of these wounded soldiers led to the book "Gunshot Wounds and Other Injuries of Nerves" which was published in 1864 and in which the first reference is made to causalgia. This was later more thoroughly described in "Injuries of Nerves and Their Consequences", another book written in 1872. He noted that a soldier in continuous pain becomes a coward and the strongest man may become hysterical. In it he refers to the psychology of amputation and phantom limbs. Other findings of his included the first description of erythromelalgia, post paralysis chorea and the role of the cerebellum in co-ordination, in which he supported the view that the cerebellum augments and re-inforces movements. In 1860 he produced cataracts in frogs by feeding them sugar.

Perhaps he is best known for the establishment of his rest cure for psychoneurosis which became the standard treatment for many decades, particularly in England. His failure to become Professor of Physiology at Jefferson Medical College or at the University of Pennsylvania caused Hammond to write "I am disgusted with everything and can only say that it is an honor to be rejected by such a set of apes!" It is said that one of the reasons for his rejection at Jefferson was that he was a Republican and the trustees were Democrats.

Mitchell was a legendary character whose portraits show him as a handsome man whose rather gaunt features and bearded face make one readily understand why he was likened by many people at the time to "Uncle Sam". He was a superb conversationalist and his personality and humor gave him a wide range of friends including William Osler, Oliver Wendell Holmes, William James, Walt Whitman and Andrew Carnegie. He actively promoted young people who he thought were outstanding, e.g. J.S. Billings and Hydeio Noguchi.

Later in life, from the 1880s onwards, he devoted his attention to writing and wrote two novels which achieved great popular success at the time ("Hugh Wynne" in 1897, and "The Adventures of Francois" in 1898). A novel entitled "Westways" was written after he was 80 and it describes his memory of the horrors of the battle of Gettysberg and its consequences.

He was famous for his sometimes eccentric approaches to patients with functional illnesses. He was asked to see a patient who was thought to be dying, and soon sent all the attendants and assistants from the room, emerging a little later. Asked whether she had any chance of recovery, he said "Yes she will be coming out in a few minutes, I have set her sheets on fire. A clearcut case of hysteria!" Another story is that he was confronted by a lady with a similar problem and having tried all the tricks he knew to induce her to leave her bed, threatened her with rape and commenced to undress – he got down to his undergarments when the woman fled the room screaming! These stories may have grown with the years since in many ways he was rather prim, and Freud's writing shocked him. He is said to have thrown a book on psychoanalysis into his fire, exclaiming "Where did this filthy thing come from?" Harvey Cushing said "He was vain but he had much to be vain about".

He contracted influenza and during the illness read the proof of his poem Bar Abbas, then lapsed into a delirium in which he is said to have reenacted operating on the wounded at Gettysberg. So died an extraordinary man who had had no experience in neurology when he enlisted in the U.S. army in 1862, but became the doyen of American neurology. Mitchell wrote of these days "Keen, Morehouse and I worked on at note-taking often as late as 12 or 1 at night, and when we got through walked home, talking over our cases ... I have worked with many men since, but never with men who took more delight to repay opportunity with labour ... the cases were of amazing interest. Here at one time were 80 epileptics, and every kind of nerve wound, palsies, choreas, stump disorders ... thousands of pages of notes were taken ... about midway we planned the ultimate essays which were to record our work." There resulted a small book on neural injuries full of novelty, a short essay on reflex palsies, etc. One of the most notable was Keen's essay on malingering. Others on epilepsy, muscular disorders and on acute exhaustion were never written because of accidental destruction of the notes by fire. These original descriptions of the results of nerve injuries still warrant re-reading. Weir-Mitchell's son John made a follow up report of 20 of the original patients.

WELCH BACILLUS

Clostridium welchii – the organism causing gas gangrene.

William H. Welch (1850–1934) He was born in Norfolk, Connecticut, the son of a physician, and went to college at Yale, graduating B.A. in 1870. His initial ambitions were to become a professor of Greek, but he was unable to obtain a suitable post and entered medicine at the College of Physicians and Surgeons, New York, where he graduated in 1875. He interned for one year at Bellevue Hospital and then went to Germany where he studied with Hoppe-Selyer, Waldeyer and von Recklinghausen in Strasburg, with Wagner and Ludwig in Leipzig and Cohnheim in Breslau (Wroclaw, Poland). There he worked on pulmonary edema by increasing left ventricular pressure and heard Koch present his work on the Anthrax bacillus. He returned to America thoroughly grounded in pathology and determined to develop experimental pathology. He commenced practice in New York in a small laboratory at the Bellevue Hospital where he gave courses in pathology.

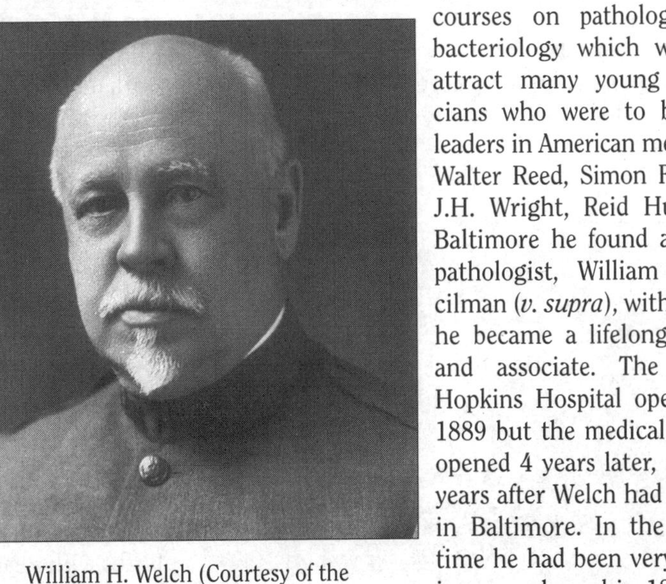

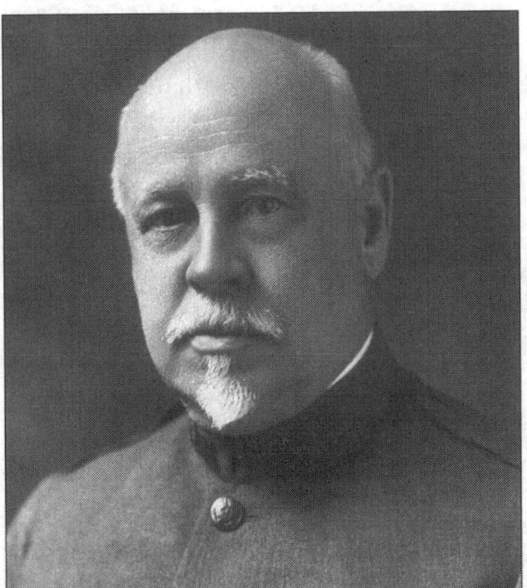

William H. Welch (Courtesy of the Royal Society of Medicine, London, UK)

In 1876 Billings (*v.* WEIR-MITCHELL) went to Europe on behalf of the Johns Hopkins Hospital to examine developments in medical science and care. In Leipzig he met Welch whilst visiting Ludwig's laboratory and was most impressed by him, so that on his return he remarked to F.T. King, the Chairman of the Hospital Board, "That young man should be, in my opinion, one of the first men to be secured when the time comes to begin the medical school." In 1884 after most favorable reports from Billings and Cohnheim, Welch was appointed Professor of Pathology at Johns Hopkins, the first clinical professor at the University. There he commenced his courses on pathology and bacteriology which were to attract many young physicians who were to become leaders in American medicine, Walter Reed, Simon Flexner, J.H. Wright, Reid Hunt. In Baltimore he found another pathologist, William Councilman (*v. supra*), with whom he became a lifelong friend and associate. The Johns Hopkins Hospital opened in 1889 but the medical school opened 4 years later, some 8 years after Welch had arrived in Baltimore. In the meantime he had been very active in research, and in 1892 had discovered the *Clostridium welchii*. His role in the development of the Johns Hopkins School is well known, he was the first Dean and held the chair of Pathology until 1916, when he vacated it to become the Director of the School of Hygiene and Public Health. In 1926 he was appointed Professor of the History of Medicine retiring in 1932. Largely due to the efforts of Welch, a Faculty was attracted to Johns Hopkins of an excellence that had never before been seen or possibly equalled in the United States with Osler as Professor of Medicine, Hallstead, Surgery and Kelly Obstetrics and Gynecology. These men established a school which was equal or superior to any in Europe. Welch was a superb teacher, an excellent lecturer and above all else a person who inspired young people to attempt to achieve the highest ideals of medicine.

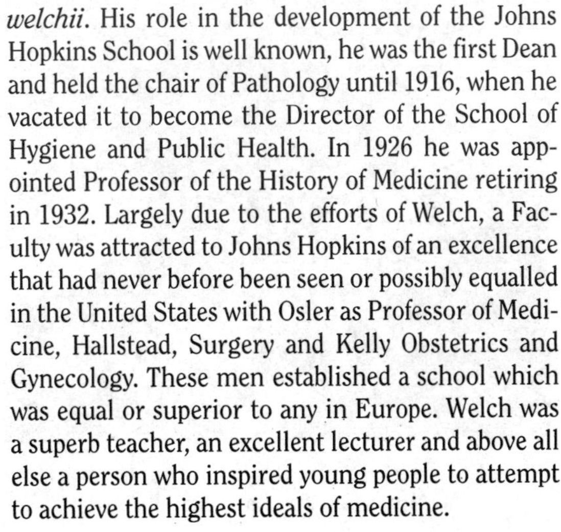

WELLS SYNDROME

Eosinophilic cellulitis – recurrent acute cutaneous swelling, sometimes with blister formation followed by indolent infiltration.

G.C. Wells Contemporary English dermatologist who worked at St. Thomas's Hospital, and St. John's Hospital for Diseases of the Skin in London. He is a keen guitarist and an enthusiastic skier.

WENCKEBACH PHENOMENON

Form of secondary atrio-ventricular heart block with progressive prolongation of the P-R interval, resulting finally in a non-conducted P wave and a dropped beat.

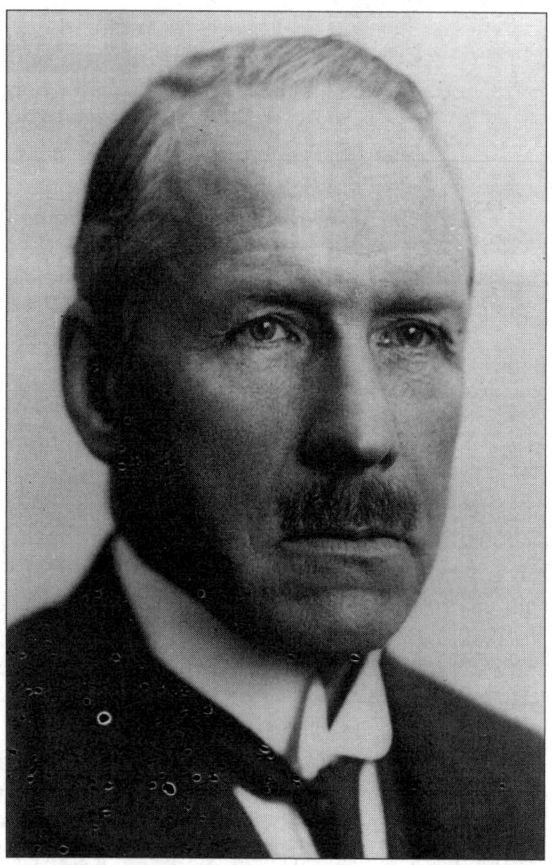

Karel F. Wenckebach (Courtesy of Institut für Geschicte der Medizin an der Universität, Vienna)

Karel F. Wenckebach (1864–1940) He was born in the Hague and graduated M.D. from Utrecht in 1888. In 1901 he was appointed Professor of Medicine at Gröningen and in 1911 in Strasburg. In 1914 he moved to Vienna and remained Professor there until he retired in 1929. Apart from his well known phenomenon, he wrote one of the first descriptions of the beneficial effects of the quinine alkaloids on arrhythmias and that its successful use was mainly in patients with auricular fibrillation of recent onset (1903–1904). He wrote an important monograph on beriberi in 1934. He loved the more traditional types of art being an ardent admirer of Franz Hals and was particularly fond of the English countryside which he visited on many occasions. In his own work he combined clinical skills with laboratory investigation but was modest of his own achievements saying "No, I am not a great man: I am a happy man" and "I owe my reputation to the fact that I use digitalis in doses the textbooks say are dangerous and in cases the textbooks say are unsuitable".

WERDNIG-HOFFMAN ATROPHY, DISEASE, PARALYSIS OR SYNDROME

Infantile spinal atrophy manifested as a "floppy infant". It is the second or third most common autosomal recessive disease in childhood (1 in 20 000 births with a carrier frequency of 1 in 60). The acute form presents with delayed milestones and weakness, at 3–4 months of age, and is usually fatal by 3. Sibling involvement is 1 in 4. In the chronic form the age of onset is 1–2 years and first involves the proximal muscles of the lower limbs. Cranial nerves are less affected but there is often facial weakness and involvement of the cervical muscles and wasting of the tongue with fasciculation. Progression is slow, but they are usually unable to stand by the age of 10.

Guido Werdnig (1844–1919) Austrian neurologist who worked in Graz when he described this syndrome but later returned to work in Vienna. He was born in the Austrian town of Ratschasch and after graduating in medicine joined the Army and took part in the suppression of a revolution in Southern Dalmatia and was in the army of occupation in Bosnia. On discharge he worked briefly in Vienna before moving to Graz. He developed a spastic paraplegia and was bedridden for the last decade of his life.

J. Hoffman (*v. supra*).

WERLHOF DISEASE

Idiopathic thrombocytopenic purpura (ITP) or autoimmune thrombocytopenia (ATP).

Paul G. Werlhof (1699–1767) He was born in Helmstedt and studied medicine at the University of Helmstedt, graduating in 1723. He became physician to the court of Hannover in 1760 and was one of the best known physicians in Europe being consulted in far away Moscow and Rome. He wrote poetry and hymns. He described Purpura Hemorrhagica (ITP) in 1735. He wrote his poetry in German but all his medical works were in Latin.

WERMER SYNDROME

Multiple endocrine adenomatosis Type 1 or multiple endocrine neoplasia Type 1 (MEN1) (*v.* SIPPLE SYNDROME). Tumors of the anterior pituitary, parathyroid and pancreatic islets. It is an autosomal dominant. The most common manifestation is hyperparathyroidism. More rarely there may be tumours of the thyroid or adrenal cortex, multiple lipomata or other tumors. Zollinger-Ellison syndrome is also common.

Paul Wermer (1900–1975) U.S. physician in the Department of Medicine, Columbia University, Presbyterian Hospital, New York.

WERNER SYNDROME

Multisystem disorder, autosomal recessive, premature senescence, dwarfism, cataracts, scleroderma like skin changes, osteoporosis, multiglandular dysfunction, particularly hypogonadism and an increased incidence of neoplasia. Except for the short stature other features develop in adult life.

Otto Werner (1879–1936) German physician. He was born in Flensburg and went to medical school at Kiel, graduating from the Christian-Albrechts University in 1904. He served with the German Navy in World War I and then returned to practice in a small town near the Danish border, dying of cancer of the liver.

WERNICKE ENCEPHALOPATHY

Confusion, ophthalmoplegia, usually lateral rectus palsy, nystagmus, ataxia and peripheral neuritis. First described in 1881 it is primarily due to thiamine deficiency secondary to alcoholism and/or starvation.

Karl Wernicke (1848–1904) He was born in a small town in Upper Silesia, Tarnowitz, which at the time was German. His father was a civil servant. He graduated in medicine from Breslau (Wroclaw), Poland and worked as an assistant to Neumann there, and whilst with him was allowed to study with Meynert in Vienna for 6 months. Meynert influenced him greatly and he was virtually the only name he mentioned in lectures and only his portrait hung on the wall in Wernicke's clinic.

When only 26 he published a book on aphasia in which he described sensory aphasia for the first time as well as alexia and agraphia. This made him internationally famous. In 1877 he observed that lesions which were relatively limited to the 6th nucleus resulted in paralysis of conjugate gaze to the side of the lesion and he was the first to postulate a centre for conjugate gaze in the pontal tegmentum. His interest in anatomy stemmed from Meynert's influence and in 1881 he published a 3 volume book which admirably summarized what was known about cerebral localization. This included a postulate of the symptomatology which would result from a thrombosis of the posterior inferior cerebellar artery, later confirmed by Wallenberg. He also predicted pseudo-ophthalmoplegia in which patients are unable to move their eyes voluntarily or fix their gaze on objects in the peripheral visual field but can follow slowly moving objects. They therefore read by letting their eyes wander aimlessly until finally all the words are perceived. In these 3 volumes he described the syndrome

Wernicke's encephalopathy and although he was aware of a toxic factor being important in its etiology, did not realize that this was nutritional. He was a rather withdrawn person with whom it was difficult to relate. He was an ardent adversary of Kraepelin, he believed that the time had not yet arrived when there should be distinction between separate psychiatric illnesses and he regarded the latter's classification as not being sufficiently scientific. In 1890 he was appointed Ordinariat in Psychiatry at Breslau and left the private practice he had in Berlin. In 1904 he moved to a similar appointment at Halle but had only been there a short time when he was killed in an accident while riding a bicycle in the Thuringian forest.

WEST SYNDROME

v. LENNOX-GASTAUT SYNDROME

Infantile spasms (Salaam attacks) in the first year of life with associated mental retardation in 80% of cases. There is a propensity to infections with a high mortality due to bronchopneumonia. A reduced cellular immunity and immunoglobulin level have been reported.

W.J. West British physician who described the condition in 1840 in one of his children in a letter to The Lancet.

WESTPHAL SIGN

Absence of the quadriceps (patellar) reflex in particular reference to tabes dorsalis.

WESTPHAL-PILCZ REACTION

Contraction of the pupil with closure or attempt to close the eye.

Alexander Pilcz (*v. supra*)

WESTPHAL-STRÜMPELL PSEUDOSCLEROSIS

v. WILSON DISEASE

v. EDINGER-WESTPHAL NUCLEUS

Carl F.O. Westphal (*v. supra*).

Ernst A.G.G. Strümpell (*v. supra*).

WHARTON DUCT

Submandibular salivary duct.

WHARTON JELLY

Mucoid substance which is the matrix of the umbilical cord.

Thomas Wharton (1614–1673) Born in Durham, he studied at Pembroke College, Cambridge, London and Oxford and at the outbreak of the Civil War went to London where he worked with John Bathurst, the physician to Oliver Cromwell. After Oxford

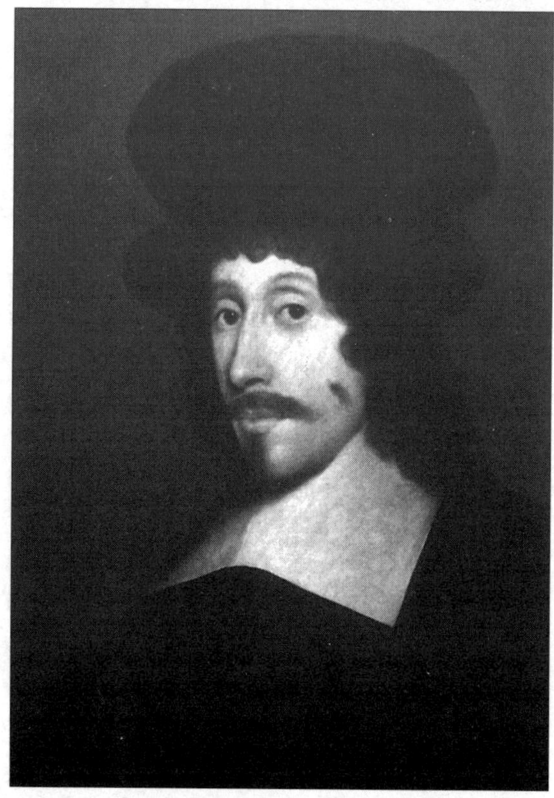

Thomas Wharton (Reproduced from *"The Royal College of Physicians of London Portraits"* by G. Wolstenholme and D. Piper [Published by J & A Churchill Ltd., London, 1964])

surrendered to Cromwell's army he gained his M.D. there. He commenced practice in London and was most successful, remaining there during the plague (1665–1673). He carried out a number of anatomical investigations, and wrote a book on the glands of the body and described the submandibular duct in 1656. He was a physician at St. Thomas's Hospital and a censor for the Royal College of Physicians.

WHIPPLE DISEASE

Steatorrhea, pigmentation, arthralgia, clubbing of the fingers, with low grade fever and sometimes pleurisy, most commonly seen in men. Glycoprotein inclusion bodies are present in macrophages in lymph nodes, intestinal mucosa and sometimes bone marrow. It is thought to result from an unidentified infection and usually responds to antibiotic therapy.

George H. Whipple (1878–) He was born in Ashland, New Hampshire, educated at Andover Academy and Yale, and graduated from Johns Hopkins in 1905. He was a pupil of Welch and worked in the pathology department at Johns Hopkins from 1905 to 1914. During that time he spent one year at the Ancon Hospital in Panama. He wrote up a patient who was a 37 year old medical missionary who succumbed to the disease. His report appeared in the Johns Hopkins Bulletin entitled "A hitherto undescribed disease characterized anatomically by fat and fatty acids in the intestinal and mesenteric lymphatic tissue". He reported the presence in lymph nodes of rod shaped organisms.

In 1914 he was appointed Professor of Research Medicine at the University of California and the Director of the Hooper Foundation for Medical Research. In 1920 he commenced his study on the effects of various foods on blood regeneration. The experimental model he used was to bleed the dogs to make them anemic and then to feed them on diets that were restricted to food from one particular organ, e.g. kidney, liver, brain, etc. Using this approach he found that liver was the most effective followed by kidney and then muscle. These experiments led Minot and Murphy to use raw liver in the treatment of patients with pernicious anemia (*v. supra*) and led to his Nobel Prize in 1930.

Whipple became the Professor of Pathology and the Dean at the University of Rochester. He showed that histiocytes broke red cells down into bilirubin and bile pigments and by exclusion of the liver that histiocytes in other organs could also do this. He demonstrated that fibrinogen was made in the liver and proposed the term Thalassemia for Cooley Anemia (*v. supra*).

WHIPPLE OPERATION

Radical pancreatico-duodenectomy for carcinoma of the ampullary area and head of the pancreas.

WHIPPLE TRIAD

Diagnostic features of an insulinoma of the pancreas.

1. Fasting blood sugar of less than 50 mg/% (2.8 mmol/l).
2. Recovery from an attack following the administration of glucose.
3. Initiation of an attack by fasting.

Allen O. Whipple (1881–1963) U.S. surgeon who was born in Iran. He commenced surgical practice in 1910 and became Professor of Surgery at Columbia, New York, and director of the surgical service at the Presbyterian Hospital in 1921, retiring in 1946. Apart from his contributions to disorders of the pancreas, he was an authority on literature and ancient cultures and was especially interested in the orient and in medical history. This is exemplified by his book "The Story of Wound Healing and Wound Repair" which was published shortly before he died. He commenced a clinic to examine problems with the spleen in his department which led to portosystemic vein shunting to treat portal hypertension by his colleague, Arthur Blakemore. He was the brother of George Whipple.

WHITFIELD OINTMENT

Ointment for fungal infections containing benzoic acid and salicylic acid.

Arthur Whitfield (1867–1947) English dermatologist, who was born in London and graduated from the King's College Hospital in 1892. He studied in Berlin and Vienna and in 1899 was appointed to the King's College Hospital as Assistant Physician to the Skin Department. Here he restricted both his public and private practice to dermatology and in 1906 was appointed Professor of Dermatology at King's College. Although dogged by ill health, he was particularly productive and published a book "Handbook of Skin Diseases and their Treatment". He was interested in mycology and was one of the first to use X-rays in the therapy of ringworm of the scalp. He used to say "Always examine your cases thoroughly, thoroughly, thoroughly. Re-examine them. Re-examine your own deductions".

He was an attractive man and people from all over the world came to work with him.

WICKHAM STRIAE

Striation seen on the top of the pruritic papular rash of lichen planus. They may appear as lines or small white dots among the classically itchy and shiny polygonal papules.

Louis F. Wickham (1860–1913) French dermatologist who practised in Paris and designed a multi-bladed knife for scarification treatment of lupus vulgaris. In 1888 he was commissioned to report on the methods of teaching dermatology in England. Whilst admiring some aspects he was critical of the lack of centralized facilities and the difficulty in follow up of the patients by students under instruction and the lack of museums, libraries, and laboratory facilities to study skin disorders. He later on promoted the use of radium particularly in the treatment of cancer.

WIDAL TEST

Agglutination test for typhoid fever.

Georges F.I. Widal (1862–1929) He was born in Dellys, Algeria, the son of an Army surgeon. He studied medicine in Paris graduating in 1889, and remained in that city for all his professional life. In 1894 he became Agrégé and in 1911 a Professor. His early work concentrated on bacteriology and noted the relationship between the streptococcus and puerperal thrombophlebitis. He discovered typhoid bacillus agglutinins in 1896 in patients with typhoid fever. In 1906 he reported sodium chloride's role in the production of edema and the use of a salt free diet in its control. In 1907 he described increased red cell fragility in familial hemolytic jaundice. He was a brilliant speaker and lecturer who took great trouble in preparation. He was described as a precise man who was not self centred and greatly admired his colleagues' abilities. Together with G.H. Roger and P.J. Teissier he edited 22 volumes of a medical textbook. He first described acquired hemolytic anemia.

The story is told by Clovis Vincent, the famous French neurosurgeon, that he approached Widal with the intention of spending a year with him when he was an intern at the Salpêtrière. The reply he got was "Not until you have won the gold medal". Vincent won the medal but when he was asked whether he still wished to work with Widal replied, "Oh, no, they say you are too much of a rabbit doctor. I want to get a job where I can learn something of general medicine; the neurologists just talk and do nothing." He died of a cerebral hemorrhage after an acute attack of gout.

WILDERMUTH EAR

Congenital deformity of the ear in which there is a turned down helix and a prominent anti-helix.

Herman A. Wildermuth (1852–1907) German psychiatrist who worked in Stuttgart.

WILKINS DISEASE

Congenital hyperplasia of the adrenals causing precocious puberty in boys and pseudohermaphroditism in girls with hypertension and episodic hypoglycemia.

WILKINS SYNDROME

v. DEBRÉ-FIBIGER SYNDROME

Lawson Wilkins (1894–1963) He graduated M.D. in 1918 in France whilst serving with the Johns Hopkins unit there. After the war he established a pediatric endocrine unit at Johns Hopkins whilst he was still in private practice. He became Professor of Pediatrics and wrote a definitive textbook on pediatric endocrinology in 1950. He promoted the use of graphs to follow growth and pioneered the use of glucosteroids in the treatment of adrenal hyperplasia.

WILKS DISEASE

1. Subacute glomerulonephritis.
2. Verruca necrogenica (dissecting room warts) or subcutaneous tuberculosis.

WILKS SYNDROME

Myasthenia gravis.

Sir Samuel Wilks (1824–1911) Born in Camberwell, London, he studied medicine at University College and received his M.D. from the University of London in 1850. He was appointed physician to Guy's Hospital in 1856. He remained connected with it for the rest of his life. He introduced the term enteric fever for typhoid fever and was one of the earliest to study visceral lesions of syphilis as well as osteitis deformans (Paget disease) and bacterial endocarditis in 1868. In 1869 he described acromegaly. His book "Lectures on the Pathological Anatomy" in 1859 was a standard work in its time, and contained one of the earliest descriptions of chronic ulcerative colitis. He wrote an historical account of Guy's Hospital with G.T. Bettany. Sir William Osler described Wilks as one of the most handsome men in London.

WILLI-PRADER SYNDROME

v. PRADER-WILLI SYNDROME

WILLIAMS SYNDROME

Infantile elfin facies with hypercalcemia and supraventricular aortic stenosis.

J.C.P. Williams New Zealand physician who graduated in science and medicine from the Otago Medical School. Nicknamed "Slim" he was a registrar when this case report was made at the Green Lane Hospital in Auckland.

WILLIAMSON SIGN OR TEST

Blood pressure in the leg is lower than the arm on the same side of the body in a pneumothorax or a large pleural effusion.

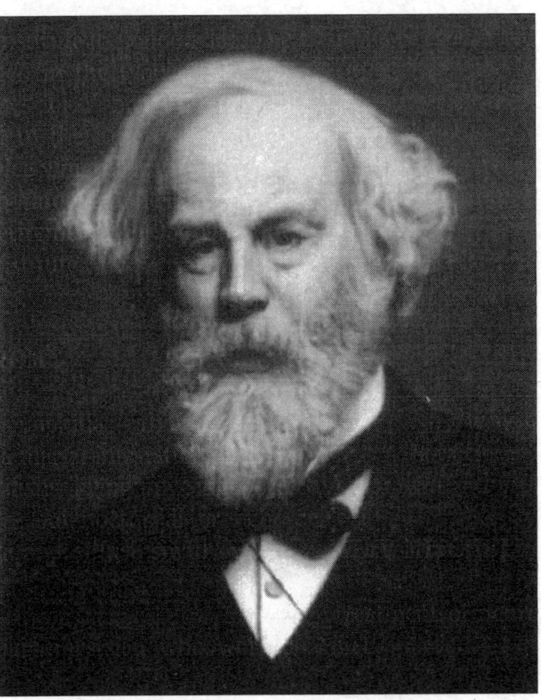

Sir Samuel Wilks (Reproduced from *"The Royal College of Physicians of London Portraits"* by G. Wolstenholme and D. Piper [Published by J & A Churchill Ltd., London, 1964])

Oliver K. Williamson (1866–1941) English physician.

WILLIS, CIRCLE OF

Arterial anastomosis at the base of the brain with the posterior communicating artery on either side joining posterior cerebral (branches of the basilar artery) to the anterior cerebral (branches of the internal carotid artery) arteries.

Thomas Willis (1621–1675) English anatomist born in Great Bedwin. The son of a Wiltshire farmer, he graduated from Oxford in 1646 (Christ Church College). An ardent Royalist, he served with Charles I's army until the latter was defeated, when he commenced practice in Oxford and was one of a small group which met at Wadham College and eventually became the Royal Society. After the Restoration in 1664 he was appointed Professor of Natural Philosophy at Oxford and in 1666 at the invitation of the Archbishop of Canterbury went to London. A rival to Sydenham as a clinician, he wrote descriptions of the intercostal and spinal nerves and a classical complete account of the nervous system, helped by Richard Lower and illustrated by Christopher Wren. His students included Robert Hook, John Locke, Richard Lower, and Edmund King who performed the first blood transfusion. He first described the 11th cranial nerve but was not the first to recognize or describe the Circle of Willis (Weffer). He wrote many treatises on headache and hearing and described paracusis. He considered asthma a nervous complaint. He noted the sweetness of urine in diabetes mellitus and distinguished it from insipidus. He described epidemic typhus and typhoid, whooping cough, meningitis, narcolepsy and general paralysis of the insane. He recognized that hysteria was not a disease of the uterus but was cerebral in origin. He described myasthenia gravis in 1672 and it was only redelineated by Erb in 1879, and by Gowers in his manual in 1886–1888. He described cardiospasm and its successful management in a patient by passing a whalebone rod with a sponge on the end to push the food down after meals. He became a Fellow of the Royal Society and the Royal College of Physicians, was financially very successful and treated members of the Royal family. He died of pleurisy and was buried in Westminster Abbey.

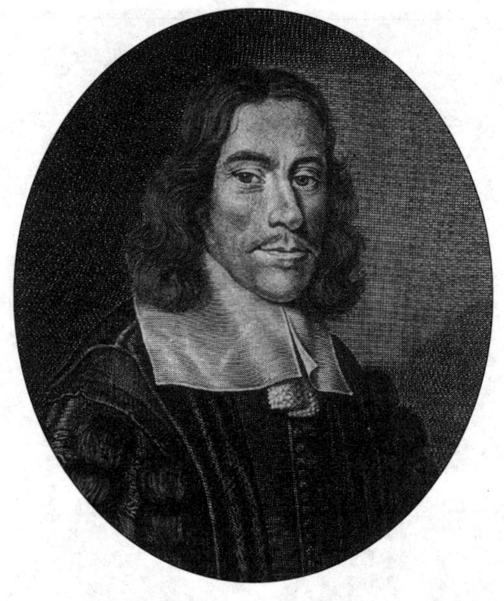

Thomas Willis (Courtesy of the Royal Society of Medicine, London, UK)

WILMS TUMOR

Kidney tumor composed of malignant epithelial and mesodermal cells in children. A small number have an autosomal dominant inheritance with hypoplasia of the iris and abnormality of chromosome 11.

Max Wilms (1867–1918) Born in Hünshoven /Geilenkirchen, Germany, he became Professor of Surgery at Leipzig, Basel and finally (1910) Heidelberg and described the tumor in 1899. He devised surgical approaches to the treatment of tuberculosis of the lung and introduced paravertebral rib resection.

WILSON DISEASE

Hepatolenticular degeneration associated with copper deposition, cerebellar signs and cirrhosis. Sometimes hemolytic anemia may be a presenting feature.

WILSON PRONATOR SIGN

Extension of the arms above the head will result in the palms facing outward in Sydenham Chorea due to pronation of the forearms.

WILSON SIGN

Eccentric pupil in neoencephalic disease.

Samuel A.K. Wilson (1877–1937) He was born in Cedarville, New Jersey, the son of an Irish clergyman, but in his early years the family returned to Scotland. He studied medicine at the University of Edinburgh and graduated M.B. in 1902 and gained a B.Sc. in 1903 in physiology. He became house physician at the Royal Edinburgh Infirmary with Byron Bramwell, and as a result commenced his lifelong involvement with neurology. He spent a year in France with Pierre Marie and Babinski. Following a brief journey to Leipzig, he returned to London, where in 1904 he became house physician at the National Hospital, Queen's Square. Here he spent most of his professional life with a group of neurologists that included Gowers, Hughlings Jackson, Bastian, and Horsley. He published his M.D. thesis on "Progressive lenticular degeneration: a familial nervous disease associated with cirrhosis of the liver". Although Westphal-Strümpell pseudosclerosis had already been described, as Wilson himself pointed out, they did not discuss the lenticular or hepatic aspects, thus they failed to recognize the two major signs of the disorder. Denny Brown once asked Wilson his opinion on the essential criteria of "hepatolenticular degeneration". Wilson eyed him with some circumspection and starting to walk away, asked "Do you mean Kinnier Wilson's disease?" He was the epitome of Queen's Square neurology, being a quick witted man with a keen if ironic sense of humor, and possessing that element of "hamishness" which seems to be essential in demonstrating neurological problems. When making rounds with Foster Kennedy at the Bellevue Hospital, New York, he spent an inordinate time examining a patient with lateral medullary syndrome but with signs that were inconsistent with the anatomy – he turned suddenly to the patient and asked "Will you see to it that I get your brain when you die?" Only someone like Wilson could get away with that type of behavior. At times he seemed distant but his humor and judgement are illustrated by this advice he gave based on his experience:

1. Never show surprise.
2. Never say the same thing twice to a patient.
3. Never believe what the patient says the doctor said.
4. Be decisive in your indecision.
5. Never take a meal with your patient.

An extremely eloquent and lucid lecturer and writer he had all but finished a textbook of neurology when he died of cancer. The world had lost a keen gardener, a left handed golfer and a great clinician.

WILSON-MIKITY SYNDROME

Neonatal respiratory distress with rib retraction, and cyanosis in premature infants with cyst-like lung lesion on X-ray.

Miriam G. Wilson (1922–) U.S. pediatrician.

Victor G. Mikity (1919–) U.S. radiologist.

WINCKEL DISEASE

Neonatal sepsis with jaundice, hemolytic anemia, hemoglobinuria and often central nervous signs.

Franz K.L.W. von Winckel (1837–1911) German physician who wrote an excellent historical account of gynecology in 1903 and worked in Munich.

WINSLOW FORAMEN

Foramen of Winslow. The epiploic foramen.

Jacob B. Winslow (1669–1760) Born in Odense, Denmark, he studied in Holland and France and graduated from the University of Paris in 1705, being greatly influenced by Duverney (v. Bartholin). In 1707 he became Professor of Anatomy at Paris and from 1743–1750 he was the Professor in the Jardin du Roy. His great uncle was N. Stensen (*v. supra*). He was a famous teacher and Albrecht von Haller was one of his students. He wrote a textbook of anatomy which simplified important aspects such as the origin and insertion as well as the nomenclature of muscles. This work was the authoritative text for almost half a century. He converted to Catholicism and was disowned by his family (Lutheran) and never returned to Denmark.

WINTERBOTTOM SIGN

Enlargement of the posterior cervical lymph nodes in sleeping sickness.

Thomas M. Winterbottom (1766–1859) Born in South Shields and graduated from the University of Glasgow in 1792. After graduation he practiced for 4 years in Sierra Leone in Africa and then returned to his native town where he practiced until his retirement 20 years later. In 1803 he published an article entitled "An account of the native Africans in the neighbourhood of Sierra Leone" in which he gave the first account of sleeping sickness in English.

WINTROBE HEMATOCRIT

A technique in which the hematocrit and the erythrocyte sedimentation rate can be measured using one tube.

Maxwell M. Wintrobe (1901–) U.S. physician and hematologist who was born in Halifax, Nova Scotia, Canada, but moved to Winnipeg when he was 10. He graduated in medicine from the University of Manitoba in 1926, the year that Minot and Murphy had reported the cure of pernicious anemia with liver. Since he had seen a number of patients die with this disorder when an undergraduate he commenced investigating this area. In 1927 he went to Tulane as an instructor and continued his research. He discovered that normal blood standards were virtually non-existent, and so devised his hematocrit tube and from this set out the calculation of indices of red blood cells which is now a routine technique in hematology. These studies were reported by him in an article "The erythrocyte in man" in Medicine. After many years at Johns Hopkins where he wrote his textbook which rapidly became and has remained a bible for hematologists, he was appointed Professor of Medicine at Salt Lake City, Utah.

WISKOTT-ALDRICH SYNDROME

Sex linked recessive disorder characterized by recurrent infections, eczema, mild bleeding disorder and thrombocytopenia. There are low levels of IgA and IgM with decreased lymphocytes in spleen and lymph nodes but not in the marrow.

Alfred Wiskott (1898–1978) German pediatrician. He was born in Essen the son of a colliery manager. He served in the German Army in World War I and was wounded at Verdun. He then studied medicine and became a pediatrician, co-authoring a successful German book on pediatrics.

Robert A. Aldrich (1917–) U.S. pediatrician who graduated from Northwestern University, Chicago and became Professor of Pediatrics at the University of Colorado in Denver.

WISTAR RAT

Strain of rats bred at the Wistar Institute in Philadelphia, U.S.A.

General Isaac Wistar He presented the University of Philadelphia with the funds to endow anatomical research and for a building to house anatomical preparations. This was opened in 1894. He was the grandson of Caspar Wistar (1760–1812) who graduated in medicine from the College of Philadelphia in 1782, and then went to Edinburgh University and gained his M.D. there in 1786. He became the first Professor of Chemistry at Philadelphia and on the death of Shippen, the Professor of Anatomy in 1808 until his own death. His textbook "Systems of Anatomy" was one of the earliest anatomical books published in the U.S.A. His friend the botanist Nuttal named the *Wistaria* vine after him.

WOHLFART-KUGELBERG-WELANDER SYNDROME

v. KUGELBERG-WELANDER SYNDROME

Gunnar Wohlfart (1909–1961) Professor of Neurology, University of Lund, Sweden.

Lisa Welander (1909–) Swedish neurologist.

WOLFE GRAFT

Full thickness skin graft.

John R. Wolfe (1824–1904) Born in Breslau but graduated from Glasgow in 1856 and later served with Garibaldi in Sicily as his surgeon. He was ophthalmic surgeon to the Royal Infirmary, Aberdeen, between 1860 and 1868. He then returned to Glasgow where he founded the Ophthalmic Institute. He resigned around 1892 to migrate to Australia to practice as an ophthalmologist in Melbourne, Victoria, where he became surgeon oculist to the Governor of Victoria. He returned to Glasgow around 1900. He first described the use of a full thickness skin graft (taken from behind the ear) to correct ectropion and other eyelid deformities caused by loss of skin. He has been described as "without doubt a very flamboyant character and in the eyes of many people a charlatan". Some people also credit him with having undertaken the first human corneal transplant, but there seems to be no firm evidence for this.

WOLFF-CHAIKOFF EFFECT

Impaired T3 and T4 formation after exposure to a high dose of iodide (over 150 mg/day), due to the inhibition of the conversion of iodide to iodine. The effect is usually transitory (less than 48 hours) because of diminishing uptake of excess iodide from the plasma. In chronic thyroiditis, or after previous treatment with radio-iodine for Graves disease, the effect may persist, resulting in iodide induced hypothyroidism. The effect may serve as a defence against a sudden increase in hormone synthesis after large increases in plasma iodide.

J. Wolff U.S. investigator at the National Institutes of Health.

I.L. Chaikoff U.S. physiologist at University of California Medical School, Berkeley.

WOLFF-PARKINSON-WHITE SYNDROME

This disorder most often presents with a supraventricular tachycardia and is due to abnormal conduction in the heart so that atrial impulses pre-excite the ventricles via accessory bypass fibres called the Bundle of Kent (*v. supra*), so that impulses reach the ventricles before those conducted by the normal His-Purkinje (*v. supra*) conducting system. The ECG has a characteristically short PR interval and wide abnormal QRS complexes.

Louis Wolff (1898–) U.S. physician who worked in Boston.

Sir John Parkinson (1885–) English physician.

Paul D. White (*v. supra* BLAND-WHITE-GARDNER SYNDROME)

WOLFFIAN CYST

Mesonephric cyst near the ovary or the uterine tube.

WOLFFIAN DUCT

Mesonephric duct.

Kaspar Wolff (1733–1794) He was born in Berlin, the son of a tailor, and graduated in medicine from Halle in 1759. In 1761 he was appointed to the anatomy department at Breslau (Wroclaw) and his work became widely known. He returned to Berlin in 1763 and there was a controversial figure and had many opponents in the faculty based on religious opposition to his theories on generation and perhaps jealousy. He spent several years in Berlin, teaching physiology and pathology but was never given professorial status and in 1767 went to St. Petersburg. He became a member of the Academy of Sciences and remained there until his death. Wolff revived Harvey's doctrine of epigenesis (gradual building up of structures), and opposed the current theory of the day that the embryo was already preformed and encased in the ovary. Wolff put forward the view that organs were formed from leaf-like layers which came close to the germ layer theory of von Baer. He described the ducts in his doctor's thesis in 1759. He founded the modern concepts of embryology and his report on the development of the chick's intestine was regarded by the embryologist von Baer as "the greatest masterpiece of scientific observation".

WOLFRAM SYNDROME

Diabetes mellitus, diabetes insipidus, optic atrophy and nerve deafness. An autosomal recessive it is sometimes associated with ureter and bladder atony.

Donald J. Wolfram (1910–) U.S. physician at the Mayo Clinic who published this description in 1938. He was born at Hamlet, Indiana and graduated M.D. from the University of Indiana in 1934. He came to the Mayo Clinic as a Fellow in 1935 leaving three years later and served in the U.S. Army in World War II.

WOLMAN DISEASE

Inborn error of lipid metabolism with deposition of cholesterol and triglycerides in the liver. Presents in the first few weeks of life with vomiting, diarrhea, hepatosplenomegaly, intestinal malabsorption, and enlargement and calcification of the adrenals. Often death occurs within 6 months. Foam cells are seen in the bone marrow and inclusion bodies of lipid droplets can be seen in the circulating white cells. Adrenal failure may occur.

M. Wolman (1914–) Israeli pathologist who was born in Warsaw, Poland, and studied at the Universities of Florence and Rome, graduating M.D. from Rome in 1938. He became Professor and Chairman of Pathology at the University of Tel-Aviv in 1964.

WOLTMAN-KERNOHAN SYNDROME

v. KERNOHAN-WOLTMAN SYNDROME

WOOD FILTER, LAMP OR LIGHT

U.V. light which causes fungal infections such as tinea to fluoresce.

Robert W. Wood (1868–1955) U.S. physicist. He was born in Concord, Massachusetts, and studied at Johns Hopkins University, the University of Chicago and Berlin. He became Professor of Experimental Physics at Johns Hopkins in 1901, retiring in 1938. He wrote on physical optics and authored some non-scientific books and nonsense verse. He invented a method for thawing frozen water pipes using electrical current.

WOOLNER TIP

The apex of the helix of the ear.

Thomas Woolner (1825–1892) English sculptor.

WORINGER-KOLOPP DISEASE

This is also called Pagetoid reticulosis and is an unusual skin disorder which consists of a solitary cutaneous plaque which is often hyperkeratotic and is most commonly located on one of the lower limbs. Its disseminated form has been called the Ketron-Goodman Variant (*v. supra*). It appears to occur more commonly in young adults.

Frédéric Woringer (1903–1964) French dermatologist. He was born in Strasburg into a family of clergymen and doctors. Educated at a Protestant school, he commenced his medical studies in 1922, firstly at Strasburg and finally in Paris. He returned to Strasburg and worked in Pautrier's dermatological clinic. Coming under Pautrier's influence he devoted the rest of his life to dermatology with a special emphasis on the application of histopathological changes in various skin conditions. He became Professor of Dermatology in Strasburg in 1957, the same position previously held by his teacher, Pautrier. Here he exerted a considerable influence on the development of dermatology and had 500 articles to his credit. Widely read, he had a particular interest in the arts and music and was a regular member of a musical quartet before the 2nd World War. He travelled widely but especially enjoyed Greece and Palestine.

P. Kolopp French dermatologist who worked with Woringer in Strasburg.

WORMIAN BONES

Sutural bones of the skull.

Ole Worm (1588–1654) Danish anatomist. He was born in Jutland and was a pupil of Fabrizio in Padua and Bauhan in Basel. He became Professor of Anatomy in Copenhagen and was physician to Christian IV and Fredrick III.

WRIGHT STAIN

Romanovsky (*v. supra*) type stain for peripheral blood and bone marrow films.

James H. Wright (1870–1928) U.S. pathologist. He worked with Welch at Johns Hopkins and developed the technique for reticulocyte counting which was crucial in following the response of patients with pernicious anemia to liver therapy and evidence of blood regeneration after blood loss or during hemolysis.

WRIGHT SYNDROME

Combined occlusion of the subclavian artery and stretching of the brachial plexus due to hyperabduction of the arms resulting in numbness and tingling in the hands and even gangrene.

Irving S. Wright (1901–) U.S. physician. He was born in New York City and graduated M.D. from Cornell University in 1925. He specialized in vascular disease and was one of the pioneers in the use of oral anticoagulants.

WUCHERIA

Filarial worms.

WUCHERIA BANCROFTI

The cause of filariasis in man.

Otto E.H. Wucheria (1820–1874) Portuguese physician. He was born in Oporto, Portugal, and practiced as a physician in London at St. Bartholomew's Hospital as well as in Lisbon. He discovered the filaria larvae whilst working in Bahia, Brazil.

J. Bancroft (*v. supra*).

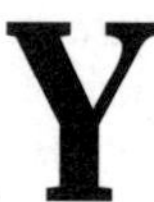

YERSINIA ENTEROCOLITICA

Organism which produces enterocolitis, fever, mesenteric adenitis, erythema nodosum and acute terminal ileitis. It may be confused with appendicitis or Crohn disease and is sometimes followed by arthritis.

Alexandre E.J. Yersin (1863–1943) Swiss (naturalised French) bacteriologist born in La Vaux (Lausanne). He carried out investigations on diphtheria with Roux and discovered diphtheria toxin in 1888 and then became surgeon in the French Army and Director of the Pasteur Institute at Nher-trang (Amman). He introduced the rubber tree into Indo-China. In Hong Kong he independently discovered the cause of plague, *Bacillus pestis,* in 1894.

YOUNG SYNDROME

Epididymal/vas obstruction with azoospermia but normal testes with abnormal secondary sexual development.

W.G. Young (1899–1965) American anatomist and endocrinologist who was Professor of Anatomy, University of Kansas 1946–1963, when he moved to the University of Oregon Medical School as Professor of Anatomy and Chairman of the Department of Reproductive Physiology and Behaviour.

Z

ZAHN INFARCT

Infarct of the liver by occlusion of portion of the portal vein.

ZAHN, LINES OF

The cut surface of an *in vivo* thrombus may show alternating red and thin white bands representing layers of platelets and white cells as succeeding episodes of clotting occur.

Friedrich W. Zahn (1845–1904) Swiss pathologist in Geneva who made the first systematic investigation of the pathogenesis of thrombosis in 1875.

ZELLWEGER SYNDROME

Autosomal recessive disorder with abnormal skull, hypotonia, mental retardation, biliary maldevelopment and cystic dysplasia of the kidneys with hepatomegaly. The characteristic lesion is a lack or absence of peroxisomes in many tissues. Patients so far reported are males ? X linked recessive – early death results.

Hans V. Zellweger (1908–) Swiss pediatrician who was born in Lugano and graduated M.D. University of Zurich in 1934. He worked with Albert Schweitzer in Africa and was Professor of Pediatrics at the University of Lebanon and migrated to the U.S.A. becoming Professor of Pediatrics at the University of Iowa, Iowa City, 1959.

ZENKER DIVERTICULUM

Diverticulum of the upper part of the esophagus which may cause swelling in the lateral part of the neck and is diagnosed by X-ray. Most commonly seen in elderly males. Sometimes present with dysphagia, characteristically occurring with first swallowing attempt.

ZENKER FIXATIVE

Mixture of salts and glacial acetic acid.

ZENKER PARALYSIS

Peroneal nerve palsy.

Friedrich A. Zenker (1825–1898) German physician and pathologist who described trichinosis in 1860 and wrote the first description of fat embolism in man in 1862 and described Charcot-Leyden crystals in asthma in 1851. He became a Professor of Pathology in his native city, Dresden.

ZIEHEN-OPPENHEIM DISEASE

v. OPPENHEIM-ZIEHEN DISEASE

Dystonia musculorum deformans with a classical dromedary gait.

Georg T. Ziehen (1862–1950) German psychiatrist.

H. Oppenheim (*v. supra*).

ZIEHL-NEELSEN METHOD OR STAIN

Acid fast staining of tubercle bacilli.

Franz Ziehl (1859–1926) German bacteriologist and physician. He was born in Wismar and while an assistant in the medical clinic in Heidelberg (1882–6) wrote up the staining technique. He worked in Lubeck as a neurologist.

Friedrich K.A. Neelsen (1854–1894) German pathologist, born in Holstein. He studied medicine in Leipzig, joined the Pathology Institute as an assistant and was later appointed as Professor in

Rostock (1878–1885), from where he returned to Dresden as Prosector in the Stadt-Krankenhaus. He wrote extensively on pathological and bacteriological subjects and was the actual inventor of the Ziehl-Neelsen technique.

ZIEVE SYNDROME

Transient hemolytic anemia associated with hyperlipoproteinemia, jaundice and liver disease.

Leslie Zieve (1919–) U.S. physician. He was born in Minneapolis, Minnesota and went to medical school at the University of Minnesota, graduating M.D. in 1943, interning at the Philadelphia General Hospital and then served in the U.S. Army as a battalion surgeon until 1946 when he became a resident at the University of Minnesota's Veterans' Hospital. Here he described the above syndrome and this initiated his interest in liver disease and phospholipids which he pursued throughout his career. He became Head of Gastroenterology (1960–1972) and also the radioisotope service (1950–1972) at the Veterans' Hospital and was appointed Professor of Medicine in 1962. In 1978 he was appointed Director of Research at the Hennepin County Medical Centre and continues to be Professor of Medicine at the University of Minnesota.

ZIMMERLIN TYPE OF MUSCULAR DYSTROPHY

Scapulohumeral muscular dystrophy.

Franz Zimmerlin (1858–1932) Swiss physician.

ZINN CENTRAL ARTERY

Central artery of the retina.

Johan G. Zinn (1727–1759) German anatomist and botanist, born in Ansbach, Bavaria. He produced a fine anatomical atlas of the eye. He became Professor of Medicine and became Director of the Botanical Gardens in Göttingen in 1753. Linnaeus named the plant *Zinnia* after him.

ZINSSER-ENGMAN-COLE SYNDROME

Dyskeratosis congenita. A rare sex-linked recessive disorder characterized by nail dystrophy, leukoplakia of mucous surfaces and reticulated telangiectatic hyperpigmentation with pancytopenia.

Ferdinand Zinsser (1865–1952) He was born of German parents in New York but went back to Germany to school and studied medicine at Bonn, Munich and Heidelberg. He worked with Curschmann (*v. supra*) in Leipzig and later became Professor of Dermatology and later Rector of Cologne University.

Martin F. Engman (1869–1953) U.S. dermatologist. He worked throughout his career in St. Louis, Missouri. After the 1897 tornado which destroyed a portion of the City Hospital in St. Louis, he gathered together doctors and businessmen to collect funds to rebuild a hospital to care for dermatological and cancer patients. His efforts attracted the attention of George Barnard who gave a new building, subsequently called the Barnard Free Skin and Cancer Hospital, as well as contributing to a maintenance fund. In it he became one of the pioneers in the use of radium and X-ray treatment of skin disease.

Harold N. Cole (1884–1966) U.S. dermatologist

ZOLLINGER-ELLISON SYNDROME

Recurrent atypical peptic ulceration due to excessive production of gastrin by the pancreas resulting in gastric hyperacidity and hypersecretion.

Robert M. Zollinger (1903–) U.S. surgeon. He graduated M.D. from Ohio State in 1927 and interned at the Peter Bent Brigham in Boston. He remained at Harvard until 1946 when he returned as Professor of Surgery at Ohio State University, Columbus, Ohio.

Edwin H. Ellison (1918–1970) U.S. surgeon who was an associate Professor in the Department of Surgery, Ohio State.

ZOON BALANITIS

A benign condition of the foreskin which causes irritation and some fixation with reddish brown discoloration. It is cured by circumcision.

Johannes J. Zoon (1902–1958) Dutch dermatologist. He was born in Wijk, Aalberg the son of a headmaster of the local school. He graduated M.D. from Utrecht in 1928 where he wrote his dissertation on a complement fixation test for gonorrhea under the direction of Theodor Van Leeuwen, in whose dermatological clinics he continued to train, becoming the head of the clinic and on his chief's death became Professor in 1946 giving an inaugural address "Reflections on Syphilis". He was very conscious of the social issues of venereal disease and the importance of not denigrating the afflicted patient. He even forbade the use of rubber gloves in examining patients with syphilis!

ZUCKERKANDL BODIES

Para-aortic bodies of adrenal medullary tissue at the bifurcation of the aorta. They are the commonest site of extra-adrenal pheochromocytomas.

ZUCKERKANDL, FASCIA OF

Retrorenal fascia.

Emil Zuckerkandl (1849–1910) Austrian anatomist who wrote an imporant monograph on the anatomy and pathology of the accessory sinuses (1882–92). He was a student of J. Hyrtl of whom he said "he spoke like Cicero and wrote like Heine". He was Professor of Anatomy in Graz and finally in Vienna.